THIRD EDITION

Philosophies *and* Theories

FOR ADVANCED NURSING PRACTICE

EDITED BY

JANIE B. BUTTS, PhD, RN

Professor
College of Nursing
The University of Southern Mississippi
Hattiesburg, Mississippi

KAREN L. RICH, PhD, RN

Associate Professor
College of Nursing
The University of Southern Mississippi
Long Beach, Mississippi

JONES & BARTLETT
LEARNING

World Headquarters
Jones & Bartlett Learning
5 Wall Street
Burlington, MA 01803
978-443-5000
info@jblearning.com
www.jblearning.com

Jones & Bartlett Learning books and products are available through most bookstores and online booksellers. To contact Jones & Bartlett Learning directly, call 800-832-0034, fax 978-443-8000, or visit our website, www.jblearning.com.

Production Credits

VP, Executive Publisher: David D. Cella
Executive Editor: Amanda Martin
Associate Acquisitions Editor: Rebecca Stephenson
Editorial Assistant: Christina Freitas
Production Manager: Carolyn Rogers Pershouse
Production Editor: Lori Mortimer
Director of Marketing: Andrea DeFronzo
VP, Manufacturing and Inventory Control: Therese Connell
Product Fulfillment Manager: Wendy Kilborn

Senior Marketing Manager: Jennifer Scherzay
Composition: S4Carlisle Publishing Services
Cover Design: Kristin E. Parker
Director of Rights & Media: Joanna Gallant
Rights & Media Specialist: Wes DeShano
Media Development Editor: Troy Liston
Cover Image: © pop_jop/DigitalVision Vectors/Getty
Printing and Binding: Edwards Brothers Malloy
Cover Printing: Edwards Brothers Malloy

Library of Congress Cataloging-in-Publication Data
Names: Butts, Janie B., editor. | Rich, Karen L., editor.
Title: Philosophies and theories for advanced nursing practice / edited by
   Janie B. Butts, Karen L. Rich.
Description: Third edition. | Burlington, MA : Jones & Bartlett Learning,
   [2018] | Includes bibliographical references and index.
Identifiers: LCCN 2017000157 | ISBN 9781284112245
Subjects: | MESH: Nursing Theory | Advanced Practice Nursing | Evidence-Based
   Nursing | Models, Nursing
Classification: LCC RT84.5 | NLM WY 86 | DDC 610.7301--dc23
LC record available at https://lccn.loc.gov/2017000157
ISBN: 978-1-284-11224-5

6048

Printed in the United States of America
21 20 19 18   10 9 8 7 6 5 4

Contents

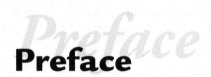

Preface

*P*hilosophies and Theories for Advanced Nursing Practice, Third Edition, edited by Janie B. Butts and Karen L. Rich, is an essential resource for advanced practice nurses and for students in graduate programs, including DNP, PhD, and master's-level programs. The cover for this third edition illustrates a road map that provides directions for a person to reach a destination. Philosophies and theories function in the same way. They provide a route or orientation to arrive at one's desired goal or outcome. Favored philosophies and theories guide nurses both personally and professionally, probably more than they realize. Philosophies and theories are not esoteric conjectures; they are meaningful guideposts integral to everyday life.

ARRANGEMENT OF THE BOOK

The book consists of 26 chapters presented in the following 5 parts:

- Part 1: Foundations of Nursing Science
- Part 2: The Structure and Function of Theory
- Part 3: Interdisciplinary Philosophies and Theories
- Part 4: Select Nursing Models and Theories
- Part 5: Tools for Integrating and Disseminating Knowledge in Advanced Nursing Practice

The chapters in Parts 1 and 2 provide a conceptual foundation, exploring the philosophy of science, the development of nursing knowledge, and the application of theory to nursing. Advanced practice nurses and nursing students can use Parts 1 and 2 as preparation for the information in Part 5, which covers theory evaluation, testing, and integrating, translating, and disseminating evidence-based findings from research to practice.

Part 3 focuses on a selection of interdisciplinary philosophies and theories relevant to advanced practice. Part 4 presents select conceptual models, grand theories, and middle-range theories of nursing. Conceptual nursing models and grand nursing theories both bring advanced practice nurses a certain reality of conceptual arrangements, theoretical variables, and propositions used for deriving middle-range theory. Middle-range nursing theories derived from conceptual models and grand theories of nursing translate theory and research findings directly into practice.

Acknowledgments

We would like to thank the Jones & Bartlett Learning staff, editors, and administrators for their diligent work and support. We also thank our colleagues who enthusiastically shared their expertise with us. The authors who contributed to this text are distinguished nursing and interdisciplinary scholars with expertise in theory. Without their contributions, we could not have completed this book. For these reasons, we extend to them a big thank-you!

Janie B. Butts and Karen L. Rich

About the Editors

Janie B. Butts, PhD, RN, The University of Southern Mississippi, College of Nursing, Hattiesburg, Mississippi

Janie B. Butts, PhD, RN, is a professor at the University of Southern Mississippi College of Nursing in Hattiesburg, Mississippi, and teaches classroom and online nursing courses at the doctoral, master's, and baccalaureate levels. Courses include ethics, advanced theory, advanced practice issues, professional development, research, and professional nursing practice. From 2008 to 2015, Dr. Butts served as a consultant editor for *Nursing Ethics* journal, an international journal with headquarters in England. Current specific research interests include death and dying ethical issues. Dr. Butts's journal articles and book chapters include topics on ethics, her research, theory, education, professional issues, and home care ethics, and she reviews for top nursing journals and book publishers. Dr. Butts's doctoral degree, with an emphasis in nursing education and nursing science, is from the University of Alabama at Birmingham, and her master's degree, with an emphasis in adult health nursing and nursing management, is from the University of Mississippi Medical Center in Jackson, Mississippi.

Karen L. Rich, PhD, RN, The University of Southern Mississippi, College of Nursing, Long Beach, Mississippi

Karen L. Rich, PhD, RN, is an associate professor at the University of Southern Mississippi College of Nursing in Long Beach, Mississippi, where she teaches public health nursing, ethics, and professional development. Dr. Rich's doctoral degree in nursing, with an emphasis in ethics, is from the University of Southern Mississippi. She has a master's degree in public health nursing from Louisiana State University and a post-master's in psychiatric–mental health nursing, nurse practitioner emphasis, from the University of Southern Mississippi. Dr. Rich serves as a consultant editor for the international *Nursing Ethics* journal. She serves on the ethics committees of a large county hospital in Gulfport, Mississippi, and a private hospital in Biloxi, Mississippi. Dr. Rich has written numerous articles and book chapters about ethics and philosophy. Her special interests are communitarian ethics, virtue ethics, ethics in public health, Eastern philosophy and ethics, and critical thinking in nursing.

Contributors

Patsy Anderson, DNS, RN
Associate Professor
DNP Assistant Coordinator, College of Nursing
The University of Southern Mississippi, Gulf
  Coast Campus
Long Beach, Mississippi

Victoria Baker, PhD, CNM, CPH
Associate Professor of Midwifery and Women's
  Health
Frontier Nursing University
Hyden, Kentucky

Sandra Bishop, DNS, RN
Assistant Professor
Academics Coordinator, College of Nursing
The University of Southern Mississippi, Gulf
  Coast Campus
Long Beach, Mississippi

Margaret M. Braungart, PhD
Professor Emeritus, Psychology
Center for Bioethics and Humanities
SUNY Upstate Medical University
Syracuse, New York

Richard G. Braungart, PhD
Professor Emeritus, Sociology
Maxwell School
Syracuse University
Syracuse, New York

Lora E. Burke, PhD, MPH, RN
Professor
School of Nursing and Graduate
  School of Public Health, Department
  of Epidemiology
University of Pittsburgh
Pittsburgh, Pennsylvania

Janie B. Butts, PhD, RN
Professor
Assistant Coordinator, College of Nursing
The University of Southern Mississippi
Hattiesburg, Mississippi

Peggy L. Chinn, PhD, RN, FAAN
Professor Emerita
School of Nursing
University of Connecticut
Storrs, Connecticut

Lisa Astalos Chism, DNP, APRN, BC
Nurse Practitioner
Department of Internal Medicine
Beaumont Hospitals
Woodhaven, Michigan

Joanne R. Duffy, PhD, RN, FAAN
Professor
Department of Environments for Health
Indiana University–Purdue University
    Indianapolis
Indianapolis, Indiana

Joan C. Engebretson, DrPH, RN, AHN-BC
Professor
The University of Texas Health Science Center
    at Houston
Houston, Texas

Jacqueline Fawcett, PhD, FAAN
Professor
College of Nursing and Health Sciences
University of Massachusetts, Boston
Boston, Massachusetts

Karen Glanz, PhD, MPH
Faculty
Rollins School of Public Health
Emory University
Atlanta, Georgia

Yolanda M. Gonzalez, DNS, MSN
Nursing Faculty
Universidad de Panama
Panama, Republic of Panama

Patricia Goodson, PhD
Professor
Department of Health and Kinesiology
Texas A&M University
College Station, Texas

Sherry Hartman, DrPH, RN
Professor Emeritus of Nursing
The University of Southern Mississippi
Hattiesburg, Mississippi

Joanne V. Hickey, PhD, RN, ACNP-BC, FAAN, FCCM
Professor, Patricia L. Starck Professor of
    Nursing
Director, Doctor of Nursing Practice
    Program
University of Texas at Houston, School of
    Nursing
Houston, Texas

Violet M. Malinski, PhD, RN
Associate Professor
Hunter-Bellevue School of Nursing
New York, New York

Kathleen Masters, DNS, RN
Associate Professor
Associate Director, College of Nursing
The University of Southern Mississippi
Hattiesburg, Mississippi

María Elisa Moreno-Fergusson, MSN, RN
Nursing Faculty
Universidad de La Sabana
Bogotá, Columbia

Janice M. Morse, PhD, RN, FAAN
Professor
College of Nursing
University of Utah
Salt Lake City, Utah

Sandra Nelson, PhD, APRN-BC
Associate Professor
Psychiatric Mental Health Nursing
Eastern Michigan University
Ypsilanti, Michigan

E. Carol Polifroni, EdD, CNE, NEA-BC, RN
Associate Professor
School of Nursing
University of Connecticut
Storrs, Connecticut

Larry Purnell, PhD, RN, FAAN
Professor
Department of Nursing
The University of Delaware
Newark, Delaware

Karen L. Rich, PhD, RN
Associate Professor, College of Nursing
The University of Southern Mississippi
Gulf Coast Campus
Long Beach, Mississippi

Barbara K. Rimer, DrPH
Dean and Alumni Distinguished
    Professor
UNC Gillings School of Global
    Public Health
Chapel Hill, North Carolina

Beth L. Rodgers, PhD, RN, FAAN
Professor
College of Nursing
University of Wisconsin, Milwaukee
Milwaukee, Wisconsin

Mary W. Stewart, PhD, RN
Associate Professor
School of Nursing
University of Mississippi Medical Center
Jackson, Mississippi

Rosemarie Tong, PhD
Director, Center for Professional and Applied
    Sciences
Distinguished Professor of Healthcare Ethics,
    Department of Philosophy
University of North Carolina at Charlotte
Charlotte, North Carolina

Steven J. Vanderheiden, PhD
Assistant Professor of Political Science
Department of Political Science
University of Colorado at Boulder
Boulder, Colorado

Martha V. Whetsell, PhD, RN, ARNP
Faculty
Department of Nursing
Lehman College, CUNY
Bronx, New York

I

Foundations of Nursing Science

Chapter 1

Philosophy of Science: An Introduction and a Grounding for Your Practice

E. Carol Polifroni

INTRODUCTION

Philosophy of science is a perspective—a lens, a way you see the world, and, in the case of advanced practice nurses, the viewpoint the nurse acts from in every encounter with a patient, family, or group. A person's philosophy of science creates the frame on a picture—a message that becomes a paradigm and a point of reference. Each individual's philosophy of science will permit some things to be seen and cause others to be blocked. It allows people to be open to some thoughts and potentially keeps them closed to others. A philosophy will deem some ideas correct, others inconsistent, and some simply wrong. While philosophy of science is not meant to be viewed as a black-or-white proposition, it does provide perspectives that include some ideas and thoughts; therefore, it must unavoidably exclude others. The key is to ensure that the ideas and thoughts within a given philosophy remain consistent with one another, rather than being in opposition.

Discussions of science, philosophy, and the philosophy of science can fill entire books. This chapter introduces readers to these topics. It is constructed in the form of a survey and is designed to launch inquiry in myriad ways. The purpose is to encourage you as a nurse to think in ways that you may not yet have discovered and to examine your assumptions and actions in your role as advanced practice nurses. If you leave this chapter without questioning your assumptions, the author has not done her job! One must appreciate the personal assumptions used in everyday professional life. Nurses, for example, must question their assumptions and reaffirm (appreciate and understand) what it is they believe.

SCIENCE

Before the concept of a philosophy of science is examined in greater depth and particular philosophies of science are specifically explored, it is important to begin by developing an appreciation of the meaning of the terms *science* and *philosophy*. Science, which comes from the Latin word *scientia*, meaning "knowledge," traditionally refers to both processes and the outcomes of processes, such as general laws and observations. General laws are the laws of nature that guide physical life, such as the laws of gravity, energy, and motion. Generators of science use these laws in a systematic way to create a body of knowledge about a specific topic. The culmination of using the scientific method (systematic process) provides a set of data (evidence) supported by propositions about an area of study (Boyd, Gasper, & Trout, 1991).

Natural (Hard) Sciences

As an outcome, science is a body of knowledge. Physics, mathematics, and chemistry are three examples of scientific disciplines composed of unique bodies of knowledge. These sciences are often classified as *natural sciences* because they employ the general laws of nature and begin with the physical notion of the world. These natural sciences (which are also sometimes referred to as the *physical sciences*) are also known as *pure sciences*. "Pure," in this context, means a unique definitive body of knowledge. A pure science is independent of others; it is able to stand alone, and it may be developed and furthered for the abstract cause of the knowledge itself. Pure science is not pursued for its utility or value or application per se.

Natural and pure sciences are based on the assumption that reality is objective, rather than subjective. As a result of this objectivity, natural science is consistent; in other words, it is reproducible and reliable. Natural science further encompasses the assumption that human beings have the capacity to be accurate and consistent in their objectivity.

Natural scientists believe that explanations (obtained using the method described later in this chapter) are present within the natural or real world. As a consequence, explanations are reasonable, constant and consistent, accurate, objective, discoverable, and understandable. Owing to its basis in objectivity, natural science is predicated on the belief that there is an external world structure independent of self that is grounded in reliability.

Natural physical sciences are referred to as *hard science*. In recent years, quantum physicists have begun to integrate the role of the observer into their discipline, which is still categorized as a hard science. This conundrum will be addressed as part of the discussion of complexity science found later in this chapter.

Examples of the physical sciences present in health care include the biophysical and biochemical processes related to diabetes, cardiovascular disease, and cancer. Using the physical sciences in health care involves assuming a disease focus, rather than a person focus. The science is about diagnosis, treatment, and outcomes of treatment. It is about side effects and it is about pathology. The concentration is on objectivity, consistent application, and the creation of algorithms of predictability.

Applied (Soft) Sciences

Sociology, psychology, and anthropology are three examples of applied sciences. *Applied sciences* have their own unique body of knowledge, albeit a different one than is found in the natural sciences category, and in combination with others. They are known as applied sciences because the focus is on the application of related knowledge, usually to meet some human need (and not to generate knowledge for the sake of knowledge). Additionally, the word "applied" is used to convey the understanding that, in the development of their own knowledge, applied scientists use the knowledge from the pure sciences. Sociologists, who study people and behavior, rely on and use the natural sciences and their inherent assumptions to further their work. Thus sociology is an applied science. Mathematicians and physicists do not use psychology or sociology to add knowledge to their scientific disciplines because mathematics and physics are pure sciences, whereas psychology and sociology are applied sciences.

Although applied scientists use what they deem accurate and appropriate from the natural sciences, they do not subscribe to the rigid belief of objectivity and reliability. In applied science, the focus is on human beings and the utility of the science to them and for them. Consequently, objectivity, observation, and reproducibility are diminished or perhaps not present at all. Therefore, the applied sciences are sometimes referred to as *soft science*.

Inherent in the distinction between hard and soft science are certain assumptions and beliefs. Hard scientists assume objectivity, whereas soft scientists do not. Hard scientists operate from a belief in an external world structure independent of self, whereas soft scientists do not. The hard sciences are grounded in a worldview based on reliability and consistency as contrasted with the soft sciences, which allow for individuality and originality. These distinctions are not minor semantics, but rather indicators of major differences in philosophy and perspective.

Examples of using soft applied sciences in health care can be found in social work, the work of a psychotherapist, and the examination of healthcare disparities between people of color, those of wealth, and fragile elders. Some state practice acts define nursing as specialized knowledge integrating both physical and social sciences. In these instances, the acts combine the concepts of hard, soft, pure, and applied sciences.

Human Science

In addition to the categories of science discussed previously, human science is an important type of science. Few scholars would choose to classify human science as either hard or soft, but rather might prefer to classify it as something totally different. *Human science* is not a new term. It was introduced by Wilhelm Dilthey in the late 1800s (Ermarth, 1978). As a German philosopher, Dilthey was perplexed by the concepts of objectivity and value-free science, which left the person out of the process. He expressed concern about a science and a subsequent knowledge base that did not include the everyday lived reality of individuals. Along the way, Dilthey created the discipline of human science, which captures human beings and their experiences as the source for knowledge.

With this understanding of human science, the scientist becomes as much a part of the experience as does the participant. This view is in direct opposition to the neutral or value-free experience of the physical scientist, whose life is irrelevant to his or her work. Thus the nature and focus of the science and the process and role of the scientist are different when the subject area is viewed as a human science. In the physical sciences, the scientist and the subject are not one. In the applied sciences, the science and the scientist are not necessarily one. In contrast, in human science, they are one; they cannot be separated from each other.

Is nursing a human science? Is the work of the advanced practice nurse inextricably interwoven with the population served? When nurses speak of patients and families, is this a function of a human science view or of something else? For nursing to be a human science, nurses must recognize themselves as scientists. The work they do in the provision of care to individuals, families, and communities may be viewed from a lens of science that is simultaneously physical (hard), applied (soft), and human.

SCIENTIFIC METHOD FOR THE PHYSICAL SCIENCES (TRADITIONAL)

As an approach or a method, traditional physical science uses a process of linear steps to solve a problem. Most nurses are familiar with the term *scientific method*, but few appreciate the assumptions inherent within the method itself. An assumption is a notion or fact that one takes for granted as true and right. The scientific method is based on the assumptions that observation is universal, that laws of nature guide every action, and that the outcome of an experiment will be useful in predicting and, therefore, controlling the object of the experiment. Being *universal*, as the term is used in relation to the scientific method and science, means that all essences are the same and that individuality does not apply. The laws of nature are those that are connected to the physical world structure independent of human consciousness, such as the laws of thermodynamics and gravity. Control through prediction is the ultimate aim of the scientific method. Control occurs through the accurate and reproducible prediction of events.

The scientific method is more than a linear process to conduct an experiment. Although hard scientists would say that it is value neutral, the scientific method is an interwoven and value-laden approach to the solution to a problem. Objectivity is a key factor that is used to validate the scientific method, yet what the scientist considers to be part of the process is a value-laden decision, regardless of whether objectivity is used later. Arguments about science being value neutral versus value laden color the aims of the two categories of science: pure and applied.

AIM OF SCIENCE

The pure hard sciences have a single aim of knowledge development for the sake of knowledge development and the search for truth. To the hard scientist, a single truth exists that can be discovered once human beings have the physical capacity to make the necessary discovery. This "single truth" approach is based on a belief that an objective world exists independent of human consciousness. Traditional science aims to describe and explain this external world structure. Another aim of the physical pure sciences is to control phenomena through an empirical approach to scientific inquiry. Control is achieved as a result of the accurate prediction of universal descriptions of outcomes. When it is known, the world can be controlled.

The aim of the applied sciences, by comparison, is the application of knowledge for a specific purpose, thereby yielding utility. Applied science is not focused on generating knowledge for the sake of having knowledge, but rather for the development of applications that can better a situation, improve a process, or change the way situations are viewed.

In human science, the aims focus on individuals, families, and communities. Aims of human science may be to improve quality of life, ensure dignified beginnings and ends to life, uncover meaning in everyday life, and highlight the roles of individuals within this examination. The aims of human science may be simply stated as *to know and understand what works for people to maximize their ability to be fully functioning individuals, families, and communities at whatever level they are able to function.*

SCIENTIFIC METHODS IN HUMAN SCIENCE

Human science requires different methods. While the scientific method may be applied in the abstract, the end for the human scientist is greater than the sum of the parts. Thus varied methods are needed. In human science, the scientists and the subject (content area) being studied are treated as parts of the same whole. Therefore, the methods used can be neither linear nor constant. Instead, the methods need to be dynamic, while still meeting the same expectation of rigor found in the hard sciences. Rigor—a notion usually associated with randomized control studies, reliability, and validity in the hard sciences—is not the goal in human science. Rather, contextual consistency, purposive sampling within the population experiencing the essence to be described, validity of questions, a detailed audit trail of data collection and data analysis, and a return to the participants for validation of the message sent and received are emphasized.

CRITERIA FOR SCIENCE

An important distinction to address is the difference between science and nonscience. This discussion has been going on for centuries. Some scholars may look at human science as nonscience. Pseudoscience—comprising theories that are presented as scientific but not proven with the scientific method or supported by data—is the bane of existence for the hard physical scientist, even though it clearly has popular appeal. Therefore, it is important for the hard physical sciences to demarcate themselves from pseudoscience and, perhaps, applied and human sciences. Five criteria are used for this purpose: (1) intersubjective testability, (2) reliability, (3) definiteness and precision, (4) coherence, and (5) comprehensiveness and scope (Feigl, 1988).

Intersubjective Testability

Intersubjective testability is based on a belief in the value of corroboration and on the idea that two people who view the same entity in the same manner should obtain the same results; if this criterion is met, the method is objective. Using the word "objective" as a synonym for intersubjectivity means that "the belief is not based on hallucination or deception and it is not a state of mind but truly exists . . . the belief is neither private nor unique. It can be and must be verified . . . and be empirically tested" (Polifroni & Welch, 1999, pp. 3–4).

Reliability

Reliability, the second criterion, means that researchers achieve the same result time and again when the circumstances of their study have not changed. If findings demonstrate reliability, then the same outcomes are achieved with repeated tests, thereby confirming the beliefs and premises set forth by the scientist. Reliability is the basis for prediction and subsequent control.

Definiteness and Precision

Definiteness and precision, which collectively constitute the third criterion, are words used to convey exactness and rigid adherence to objectivity. Precision is not about approximation, but rather exactness; it is about specifics, not generalities. If experimentation meets the criterion of definiteness and precision, creating the same circumstances for repeated experimentation leads to a reasonable expectation that the same results will be achieved. Definiteness and precision are not about inclusion of the researcher or fluidity of ideas; indeed, they focus on the opposite goal.

Coherence

Coherence or systematic character, the fourth criterion, addresses connectedness and wholeness. How do the parts relate to one another to form a unique body of knowledge? The connectedness (the sense of a whole with integrated parts, not disparate ideas) is the coherence required in science that is not necessarily present in pseudoscience. It is important to distinguish the wholeness of coherence from holism in human science. In coherence, the focus is on the parts and their relation to one another. In contrast, holism in human science focuses on the whole from the outset, not the parts.

Comprehensiveness and Scope

The fifth criterion, comprehensiveness and scope, encompasses the ability of the science to be used for something other than its intended purpose. Comprehensiveness and scope define applications beyond the basis of the planned study and achieving the expected outcome through appropriate utilization. Polifroni and Welch (1999) explain this concept as follows:

> The thrust of this criterion is the maximum explanatory power of the science and its related theories. . . . A science is not a science if it does not explain and address events and related concerns beyond the issue under study at the present time. (p. 4)

QUESTIONS FOR THE PRACTITIONER

The five criteria—intersubjective testability, reliability, definiteness and precision, coherence, and comprehensiveness and scope—serve to separate science and pseudoscience, as well as common sense. It is important for advanced practice nurses to understand the scientific nature of their work. They should consider the following: Is nursing a science? If so, is nursing work that of pure science or applied science? Is the care provided to patients, families, and communities done for the purpose of prediction and control? Are there universals within patient care provision? Is there an external world independent of human consciousness that colors the care delivered? Does nursing as a science satisfy the five demarcation criteria? Is nursing practice objective? (See **Box 1-1**.)

Box 1-1   Questions for Advanced Practice Nurses

1. Is nursing a science?
2. Does your practice meet the five criteria of a science?
3. How do you use the concept of universals in your care while making the care individualized?
4. How do algorithms of treatment embrace person-centered care?
5. As population-based care comes to the forefront, what assumptions are needed to provide state-of-the-art care?

PHILOSOPHY

Whereas science is about knowledge, the term *philosophy* (originally from the Greek word *philosophia*) means "love of wisdom." Enjoyment of the thought process, the notion of thinking for the sake of thinking (How often have you said, "If only I had time to think . . ."?), the examination of ideas, and the search for truth are all part of philosophy. Philosophy also involves a search for meaning; it represents a perspective, and it is a set of beliefs. Philosophy, like science, is both a process and an outcome. The process of philosophy is the critical inquiry and examination of meaning and the method one undertakes when beliefs are examined, ideas are proposed, and assumptions are challenged.

Philosophy encompasses more than rhetoric; it is the guide by which situations are approached, the viewpoint used to see what is before one, and the method by which one searches for truth, as well as an understanding of what truth is. Philosophy is contextually grounded; it relies on the present but is embedded in the historical past. Philosophy is dynamic, it evolves, and it is subtle while simultaneously being overt.

Philosophy captures the essence of a human being, such as the essence of what it means to be a provider in a caring profession. The deliberate use of the word "caring" here indicates a philosophical belief based on the author's experience, gender, and role as a scientist. Philosophy is more than just a belief; it is the *application* of that belief to situations known and unknown. Philosophy is epistemology *and* ontology, the knowledge of and the belief about something. Epistemology is the study of knowing, of determining what knowledge is and how that knowledge is relevant and related to extant knowledge. Ontology is the study of being and of meaning.

All schools of philosophical thought cannot possibly be explored in a single chapter. One way to undertake a large survey of philosophical thought is to examine the various perspectives in terms of two major schools of philosophical thought: analytical and continental. Analytical philosophers originally were those primarily located outside of Europe, whereas advocates of continental philosophy originally emanated from Europe. While the two schools are often discussed in opposition to each other, their discordant viewpoints are actually simply a matter of the philosophers using a different lens, differing approaches, and differing subjects. Analytical philosophy is wedded to objectivity and reproducibility, whereas continental philosophy is about essence and experience.

Continental philosophy is grounded in the viewpoint that the phenomena of interest are deeply embedded in the human experience. *Analytical philosophy*, by comparison, focuses more on the use of the process of logic and rational discourse than on the subject itself. Analytical philosophies include positivism, empiricism, instrumentalism, pragmatism, and rationalism, whereas continental philosophies include phenomenology, hermeneutics, critical social theory, feminism, structuralism, post-structuralism, and postmodernism. Some of these views will be discussed later in this chapter. (See **Box 1-2**.)

Box 1-2	Essential Terminology in Philosophy	
Analytical philosophy	Epistemology	Phenomenology
Antirealism	Essence	Positivism
A priori	Experience	Post-structuralism
Chaos	Hermeneutics	Pragmatism
Complexity science	Idealism	Priori
Continental philosophy	Logical positivism	Realism
Empiricism	Ontology	Truth

PHILOSOPHY OF SCIENCE

Philosophy of science exists at the intersection of philosophy and science—where the two meet to form a new perspective that aims to examine the body of knowledge *and* the approaches to the study of the body of knowledge. Philosophy of science in nursing is an "examination of nursing concepts, theories, laws and aims as they relate to nursing practice. Through such an understanding and deliberate thought, praxis evolves" (Polifroni & Welch, 1999, p. 5). Praxis is the planned, deliberate, and thoughtful creation of a plan of action to achieve a set goal. Philosophy of science in nursing explores the meaning of truth, the meaning of evidence, and the meaning of life through praxis.

It is nurses' responsibility to view science from a multitude of perspectives: as nurse scientist; as care provider; and from the perspective of the patient, family, and society. Each perspective potentially offers a different lens for examining the same concept. Each lens brings certain assumptions to the forefront that color both the lens and the object of review.

Analytical philosophers, who are often physical scientists, examine the nature of truth using a lens of objectivity, linear thinking, and rationality. Continental philosophers explore the meaning and nature of truth from an individual lens focusing on the experience of truth from the perspective of the person (including the perspective of the scientist), which leads to some subjectivity in the results. These two lenses or perspectives require practitioners to examine their own perspective of truth and ask, "Is there only one truth? Does truth reside in the external world structure independent of human consciousness, or is truth found within the individual and highly contextual? Is there more than one truth? Is truth even a relevant subject for discourse, or should the focus of practice be on the outcomes of treatment modalities?" The answers to these questions enable providers to become comfortable with the assumptions and underpinnings of the various philosophical perspectives.

HOW DO WE KNOW?

Answering the question "How do we know?" is key to helping anyone understand philosophy of science. This question can be pondered by considering where knowledge and knowing originate. A first thought is that people know because of tradition: Experiences that happened yesterday color and shape what is known about today. Tradition often shapes experiences into a repetitive pattern of behavior. Authorities also inform what is known. An authority may be a person, a role, or an institution. A police officer is an authority; a college professor is an authority; an institution of higher learning is an authority, as is a church. In addition, doctrine can shape what is known. Without evidence or in the face of contradictory evidence, those who believe in and practice a religion profess it as their knowing. Reason, without regard for religion or tradition, is yet another realm of knowing. Reason may lead to a path that contradicts religion or tradition; thus individuals must decide what to believe.

Common sense is a form of knowing also: People know that they become wet when it rains and, therefore, they should seek shelter. If people do not eat, they know that they will become hungry and should find food. These are two examples of common sense.

Finally, there is science as a way of knowing (*to know = science*). Science is knowledge derived from methods that may be linear or complex (chaotic) depending on the view and approach. Science could be physical science, social science, human science, or nursing science. Science is how people know, regardless of the type of science.

ANALYTICAL PHILOSOPHY OF SCIENCE

Reviewing the analytical and continental categories is merely one way to examine philosophical schools of thought. Other options include using received and perceived views (Suppe, 1977), a historical timeline, a context of major events in history, and many others. Choosing the analytical and continental categories as criteria implies nothing more than a framework choice for examination. It is important to note that continental philosophers analyze and analytical philosophers examine applications.

The analytical perspective is closely associated with positivism and, more specifically, with logical positivism. Given that a significant amount of what can be read about philosophy today is contrary to logical positivism, it is important to understand that base. Logical positivism is a school of thought that originated in the early 20th century under the aegis of the Vienna School in Austria. That geographic location, while on the European continent, does not mean that the analytical perspective is necessarily associated with continental philosophy, however.

Logical positivism actually began earlier than the 20th century, with Auguste Comte's (1798–1857) view of positivism. Comte, the father of positivism, asserted that human history progresses from the theological to the metaphysical to the positivistic. By the last term, he asserted the *positive* role that the universal laws of nature provided. Following in Comte's footsteps, Kolakowski (as cited in MacKenzie, 1977) suggested four characteristic rules of positivism: (1) phenomenalism, (2) nominalism, (3) the denial of cognitive value in value judgments and normative statements, and (4) the essential unity of the scientific method.

The major tenets of logical positivism, consistent with the use of an analytical approach to problem solving, require a rigid adherence to the scientific method (deductive nomological approach), a belief in cause and effect, a solid underpinning of replicability, and an unwavering belief in an external world structure that remains independent of self. It is the final point that provides the platform for the cause-and-effect relationship and the needed objectivity divorced from humans and subjectivity.

Noted philosophers Rudolf Carnap, Herbert Feigl (demarcation criteria), Carl Hempel and L. F. L. Oppenheim (1948), and Karl Popper (2002) developed logical positivism with an aim to affirm the external world structure, solidify a reliance on the inherent laws of nature, and promote the deductive method of analysis to achieve a problem's solution. These logical positivists believed in the verifiability principle—the belief that a statement is meaningful only if it is proven true or false through the means of experience (experiment). They suggested that there is a logical structure of scientific theories, probability is meaningful in science (as opposed to possibility), science is a deductive experience, and the sources of knowledge are twofold (logical reasoning and empirical experience).

A large amount of literature in the nursing field has criticized logical positivism as being too rigid, too deductive, and lacking an appreciation or recognition of the human experience. To overcome these objections, logical positivism eventually segued into empiricism. Empiricism, which relies on the scientific method for the production of truth, held to tenets similar to those underlying logical positivism, except that the empiricist required actual experience. The logical positivist accepted the external world structure, whereas the empiricist, while neither accepting nor dismissing the existence of the external world's structure, required that science be generated through the senses of experience. Empiricism is what is commonly called science in today's world.

Over time, both empiricism and logical positivism were incorporated into the received view described by Suppe (1977). The received view of science states that a theory is either right or wrong, that mature or developed theories must be formalized, that a theory must be axiomized (taken apart into propositions and independently tested), that all sciences should be patterned after physics, and that there is a clear separation between theoretical and empirical understandings.

The received view is strongly supportive of the prominence and dominance of physical sciences. It is based on the search for truth, wherein a single truth is desired and possible to identify. Put simply, empirical (scientific) methods lead the knower to *the* answer.

This view of empiricism, which is embedded in analytical philosophy, is commonly known as traditional science. It is how most people are taught in elementary and high schools throughout the United States. Learning physical science by having opportunities to experience through observation is the gold standard of science, knowledge, and truth. Prediction, using descriptive laws and understanding initial conditions, is the purpose of science for scientists who advocate a received view. Such value-free science relies on a single universal scientific method. The received view is sometimes known as *realism*.

CONTINENTAL PHILOSOPHY OF SCIENCE

Whereas the analytical philosophy of science focuses on the search for a single truth through a scientific process of controlled experimentation, the continental philosophy of science is concerned with the connection of an idea to the world around the idea and its historical context. Continental philosophy is not about theories or truths, but rather about the relationships between people, ideas, meaning, and their historical connectedness.

Georg Hegel, Wilhelm Dilthey, Pierre Duhem, Paul Thagard, Philip Kitcher (2001), Edmund Husserl, and Martin Heidegger (1962) all have written from the continental philosophy-of-science perspective. Their works focus on the applied sciences of sociology and psychology, the historical approach and context, the understanding of power (Foucault, 1976), and the lived experience of the subject and scientist (philosopher).

Human science is the domain of the continental philosophy of science. As described earlier, human science deals with persons and their connectedness to the world in which they live and the lived experiences of their life. Continental philosophers examine this lived experience in the past as well as the present. Using continental philosophy requires an examination of historical context as much as it does what is happening in the present time. Continental philosophers of science believe not in cause and effect, but rather in connectedness and the often used proverb "Past is prologue."

Phenomenology is an example of a philosophy that emanates from the continental philosophy-of-science perspective. In phenomenology, as in philosophy, value is placed on universal experiences. Husserl (1990), a continental philosopher, believed that while human experience is personal, the essence of it is universal. For example, the essence of grief is strikingly similar whether one is grieving the loss of a limb, a loved one, a home, or a pet. For Husserl, phenomenology entails a focus on examining phenomena that appear in the consciousness of the subjects. It is about personal experience; from an examination of such experience, the essences of the phenomena are drawn.

Hermeneutics is another continental philosophy. As a philosophy, hermeneutics deals with the interpretation and understanding of a message that is being delivered. The name of this school of thought derives from Hermes, the messenger of the Greek gods. Hermeneutics is characterized by the assumptions that people are social and dialogical beings; that culture, language, skills, and experiences create shared understandings; that there is a continual circle of connectedness and understanding; that understanding precedes interpretation; and that the interpreter and the interpreted are seen as one. In hermeneutics, meaning and understanding are identified as the aims of the philosophical inquiry.

Post-structuralism, another philosophy that falls under the broad rubric of continental philosophy, speaks to the premise that the study of structures (above and below the surface of relationships and contexts) must be viewed as a cultural phenomenon. As a result, the analysis is open to a variety of interpretations and likely misinterpretations. Post-structuralism conveys the message that both the object and its context for creation, development, and evaluation must be studied. This view is similar to that taken by all the continental philosophies, which are based on a contextual grounding for analysis. The assumptions of post-structuralism are typically that the meaning of a message is based on the perception of the receiver and that the person who conveys the message is not necessarily significant in terms of the message itself. For example, this view would suggest that an advanced practice nurse is not the important component in the delivery of a message; rather, what is important is what the patient hears and interprets the message to be. This approach serves to equalize the imbalance of power between healthcare providers and patients noted in the healthcare field today.

Although the three varieties of continental philosophy described in this section certainly demonstrate some differences, all revolve around context, meaning, and the knowing subject of the discourse or action. Collectively, continental philosophies may also be called the *perceived view*, *antirealism*, or *idealism*. These terms are meant to intrigue the reader and encourage further exploration because the space limitations here do not permit an adequate discussion of them.

Perceived View

Suppe (1977) examined the perceived view with a different lens. As with the view evinced by the continental philosophers, who engaged the notion of human science and the human experience in the search for truth and knowing, the perceived view is more fluid and dynamic than the received view. Within the perceived view, theories are neither right nor wrong. This position stands in stark contrast to the verification approach of the received view.

In the perceived view, observation leads to the generation of theory, which in turn is value laden. Both the received and the perceived views rely on observation, but the meaning of this term and the process by which observation is achieved differ for the two views. Observation for the received, analytical philosopher is precise, detailed, physical, objective, and inherently value neutral or value free. For people subscribing to the perceived view, observation involves the use of the senses and the mind. Observation is accurate but is not reliant on precision; it is both physical and mental. Observation is detailed but not necessarily measurable, and it is subjective. Therefore, observation from the perceived-view perspective is inherently subjective. What one chooses to observe is as much a part of the process as is the observation itself.

The received view supports the beliefs that progression in science leads to a deeper understanding and that this understanding leads to theories for examination. Perceived-view proponents believe in using different kinds of theories and many methods to obtain truth, although some do not seek truth at all, only understanding. Whereas following the tenets of the received view requires use of the scientific method, exploration, and experimentation, proponents of the perceived view use varied approaches to science and seeking truth, such as phenomenology, grounded theory, case method, and hermeneutics. Received-view scientists use the quantitative method in their pursuit of science, whereas perceived-view scientists use methods appropriate to the question asked, which may be either quantitative or qualitative, or a mixture of the two.

CHAOS AND COMPLEXITY SCIENCE

Contemporary philosophers of science synthesize the work of both the analytical and continental philosophers into a new and emerging philosophy of science. The emerging philosophy incorporates chaos and complexity science, which is closely aligned with quantum physics. Truth, the domain of the analytical scientists and philosophers, and understanding, the realm of the continental philosophers and scientists, come together in a different and dynamic way in chaos and complexity science. Complex adaptive, dynamic systems (organic or inorganic) are connected to environments and are influenced by what has come before and what will come after; these systems are irreducibly whole.

Complexity science and a view of complex adaptive systems with the language of fluidity and dynamicism push the scientist to look at things differently. Is there a real difference—not just a semantic difference—between the images conjured up by the terms "fine-tune" and "emergent" or "work up" and "evolve"? (See **Box 1-3**.)

Bohm (1980) stated that the "universe is no longer seen as a machine, made up of objects, but rather pictured as one indivisible whole whose parts are essentially interrelated and can only be understood as patterns of a cosmic process" (p. 29). The assumptions about complex adaptive systems are many, and they include the characteristics of embeddedness (meaning patterns that can be traced backward and forward), distributed control (an equalization of power bases), nonlinearity, multidirectionality, emergence

Box 1-3 What Image Do These Terms Conjure?			
Work up	Industry	Control	Emergent
Diagnose	Engineer	Check	Self-organize
Fine-tune	Design	Evolve	Diversity
Prescribe	Operate	Adapt	Ecology

Box 1-4   Provider Questions

1. What is my view of truth?
2. Are there multiple truths?
3. What if my patient and I do not agree on the truth or the view of truth?
4. Is the lived experience important?
5. Is the lived experience more important than lab values and blood gases?
6. How do I justify/juggle evidence-based practice guidelines and individuality?

in the dynamic diversity of subjects and objects, a simultaneous coexistence of order and disorder, and outcomes that are inherently unpredictable. This perspective stands in direct contrast to the notion of traditional science, which aims to explain and predict in order to control.

SUMMARY

There is more to philosophy of science than what is presented here. Nurses embody philosophy in their actions when they enact their knowledge, ethics, and whole being in the care of others (Bruce, Rietze, & Lim, 2014, p. 70). Whole schools of thought have not been addressed because the purpose of this chapter is to offer a landscape view to appreciate the role of philosophy of science in your everyday work.

Throughout the chapter, several underlying questions have colored all else: What are the assumptions of each nurse's philosophy of science? Do nurses aim to diagnose and treat illness, or to diagnose and treat human responses? Do nurses aim to control through prescription, or do they aim to understand and co-create meaning and action? Is there a single way to resolve a problem, or are different views and approaches permissible? Is one's praxis dynamic and wedded to a guideline, a critical path, or a set of standing orders? What do nurses need to be the best practitioners they can be? What do patients, families, and communities need? Finally, each nurse is encouraged to ask, "Am I the nurse that I want to be?" (See **Box 1-4**.)

DISCUSSION QUESTIONS

1. What are the assumptions that color/shape my approach to care?
2. Describe the disruptive change needed within health care to address the major issues facing us today.

REFERENCES

Bohm, D. (1980). *Wholeness and the implicate order*. London, UK: Routledge.

Boyd, R., Gasper, P., & Trout, J. D. (Eds.). (1991). *The philosophy of science*. Cambridge, MA: Blackwell.

Bruce, A., Rietze, L., & Lim, A. (2014). Understanding philosophy in a nurse's world: What, where and why? *Nursing and Health, 2*(3), 65–71.

Ermarth, M. (1978). *Wilhelm Dilthey: The critique of historical reason*. Chicago, IL: University of Chicago Press.

Feigl, H. (1988). The scientific outlook: Naturalism and humanism. In E. D. Klemke, R. Hollinger, & A. D. Kline (Eds.), *Philosophy of science* (pp. 427–437). Buffalo, NY: Prometheus Books.

Foucault, M. (1976). *The will to know*. Paris, France: Gallimard.

Heidegger, M. (1962). *Being and time* (J. Macquarrie & E. Robinson, Trans.). New York, NY: Harper & Row.

Hempel, C., & Oppenheim, P. (1948). Studies in the logic of explanation. *Philosophy of Science, 15,* 135–175.

Husserl, E. (1990). *The idea of phenomenology* (W. Altson & G. Nakhnikian, Trans.). Boston, MA: Kluwer Academic.

Kitcher, P. (2001). *Science, truth, and democracy*. Oxford, UK: Oxford University Press.

MacKenzie, B. D. (1977). *Behaviourism and the limits of scientific method*. London, UK: Routledge & Paul.

Polifroni, E. C., & Welch, M. (1999). *Perspective on philosophy of science in nursing: An historical and contemporary anthology*. Philadelphia, PA: Lippincott.

Popper, K. (2002) [1959]. *The logic of scientific discovery* (2nd English ed.). New York, NY: Routledge.

Suppe, F. (1977). *The structure of scientific theories*. Chicago, IL: University of Illinois Press.

Chapter 2

The Evolution of Nursing Science

Beth L. Rodgers

INTRODUCTION

In discussions of nursing, images that commonly come to mind are those of the nurse performing certain acts such as listening to blood pressure sounds, changing a dressing for a wound, assisting someone with ambulation, giving medication, or starting an intravenous line. Undoubtedly, people who have been registered nurses for some time recall their early days in school and the tremendous anticipation of performing the first immunization or urinary catheterization, or the excitement the first time an intravenous catheter was inserted smoothly and successfully.

Nurses who have been engaged in the broad professional role of the registered nurse recognize that there is a great deal more to nursing than the performance of those skills. Nonetheless, when talking about nursing, discussion often turns to a focus on what nurses *do*—the skills, tasks, and functions that are associated with the actions and behaviors of nurses. Much less common is an emphasis on what nurses *know*—the knowledge base that underlies the performance of those acts—as well as the many more things that nurses do beyond obvious physical functions. No doubt it is much easier to describe the mechanics of listening to breath sounds than it is to describe the detailed thinking that goes into formulating a holistic portrayal of an individual patient for whom those breath sounds are only a small part of his or her scenario.

Nurses engage in a variety of actions that are far subtler than those involving the common skills that are directly observable. For example, they form important relationships with patients to help them achieve their health and wellness goals; they counsel, educate, guide, facilitate, assess, plan, relate, evaluate, and engage with people as individuals or in groups or communities on a variety of levels consistent with a holistic approach to health concerns and health promotion. Nurses also engage in activities such as arranging for referrals, managing various stages of care, and facilitating access to necessary resources. This list is in no way exhaustive, but it provides some indication of the tremendous number of cognitive activities associated with nursing. These actions also are done not as simple tasks, but as the result of complex decision making based on the intricate details determined through comprehensive assessment of each situation. Because these activities lack implements or other tangible equipment, the cognitive work of the nurse may be recognized less readily by the public. This lack of recognition is compounded by the fact that nurses are not typically thought of in terms of their knowledge base, unlike other professions where there is more awareness of education and knowledge. Nurses have perpetuated that lack of awareness by being less quick to describe their knowledge, possibly because of the difficulty associated with articulating the specific thought processes that are essential for effective and appropriate care. Many nurses seem to give themselves less credit than is warranted for the cognitive capabilities and knowledge that go into nursing. When asked why they reacted to a situation in a particular way or what prompted them to intervene, it is not uncommon to hear the nurse say, "I just knew," referring to a gut feeling or intuition as the basis for significant action.

These responses on the part of nurses fail to give credit to the vast amount of knowledge that nurses carry with them every day. It is not the tasks and skills that nurses perform that make them such an indispensable part of health care, but rather what they "know." The knowledge of nurses not only lies at the root of competent and effective care, but it also provides the foundation that makes nurses essential contributors to broader decision making and planning. When nurses argue that they should be involved in committees, on boards, or in other influential positions, and when they discuss why certain concerns or problems clearly could benefit from nursing involvement, it is the knowledge of nurses that makes these arguments so meaningful. Although nurses often find themselves in a position of needing, or at least wanting, to articulate what is unique about their particular level of preparation, discussion of the knowledge base of nursing can be a challenging undertaking. It is much easier to describe what nurses do than what they know.

THE IMPACT OF THE DOCTOR OF NURSING PRACTICE DEGREE

As nurses have achieved higher levels of education (particularly doctoral degrees), the need to understand the knowledge base of the discipline has become even more imperative. Nurses with doctoral-level education are likely to be perceived as leaders both in the discipline and in the broader community, and they should be prepared and willing to assume roles as leaders in a number of contexts. They often are confronted with both the opportunity and the need to explain what constitutes nursing at that level. No doubt this need will persist and most likely will expand greatly as more nurses with doctor of nursing practice (DNP) degrees work within a variety of settings. The DNP is an advanced degree, which surely will grab the interest of the public, whose familiarity with nursing is most likely limited to personal experience with hospital or clinic nurses (i.e., nurses who have completed shorter programs leading to the ability to obtain a license as a registered nurse). In addition, it is a relatively new degree that carries with it credentials and titles that are not known to the broader public, and that are perhaps also not well understood within nursing. At the same time, nurses with the DNP degree are in an important position to serve as leaders in the continuing articulation of the discipline, as well as contributors on multiple levels to the development of the knowledge base for nursing.

All of these factors create a tremendous need for nurses at all levels of preparation to articulate with clarity the nature of nursing knowledge and what nurses are capable of contributing to health in all realms—individual, family, local, community, and global. DNP-prepared nurses have particular responsibility to assume leadership roles to represent the discipline and profession of nursing well and to identify and discuss the particular expertise and advanced knowledge of the DNP-prepared nurse. In addition, nurses with the DNP degree often are in important positions to collaborate with researchers and to identify both needs for research and innovations that add to the knowledge base of nursing as it continues to develop as a discipline. Similarly, they have a key role in implementing new knowledge for the improvement of healthcare access and delivery. All of these responsibilities point to the importance of the DNP-prepared nurse's understanding the nature of nursing and the knowledge base of the discipline.

SCIENCE AND KNOWLEDGE

Without an understanding of the overall discipline, including the knowledge that underlies the thoughts and actions of the nurse, both practice and research can become isolated, individualistic, situational endeavors. Science is the general term used to refer to the knowledge base of a discipline that has been developed rigorously and systematically. The idea of "science" has an interesting history, however, and science was not always the dominant term used to refer to credible knowledge. As evidenced by the writings of Aristotle, for example, and in the work of many others continuing into the 19th century, the terms *science* and *knowledge* were used almost interchangeably for much of recorded history. It is only in modern times that science has been recognized as a rather specialized form of knowledge, replete with specific methodologies and means to evaluate credibility. In exploring the underpinnings of nursing work, especially those elements that provide nurses with valuable and trustworthy information as a foundation for practice, it is helpful to look at not just science but also the broader realm of nursing knowledge.

The discipline of nursing includes components other than just the knowledge base. Disciplines also involve a human component in that judgments are made about what is acceptable science and what are current priorities. This component necessarily involves the expression of the values embodied in the discipline in regard to what is needed for knowledge development. The human component, what Toulmin (1972) referred to as the "profession," works with and develops the knowledge base of the discipline and develops mechanisms for the sharing of ideas through debate and dialogue, both oral and in the form of publications. Organizations within the discipline provide leadership, whether through societies that have bestowed honors upon esteemed nurses, research organizations that promote the conduct of research and dissemination of results, or specialty organizations that shape practice. Those organizations also have important roles in the ongoing development of nursing as a discipline. Discussion of the science of nursing, or the knowledge base, cannot be carried out without recognition of the context that exists for that knowledge in the discipline. In addition, this nursing context exists within a larger societal context that includes expectations for nurses, as well as standards for what is considered to be knowledge or science, and especially "good" science.

It is easy to identify examples of how knowledge has changed, sometimes rapidly, and just as often in radical ways. Recent discoveries related to genetics are stimulating revolutionary developments in treatment as well as renewed efforts at prevention as that genetic knowledge evolves. Dietary guidelines are evolving as awareness develops that blood lipid profiles are not inextricably linked to dietary intake of fats, with new information being in substantial opposition to prevailing ideology about nutrition and illness. Awareness of the effect of environmental conditions and artificial substances on health and the development of health problems has raised questions in areas that were not given much consideration in the prior germ theory–oriented approach to medicine, questions ranging from food production to vaccination guidelines. In such a context of ever-changing science, often accompanied by competing values and priorities, significant challenges are presented for nurses who not only provide "best practice" in their realm of work, but who also must defend those practices in the face of changing knowledge.

It is clear that context has considerable influence on the discipline of nursing and the development of the corresponding knowledge base. Because of that influence, it is reasonable to look at the evolution of nursing knowledge using a chronological approach; in fact, many aspects of context are associated with historical events and timing. One limitation associated with such a chronology is that it gives the impression that change is linear. That would be quite a naïve view, however. Science is inextricably tied to human behavior and attitudes; given that science is a human enterprise, and multiple stakeholders and influences exist, the development and change of knowledge over time is far from linear. In contrast, the movement of knowledge often involves multiple and simultaneously existing and competing areas of focus influenced by diverse philosophical systems and sets of values.

Nonetheless, early ideas do provide the impetus for later ideas; societal needs and expectations at one period of time eventually lead to other sets of ideas. As such, there is continuity in the progression of ideas, and that continuity provides a useful framework for studying the history of ideas about nursing science. It is important to keep in mind that changes in ideas and emphasis must be considered as an evolutionary process and not necessarily a progression. Progression implies movement toward some specified point or goal, such that it is possible to say that nursing knowledge or science is getting closer to whatever that goal might be. Because of the fluidity of the context of nursing, as well as the context of the greater society, that endpoint or goal must be amenable to change as well. Although the evaluation of progress in regard to knowledge is a difficult task, nurses can say with certainty and, perhaps, with pride that there have been incredible improvements in educational preparation, in leadership and organization within the discipline, and in the ability to address the changing needs of the people who are the beneficiaries of nursing care.

This element of continuity also needs to be examined from the standpoint of ideas about nursing. Nursing, in various forms, has existed, depending on how it is defined, since the beginning of time. Nursing also exists in a global context despite the variation that might exist from one setting to the next, even within general geographic regions. It is tempting sometimes to avoid defining nursing, or making clear statements about what nursing "is" because of this variation. However, there are some things that enable all of these disparate situations to be thought of as nursing. Despite all the differences, there are some things that hold nursing together as a distinct type of knowledge and work; some essence persists across time and contexts and makes it proper to call these things nursing. Leaders and scholars in nursing have the obligation to be able to discuss nursing with others who may have different perceptions of nursing and be able to articulate to others the nature of nursing and the incredible contributions to human health that can be made by those who are registered nurses.

NURSING AS A DISCIPLINE

Despite the tremendous contributions of nurses to meeting the healthcare needs of individuals, groups, and populations, and despite the pervasiveness of nursing throughout much of history, it can be difficult to delineate clearly what constitutes nursing as a discipline. Problems articulating the nature of the knowledge base of nursing can give the impression that there is not a specific, unique substance of knowledge or science that underlies the practice of nurses. Such claims might seem absurd to any nurse who has been carrying out acts of nursing for an entire career. While it should be self-evident that nurses cannot act without some base of knowledge—otherwise, their actions would be totally without reason—significant challenges have arisen as they have tried to articulate precisely what constitutes that knowledge base.

This desire to define the knowledge base of nursing has been enhanced by some authors who have argued that it is essential for nursing's continued viability to distinguish its knowledge base from that of other disciplines (Feldman, 1981; Smith & McCarthy, 2010;

Visintainer, 1986). While such concerns are not voiced in nursing as frequently today as they were a few decades ago, lingering questions persist about precisely what constitutes nursing and what reflects or represents some other field of knowledge or inquiry.

To respond to these concerns, unique languages have been created in the form of nursing diagnoses and other taxonomies, and research has been conducted rather extensively on intuition and clinical decision making in nursing. Nurses have focused on aesthetics, empathy, and "caring" as a way to capture what some consider to be the unique essence of nursing knowledge. These and more themes evident in the evolution of nursing science reflect the ongoing quest by nurse scholars to answer questions about the nature of nursing and, especially, the knowledge base or science that constitutes the discipline.

THE EDUCATION OF NURSES

As noted previously, concern has been expressed in nursing literature, especially during the period of the late 1960s through the late 1980s, about the apparent lack of a unique knowledge base for the discipline. At other times, critics noted a failure to articulate what makes up that unique knowledge. No doubt the history of the development of nursing supports concerns about the existence of a distinct, unique knowledge base in the discipline. Education for nurses has been referred to historically as training, a term that was particularly relevant during the apprentice-type model of early nursing preparation. Despite Florence Nightingale's revolutionizing the preparation of nurses for her day, even well into the 20th century a substantial portion of the preparation of nurses occurred through on-the-job apprenticeships.

Nurses educated as recently as the 1970s (and sometimes even more recently) may still refer to their preparation as training rather than as education. While these semantics might seem like a minor point, terminology can be quite powerful in its ability to convey unintended messages, as well as those desired by the speaker or writer. The term *education* carries a different connotation than the term *training*; the latter is focused on the ability to perform certain actions, not on the knowledge and understanding that precede reasoned action. In addition to this distinction, the emphasis in early nursing training was placed on selecting the best candidates to be nurses on the basis of personal characteristics that were presumed to be appropriate; the focus was not on the intellectual capacity or aptitude for gaining the knowledge needed to be an effective nurse. A review of conditions for nurse preparation in the early days of the discipline clearly reveals that fortitude and persistence were valued as characteristics essential to successful completion of these preparatory programs. At the same time, rules for nurses mandated subservient behaviors rather than critical thinking.

At the time that nurses began to receive formal education through actual involvement in classroom work and didactic presentations, much of the content of nursing programs was taught by physicians. Programs were associated with hospitals rather than colleges and universities, and the learning of the skills associated with nursing continued to occur primarily by actually doing the work of the nurse. Nursing was not associated closely with academic settings until 1909, when Richard Olding Beard successfully integrated the nursing program into the formal academic structure of the University of Minnesota. This program led to a 3-year diploma and was subsumed under the medical school, yet it was the first instance of nursing education as an official part of a university structure. Yale School of Nursing, which opened in 1924, was the first autonomous school of nursing with its own dean and budget (Kalisch & Kalisch, 1995).

Education at the graduate level developed slowly within the context of academic settings. Master's degrees were available in the early 1930s, yet by 1962 data revealed only 2,472 students pursued the master's degree in nursing; for the period 1961–1962, only 1,098 graduates were enrolled in master's degree programs (U.S. Public Health Service, 1963). Opportunities for doctoral-level education were severely limited in nursing, and nurses who wanted such preparation typically pursued their degrees in the discipline of education rather than nursing per se. The first programs that enabled nurses to pursue doctoral degrees were established in schools of education at Teacher's College, Columbia University, and at New York University, both developed in the 1920s and 1930s.

As nursing evolved as a discipline, recognition of the need for nurses with doctoral-level preparation as researchers grew, yet there was almost no opportunity to obtain such education within the discipline of nursing. In 1962, the U.S. Public Health Service began the Nurse Scientist Program to support advanced education to prepare nurses as researchers. Because of the absence of doctoral programs in the discipline of nursing, nurses who pursued their education as a part of this program had no choice but to receive their education in other fields. As a result, they typically were socialized into those other disciplines, bringing the perspective of physiologists, sociologists, and educators to bear on their ideas about nursing.

Nurses with doctoral preparation in nursing and increased nursing research activity are fairly recent developments. The first doctoral nursing program was established at the University of Pittsburgh in 1954 and was limited to maternal–child health, with a doctor of nursing science (DNS) program being established at Boston University 6 years later in 1960 (Kalisch & Kalisch, 1995). Because many universities did not support doctoral-level preparation in nursing, doctoral programs often had to offer a distinct degree, typically the DNS or DNSc. Journals devoted to nursing research did not emerge until the 1950s, with an additional surge of activity in this area occurring in the 1970s. It is only within the last 30 years or so that a preponderance of people teaching in programs that lead to a doctoral degree in nursing also have had their own doctoral-level preparation in nursing.

Awareness of this historical development in nursing helps to explain the nature of research that has been done and, similarly, the development of the discipline over the last several decades. It is only within the last two or three decades that the individuals conducting research within the field of nursing were likely to have been educated with degrees in nursing and socialized primarily as researchers and scholars in nursing. As a result, there has been an increase in research conducted by nurse investigators with a viewpoint that has been derived from and has reflected a nursing perspective toward the problems addressed by the research.

This brief glimpse into a significant aspect of the history of nursing education makes it easy to see why concerns about borrowed knowledge have had a prominent role in the evolution of nursing as a discipline. This lack of clarity in regard to a unique knowledge base for nursing was compounded by prevailing ideas about the nature of disciplines. Prominent nurse scholars in the 1960s through the late 1970s brought to nursing ideas from education about the nature and structure of disciplines.

DELINEATING THE DISCIPLINE

Underlying all of this historical activity was a variety of theoretical thinking about knowledge in nursing, including nursing as a discipline, the role of theory in nursing, mechanisms for theory development, and, in more recent years, a broad interest in nursing science and its development. In the early stages, attention was focused on the delineation and development of nursing as a discipline, motivated to some extent by the need to demonstrate the unique aspects of nursing. Early efforts were focused particularly on knowledge development consistent with prevailing ideas about the way disciplines were structured. This focus on structure likely was a result of, at least in part, close connections between nursing and the discipline of education, and the structure of disciplines was an area of considerable theoretical interest and emphasis in education, particularly in the 1960s. The premise in the literature that promoted this focus in nursing was that the determination of the nature of nursing as a discipline, including its structure and boundaries, would provide direction for continuing development. Donaldson and Crowley (1978) pointed out the need for work on the discipline of nursing, indicating that such investigation would determine "the essence of nursing research and of the common elements and threads that give coherence to an identifiable body of knowledge" (p. 113).

Invoking ideas about borrowed versus unique knowledge, Donaldson and Crowley (1978) argued that much of the basis for nursing was "tacit rather than explicit" (p. 113), and they emphasized the need to ensure that nursing research was actually research in the discipline of nursing and not merely research that was conducted by nurses. Donaldson and Crowley described a *discipline* as "characterized by a unique perspective, a distinct way of viewing all phenomena, which ultimately defines the limits and nature of its inquiry" (p. 113). Developing nursing knowledge consistent with this idea of disciplinary structure would make it possible to demonstrate what knowledge was unique to nursing in contrast to knowledge that might be considered borrowed. Donaldson and Crowley's (1978) work was seen as providing some important direction for continuing knowledge to develop what ultimately could be seen as a distinct discipline of nursing.

As part of their work, Donaldson and Crowley (1978) used an approach to disciplines based on the writings of Schwab (1962) to provide guidance for development of the discipline. Schwab (1962) and others who worked in the area of disciplinary structure (Shermis, 1962) argued that disciplines comprised two components: a *substantive structure* and a *syntax*. The content of the discipline constitutes the substantive structure; it includes concepts, theories, and other knowledge, principles, and ideas that make up the knowledge base of the discipline of nursing. Research to develop the discipline, therefore, should focus on content according to this idea of the disciplinary structure. The syntax includes the methods used in inquiry, as well as means to evaluate the value, credibility, or usefulness of inquiry done in the discipline. A general perspective, or worldview, provides the context for the substantive structure and the syntax to be brought together as characteristic of the particular discipline. Overall, these authors argued for the importance of delineating a distinct discipline of nursing, ensuring that the substance of the discipline served as a guide for practice, and establishing clear connections between research, the development of the discipline, and nursing practice.

It is worth noting that the approach to disciplinary structure that was advocated in nursing was that of the natural sciences. While this strategy may seem appropriate, it is important to consider how nursing might have developed differently if an idea relative to social sciences or humanities had been employed. This placement of nursing within the ranks of natural sciences became evident again when the philosophy of science known as *logical positivism* began to influence nursing knowledge development beginning in the 1970s, such that greater use of references in the area of natural, rather than social, sciences (although such works existed within philosophy of science) continues to be found throughout the nursing literature.

THE IDEA OF A "PROFESSIONAL" DISCIPLINE

The focus on disciplines occupied the nursing knowledge literature for some time, providing a framework for discussion of the uniqueness of nursing. This discussion encompassed topics such as the differences between basic and applied sciences, with nursing being held out as distinct from the basic sciences through its focus on application (Donaldson & Crowley, 1978; Johnson, 1959). The notion of applied science as a key aspect of nursing was captured sometimes through the references to nursing as a *professional discipline*. Professional or practice disciplines were thought to have specific characteristics that set them apart from those without a clear practice component. Thus professional disciplines, such as nursing, were viewed as different from the academic disciplines. A unique characteristic of the professional discipline is the delivery of service of some sort by those engaging in practice.

It is easy to argue that all disciplines have individuals who carry out the work of the discipline, who teach its substance, and who contribute to its ongoing development.

Anyone who applies the knowledge of a discipline is engaging in practice related to that knowledge. The mere existence of people who engage in practice is not sufficient to differentiate a field from other disciplines whose members lack such a component. Nurses have used the argument that nursing is a "practice discipline" or a "professional discipline" to delineate nursing from other disciplines and to rationalize certain constraints or other challenges that set nursing apart from more traditional disciplines. However, describing nursing as a practice discipline is misleading because all disciplines have individuals who apply the knowledge. Without such application, there would be no opportunity for testing, studying, enhancing, refining, or sharing the knowledge of the particular discipline. What is important in regard to nursing, however, is that there are social constraints, licensing requirements, and means of public oversight that create a special context for nursing. These aspects are critical to the development of nursing and do require important considerations about the process of knowledge development. These characteristics also translate into specific needs for the nursing knowledge base (Dickoff, James, & Wiedenbach, 1968a, 1968b). Merely referring to nursing as a practice discipline may not draw sufficient attention to these aspects that affect its development. Despite these social and legal constraints, however, it may not be beneficial to the development of nursing to emphasize these differences. It is not self-evident that nursing as a discipline is sufficiently distinct from other disciplines in its organization and development, and a focus on similarities may bring greater progress to understanding and valuing nursing than a continuing emphasis on differences. Indeed, failure to recognize the academic basis for nursing practice and the need for ongoing knowledge development may have contributed to the slow acceptance of nursing and valuing of nursing knowledge within university and healthcare settings.

The idea of a discipline having a unique substance, as advanced by scholars in nursing during the 1970s and 1980s, contributed to concerns mentioned previously about whether knowledge can be borrowed. This idea of borrowing knowledge from one discipline to the next does not hold up to further scrutiny. First, for something to be borrowed, it must belong to someone, yet it is not reasonable to think of knowledge as the possession of any one person or group of people. Researchers in the field of psychology may have created much of what is known about stress or behavior change, for example, yet it is clear that there are important connections to physiology, medicine, nursing, and sociology, in addition to other disciplines. Similarly, the members of other disciplines use, expand, critique, revise, and refine what is known on an ongoing basis, often with minimal regard for the origin of the knowledge.

There is some legitimate reason to be concerned about the perspectives that are represented in existing knowledge. To that end, nursing's holistic viewpoint and focus on relationships and contexts could be overlooked if nurses are not involved in the generation of that knowledge. Looked at another way, knowledge developed within other disciplines could fail to address the problems that nurses confront and that are important to their work with their populations of interest. Borrowing and the viability of the discipline of nursing are not the concerns here; rather, there is a legitimate concern that knowledge be generated that addresses the epistemic (knowledge-oriented) needs of nurses.

The idea of borrowed versus unique knowledge may not have much utility or support at this time, yet the need to pay attention to the knowledge base of nursing still has considerable merit. Nurses need to have an understanding of their discipline, particularly nurses who are in positions to help shape that knowledge. Nurses with DNP-level preparation will be in roles that enable them to have a significant influence over which knowledge development activities are pursued, and they should be engaged as members of research teams to ensure that the knowledge generated addresses areas of need. Because of the advanced practice focus of DNP education, DNP-prepared nurses are especially likely to have meaningful interaction with the public—the recipients of care—and, therefore, are in important positions to influence public perceptions of nursing. Understanding the current status of the discipline, and particularly the evolution of nursing to the present day, helps to create an understanding of the discipline that can be shared with others, can guide continuing research, and can shape the individual nurse's own perception of the role of nursing and the area of practice.

The earlier brief mention of nursing history points to the continuing emergence of nursing as a discipline with a body of what can be called nursing knowledge. While there are occasional references to nursing as being in an early stage of development, particularly in reference to other disciplines, such a characterization does not do justice to the long history that exists, especially in connection with religious orders or the military, of people providing essential health services to those in need. Human beings have always needed individuals to whom they could turn for support with health and illness situations, whether that support has taken the form of the recommended cures of the day or more long-term care. To the extent that certain humans were identified as being particularly adept at providing such care, nursing has existed. As early as the time of the Crusades (the 11th century CE), efforts were made to provide a means for placing the work of tending to ill individuals in the hands of those skilled at providing needed care. These early efforts served as a harbinger of nursing that would develop in a more formal sense in later centuries, making it clear that nursing care in some form has been available to people for an exceptionally long time. Although the nursing of centuries ago bears little resemblance to the nursing of modern times, it does support the idea that the practice of nursing is not new or embryonic—a characterization occasionally used to describe nursing's state of development. Contemporary nursing involves formal education with complex substantive content reflecting a variety of disciplines, yet integrated into an approach to health and illness situations that represents the special influence of nursing. Arriving at this point in nursing education and practice reflects centuries of ongoing development.

THE EMERGENCE OF NURSING SCIENCE

As emphasis increased on nursing as a discipline, there emerged a concomitant drive to develop what can be referred to as *nursing science*. This emphasis became the specific focus of theory development for nursing and was the primary consideration in the development of the discipline from the 1960s through the 1980s. This section and subsequent sections of this chapter describe the major traditions in epistemology that have influenced the development of theory and nursing science (see **Box 2-1**).

A review of nursing knowledge development over the latter half of the 20th century shows the steady and profound influence of logical positivism. Logical positivism produced a lasting impact on nursing knowledge development, with one particularly strong example of its influence being extensive theory development activities demonstrated from the late 1960s into the 1990s. Nurses who received their doctoral-level education in fields other than nursing were influenced by the dominance of this ideology at the time, a factor that helped to ensure its translation to a nursing context. Logical positivism, in fact, was pervasive throughout all of the sciences and has had a lasting impact on broad societal ideas about science and what constitutes appropriate or acceptable scientific activity. Logical positivism no longer occupies the forefront of philosophical thought about science; in fact, Webster, Jacox, and Baldwin (1981) declared it dead in the early 1980s. It is questionable, however, whether any philosophical movement ever dies completely, and there can be no doubt that the influence of logical positivism persists and has had a major role in shaping current ideas about science.

Logical positivism placed great emphasis on the demarcation of science from other forms of knowledge. Science was characterized as developing in a cumulative and linear fashion, with successive studies building on prior research. This process was oriented toward continuously refining and building theory in the quest for parsimonious statements that accurately corresponded with reality. Science, in essence, was seen as a theory-building activity, with the ideal theoretical statements being those that were capable of expression using the rules of logic and mathematics. Theory formed the core of scientific activity, and investigations represented an attempt to further develop, refine, or verify existing theory. With this emphasis on theory, it is easy to see how a discipline that lacked specific theoretical

Box 2-1 Epistemologies in Nursing Science Development
Logical positivism
Historicism
Postmodernism
Phenomenological philosophy
Hermeneutics
Feminist epistemology
Pragmatism and neopragmatism

statements and clearly delineated bodies of theory might have been hindered in its efforts to gain recognition as a scientific discipline. If science was a theory-building activity, then nurse scholars suggested that there must be a theoretical foundation for nursing knowledge and practice for the discipline to be considered a science.

THE THEORY MOVEMENT IN NURSING

Nurse scholars and leaders devoted considerable effort to identifying the core or essence of nursing, to constructing theoretical formulations that would reflect this core, and to promoting further inquiry, as well as theory-based nursing practice. Federal funding was provided during the 1960s to support a series of conferences on theory development. The first conference was held at Case Western Reserve University in 1968; the second was held at the University of Colorado in 1969. Papers and discussion at these conferences clearly revealed the focus on the science of nursing and the influence of the philosophy of logical positivism on such activities during this time. The theoretical activity that took place under this influence amply illustrates the impact of logical positivism and this philosophical movement in the evolution of nursing as a discipline. Early nursing theory development activities, reflected in the work of Orlando (1961), Rogers (1970), Roy (1970, 1971), and others, served as important milestones in the effort to develop a theoretical basis for nursing.

Developing status as a science required not only the identification or development of theory for nursing, but also the use of existing theory as a basis for research. Logical positivism, after all, required that scientific activity focus on development and further articulation of theory. Descriptive research—that is, inquiry intended to discover or document events or conditions—did not meet the criteria for science that were espoused by philosophers and the dominant thinking of the period. As a result of this emphasis, the literature of nursing during this time includes a number of articles and ongoing discussion about the necessary connection between theory, research, and practice, with Fawcett's "double helix" metaphor being a particularly poignant example of this focus (Fawcett, 1978, 1985). Writings related to the role of theory in science reflected the tenets of logical positivism; theory development was viewed as a very formal activity with a focus on axioms and propositions in the construction of theory. Reynolds's (1971) *A Primer in Theory Construction* is referenced frequently in the nursing literature of this era and shows the emphasis on the development of formal theory, the importance of concepts being defined in operational terms to show their means of empirical testing, and a focus on quantitative testing of hypotheses derived from the theories. Research with an emphasis on describing situations or phenomena was possibly of some value, but only to the extent that it provided baseline data for further theory development (Fawcett, 1978, p. 60).

Science that was developed according to the tenets of logical positivism represented what is sometimes referred to as *hard science*, yet nurse scholars and leaders in the area of knowledge development encountered considerable difficulty with this philosophy in that a significant amount of nursing was not amenable to this conception of science. Despite the great strides that were made during this time in developing the scientific and theoretical foundations of nursing, some aspects of nursing just could not fit these specific criteria. Nursing had maintained a long history of being regarded as holistic, humanistic, and relational, with an emphasis on psychological and social aspects of health and wellness as much as physiological and biological aspects. Concepts such as dignity, empathy, presence, and caring could not be forced into the mold of logical positivism without tremendous difficulty and, as nurses readily recognized, without considerable disservice to those crucial aspects of the human condition.

The lack of fit between nursing and prevailing ideas about science left nurses with some difficult choices. One option was for nurses to strive to meet the criteria of science as defined by the logical positivist philosophers. This endeavor would, however, require forcing some elements of nursing knowledge to meet the requirements of the prevailing ideology. Needless to say, this option was akin to the "square peg and round hole" metaphor, and it is debatable whether some of the highly valued aspects of nursing could ever be recast in this fashion without significantly changing their nature.

As a second option, nurses could argue that some components of nursing fit the idea of science, maintaining the logical positivist idea of science, while acknowledging that other aspects did not fit this ideology. Those other aspects are referred to as art: The dogma of nursing as "an art and a science" (Rodgers, 1991) persists throughout the history of modern nursing thought.

As a third option, nurses could accept that the knowledge base of the discipline, in its totality, did not meet the requirements of logical positivism. Carper's (1975, 1978) widely cited work identifying patterns of knowing in nursing addressed some of these concerns, identifying the empirical knowing that is consistent with traditional ideas of science as only one of four types of knowing inherent in nursing. Personal knowing, aesthetic knowing, and ethics were the terms used to label other forms of knowing that she argued were essential in nursing. This schema went beyond the mere separation of knowledge into science and everything else (e.g., art) and emphasized the existence of numerous ways of knowing, all of which are essential to the work of nursing.

THE IMPORTANCE OF EVALUATING PHILOSOPHICAL IDEOLOGY

The fact that nurses largely failed to raise questions about the legitimacy of logical positivism as a useful and acceptable definition of science regardless of discipline is notable. The challenge for nurses should not have been viewed as only the determination of how to adopt and follow a particular line of activity or thought. In the case of logical positivism, nurses could have argued—as some did—that this philosophical approach just was not an acceptable or legitimate approach for nursing. In fact, there are significant problems with this philosophy regardless of discipline, even for those that seem to be a more reasonable fit with this idea of traditional science.

Although logical positivism was not an appropriate view for the development of the discipline of nursing, looking only at whether this philosophy "fit" nursing (rather than evaluating its merits overall) has two strong detrimental effects. First, it sets nursing apart as different, and not necessarily in a good way, but in a way that indicates nursing cannot, or will not, conform to prevailing standards for science. Second, and particularly significant in the case of logical positivism, it fails to address the crucial question of the legitimacy of the philosophy. Without that challenge, a philosophical tradition can continue to be held as an ideal, and progress in disciplines can be evaluated relative to its major tenets regardless of whether a particular discipline accepts that view. Those who rejected logical positivism as a suitable guide for the development of nursing without assessing the philosophy's inherent value created a situation where nursing could easily be viewed as "different," or as a lesser science than others that appeared to follow prevailing standards. The situation that resulted from this rejection (perpetuated in the argument that nursing is an art and a science) is similar to criticisms that continue to be levied against qualitative research—that it is "soft" and fails to meet the criteria of real science.

Trends and paradigm shifts are always occurring, and the critical questions asked by nurses cannot be limited to whether to follow along as viewpoints shift. The most important questions that need to be asked by nurses in regard to the knowledge base involve two things. First, is the latest ideology sound, not just for nursing but for any discipline? Second, does it enable progress in nursing? In other words, is it an ideology that will help nurse scholars and researchers to make sound moves toward achieving the goals of the discipline? Applying such questions to logical positivism reveals quite quickly that the answer is *no* in regard to both aspects. Indeed, the shortcomings of logical positivism led to its demise as the dominant ideology of science by the mid-1900s.

The ideal put forth by the philosophers of this genre, however, continues to influence expectations and desires in the creation of science in nursing and elsewhere, ideals that persisted long after logical positivism lost its favored status. Science continues to be seen by society at large, as well as in many of the academic disciplines, as a special or unique form of knowledge with greater credibility than other forms of knowledge. Expectations for widespread generalizability of results, for statistical significance as the measure of meaningful results, for theory development as a focus of scientific activity, and for objectivity and a value-free orientation to inquiry continue to shape both the conduct of research and the needs of the public and others who will apply the results of scientific endeavors.

Webster and colleagues (1981) clearly pointed out the effects of "undue adherence to the positions and ideas of the received view" and noted how that perspective "stilted the development of nursing theories" (p. 34). *Truth*, as a criterion for evaluating theory, particularly in the form of correspondence with facts, presented other problems in the logical positivist viewpoint. The correspondence theory requires that phenomena be objectified—that is, measured in some way that is precise, repeatable, rigorous, and, as is evident in any research methods text, a valid measure of the phenomenon being studied. As a result, the phenomenon is believed to be captured successfully through the collection of empirical data.

Although this goal of precision and high validity certainly is an admirable one, it ignores elements of phenomena that can be the source of important information but are not reducible to means of measurement. With this approach, grief, for example, could be understood only as "grief as measured by a score on the grief instrument" because that is the only means for assigning numbers to grief to quantify and validate its existence. An individual's description of grief, including its emotional impact, its effect on daily life, and feelings that are often expressed by people using metaphors rather than checklists or Likert scales, could not be included under the heading of scientific.

It is easy to see how social or psychological phenomena are particularly troublesome to study from the perspective of logical positivism because these phenomena have strong personal—or what might be called subjective—components. Physiological phenomena, however, are not immune to these difficulties either. Consider, for example, hypertension, measured as the pressure of the blood against vessel walls, or diabetes control, measured with glucose or $HgbA_{1c}$ levels. While these methods clearly are meaningful measures of these physical phenomena, they do not provide a broad or holistic perspective on how these conditions affect individuals with these diagnoses or what it is like to live with and try to maintain control of these physiological challenges. There are many challenges with the logical positivist philosophy of science. For purposes here, the significant point is to note the barriers to progress in the discipline of nursing that were confronted as a result of the rise in popularity of logical positivism and a staunch adherence to empirical ways of knowing, particularly within the context of a discipline that derives a significant amount of its identity from a holistic approach to human beings. These challenges also led to difficulties with the adoption of logical positivism in other disciplines. Despite these barriers, however, logical positivism had a profound and lasting role on shaping views of science through the 20th century and beyond. Specifically, the philosophy created expectations for science in both academic settings and society at large that continue to influence the evaluation of knowledge for its applicability and meaningfulness.

Before moving on to address the changes that have arisen since the logical positivist approach became prominent, it is appropriate to reiterate some important points. Methods and philosophy are linked inextricably: The choice of method that a nurse or any scientist takes in regard to knowledge development has strong philosophical underpinnings that need to be recognized as an inherent part of the science or knowledge development enterprise. These foundations are not always obvious, yet the philosophical position taken by a researcher can be determined by assessing the approach to inquiry that is taken. It also is possible to use similar strategies for inquiry despite different philosophical positions.

When a researcher measures some phenomenon, the researcher is indicating that it is possible and appropriate to measure the phenomenon of interest. Yet, one researcher using a quantitative instrument to measure a phenomenon may believe that those measurements reflect true and meaningful data, whereas another may believe that the results are meaningful, but only a piece of a complex human situation, and that the answer to the research question is just one of many possible answers. Logical positivism, for example, undoubtedly leads to a quantitative approach to science, but, conversely, not all quantitative science is necessarily based on logical positivism.

From a philosophical or disciplinary standpoint, it is important to look at assumptions about the nature of reality, truth, the goals and purpose of science, and the criteria that are used for differentiating good science as reflective of the philosophical viewpoint of the researcher or scientist. Those underpinnings are reflected in the methods used, but the methods essentially are tools, and they can be used with perspectives that have some perhaps subtle—but important—variations. Failure to distinguish method from philosophical underpinnings can lead to wholesale rejection (or, conversely, blind adoption) of alternatives to knowledge development without appropriate thought being given to the choices that are being made. The responses of nurses to various trends as evidenced in the literature of nursing do not always capture this subtle yet important difference. Without that understanding, however, there is a tendency to abandon useful aspects of some approaches to knowledge development or to develop a bandwagon mentality when new trends emerge and either become popular or later are found to be insufficient to meet the needs of the discipline.

As noted earlier, the logical positivist approach to knowledge had significant limitations as a focus for the development of knowledge, especially within the narrower realm of scientific knowledge. As a philosophy of science, it not only presented challenges within the philosophy itself with regard to views of the nature of reality, truth, and the proper goal of science, but it was also created as a prescriptive view—in other words, a directive dictating how science should be done. In essence, logical positivism was not comprehensive in terms of how science actually was conducted. Prescriptive approaches can be of great value, of course; this point is clearly seen in health care where prescriptions for all sorts of things are intended to set people on a healthier and more productive path, just as a prescriptive view of science could have the same intention. This prescriptive focus likely added to the strength of its influence because it was put forth as a directive for how science should be carried out.

THE SEARCH FOR A NURSING PARADIGM

An obvious problem raised by this prescriptive focus was the fact that it ignored much of how science actually was carried out. An insider view of science would provide great insight into how science worked, not just on the level of particular methods but also in regard to the broader enterprise of science—an enterprise consisting not only of theories and ideas but also of scientists (the people who do the work of science) and the context in which their work takes place. Thomas Kuhn (1970, 1974) provided just such insight into not only the workings of science but the people who did that work. Because logical positivism was found to be lacking for nursing, Kuhn's views quickly gained the attention of nurses looking for a useful understanding of science.

One of the major shifts presented in Kuhn's writing was the change in the philosophy of science from a focus on product to a focus on process—in other words, the way in which science was done. Kuhn's view of science was organized around the idea that a central paradigm provided a focal point for activity in a discipline. The paradigm served as a disciplinary matrix and included the values and aims inherent in the major substantive content of the discipline. The work of scientists, according to Kuhn, was to articulate this paradigm. Progress, truth, and theory, among other aspects of science, were determined by viewing these developments from the perspective of the paradigm. This was a radically different approach to science than the view of the logical positivist because it allowed judgments about science to be made relative to a viewpoint—in this case, the disciplinary matrix or paradigm—rather than in reference to an objective reality.

Although there were some limitations to this new perspective, nurses writing during this period gave a great deal of attention to Kuhn's views and argued for the relevance of this philosophical position for knowledge development in nursing. Kuhn's discussion of scientific revolutions and the term *paradigm*, derived from his work, became common features in discussions of nursing as a discipline and, especially, as a science. Writers in nursing during this period ultimately concluded that nursing had a *metaparadigm*, a broader worldview and conceptualization or important elements of the discipline, yet evidence of a paradigm as required by Kuhn was presented as lacking (Hardy, 1983; Kim, 1989). Kim (1989) identified a number of distinct paradigms that were used in nursing but acknowledged the lack of a single overriding paradigm that would characterize nursing as a discipline in accordance with Kuhn's position.

Interestingly, while logical positivism experienced a relatively long life in nursing, Kuhn's view was quite short-lived in comparison. Nurse leaders and theorists during this time had become more familiar with philosophy and philosophical principles through their advanced education. As a result, there may have been a greater level of sophistication employed in evaluating ideology such as that presented by Kuhn. Limitations of Kuhn's view were quite obvious in nursing and perhaps contributed to acceptance of this tradition being less widespread, as well as shorter in duration in nursing. Although the term paradigm still has a prominent place in discussions about science, Kuhn's view overall was supplanted rather quickly by the views of other historicists and the rise of postmodernism, which followed shortly after the popularity of his work faded.

It is important to acknowledge the work of other historicist philosophers and the connection of such ideas to the development of nursing science. Larry Laudan was another noted philosopher of the late 1970s and a historicist whose work received some attention from nurse scholars. Laudan's (1977) philosophy was particularly noteworthy because he provided a view of science that addressed both conceptual and empirical problems in the conduct of science and the determination of progress. In general, Laudan focused on science as a problem-solving activity and assigned some weight to both conceptual and empirical work. Relatively few nurse authors (articles such as Fry, 1995, and Tinkle & Beaton, 1983, are good examples) described positions in support of Laudan's viewpoint and the practicality of his approach for nursing, and his work, like that of Kuhn, received far less attention than did the positions advocated by the logical positivists. Two significant aspects of the time could have contributed to this lack of attention. First, there was a continuing dominance of logical positivism and its influence on views of science, even as historicist viewpoints were being articulated; this entrenched view would not be supplanted easily. Second, the philosophy of postmodernism emerged, developing particularly in the social sciences and then gradually spilling over into a number of other fields. Postmodernism served as a direct counterpoint to the rigidity of logical positivism, its emphasis on foundationalism, and its adherence to a belief in objective reality. This perspective represented quite a radical departure from both positivism and historicism, although it overlooked what might be considered the more moderate or intermediate position presented by historicist philosophers.

CONCEPTUAL PROBLEMS AND CONCEPT DEVELOPMENT

The potential contributions of historicism to nursing knowledge development are evident when reviewing the emphasis placed on concepts during the 1970s and 1980s. Although concepts and conceptual problems received attention during this time, the focus was not totally consistent with a historicist or postmodern perspective; in fact, discussion of concepts during this time had a strong positivist orientation. Concepts were valued primarily as elements of theory or, to use a popular phrase in nursing, as the "building blocks of theory," and not in a broader philosophical sense as ways to reflect, describe, and navigate through existence. Nonetheless, at least some attention was being paid to concepts, an occurrence that stands out in the history of the development of nursing science and points to the significance of concepts within the knowledge base.

Catherine Norris (1982) gave conceptual activity an important emphasis with the publication of a detailed book on concept clarification in nursing. Walker and Avant (1983, 1988) drew on the work of John Wilson (1969) to bring a method of concept analysis to nursing. This method remains popular in nursing and has been used in the analysis or clarification of a wide range of concepts. The text by Walker and Avant (1983, 1988) that addressed a method of concept analysis actually was focused on strategies for theory development in nursing, consistent with that common focus during the time of its initial publication. Content included analysis, synthesis, and derivation in the three categories of concepts, statements, and theories, all discussed as strategies for theory development. Perhaps as a remnant of logical positivism, or perhaps merely as recognition of the role of theory in science, work continued to be focused on theory development through much of the 1990s.

More recent work emphasizing concepts in nursing has been focused on developing useful concepts and resolving conceptual problems without being limited to theory development as the only relevant context for such work. Numerous philosophers addressed the role of concepts in cognition and, to a lesser extent, in science, yet their work has not received much of a reception in nursing. Rodgers (1989) constructed a view of concepts that emphasized concept development, not merely analysis, with analysis being a component of a broader process to generate meaningful and useful concepts. This work was informed by philosophers such as Laudan (1977), Toulmin (1972), Price (1953), and others and was oriented toward providing a solid foundation for conceptual work as part of the development of science and the discipline. Since that time, increased attention has been paid to concept development rather than merely to analysis, or to analysis as a strategy oriented more broadly to the development of useful and effective concepts (Rodgers, 2000a, 2000b; Rodgers & Knafl, 2000). Despite this development, a great deal of conceptual work in nursing continues to follow the techniques described by Walker and Avant, being empirical in orientation and poorly linked to resolution of conceptual problems. Although sound philosophy and techniques for improving the conceptual base of nursing are readily available, this aspect of knowledge development is not well utilized in nursing. This is an unfortunate situation because a number of the significant problems regarding nursing knowledge are conceptual in nature rather than empirical. Even for problems that are clinical in nature, clear and sound concepts are needed to ensure that empirical problems are articulated with clarity and relevant variables are understood, defined, and measured appropriately.

There is a need for additional work in concept development because many of the problems that are paramount in nursing are conceptual in nature and because methodological advances in concept development are not well integrated into nursing inquiry. In addition, concepts are important in delineating the identity and scope of the discipline. Consistent with the earlier effort to identify the essence of nursing, fundamental concepts were stipulated as constituting the core of nursing knowledge. Kim (1987), Flaskerud and Halloran (1980), and others identified nursing, person, health, and environment as the key concepts in nursing, with Flaskerud and Halloran referring to the centrality of these concepts as an important area of agreement in nursing. Other writings around this time were consistent with this focus, specifying that these concepts could provide a foundation for theory development in the discipline (Hardy, 1978; Johnson, 1968; Newman, 1972). As noted previously, although work conducted during the 1980s and 1990s reveals attention to the role of concepts in developing the knowledge base, a significant part of this effort, particularly in the early phases, was consistent with the positivist focus on theory development. More recently (Rodgers, 1989, 2000b), concepts have begun to take on a role as significant parts of knowledge outside of theory development. There is a continuing need for attention to concept development that goes beyond the basic level of analysis to modes of inquiry that result in better ways to conceptualize important phenomena in nursing (Rodgers, 2000a, 2000b). The analysis of concepts should not be seen as an endpoint to inquiry; instead, the results of any analysis should be tied to a continuing process of developing knowledge that addresses significant problems in the discipline.

THE POSTMODERN TURN

The historicist tradition (*historicism*) presented a stark contrast to the major tenets of logical positivism. Historicism provided an emphasis on problem solving as evidenced by the work of Laudan (1977), conceptual repertoires as discussed by Toulmin (1972), the notion of science as an enterprise with work conducted by people with their own values and perspectives, and a focus on science as a process rather than the product—all of which prompted questions about appropriate ways of doing and evaluating science. The historicist tradition offered substantial advantages over the rigid requirements placed on science by logical positivism. The potential contributions of historicist philosophy, however, received relatively scant attention in nursing. A review of the literature for nursing knowledge development and nursing science in the 1980s and 1990s reveals few works that address the work of historicist philosophers. This lack of attention likely is related to the development of yet another philosophical tradition, *postmodernism*, which garnered substantial attention in nursing shortly after the peak of historicism.

Postmodernism involves an emphasis on hermeneutics, narrative traditions and discourse, and philosophies of critical social theory and feminism. The emergence of this array of ideologies overshadowed discussions of historicism and quickly became a major focus of interest in nursing. Postmodernism, to many nurse authors at the time, seemed to closely approximate many of the values and purposes of nursing knowledge. This philosophical tradition was based on ideas of relativism, or viewpoints that truths existed on an individual level. This orientation was consistent with a longstanding emphasis in nursing on the whole person and the uniqueness of each individual. Nursing had developed around a focus on individualized care, and postmodernism was wholly consistent with that idea, not only allowing for but requiring recognition of uniqueness related to gender, culture, social status, and other characteristics inherent in the individual. Postmodernism also captured the idea that power differentials present in society are reflected in the healthcare system and interactions with care providers. In contrast to the idea that one single, central, fundamental overarching reality exists, with the purpose of science being to discover that reality, postmodernism was founded on uniqueness, diversity, power structures, and multiple realities as a result of human and social variation. This notion that there is not one single, central truth or story that is applicable to everyone is a defining feature of postmodernism and is referred to as the rejection of metanarrative, overarching narratives that are broadly generalizable.

Feminism, in particular, received a tremendous amount of attention, and it was not uncommon for authors to stipulate that feminism was a natural fit for nursing given that the majority of nurses were female. Feminism provided a clear example of postmodernism and was seen by many nurse leaders as exemplary of the postmodern emphasis on the uniqueness of each individual; the importance of individual realities with their gender, class, social, economic, and other influences; recognition of cultural relativism; and awareness of the role of power differentials in health care as in the rest of society. As a result, postmodernism garnered considerable attention as a good fit as a philosophical system for nursing knowledge development.

Postmodernism represented a radical departure from earlier philosophies dealing with science and knowledge. As a result of its emergence, new modes of inquiry and new methodologies began to receive attention in nursing. The emphasis on individual beliefs, cultural and social contexts, multiple realities, power differentials, and so on required the development of methods that were able to capture these aspects of existence through research. With such significant philosophical differences, it was clear that traditional scientific principles could not be applied to the study of human beings given their individual and social contexts. At the very least, a pluralistic approach to inquiry would be necessary, balancing the supposedly objective and quantifiable facets with the more personal and individual aspects of human beings. A more extreme form of ideology at the time held that reduction and quantification could be rejected in their entirety and replaced with more holistic traditions of inquiry. Techniques for deconstruction could be applied to language, as well as images, and reveal power differentials and biases implicit in communication. Similarly, narrative or text, including the idea that action constitutes a text as described by Ricoeur (1981, 1984), provided a means to identify precepts, values, hidden meanings, and other contextual elements of experience. During this time there was an increasing emphasis on language and communication, with the development of narrative modes of inquiry that focused on individual story rather than attempts to uncover any form of truth.

Qualitative research began to emerge as a viable option for inquiry in nursing and in other disciplines. Philosophical methods such as phenomenology and hermeneutics had existed for a long time, with hermeneutics having a particularly long history dating back to the early study of biblical texts. Despite this extensive history, however, these philosophical methods had not been compatible with traditional ideas of science. Acceptance of qualitative research grew slowly and continues to meet resistance in some disciplines and by some researchers even in nursing. Nonetheless, the rise of postmodern philosophy opened the door for, and subsequently fueled rapid growth in, qualitative methodologies to develop knowledge for the discipline. In fact, the popularity of qualitative research grew so quickly that it appeared at times to be a sort of bandwagon, drawing significant attention and support simply because it offered such a stark contrast to the method supported by the quantitative methods of logical positivism. The quality of studies was variable, and there was evidence of some confusion regarding the various specific methods, resulting in awkward piecemeal combinations of different, and sometimes incompatible, methodological traditions. This blending of perspectives and methods was referred to as "method slurring" by Baker, Wuest, and Stern (1992). Over time, an increasing number of publications dealt with aspects of quality in qualitative research, and the initial excitement about qualitative methods gradually evolved to leave a variety of distinct, clear, and highly rigorous approaches for the conduct and the evaluation of such forms of inquiry.

Postmodernism led to the emergence of a particular form of qualitative inquiry referred to as *interpretive approaches*. These approaches focus on experiences as people live them with all their individual interpretations and reactions; consistent with this view is the idea that actions represent values and an emphasis on the primacy of dialogue and language as means to share realities. As a result, actions, dialogue, and language provide a mechanism for the investigator to gain a greater understanding of those unique realities. Hermeneutical, phenomenological, narrative, and other interpretive approaches have been used to explore a variety of experiences of interest to nurses, including suffering (Steeves, Kahn, & Benoliel, 1990), race and attrition in nursing programs (Jordan, 1996), the care provider–patient relationship (Sundin, Jansson, & Norberg, 2002), and nurses in various roles, such as nurse consultant (Walters, 1996).

The philosophy of postmodernism reflects another unique turn in ideas about the development of knowledge by raising significant questions about the presumption of objectivity in the conduct of science. In postmodernism, the separation of what is known from who is doing the knowing no longer exists; moreover, social elements not only have an effect on knowledge, but they also are viewed as an appropriate focus for inquiry. As noted previously, feminism and feminist epistemology gained considerable attention in relation to the growth of postmodernism. Postmodern philosophy makes it clear that social elements, such as class and gender, are important in regard to knowledge development; in feminism, the specific emphasis is on gender.

Feminism exists in numerous forms, ranging from a moderate view that gender is important when looking at ways of interacting with the world to a more extreme version that holds gender to be the most important factor in interactions. In the extreme view, political action to counteract the dominant patriarchy is crucial to social progress (Harding, 1986, 1991). Some of the roots of feminism can be traced to historical events in which women were denied what are now considered to be basic social and civil rights.

Adding to this historical origin is a considerable body of research that was biased against women. Kohlberg's (1981) research on moral development, for example, was groundbreaking, but the stages of moral development that were identified, when used in research with female subjects, led to the conclusion that females functioned at a considerably lower level of moral development than their male counterparts. Subsequent research using a different frame of reference, such as the work conducted by Carol Gilligan (1982), revealed the gender bias inherent in Kohlberg's work. The differences between male and female subjects in regard to development was argued by Gilligan to be not a matter of more or less of something, or one group being more developed than the other, but rather an altogether different way of approaching ethical problem solving. Gilligan's work was foundational in supporting the idea that females have a different frame of reference and a different way of working through ethical problems than do males. Such differences do not equate to higher or lower levels of moral development. Additional work in this area was carried out by Belenky, Clinchy, Goldberger, and Tarule (1986), who interviewed a group of 135 women; their study revealed that women interact with the world and have ways of knowing that appear to be substantially different from how men interact with and know the world.

The recognition of gender differences evident in research, along with the postmodern emphasis on individual realities rather than grand narratives, made it easy to see how feminism could be viewed as a philosophy with a good fit for nursing. In addition, a number of noted scholars in nursing recognized the consistency between a feminist view and the professional status of nurses. History is replete with references to nurses as the handmaidens of the physician, and it is likely that most nurses have heard stories of nurses giving up their chairs or handing over patient charts to the physician whenever he was present (and, of course, in early years, physicians were *he* rather than *she*, as the discipline of medicine demonstrated a similar bias against women). From a political standpoint, then, feminism was seen as offering some potential benefit to a predominantly female profession such as nursing.

Feminist ideology, however, often results in assigning a gender orientation to knowledge, labeling some approaches as distinctly feminine. This can create awkwardness in regard to thinking of knowledge claims as having a particular gender and presenting some views as superior to others based on a gender orientation. Rather than offering a means to overcome problems with bias that are presumed to be present in science, this approach sometimes seems only to offer yet a different form of bias in knowledge development. Some authors have justified this development, arguing that the masculine, patriarchal orientation is so strong that it is necessary to promote an equally strong feminist orientation as a counterpoint to the male hegemony. Others see feminism as opening the door to more diversity in a broad scope of perspectives that can be considered. Chinn (1989) described nursing as emphasizing wholeness, with any singular perspective—masculine or feminine—being insufficient to accomplish this idea of wholeness in health. According to Chinn, nurses see the world through the lens of integration and wholeness. We cannot conceive of knowing sufficiently in any way nor can we rely on any one way of knowing that disregards another dimension of experience. We know we experience reality in a whole way.

It seems essential that myriad viewpoints be considered in the development of a view that meets the expectations of being holistic and values the uniqueness of individuals. As societies and cultures evolve, the viewpoints to be considered and included in knowledge development have evolved as well, a situation evident in the development of viewpoints based on voices of many unique groups including immigrants and gay, lesbian, and trans-gendered persons.

The relationship between nursing and feminism as a political movement has been a difficult one in many regards. Historically, men had positions of prominence in nursing because of the association of nursing with the military and with religious orders. In addition, women who in earlier times had worked to advance the professional status of nursing did not always see this work as connected to promoting the status of women in general. The American Nurses Association, for example, was not a supporter of women's right to vote in the early years of the organization. At the same time, as opportunities for women have expanded throughout recent history, there has been a tendency for women in traditionally female occupations to feel disenfranchised for choosing those occupations rather than new ones that have become available to them. The tensions surrounding nurses in relation to feminism as a political movement in nursing, therefore, emanated from both the feminist action side and the nursing professional side.

Despite political tensions and debates regarding the merits of gender as a specific focus in knowledge development, feminism has had a significant role in the development of nursing knowledge. Leaders in this movement in nursing brought energy to workplace issues that affect both nursing practice and the nursing workforce. Awareness of bias in scientific research—particularly the historical exclusion of women from a large body of medical research—raised questions about the applicability and generalizability of scientific findings to the care of patients. Recognition of the role of gender and science and what Lather (1991) referred to as the failure of traditional science increased awareness of numerous factors in the development of nursing knowledge and the ways in which knowledge is applied in practice.

The postmodern movement, including feminism, led to considerable research in nursing dealing with cultural and unique individual factors and helped to illuminate on a much broader scale the spectrum of human health and illness as lived by real people in their natural social and cultural settings. Through developments consistent with this ideology, meaningful work has been used not only to understand but also to empower people in their interactions related to health and health care. Philosophies of the postmodern, critical social theory, and feminist traditions continue to evolve and stimulate new ideas for research methodology and criteria for evaluating the quality and range of application for research results.

Work remains, however, to explore ideas of postmodernism and the methodologies consistent with these ideas in a context of contemporary science. Prevailing notions of quality and what constitutes science still tend to be consistent with a positivist or logical positivist philosophy. To date, considerable effort has been devoted to articulating standards for evaluating the quality of inquiry in postmodern traditions (Guba & Lincoln, 1989; Hall & Stevens, 1991; Rolfe, 2006), and the rules associated with such work represent a vast departure from traditional notions of science. Reconciling these disparate viewpoints is important so that the merit of each viewpoint is appreciated and the potential usefulness understood. This is an area in which continuing work can develop a cohesive body of nursing knowledge and have that knowledge valued across an array of situations and contexts.

PRAGMATISM AND NEOPRAGMATISM

The philosophical tradition known as pragmatism has received little attention in nursing but may warrant consideration for its potential to inform the development of nursing as a discipline (Mason, 2008). Pragmatism emerged in the United States in the late 19th century with philosophers John Dewey (Boydston, 2008), William James (2000), and Charles Sanders Peirce (1878) as leaders of this movement. Other philosophers carried on this work in the 1970s and later, including Hilary Putnam (1991) and Richard Rorty (1979, 1982), a particularly prominent and prolific writer in this tradition. Pragmatism had a strong influence on views of truth; thus it has significance for views of science, even though the specific approach to truth varied among the early pragmatists. More important for the early pragmatisms is the idea that understanding the nature of truth is not necessarily a desirable endpoint. Instead, it becomes meaningful when it has significant consequences in the quest for knowledge. Most writers would refer to this tenet of pragmatism in terms of the importance of "practical consequences" of truth. It is risky to do so, however, since "pragmatic" and "practical" are often considered to be interchangeable in everyday speech. To continue that trend would provide a very superficial view of pragmatism and its more recent iterations such as neopragmatism, which has a particular focus on language.

Because of differences of ideologies that fall under the heading of pragmatism, it is not possible to provide a list of basic tenets as is possible with many of the other philosophical traditions discussed in this chapter. There is, however, sufficient commonality to identify pragmatism as a distinct tradition—embodied by an idea that is typically referred to as the "pragmatic maxim" (or what should be referred to as "variations of the pragmatic maxim," as it exists in a number of versions). The pragmatic maxim, very broadly, relies on language and conceptualization and the consequences of certain beliefs. One of Peirce's (1878) most well-known works was an article titled "How to Make Our Ideas Clear." In some respects, this work involved a rejection of the skepticism of Descartes and an attempt to render science as a more meaningful and useful process, freeing it from the mental gymnastics that were so prominent in Descartes's writings. In a clear operationalization of this shunning of Cartesian ideology, Rorty openly rejected the idea that the mind is a mirror of nature, thus rejecting the notion of correspondence theories of truth and the idea that acts of cognition must necessarily relate to a veri-fiable external reality. This may seem like a simple, or perhaps even obvious turn of events, yet this shift in thinking had a significant outcome; it opened philosophy, and also science, to the possibility of developing belief systems rather than requiring strict correspondence with facts, and it allowed a renewed focus on things that are clear and that make sense in a general way. A related outcome would be the development of theory that does something, particularly that stands up to the test of time and continues to answer important questions.

This shift in thinking might look like it was in synch with other established philosophical traditions adopted in nursing inquiry. The emphasis on language, consequences, practical results, establishment of belief systems, pluralism, and rejections of single views of truth is somewhat consistent with historicism and postmodernism in their different forms. Yet, in the literature of nursing, postmodern thought and newer variations of empiricism have remained most prominent, though no tradition is without significant criticism (Garrett, 2016; Rodgers, 2005). In philosophy, pragmatism experienced renewed interest with the writings of Rorty and Putnam, though it has remained rather diffuse with numerous different forms. This lack of a single cohesive ideology may be responsible, at least in part, for this tradition not receiving the attention of nurses and researchers that the other developments have. Nonetheless, this tradition's similarities with some other established views may make it worth remembering as nurses explore the many different viewpoints that exist to inform nursing inquiry and knowledge development.

EMERGING TRENDS IN NURSING SCIENCE

The prior examination of developments and trends in the evolution of nursing science provides a glimpse into the progress made in the discipline and attempts to provide a solid foundation for nursing knowledge. Numerous approaches to knowledge relevant to nursing practice have been entertained within the discipline; some were taken as prescriptions for nursing thought, whereas others offered what was considered a closer fit with nursing as it existed. While the variety of philosophical approaches and methodologies may be appealing simply because of the diversity of perspectives offered, the plethora of philosophies also places some demands on the nurse in an advanced practice role.

One option for dealing with the myriad approaches that might be appealing to adopt is a pluralistic view, or something similar to an *anything goes* attitude. Each era in nursing history has contributed to the development of the discipline of nursing through expansion and articulation of the knowledge base and, concomitantly, a stronger identity for nurs-ing. In addition, each viewpoint has some merits, just as each has limitations. So why not selectively apply pieces of these traditions, if not the whole tradition, when addressing a problem relevant to nursing? Noted Austrian philosopher Feyerabend (1975) specifically supported an approach allowing for maximum creativity and innovation in the process of knowledge development. Numerous authors in nursing have taken such a position as well, by suggesting that there should be a variety of methods and perspectives from which nurses can choose whatever is appropriate to guide their research or practice (Baker, Norton, Young, & Ward, 1998; Coward, 1990; Schultz, 1987).

Such an approach, referred to as pluralism, requires thoughtfulness, rather than merely accepting the wide variety of options as equally meaningful. One complex issue that needs to be considered is the notion of *philosophical congruence, coherence*, and *fit* with the values and ontological perspective of the discipline. Philosophical congruence and coherence concern whether different perspectives in nursing are compatible with a philosophical basis. If nursing holds that the human being is holistic and cannot be viewed specifically in terms of parts, the viewpoints that are considered as a philosophical foundation for knowledge development need to be consistent on that point. Given this example, positions based on the philosophy of logical positivism are likely to be incompatible with nursing values and principles.

This example also points out the importance of ontological fit with nursing. In this case, the ontological view supports the position that human beings need to be considered on a holistic basis. The human being cannot be both holistic and reducible at the same time, and advocating this position would be inconsistent with nursing's expressed metaphysical position on the nature of the human being. Positions about truth, generalizability, the nature of reality, the nature of facts, the role of the investigator, and the role of ethics and values are fundamental considerations and intrinsic parts of the discipline. There is certainly a need for differing perspectives in the process of knowledge development, but whatever approaches are taken need to be consistent with the espoused values and worldview held by the discipline at large.

Arguing for coherence and congruence does not preclude the use of a variety of methodologies for developing the knowledge base for nursing. The discipline will benefit most, however, if the use of a variety of means of knowledge development relevant to nursing is based on a consistent philosophical viewpoint that supports such diversity. The purpose of nursing knowledge is to support the work of nurses and provide information critical to both the delivery of effective care and the continuing development of the discipline. These real and practical aims provide an organizing viewpoint for continuing knowledge relevance. For example, Rodgers (2005, 2007) advocated a problem-solving approach based on the philosophies of Laudan (1977) and Toulmin (1972) as a way to justify multiple approaches to knowledge development and nursing while still maintaining some consistency and identity for the discipline. These philosophers, reflecting different historicist ideas, allow for a problem-driven focus to knowledge development such that both conceptual and empirical problems are important and there are mechanisms or at least judgments involved in determining what problems are of greatest concern at any specific time in the development of the knowledge base.

From a philosophical standpoint, a focus on problem solving pertains specifically to epistemic problems in the discipline—in other words, problems of knowledge development. An epistemic problem is different from a clinical problem. A clinical problem is a problem of care delivery or system structure, such as how to document nursing care effectively in a new electronic health record. A nurse might think also of ethical problems such as those that arise from conflicts of values in end-of-life care. Epistemic problems are at the root of practice or clinical problems, and part of the important role of the DNP-prepared nurse is to help make that translation from clinical to epistemic problems. A nurse might be concerned about decreasing the incidence of catheter-associated urinary tract infections and might think about addressing the problem as one of proper equipment or education for the individual with recurrent infection. The DNP-prepared nurse, approaching this as an epistemic problem, can identify the knowledge that is lacking in terms of the body of evidence that underlies the clinical situation and be part of the development of research to uncover the reason for the infections. In clinical problems, there is a challenge relating to what care to provide; epistemic problems arise from a lack of knowledge needed to ensure that practices are built on a sound knowledge base and whatever work that is done to solve the problem also helps to expand knowledge. It requires thinking about what is known and not known and also a vision of the nurse as not just using information but of actually contributing to new knowledge.

The advanced practice nurse with a practice-focused doctoral degree is the ideal person to facilitate this process. The advanced practice nurse has clinical expertise and practical experience that enables the nurse to detect problems that need to be addressed. The DNP-prepared nurse also has sufficient knowledge of processes of inquiry and an understanding of the discipline of nursing, both of which help to ensure that attempts to expand the knowledge base are properly conducted and are relevant to the discipline. The DNP-prepared nurse can identify problems, determine what knowledge is needed, and work with others with research expertise to address the lack of science and expand the knowledge base needed for effective care delivery.

Other developments in the history of nursing helped to bring some focus and direction to knowledge development in the discipline. During the 1980s and 1990s, a series of conferences was held in the northeastern United States, alternately sponsored by schools of nursing at the University of Rhode Island and Boston College. These conferences served as a vital forum for discussion of ideas about science and knowledge development relevant to the discipline of nursing. After this period of sharing and development, it became apparent to the conference organizers that the next appropriate step would be the development of a consensus statement reflecting crucial areas of agreement about nursing as a discipline.

The purpose of the Nursing Knowledge Consensus Conference in Boston in 1998 was for the 40 participants "to discuss and synthesize various perspectives on knowledge development related to (1) the nature of the human person, (2) the nature of nursing, (3) the role of nursing theory, and (4) the links of each of these understandings to nursing practice" (*Consensus Statement on Emerging Nursing Knowledge*, 1998, as cited in Roy, 2007, p. 26). The document that resulted from this effort, the *Consensus Statement on Emerging Nursing Knowledge*, served as an important event in the history of contemporary nursing and reflected the values and knowledge that were thought by participants to be essential to the discipline, as well as the practice, of nursing.

The consensus statement was an attempt to move beyond repeated discussion of the nature of nursing and the knowledge base and provide a foundation for continuing focused development of the discipline. What this manifesto provided was a statement of agreed-upon values and perspectives that could provide some cohesiveness among nurses, a reminder of the lens through which nurses see the world and the recipients of their care. A variety of philosophical traditions, modes of inquiry, and research methods may be used to solve epistemic problems in nursing. Keeping in mind the key assumptions and values embedded in the discipline allows plurality in approaches to knowledge development while still supporting a sense of unity in the discipline and the knowledge that underlies the work of nurses. The consensus statement was disseminated through a website, and there was an opportunity for sharing and continuing dialogue.

THE FUTURE OF NURSING KNOWLEDGE DEVELOPMENT

Reference to the future of nursing knowledge development does not imply that anyone truly can make accurate predictions. It is reasonable, however, to anticipate some changes and developments based on current trends and existing priorities both in nursing and in the society in which nursing exists in the United States. The future of nursing knowledge development certainly will require nurses with strong analytical skills to clearly identify problem areas where research is needed. Nurses also are needed who can work with trends within society, as well as within the discipline, and demonstrate the leadership and interpersonal skills to address the needs on all levels. The development of a cohesive discipline with clear identity also depends on nurses who can construct approaches to nursing knowledge development and practice that are cohesive, consistent, and grounded in a clear understanding of nursing as a discipline.

Along those lines, patterns that reveal potential significance for nursing involvement can be identified. Changes in philosophy, as well as in social context, call for new methods to address pressing issues in nursing. Recognition of the role of culture and social context requires increasing development, application, and evaluation of methods effective at capturing those aspects of existence. These changes also require nurses who understand the philosophy and knowledge development enterprises well enough to articulate the value of differing approaches to inquiry. Advanced practice nurses will provide a critical link in this process through their skill and understanding of both the knowledge development and scientific enterprises, as well as the realm of application in practice. Nursing science work without that critical link to practice is likely to fail in meeting the needs of nurses who apply that science on a daily basis. Nurses at levels prior to advanced practice need leadership and guidance from advanced practice nurses to offer a few problems suitable for inquiry, as well as to help evaluate and apply new information for evidence-based practice.

Promoting continuing progress in nursing in regard to knowledge development also requires nurses who recognize that the future is something to be constructed as well as anticipated. Perhaps what the future of nursing knowledge development needs most is nurses who have a vision of what nursing can be and who have a commitment and desire to help create that idealized future. Advanced practice nurses will continue to be an essential part of the process of developing the discipline of nursing.

One area in need of increased attention in nursing is that of theory development. Theory often is poorly understood in nursing, with a common misperception being that theory is limited to the work of the grand theorists such as Orem, Johnson, and others. Exposure to theory in nursing programs unfortunately has perpetuated a gross misunderstanding about the role of theory in the knowledge base and in support of the practice of nursing. Ideas of theory need to be expanded beyond these broad narratives about nursing and also beyond the axiomatic and propositional constructions supported by the logical positivists. Theory is merely organized knowledge—knowledge that is connected and structured in such a way as to be slightly abstract, rather than case dependent, and potentially relevant to a variety of situations. Theories exist that can be immensely beneficial to nurses dealing with a wide array of topics commonly encountered in practice.

Nurses also need to recognize that knowledge changes. Just as the history of philosophical views about knowledge has changed over time, knowledge itself can and must change. Nurses need to develop skills that enable thoughtful critique of knowledge, characteristics of flexibility, a spirit of creativity, and a willingness to evaluate and embrace changes in knowledge.

Along with this approach, particularly critical for nurses in leadership positions such as those with DNP degrees, nurses need to recognize the vital connection between the knowledge base and the discipline of nursing and look beyond immediate practice implications to promote changes in the discipline and perception of nursing among the public, other health professionals, and the nursing community itself. All activities, whether administrative, clinical, or research oriented, should be undertaken with an understanding of the essential connections among the discipline; the knowledge base, including the organization of knowledge into theories; and the practice of nursing.

SUMMARY

In this chapter, the nonlinear evolution of nursing science was explored in regard to philosophical traditions in epistemology and philosophy of science, specifically logical positivism, historicism, postmodernism, phenomenological philosophy, hermeneutics, and feminist epistemology. Events in the development of nursing as a discipline were examined in light of philosophical change. Emerging trends were presented along with suggestions for continuing development appropriate to the role of the DNP nurse.

DISCUSSION QUESTIONS

1. Discuss significant historical trends that have shaped the development of nursing knowledge.
2. Describe trends in philosophy that have influenced the development of nursing science.
3. Describe the role of the DNP-prepared nurse in the development of nursing science.

REFERENCES

Baker, C., Norton, S., Young, P., & Ward, S. (1998). An exploration of methodological pluralism in nursing research. *Research in Nursing and Health, 21, 545–555.*

Baker, C., Wuest, J., & Stern, P. N. (1992). Method slurring: The grounded theory/phenomenology example. *Journal of Advanced Nursing, 17,* 1355–1360.

Belenky, M. F., Clinchy, B. M., Goldberger, N. R., & Tarule, J. M. (1986). *Women's ways of knowing: The development of self, voice, and mind.* New York, NY: Basic Books.

Boydston, J. (Ed.). (2008). *Collected works of John Dewey.* Carbondale, IL: Southern Illinois University Press.

Carper, B. A. (1975). *Fundamental patterns of knowing in nursing* (Doctoral dissertation). Teachers College, Columbia University, New York. University Microfilms Cat # 76–7772.

Carper, B. A. (1978). Fundamental patterns of knowing in nursing. *Advances in Nursing Science, 1*(1), 13–23.

Chinn, P. L. (1989). Nursing patterns of knowing and feminist thought. *Nursing and Health Care, 10,* 71–75.

Coward, D. D. (1990). Critical multiplism: A research strategy for nursing science. *Image: Journal of Nursing Scholarship, 22,* 163–167.

Dickoff, J., James, P., & Wiedenbach, E. (1968a). Theory in a practice discipline: Part I. Practice-oriented theory. *Nursing Research, 17,* 415–435.

Dickoff, J., James, P., & Wiedenbach, E. (1968b). Theory in a practice discipline: Part II. Practice-oriented theory. *Nursing Research, 17,* 545–554.

Donaldson, S. K., & Crowley, D. M. (1978). The discipline of nursing. *Nursing Outlook, 26*(2), 113–120.

Fawcett, J. (1978). The relationship between theory and research: A double helix. *Advances in Nursing Science, 1*(1), 49–62.

Fawcett, J. (1985). Theory: Basis for the study and practice of nursing education. *Journal of Nursing Education, 24,* 226–229.

Feldman, H. R. (1981). A science of nursing: To be or not to be? *Image: Journal of Nursing Scholarship, 13,* 63–66.

Feyerabend, P. K. (1975). *Against method.* London, UK: Humanities Press.

Flaskerud, J. H., & Halloran, E. J. (1980). Areas of agreement in nursing theory development. *Advances in Nursing Science, 3*(1), 1–7.

Fry, S. T. (1995). Science as problem solving. In A. Omery, C. E. Kasper, & G. G. Page (Eds.), *In search of nursing science* (pp. 72–80). Thousand Oaks, CA: Sage.

Garrett, B. M. (2016). New sophistry: Self-deception in the nursing academy. *Nursing Philosophy, 17,* 182–193.

Gilligan, C. (1982). *In a different voice: Psychological theory and women's development.* Cambridge, MA: Harvard University Press.

Guba, E. G., & Lincoln, Y. S. (1989). *Fourth generation evaluation.* Newbury Park, CA: Sage.

Hall, J. M., & Stevens, P. E. (1991). Rigor in feminist research. *Advances in Nursing Science, 13*(3), 16–29.

Harding, S. (1986). *The science question in feminism.* Ithaca, NY: Cornell University.

Harding, S. (1991). *Whose science? Whose knowledge?* Ithaca, NY: Cornell University.

Hardy, M. E. (1978). Perspectives on nursing theory. *Advances in Nursing Science, 1*(1), 27–48.

Hardy, M. (1983). Metaparadigms and theory development. In N. L. Chaska (Ed.), *The nursing profession: A time to speak* (pp. 427–437). New York, NY: McGraw-Hill.

James, W. (2000). *Pragmatism and other writings.* London, UK: Penguin Classics.

Johnson, D. E. (1959). The nature of a science of nursing. *Nursing Outlook, 7,* 291–294.

Johnson, D. E. (1968). Theory in nursing: Borrowed and unique. *Nursing Research, 17,* 206–209.

Jordan, J. D. (1996). Rethinking race and attrition in nursing programs: A hermeneutic inquiry. *Journal of Professional Nursing, 12,* 382–390.

Kalisch, P. A., & Kalisch, B. J. (1995). *The advance of American nursing.* Philadelphia, PA: Lippincott.

Kim, H. S. (1987). Structuring the nursing knowledge system: A typology of four domains. *Scholarly Inquiry for Nursing Practice, 1,* 111–114.

Kim, H. S. (1989). Theoretical thinking in nursing: Problems and prospects. *Recent Advances in Nursing, 24,* 106–122.

Kohlberg, L. (1981). *Essays on moral development.* San Francisco, CA: Harper & Row.

Kuhn, T. S. (1970/1962). *The structure of scientific revolutions* (2nd ed.). Chicago, IL: University of Chicago.

Kuhn, T. S. (1974). Second thoughts on paradigms. In F. Suppe (Ed.), *The structure of scientific theories* (pp. 459–482). Urbana, IL: University of Illinois.

Lather, P. (1991). *Getting smart: Feminist research and pedagogy with/in the postmodern.* New York, NY: Routledge.

Laudan, L. (1977). *Progress and its problems.* Berkeley, CA: University of California Press.

Mason, W. H. (2008). Constructing a "plausible narrative of progress" for nursing: A neopragmatist suggestion. *Nursing Philosophy, 10,* 4–13.

Newman, M. A. (1972). Nursing's theoretical evolution. *Nursing Outlook, 20,* 449–453.

Norris, C. M. (1982). *Concept clarification in nursing.* Rockville, MD: Aspen.

Orlando, I. (1961). *The dynamic nurse–patient relationship.* New York, NY: G. P. Putnam's Sons.

Peirce, C. S. (1878). How to make our ideas clear. *Popular Science Monthly, 12*, 286–302.

Price, H. H. (1953). *Thinking and experience.* London, UK: Hutchinson House.

Putnam, H. (1991). *Representation and reality.* Cambridge, MA: MIT Press.

Reynolds, P. D. (1971). *A primer in theory construction.* New York, NY: Bobbs-Merrill.

Ricoeur, P. (1981). *Hermeneutics and the human sciences* (J. B. Thompson, Ed. & Trans.). Cambridge, UK: Cambridge University Press.

Ricoeur, P. (1984). *Time and narrative* (2 Vols., K. McLaughlin & D. Pellauer, Trans.). Chicago, IL: University of Chicago Press.

Rodgers, B. L. (1989). Concepts, analysis, and the development of knowledge: The evolutionary cycle. *Journal of Advanced Nursing, 14*, 330–335.

Rodgers, B. L. (1991). Deconstructing the dogma in nursing knowledge and practice. *Image: Journal of Nursing Scholarship, 23*, 177–181.

Rodgers, B. L. (2000a). Concept analysis: An evolutionary view. In B. L. Rodgers & K. A. Knafl (Eds.), *Concept development in nursing: Foundations, techniques, and applications* (pp. 77–102). Philadelphia, PA: Saunders.

Rodgers, B. L. (2000b). Philosophical foundations of concept development. In B. L. Rodgers & K. A. Knafl (Eds.), *Concept development in nursing: Foundations, techniques, and applications* (pp. 7–38). Philadelphia, PA: Saunders.

Rodgers, B. L. (2005). *Developing nursing knowledge: Philosophical traditions and influences.* Philadelphia, PA: Lippincott Williams & Wilkins.

Rodgers, B. L. (2007). Knowledge as problem solving. In C. Roy & D. A. Jones (Eds.), *Nursing knowledge development and clinical practice* (pp. 107–117). New York, NY: Springer.

Rodgers, B. L., & Knafl, K. A. (Eds.). (2000). *Concept development in nursing: Foundations, techniques, and applications.* Philadelphia, PA: Saunders.

Rogers, M. E. (1970). *An introduction to the theoretical basis of nursing.* Philadelphia, PA: F. A. Davis.

Rolfe, G. (2006). Judgments without rules: Towards a postmodern ironist concept of research validity. *Nursing Inquiry, 13*(1), 7–15.

Rorty, R. R. (1979). *Philosophy and the mirror of nature.* Princeton, NJ: Princeton University Press.

Rorty, R. R. (1982). *Consequences of pragmatism: Essays 1972–1980.* Minneapolis, MN: University of Minnesota Press.

Roy, C. (1970). Adaptation: A conceptual framework for nursing. *Nursing Outlook, 18*(3), 42–45.

Roy, C. (1971). Adaptation: A basis for nursing practice. *Nursing Outlook, 19*, 254–257.

Roy, C. (2007). Advances in nursing knowledge and the challenge for transforming practice. In C. Roy & D. A. Jones (Eds.). *Nursing knowledge development and clinical practice* (pp. 3–37). New York, NY: Springer.

Schultz, P. R. (1987). Toward holistic inquiry in nursing: A proposal for synthesis of patterns and methods. *Scholarly Inquiry for Nursing Practice: An International Journal, 1*, 135–146.

Schwab, J. (1962). The concept of the structure of a discipline. *Educational Record, 43*, 197–205.

Shermis, S. (1962). On becoming an intellectual discipline. *Phi Delta Kappan, 44*, 84–86.

Smith, M., & McCarthy, P. M. (2010). Disciplinary knowledge in nursing education: Going beyond the blueprints. *Nursing Outlook, 58*, 44–51.

Steeves, R. H., Kahn, D. L., & Benoliel, J. Q. (1990). Nurses' interpretation of the suffering of their patients. *Western Journal of Nursing Research, 12,* 715–729.

Sundin, K., Jansson, L., & Norberg, A. (2002). Understanding between care providers and patients with stroke and aphasia: A phenomenological hermeneutic inquiry. *Nursing Inquiry, 9,* 93–103.

Tinkle, M. B., & Beaton, J. L. (1983). Toward a new view of science: Implications for nursing research. *Advances in Nursing Science, 5*(2), 27–36.

Toulmin, S. (1972). *Human understanding.* Princeton, NJ: Princeton University Press.

U.S. Public Health Service. (1963). *Toward quality in nursing: Needs and goals.* Washington, DC: Government Printing Office.

Visintainer, M. A. (1986). The nature of knowledge and theory in nursing. *Image: Journal of Nursing Scholarship, 18,* 32–38.

Walker, L. O., & Avant, K. C. (1983). *Strategies for theory construction in nursing.* Norwalk, CT: Appleton & Lange.

Walker, L. O., & Avant, K. C. (1988). *Strategies for theory construction in nursing* (2nd ed.). Norwalk, CT: Appleton & Lange.

Walters, A. J. (1996). Being a clinical nurse consultant: A hermeneutic phenomenological reflection. *International Journal of Nursing Practice, 2*(1), 2–10.

Webster, G., Jacox, A., & Baldwin, B. (1981). Nursing theory and the ghost of the received view. In J. C. McCloskey & H. K. Grace (Eds.), *Current issues in nursing* (pp. 26–35). Boston, MA: Blackwell Scientific.

Wilson, J. (1969). *Thinking with concepts.* New York, NY: Cambridge University Press.

Chapter 3

The Essentials of the Doctor of Nursing Practice: A Philosophical Perspective

Lisa Astalos Chism

INTRODUCTION

The doctor of nursing practice (DNP) degree has been recommended by the American Association of Colleges of Nursing (AACN) as the terminal practice-focused degree in nursing (AACN, 2004). Since its inception, the DNP degree has been met with both support and criticism (Burman, Hart, & McCabe, 2005; Chase & Pruitt, 2006; Dracup & Bryan-Brown, 2005; Hathaway, Jacob, Stegbauer, Thompson, & Graff, 2006). Despite the controversy associated with this innovative degree, approximately 272 DNP programs exist, with over 100 more currently in development (AACN, 2016). Because of the recommendations of the AACN (2004), as well as the growth in programs devoted to awarding this degree, it is necessary that graduate nursing students understand the definition and competencies of the DNP degree.

This chapter provides a definition of the DNP degree. This definition may be more easily understood from a historical perspective of nursing education; therefore, the history of doctoral education in nursing leading up to the development of the DNP degree is reviewed. The AACN's *Essentials of Doctoral Education for Advanced Nursing Practice* defines the competencies of the DNP degree (AACN, 2006a) and is also discussed. *Essential I, Scientific Underpinnings for Practice*, is extensively explored, with particular attention being paid to philosophical inquiry regarding the nature of the discipline of nursing and nursing science. The chapter concludes with a description of this author's development of a middle-range theory to exemplify bridging theory with practice.

OVERVIEW OF THE DOCTOR OF NURSING PRACTICE DEGREE

The DNP degree is defined as a practice-focused, terminal degree in nursing practice (AACN, 2004). Nursing practice is defined as follows:

> Any form of nursing intervention that influences healthcare outcomes for individuals or populations, including the direct care of individual patients, management of care for individuals and populations, administration of nursing and healthcare organizations, and the development and implementation of health policy. (AACN, 2004, p. 1)

Historically, nursing has been concerned with care of the individual. This more contemporary definition accurately describes care that focuses on the healthcare outcomes of populations from an organizational perspective, as well as nursing's impact on healthcare policy (Chism, 2016). These themes remain consistent throughout the competencies of DNP curricula as well and are reflected in *Essentials of Doctoral Education for Advanced Nursing Practice* (see **Table 3-1**).

It should be noted that the DNP degree differs from the traditional PhD in both focus and content (see **Table 3-2**). The DNP degree is a *practice-focused degree*, whereas the doctor of philosophy (PhD) is a *research-focused* degree. Both degrees share a common goal regarding a "scholarly approach to the discipline and commitment to the advancement of the profession" (AACN, 2006a, p. 3). However, the DNP degree emphasizes practice, while the PhD degree emphasizes theory and research methodology (AACN, 2004, 2006a). The DNP graduate is expected to demonstrate scholarly activity through a theory-driven research project, often termed a capstone project. This project may be guided by middle-range

Table 3-1   AACN's Essentials of Doctoral Education for Advanced Nursing Practice

Essential I	Scientific Underpinnings for Practice
Essential II	Organizational and Systems Leadership for Quality Improvement and Systems Thinking
Essential III	Clinical Scholarship and Analytical Methods for Evidenced-Based Practice
Essential IV	Information Systems/Technology and Patient Care Technology for the Improvement and Transformation of Health Care
Essential V	Healthcare Policy for Advocacy in Health Care
Essential VI	Interprofessional Collaboration for Improving Patient and Population Health Outcomes
Essential VII	Clinical Prevention and Population Health for Improving the Nation's Health
Essential VIII	Advanced Nursing Practice

Table 3-2   Key Differences Between DNP and PhD/DNS/DNSc Programs

	DNP	PhD/DNS/DNSc
Program of study	**Objectives**	**Objectives**
	Prepare nurse specialists at the highest level of advanced practice	Prepare nurse researchers
	Competencies	**Content**
	Based on AACN essentials of the DNP degree	Based on indicators of quality in research-focused doctoral programs in nursing (AACN, 2001)
Students	Commitment to a practice career	Commitment to a research career
	Oriented toward improving outcomes of care	Oriented toward developing new knowledge
Program faculty	Practice doctorate and/or experience in the area of teaching	Research doctorate in nursing or a related field
	Leadership experience in the area of specialty practice	Leadership experience in the area of sustained research funding
	High level of expertise in specialty practice congruent with the focus of the academic program	High level of expertise in research congruent with the focus of the academic program
Resources	Mentors/preceptors in leadership positions across a variety of practice settings	Mentors/preceptors in research settings
	Access to diverse practice settings with appropriate resources for areas of practice	Access to research settings with appropriate resources
	Access to financial aid	Access to dissertation support dollars
	Access to information and patient care technology resources congruent with the areas of study	Access to information and research technology resources congruent with the program of research

(Continues)

Table 3-2 Key Differences Between DNP and PhD/DNS/DNSc Programs (Continued)

	DNP	PhD/DNS/DNSc
Program assessment and evaluation	**Program Outcome**	**Program Outcome**
	Healthcare improvements and contributions via practice, policy change, and practice scholarship	Contributes to healthcare improvements via the development of new knowledge and other scholarly projects that provide the foundation for the advancement of nursing science
	Oversight by the institution's authorized bodies (i.e., graduate school) and regional accreditors Receives accreditation from a specialized nursing accreditor Graduates are eligible for the national certification exam	Oversight by the institution's authorized bodies (i.e., graduate school) and regional accreditors

Reproduced from AACN. AACN DNP Roadmap Taskforce Report, October 20, 2006 (b). Reprinted by permission of American Association of Colleges of Nursing.

nursing theory and demonstrate ways in which research affects practice. Middle-range nursing theory and the DNP degree are discussed later in this chapter.

Historical Perspectives

Doctoral education in nursing has, indeed, evolved over the past 40 years. In the 1960s, nurses' choices for doctoral education included a PhD in the basic sciences such as biology, anatomy, or physiology or an education doctorate (EdD; Carpenter & Hudacek, 1996; Marriner-Tomey, 1990). As doctoral education in nursing evolved, more nursing-related doctoral degrees emerged.

The first nursing-related doctorate degree originated at Teachers College, Columbia University, in 1924. This degree was an EdD that was designed to prepare nurses to teach at the college level. It was unique in that it was the first doctoral degree in nursing to emphasize both nursing education and the needs of the profession (Carpenter & Hudacek, 1996). Later, in 1934, the first PhD in nursing was offered at New York University, followed by introduction of a maternal–child nursing PhD program in the 1950s at the University of Pittsburgh (Carpenter & Hudacek, 1996). Importantly, the latter PhD program was the first to recognize the importance of clinical research for the development of the discipline of nursing (Carpenter & Hudacek, 1996). Throughout the United States, other PhDs continued to focus on sociological fields such as psychology, sociology, and anthropology. Actual nursing PhDs did not become popular until the 1970s (Grace, 1978).

According to Murphy (1981), doctoral education in nursing developed in three phases. The focus of these phases included nursing doctorates that emphasized the development of (1) functional specialists, (2) nurse scientists, and (3) doctorates that were "in and of nursing" (p. 646). The first phase, which emphasized the development of functional specialists, focused on preparing nurses as teachers or administrators. Throughout the second phase—the development of nurse scientists—relevant questions emerged that directly affected the third and final phase of nursing doctoral education:

- What is the essential nature of professional nursing?
- What is the substantive knowledge base of professional nursing?
- What kind of research is important for nursing? As a knowledge discipline? As a field of practice?
- How can the scientific base of nursing knowledge be identified and expanded? (p. 646)

These questions led to the development of nursing doctorates that were "in and of nursing" (p. 646), and they continue to influence nursing doctoral education today.

More recently, a fourth phase of doctoral education in nursing has evolved. This phase emphasizes nursing practice and initially began with the development of the doctor of nursing science (DNS) degree. The first DNS degree was developed at Boston University and "focused on the development of nursing theory for a practice discipline" (Marriner-Tomey, 1990, p. 135). The DNS was perceived as the first practice-focused doctorate. Cleland (1976) noted that the research doctorate should focus on contributions to nursing science and the practice doctorate should focus on expertise in clinical practice. Grace (1978) suggested that nurses be prepared as "social engineers," with attention being given to the clinical field (p. 26). Finally, Newman (1975) indicated that a practice doctorate would prepare nurses as "professional practitioners" for entry into practice (p. 705).

Although the DNS was developed to prepare nurses as practice experts, over time curricula in these programs began to resemble the PhD in nursing (AACN, 2006b; Apold, 2008; Marriner-Tomey, 1990). Given this development, the AACN has designated all DNS degrees as research-focused degrees (AACN, 2004). Hence, the challenge to develop a true practice doctorate remained.

Rozella Schlottfeldt pioneered the development of a doctorate of nursing (ND) degree in 1979 at Case Western Reserve University in Cleveland, Ohio. Schlottfeldt posited that nursing needed a practice doctorate to address several needs of nursing education:

- The need to reorient the existing system of health care toward services that enhance the health status of all people, while maintaining the existing services that focus primarily on detection and treatment of disease

- The need to reorient the nursing community in ways to hasten the emergence of nursing as a scholarly discipline and a fully autonomous practice profession
- The need to reorient nursing's approach to preparing professionals with a view toward promptly augmenting the cadre of competent, independent, accountable nursing practitioners (Schlottfeldt, 1978, p. 302)

Unfortunately, ND programs did not have the same popularity as DNS or PhD degrees. It was also noted that the curricula for these programs lacked the uniformity needed to establish their credibility as practice doctorate programs (Marion et al., 2003). Interestingly, the needs outlined by Schlottfeldt are reflected in the curricula of present DNP programs.

Development of the Doctor of Nursing Practice

In 2002, a task force was formed by the AACN to evaluate the current status of practice doctorates in nursing. The task force was charged with developing recommendations for a practice doctorate in nursing, as well as proposing practice doctorate curriculum models. This work led to the development of the *AACN Position Statement on the Practice Doctorate in Nursing*, which was published in 2004. The position statement recommended that the DNP degree become the terminal practice-focused degree for nursing by 2015 (AACN, 2004).

The University of Kentucky's School of Nursing was the first to admit students to this program in 2001. Dr. Carolyn Williams, President of AACN (2000–2002) and Dean Emeritus of the University of Kentucky's School of Nursing, was an early proponent of the practice doctorate in nursing and, along with others, helped to facilitate the development of the DNP degree. Currently, more than 272 DNP programs exist in the United States, with more than 100 in development (AACN, 2016).

Doctor of Nursing Practice Competencies

In 2006, the AACN developed the *Essentials of Doctoral Education for Advanced Nursing Practice*. The *Essentials* "address the foundational competencies that are core to all advanced nursing practice roles" (AACN, 2006a, p. 8). Also in 2006, the National Organization of Nurse Practitioner Faculties developed the *Practice Doctorate Nurse Practitioner Entry-Level Competencies*, and in 2008, the National Association of Clinical Nurse Specialists developed the *Core Practice Doctorate Clinical Nurse Specialist Competencies*. Together, these documents provide the curriculum standards for all DNP programs. The following is a summary of the *Essentials of Doctoral Education for Advanced Nursing Practice*.

Essential I: Scientific Underpinnings for Practice

Essential I describes the scientific foundations for nursing practice. These scientific foundations are derived from the natural and social sciences and may include human biology, physiology, and psychology. This foundation also includes nursing science, which adds to the discipline of nursing. Within the discipline of nursing, specific nursing middle-range theories that guide practice are also part of the foundation for nursing practice (AACN, 2006a). *Essential I* provides the scientific basis necessary for advanced nursing practice. Because of the importance of understanding the foundations for nursing practice, *Essential I* will be discussed in more depth later in this chapter.

Essential II: Organizational and Systems Leadership for Quality Improvement and Systems Thinking

Essential II describes preparation in organizational and systems leadership that affects subsequent healthcare delivery and patient care outcomes. Preparation in this area provides DNP graduates with expertise in "assessing organizations, identifying systems' issues, and facilitating organization-wide changes in practice delivery" (AACN, 2006a, p. 10). The DNP graduate is prepared to assume roles in leadership at every level, from informal leadership in the clinical setting to more formal leadership at an executive level (Chism, 2016).

Essential III: Clinical Scholarship and Analytical Methods for Evidence-Based Practice

Essential III describes competencies related to the evaluation, integration, translation, and application of evidence-based practice. DNP graduates are unique in that their practice perspective allows them to merge nursing science, practice, human needs, and human caring (AACN, 2006a). Additionally, because of their practice perspective, DNP graduates are well positioned to apply research to practice, as well as to ask pertinent questions related to practice (Chism, 2016). Potential roles related to *Essential III* include partnering with research colleges and participating in clinical research, evaluating and developing practice guidelines, critically evaluating existing literature to determine best practices, and designing and evaluating methodologies that improve patient care (AACN, 2006a).

Essential IV: Information Systems/Technology and Patient Care Technology for the Improvement and Transformation of Health Care

Essential IV prepares the DNP graduate to use information technologies in ways that improve patient care outcomes. Additionally, DNP graduates develop expertise in information technologies to support leadership and clinical decision making. Examples of information technologies important for improvement of healthcare outcomes include web-based communications, online documentation, telemedicine, and data mining. DNP graduates may employ their expertise in information technologies when evaluating programs for online documentation or data from large systems or databases as part of a search for practice outcome patterns. Graduates may also use information technologies to communicate and evaluate the accuracy, timeliness, and appropriateness of healthcare consumer information

(AACN, 2006a). Finally, DNP graduates have a role in attending to the ethical and legal issues related to information technologies (AACN, 2006a).

Essential V: Healthcare Policy for Advocacy in Health Care

Essential V describes the importance of nurses' involvement in healthcare policy and advocacy. As leaders in the practice setting, it is imperative that DNP graduates understand the relationship between practice and policy. Such graduates may be called on to analyze health policies and proposals from multiple points of view; provide leadership in the development of healthcare policies on different levels; actively participate on committees, boards, or task forces; and act as advocates for the nursing profession through organizational leadership (AACN, 2006a).

Essential VI: Interprofessional Collaboration for Improving Patient and Population Health Outcomes

Essential VI prepares the DNP graduate to understand the importance of interprofessional collaboration within a multitiered healthcare environment. Nurses frequently function as collaborators with members of other professions. This essential skill expands on the collaboration that naturally occurs among professionals by ensuring that DNP graduates will develop the expertise needed to assume leadership roles when collaborating with teams, as well as participate in the work of the team. Graduates must also be prepared to act as consultants during times of change (AACN, 2006a).

Essential VII: Clinical Prevention and Population Health for Improving the Nation's Health

Essential VII prepares DNP graduates to "analyze epidemiological, biostatistical, occupational, and environmental data in the development, implementation, and evaluation of clinical prevention and population health" (AACN, 2006a, p. 15). Nursing has traditionally been involved in health promotion and risk reduction/illness prevention. The DNP graduate is prepared to assume roles that improve health promotion and reduce risk from an advanced nursing practice perspective.

Essential VIII: Advanced Nursing Practice

Essential VIII describes the clinical specialization content from a specific domain of advanced nursing practice. Post-baccalaureate DNP degree programs "provide preparation within distinct specialties that require expertise, advanced nursing knowledge, and mastery in one area of nursing practice" (AACN, 2006a, p. 16). The DNP graduate is prepared to develop therapeutic relationships with patients and other healthcare professionals to improve patient outcomes, assess health and illness parameters, utilize advanced clinical decision-making skills and critical thinking, serve as mentor to others in the nursing profession, and educate patients (AACN, 2006a).

FOCUS ON ESSENTIAL I: SCIENTIFIC UNDERPINNINGS FOR PRACTICE

The scientific underpinnings of practice provide the basis of knowledge for advanced nursing practice. These scientific underpinnings include sciences such as biology, physiology, psychology, ethics, and nursing. Although the basic sciences are often accepted as the basis of knowledge for nursing practice, the role of nursing science may not be as readily understood. Nursing science has expanded the discipline of nursing to include the development of middle-range nursing theories and concepts to guide practice (AACN, 2006b). Graduates of DNP programs have a pertinent role in the implementation of middle-range nursing theories to guide nursing practice. Hence, understanding the scientific underpinnings for nursing practice is essential for all DNP graduates.

Basic Sciences

It is often accepted that advanced nursing practice borrows from the social and basic sciences—much as medicine does—to build a scientific basis for practice. These sciences frequently include biology, physiology, psychology, and ethics. According to Webber (2008), nurse practitioners "rely on medical research to support their practice because not enough advanced practice research and researchers exist" (p. 466). Concerns have been raised that advanced nursing practitioners "adopt the practice values of medicine rather than identifying and adopting knowledge, skills, values, meanings and experiences unique to this nursing specialty" (p. 466). This point may be well taken; however, without the basic understanding of disease, how will nursing develop an understanding of the human responses to disease? Gortner (1980) noted this paradox also and suggested that if nursing rejects the medical model, it rejects the body of knowledge that describes and explains the pathology that leads patients to nurses' care. Through development of an understanding of the fundamentals of the sciences that predict and explain disease processes, nursing can build a basis for understanding how best to care for those affected by disease. Donaldson and Crowley (1978) described professional disciplines such as nursing as "emerging *along with* rather than *from* academic disciplines" (p. 116).

The Discipline of Nursing

A discipline is characterized by a "unique perspective, a distinct way of viewing all phenomena, which ultimately defines the limits and nature of its inquiry" (Donaldson & Crowley, 1978,

p. 113). The discipline of nursing has been defined as the body of knowledge concerned with the following aspects of care:

- The principles and laws that govern all life processes, well-being, and optimal functioning of human beings, sick or well
- The patterning of human behavior in interaction with the environment in normal life events and critical life situations
- The processes by which positive changes in health status are effected
- The wholeness of health of human beings, recognizing that they are in continuous interaction with their environments (adapted from AACN, 2006a; Donaldson & Crowley, 1978; Fawcett, 2005; Gortner, 1980)

Nursing is concerned "with the whole human, with lifestyles and with health behavior" (Gortner, 1980, p. 181) and looks beyond the biological and physiological perspectives on disease. In doing so, nursing seeks to explain and predict responses to therapy, improvement in health status, and wellness (Gortner, 1980).

Nursing Science

The definition of nursing science may be somewhat more difficult to elucidate. Nursing science has been described as both a body of theoretical knowledge and the methods of reproducible modes of inquiry (Gortner, 1980; Jacobs & Huether, 1978; Jacox, 1974). Gortner (1980) defined it as "the base of knowledge underlying human behavior and social interaction under normal and stressful conditions across the lifespan" (p. 180). Interestingly, Jacobs and Huether (1978) defined nursing science as "the process, and the result, of ordering and patterning the events and phenomena of concern to nursing" (p. 65). Thus nursing science may be understood as both the "methods of inquiry specific to the discipline of nursing—the process—as well as the outcomes of that inquiry—the result" (Jacobs & Huether, 1978, p. 65). Nursing research has been differentiated from nursing science as "the systematic inquiry into problems associated with illness, health, and care" (Gortner, 1980, p. 180).

Nursing Theory

Nursing theory has been described as the product of nursing science (Jacobs & Huether, 1978; Kerlinger, 1973). Specifically, Jacobs and Huether (1978) described the dual purposes of nursing science as "to define common goals and guide the practice of nursing" (p. 64)—hence, the development of nursing theory. A *theory* is defined as a relationship between two or more concepts, whereas the term *concept* describes objects, properties, or events, and indicates the subject matter of the theory (Jacox, 1974). The concepts within a theory are related by propositions that describe the relationships between two or more concepts (Jacox, 1974). In essence, then, nursing theory attempts to describe, predict, or explain phenomena consistent with nursing's perspective (Donaldson & Crowley, 1978).

Middle-Range Theory

Nursing's body of knowledge, or discipline, includes both grand and middle-range theories (Fawcett, 2005). Grand theories are more abstract and are broader in type, whereas middle-range theories are more concrete and are narrower in type (Fawcett, 2005). For this reason, middle-range theories are more applicable to clinical practice (Lenz, 1998). Further, clinicians may use middle-range theory "situationally," or to help "direct their assessment, decision-making, and nursing interventions when cued by a particular kind of situation rather than practicing consistently according to the tenets of a given theory" (Lenz, 1998, p. 63).

Doctor of Nursing Practice Graduates and Nursing Theory

Nursing has traditionally struggled to close the theory–practice gap (i.e., the lack of use of theory in practice or the inability of nurses to use theory in practice; Kenney, 2006). Reasons for this shortcoming include lack of knowledge, understanding, belief, or applicability of nursing theory as a guide for practice (McKenna, 1997). Further, the use of medical knowledge, especially in advanced practice nursing roles, has prevailed as a guide for nursing practice (Meleis, 1993).

Because of the limited, narrower, and more applicable scope of middle-range theories, the understanding and application of such theories may be vital to closing the theory–practice gap. As a practice discipline, when nursing theories prove useful in the real world and are "logical and consistent with other validated theories, they may provide a rationale for nursing actions that lead to predictable client outcomes" (Kenney, 2006, p. 297). For this reason, DNP graduates must have an understanding of middle-range theories, as well as the skills necessary to apply those theories in practice.

In a book chapter titled "Expectations for Theory, Research, and Scholarship," Magnan (2016) suggested that it was more important for DNP students to acquire the skills needed to apply theory to practice than to simply be exposed to a number of middle-range theories. Further, Magnan noted that these skills should be "transferable" and apply to the application of other middle-range theories to practice (p. 120). To achieve this goal, DNP students will need to meet the following criteria:

- Have a foundation in the language of theory (e.g., concepts, relational statements)
- Learn how to distinguish modifiable from nonmodifiable predictors and understand the meaning they have for planning theory-based interventions
- Understand how to interpret the research literature to determine the level of empirical support for relationships between theoretical concepts (Magnan, 2016, p. 120)

As experts in the application of theory, and specifically in middle-range theory, DNP graduates are well positioned to close the theory–practice gap (Magnan, 2016). Such nurses are practice experts who combine their clinical expertise with a doctoral-level understanding of nursing science and theory. This combination prepares the DNP graduate to clearly articulate for others the importance of theory in practice. DNP graduates are ideal role models to increase the use and understanding of theory-guided practice.

DOCTOR OF NURSING PRACTICE GRADUATES AND USE OF OTHER THEORIES

Essential I of the AACN's *Essentials of Doctoral Education for Advanced Nursing Practice* clearly recommends that DNP graduates garner an understanding of the scientific underpinnings of nursing practice (AACN, 2006a). It is well understood that these scientific underpinnings include other sciences such as biology, physiology, psychology, and ethics. *Essential I* reaffirms the notion that DNP graduates must apply other middle-range theories to practice in an effort to provide patient-centered care. As Meleis (1997) noted, because nurses study many disciplines as a foundation for practice, nursing theory tends to reflect a broad range of perspectives and premises.

Donaldson and Crowley (1978) asserted that nursing is—importantly—a practice-oriented discipline. In a book chapter titled "Nursing Science for Nursing Practice," Donaldson (1995) thoughtfully emphasized the point that nursing practice, as well as society's need for nursing services, has shaped the discipline of nursing. Because of nursing's interest in societal needs and desired patient outcomes, the discipline of nursing may include many theories, and the most appropriate theory selection will depend on the patient or societal situation. Donaldson (1995) described the nurse pragmatist as a nurse who will use the most pragmatic theory to accomplish the desired patient outcome. Further, nursing science will be a source of theory to the nurse pragmatist only if that theory "fits" the desired patient outcome (Donaldson, 1995).

DNP graduates, therefore, not only have a responsibility to exemplify the application of nursing theory to practice, but they must also be "nurse pragmatists" (Donaldson, 1995) and apply various theories from other sciences to practice. The role of the DNP graduate in theory evaluation and selection may well be one of the most valuable roles that such a person fills. Hence, DNP graduates become the knowledge appliers and exhibit expertise in evaluating, applying, and supporting theory-based interventions to ensure patient-centered care.

DILUTION OF THE DISCIPLINE OF NURSING: PHILOSOPHICAL CONSIDERATIONS FOR DOCTOR OF NURSING PRACTICE GRADUATES

Although applying and integrating theories from various disciplines may add to the knowledge base considered to be part of the discipline of nursing, some practitioners have expressed concerns that this trend dilutes the discipline of nursing (Cody, 1996; McKenna,

1997). McKenna (1997) expressed concerns that combining other theories with nursing theories compromises the context of the original nursing concepts. Additionally, if theories are constantly borrowed and incorporated into the discipline, it may become difficult to differentiate nursing as its own discipline (Cody, 1996). Johnson (1968) pointedly discussed this dilemma, stating that if nursing "continues to observe behavior from the perspective of the sciences such as sociology and psychology, if we continue to study disease with the aim of elucidating etiologies, properties, or life cycles,... we may be serving the cause of science, but not necessarily the cause of nursing" (Johnson, 1968, pp. 207–208).

The dilemma ensues upon reviewing *Essential I* of the AACN's *Essentials* document. DNP graduates are frequently advanced practice nurses. Many people who fill advanced practice nursing roles identify very closely with a medical model and may be viewed as "junior doctors" (Meleis, 1993). According to Fawcett (1997), nurses are often unaware of their discrete knowledge and instead glean fragmented information from a medical model. Moreover, DNP graduates are expected to understand the scientific underpinnings of practice, including the basic sciences—sciences that are traditionally associated with the medical model. An interesting question then arises: How do DNP graduates understand and contribute to the discipline of nursing through application of knowledge if this knowledge base has been infused with theories borrowed from other disciplines, specifically the basic sciences?

This dilemma may be resolved by DNP graduates developing a good understanding of nursing as a profession, a science, and a discipline. Nursing is a practice profession whose science and body of knowledge depend on its perspective. Further, if this understanding is developed, DNP graduates will integrate the necessary knowledge from a nursing perspective, understanding what nursing is and what it is not. While the basis of knowledge may include knowledge borrowed from various sciences to explain and predict disease, nursing is concerned with the laws and principles that govern the life processes, well-being, and optimal functioning of human beings; the human behavioral responses to disease; and the processes by which positive health status is effected (Donaldson & Crowley, 1978). The ability to elucidate what defines nursing practice, while employing various "pragmatic" (Donaldson, 1995, p. 6) scientific underpinnings from a nursing perspective, may be what truly differentiates the DNP-prepared nurse.

SUMMARY

The AACN recommended that the DNP degree become the terminal practice-focused degree for nursing by 2015 (AACN, 2004). Adoption of this recommendation has implications for the advancement of nursing as a profession, a science, and a discipline. Expanding their understanding of the scientific underpinnings for practice is perhaps the most essential expectation for DNP graduates. Through the process of gaining this understanding, DNP graduates will garner expertise in the differentiation and application of nursing knowledge.

Moreover, as the practice experts and knowledge appliers, DNP graduates will be in an ideal position to bridge the theory–practice gap, an enduring ambition of nursing.

EXEMPLAR

The following discussion is a case scenario in which this author developed, tested, and applied a nursing middle-range theory, thereby bridging theory and practice.

During my doctoral study at Oakland University in Rochester, Michigan, Dr. Morris Magnan charged the advanced theory class with writing a middle-range theory paper. I had only recently been introduced to middle-range theory and was struggling to develop an understanding of nursing as a science and a discipline. However, applying middle-range theory to an actual patient scenario helped me to develop a broader understanding of nursing.

Dr. Magnan and I were having a telephone meeting one evening to discuss which middle-range theory I would use for my theory paper. My research interest was spiritual care in nursing. I was drawn to Olson's empathic process theory (Olson, 1995) as the theoretical guide for my ideas. Dr. Magnan urged me to describe in more detail why I believed that this middle-range theory applied to spiritual care in nursing.

I explained that I had recently cared for a patient whose son had attempted suicide and was now in an intensive care unit (ICU), clinging to life. My patient was struggling with what to pray for: death or healing. She was disturbed also by how she was approached by a rabbi in the ICU who whispered to her in Hebrew and touched her knee when he spoke to her. She related, "Just because I am Jewish, it doesn't mean that I speak Hebrew. And furthermore, I don't want anybody whispering to me and touching me. I will pray in my own way and on my own terms." I replied to my patient, "So, you felt that instead of asking you how you pray, or what your spiritual need was, the rabbi assumed what you needed and made you even more anxious." She immediately relaxed in the chair and exclaimed, "Yes! That's exactly how I feel." Her body language clearly exhibited an openness to further spiritual discussion. I added, "Why don't you pray for peace?" She agreed: "Yes, that's what I will pray for—peace."

I will never forget the night I shared this story with Dr. Magnan. When I had finished, he replied, "Well, I believe you have a middle-range theory here."

With Dr. Magnan's guidance, we developed my ideas into Chism's middle-range theory of spiritual empathy (MTSE; Chism, 2007). The MTSE was deductively derived from Olson's (1995) empathic process theory (middle-range theory) and Orlando's (1990) dynamic nursing process theory (grand theory). The MTSE purports that nurses' spiritual care perspectives—that is, nurses' attitudes and beliefs about spiritual care (Taylor, 2002)—will influence nurses' expression of spiritual empathy—that is, the nurse's expression of verbal understanding of a patient's spiritual concern (Chism, 2007; Chism & Magnan, 2009; Olson, 1995). Expression of spiritual empathy will then increase the patient's perception of empathy—patients feeling that they are understood by nurses (Olson, 1995). Spiritual distress—impairments in a sense of connectedness to self and others, faith and belief system, sense of purpose, inner peace, and inner strength (Villagomeza, 2005)—will then decrease. The final concept, spiritual well-being—a sense of inner peace and contentment resulting from one's perceived sense of connection to self or others (Chism, 2007)—is purported to increase at this point.

One portion of the MTSE was tested as my capstone project: the relationship between nurses' spiritual care perspectives and their expressions of spiritual empathy. The MTSE has been presented in two poster presentations, and findings from the theory testing study have been published (Chism & Magnan, 2009).

The development and testing of the MTSE during doctoral study in a DNP program was somewhat industrious and not a customary expectation of a DNP research project. This rewarding experience not only challenged me to develop my scholarship; it also exemplified the use of theory (specifically, middle-range theory) to guide practice. As a DNP graduate and advanced practice nurse, I have a responsibility to understand, from a nursing perspective, the scientific underpinnings of disease processes and the care of my patients. Moreover, the development and testing of the MTSE reinforced for me the idea that the discipline of nursing truly guides nursing practice.

ACKNOWLEDGMENT

I would like to acknowledge Dr. Morris Magnan for his expert guidance and mentorship throughout my doctoral study and beyond. He is an exemplary nurse, scholar, mentor, and friend who continues to inspire me every day.

REFERENCES

American Association of Colleges of Nursing. (2004). AACN position statement on the practice doctorate in nursing. Retrieved from http://www.aacn.nche.edu/publications/position/DNPpositionstatement.pdf

American Association of Colleges of Nursing. (2006a). Essentials of doctoral education for advanced nursing practice. Retrieved from http://www.aacn.nche.edu/publications/position/DNPEssentials.pdf

American Association of Colleges of Nursing. (2006b). DNP Roadmap Task Force report. Retrieved from http://www.aacn.nche.edu/dnp/roadmapreport.pdf

American Association of Colleges of Nursing. (2016). DNP program list. Retrieved from http://www.aacn.nche.edu/dnp/program-schools

Apold, S. (2008). The doctor of nursing practice: Looking back, moving forward. *Journal for Nurse Practitioners, 4*(2), 101–106.

Burman, M., Hart, A., & McCabe, S. (2005). Doctor of nursing practice: Opportunity amidst chaos. *American Journal of Critical Care, 14*(6), 463–464.

Carpenter, R., & Hudacek, S. (1996). *On doctoral education in nursing: The voice of the student.* New York, NY: National League for Nursing Press.

Chase, S., & Pruitt, R. (2006). The practice doctorate: Innovation or disruption? *Journal of Nursing Education, 45*(5), 155–161.

Chism, L. (2007). *Spiritual empathy: A model for spiritual well-being.* Unpublished doctoral paper. Oakland University, Rochester, MI.

Chism, L. (2016). *The doctor of nursing practice: A guidebook for role development and professional issues* (3rd ed.). Burlington, MA: Jones & Bartlett Learning.

Chism, L., & Magnan, M. H. (2009). The relationship between student nurses' spiritual care perspectives and their expressions of spiritual empathy. *Journal of Nursing Education, 48*(11), 597–604.

Cleland, V. (1976). Develop a doctoral program. *Nursing Outlook, 24,* 631–635.

Cody, W. K. (1996). Drowning in eclecticism. *Nursing Science Quarterly, 9*(3), 86–88.

Donaldson, S. K. (1995). Nursing science for nursing practice. In A. Omery, C. E. Kasper, & G. G. Page (Eds.), *In search of nursing science* (pp. 3–12). Thousand Oaks, CA: Sage.

Donaldson, S. K., & Crowley, D. M. (1978). The discipline of nursing. *Nursing Outlook, 26*(2), 113–120.

Dracup, K., & Bryan-Brown, C. (2005). Doctor of nursing practice: MRI or total body scan? *American Journal of Critical Care, 14*(4), 278–281.

Fawcett, J. (1997). Conceptual models of nursing, nursing theories, and nursing practice: Focus on the future. In M. R. Alligood & A. Marriner-Tomey (Eds.), *Nursing theory: Utilization and application* (pp. 211–221). St. Louis, MO: Mosby.

Fawcett, J. (2005). *Contemporary nursing knowledge: Analysis and evaluation of nursing models and theories* (2nd ed.). Philadelphia, PA: F. A. Davis.

Gortner, S. (1980). Nursing science in transition. *Nursing Research, 29,* 180–183.

Grace, H. (1978). The development of doctoral education in nursing: In historical perspective. *Journal of Nursing Education, 17*(4), 17–27.

Hathaway, D., Jacob, S., Stegbauer, C., Thompson, C., & Graff, C. (2006). The practice doctorate: Perspectives of early adopters. *Journal of Nursing Education, 45*(12), 487–496.

Jacobs, M. K., & Huether, S. E. (1978). Nursing science: The theory–practice linkage. *Advances in Nursing Science, 1*(1), 63–73.

Jacox, A. K. (1974). Theory construction in nursing. *Nursing Research, 23*(1), 4–13.

Johnson, D. E. (1968). Theory in nursing: Borrowed and unique. *Nursing Research, 17*(3), 206–209.

Kenney, J. W. (2006). Theory-based advanced nursing practice. In W. K. Cody (Ed.), *Philosophical and theoretical perspectives for advanced nursing practice* (pp. 295–310). Sudbury, MA: Jones and Bartlett Publishers.

Kerlinger, F. N. (1973). *Foundations of behavioral research* (2nd ed.). New York, NY: Holt Rinehart & Winston.

Lenz, E. R. (1998). The role of middle-range theory for nursing research and practice: Part 2. Nursing practice. *Nursing Leadership Forum, 3*(2), 62–66.

Magnan, M. (2016). Expectations for theory, research, and scholarship. In L. Chism (Ed.), *The doctor of nursing practice: A guidebook for role development and professional issues* (2nd ed., pp. 107–140). Burlington, MA: Jones & Bartlett Learning.

Marion, L., Viens, D., O'Sullivan, A., Crabtree, M. K., Fontana, S., & Price, M. (2003). The practice doctorate in nursing: Future or fringe. *Topics in Advanced Practice Nursing eJournal, 3*(2). Retrieved from http://www.doctorsofnursingpractice.org/wp-content/uploads/2014/08/Marion_Viens2003.pdf

Marriner-Tomey, A. (1990). Historical development of doctoral programs from the Middle Ages to nursing education today. *Nursing and Health Care, 3*(11), 132–137. Washington, DC: National Academies Press.

McKenna, H. (1997). Applying theories in practice. In H. McKenna (Ed.), *Nursing theories and models* (pp. 158–189). New York, NY: Routledge.

Meleis, A. I. (1993). Nursing research and the Neuman model: Directions for the future. Panel discussion conducted at the Fourth Biennial International Neuman Systems Model Symposium, Rochester, NY.

Meleis, A. I. (1997). *Theoretical nursing: Development and progress* (3rd ed.). Philadelphia, PA: Lippincott.

Murphy, J. (1981). Doctoral education in, of, and for nursing: An historical analysis. *Nursing Outlook, 29*(11), 645–649.

National Association of Clinical Nurse Specialists. (2008). Clinical nurse specialist core competencies. Retrieved from http://www.nacns.org/docs/CNSCoreCompetenciesBroch.pdf

National Organization of Nurse Practitioner Faculties. (2006). Practice doctorate nurse practitioner entry-level competencies. Retrieved from http://c.ymcdn.com/sites/www.nonpf.org/resource/resmgr/competencies/dnp%20np%20competenciesapril2006.pdf

Newman, M. (1975). The professional doctorate in nursing: A position paper. *Nursing Outlook, 23*(11), 704–706.

Olson, J. (1995). Relationship between nurse-expressed empathy, patient-perceived empathy, and patient distress. *Image: Journal of Nursing Scholarship, 27*(4), 317–322.

Orlando, I. (1990). *The dynamic nurse–patient relationship.* New York, NY: National League for Nursing.

Schlottfeldt, R. (1978, May). The professional doctorate: Rationale and characteristics. *Nursing Outlook,* 302–311.

Taylor, E. (2002). *Spiritual care: Nursing theory, research, and practice.* Upper Saddle River, NJ: Prentice Hall.

Villagomeza, L. (2005). Spiritual distress in adult cancer patients. *Holistic Nursing Practice, 19*(6), 285–294.

Webber, P. B. (2008). The doctor of nursing practice degree and research: Are we making an epistemological mistake? *Journal of Nursing Education, 47*(10), 466–472.

II

The Structure and Function of Theory

Chapter 4

Theory as Practice

Patricia Goodson

INTRODUCTION: DEFINING THEORY

People have a hard time understanding precisely what a theory is, what exactly it can do to guide research, and how to know which theory to use. Difficulties often begin when attempting to define theory, because uncovering a simple explanation is difficult. Scholars' conceptualizations and explanations are often abstract, convoluted, and complex. Actually, the question "What is theory?" can be an unimaginative question—on the one hand, presupposing simplistic, reduced accounts of a seemingly rich phenomenon, and on the other hand, offering abstract, complicated, and unintelligible answers. The impulse is to fill in the blank in "Theory is _____" with a quick, concise, one-sentence description. However, such concise and short definitions may render theory meaningless, lifeless, confusing, and dry.

A friend of mine enjoys reminding me that "Theory is not rocket science; it's much more complicated than rocket science." If this holds true, then it does not seem logical to define theory as one single, simple entity. As I came to understand late in my studies, theory is multifaceted and amazingly complex. To reduce it to a one-dimensional phenomenon would come close to mutilation. Theory's beauty lies precisely in its dynamic and intricate complexity (Hoffmann, 2003). Brief definitions never do it justice. If simply asking "What is theory?" leads nowhere interesting, then it may be more productive to ask a different set of interconnected questions:

- What does theory do?
- What does theory—in action—look like?
- How can one recognize theory?
- What does theory do that is uniquely "theory-*ish*"?

This chapter, which is primarily approached from a health promotion perspective, focuses on the first two questions: "What does theory do?" and "When theory is doing its 'thing,' what does it look like?" Put in simple terms, theories have at least two faces or may be found in two different varieties: *commonsense theories* and *scientific theories*. These familiar categories are covered in this chapter.

Commonsense Theories

Commonsense theories comprise explanations that people invoke on a daily basis to make sense of their lives. Suppose, in the past couple of weeks, Laura's behavior seems a little "off." She arrives late for team meetings and appears distant and broody when the team interacts. Laura is a graduate assistant and doctoral student. As her teacher, I do have a theory (or a proposed explanation) for Laura's behavior: Laura has been under considerable stress lately, taking her comprehensive exams, finalizing a manuscript to submit for publication, and teaching two freshman-level classes.

My theory is a commonsense theory because it represents a personal attempt to make meaning of a situation (a sense-making task), based on the information at hand. I may choose to test this theory of mine, for instance, by asking Laura if what I'm thinking is valid or by asking some of her colleagues about what is happening, but such testing will not go far. As soon as I understand what is going on or as soon as Laura's behavior returns to "normal," I will forget my little theory and the need to test it and will gladly move on to the next problem.

Another good example of a commonsense theory is conspiracy theory. People can certainly recognize a conspiracy theory when they see or hear about one. Such a theory tends to grab one's imagination. Conspiracy theories combine challenging questions with sometimes outlandish answers, attempting to explain why something happened. An example is President John F. Kennedy's assassination: Many explanations have been proposed to make sense of the bizarre events that ended the president's life. Among these explanations, a handful of conspiracy theories have emerged. These theories started by zeroing in on the questions that were dismissed or brushed aside by the mainstream official reports because they (the questions) were unthinkable, outrageous, or too far-fetched. The theory proposing that President Kennedy and Governor John Connally were not struck by a single bullet is only one example of the many conspiracy theories that sprang up after the event (Kurtz, 2006).

Frequently, unique perspectives or approaches are followed, and unusual solutions to difficult problems are sometimes found because of these conspiracy-type accounts. More often, conspiracy theories are unsupported by available evidence and, with time, become tales and myths that societies' members enjoy telling and retelling. Underlying both commonsense and conspiracy theories is a shared element: an attempt to make sense of reality, to explain events and circumstances so that humans can function in a world, in a reality, in a place furnished with meaning.

Scientific Theories

From the outset, scientific theories look different from commonsense theories. Definitions of scientific theories are much more elaborate, contain more clearly outlined characteristics, and have better defined purposes when compared with definitions of commonsense theories. The following are examples of these definitions as they appear, specifically, in the social sciences. In the now classic textbook on health behavior theories, *Health Behavior and Health Education*, for instance, *theory* is defined as "a set of interrelated concepts, definitions, and propositions that present a *systematic* view of events or situations by specifying relations among variables, in order to *explain* and *predict* the events or situations" (Glanz, Rimer, & Viswanath, 2008, p. 26).

Another elaborate, yet slightly clearer, definition of social science theory was proposed by Denzin (1970):

> A theory is a set of propositions that furnish an explanation by means of a deductive system. *Theory is explanation.* Durkheim's theory of suicide in Spain conforms to the above specifications. . . . It states that: (1) In any social grouping, the suicide rate varies directly with the degree of individualism (egoism); (2) the degree of individualism varies with the incidence of Protestantism; (3) therefore, the suicide rate varies with the incidence of Protestantism; (4) the incidence of Protestantism in Spain is low; (5) therefore, the suicide rate in Spain is low. (p. 34, emphasis added)

Other definitions provide additional details regarding scientific theory's main elements:

> A theory is a set of interrelated universal statements, some of which are definitions and some of which are relationships assumed to be true, together with a syntax, a set of rules for manipulating the statements to arrive at new statements. (Cohen, 1980, p. 171)
>
> Theory is a mental activity. . . . It is a process of developing ideas that can allow us to explain how and why events occur. Theory is constructed with several basic elements or building blocks: (1) concepts, (2) variables, (3) statements, and (4) formats. (Turner, 1986, pp. 4–5)
>
> Behavioral theories are composed of interrelated propositions, based on stated assumptions that tie selected constructs together and create a parsimonious system for explaining and predicting human behavior. (DiClemente, Crosby, & Kegler, 2002, p. 3)

When examined further, these definitions also refer to scientific theories' three main goals, purposes, or functions:

- *Description.* Theories should facilitate the description (and understanding) of the phenomena being studied. The scientist/social scientist must be able to "describe the phenomena he [sic] is studying so that others can repeat his descriptions with a high degree of agreement" (Denzin, 1970, p. 31).
- *Explanation.* Scientific theories allow "the construction of a system of interrelated propositions that permits the scientist to 'make sense' out of the events observed" (Denzin, 1970, p. 31).

- *Prediction.* The utility of scientific theories extends beyond mere description and explanation, however. "If a [scientist/social scientist] claims to have explained why a given set of variables occurs together, he must be able to predict the future relationships" (Denzin, 1970, p. 31).

This, in simple terms, is how scientific theories are often defined and characterized. Scientific theories explain phenomena in a logical, ordered, interconnected manner. Like commonsense theories, scientific theories represent attempts to make sense of reality through descriptions, explanations, and predictions of events and circumstances.

The definition proposed by Turner (1986, p. 4) places theory in the world of words or ideas (a mental activity), highlighting the power of language to create and shape human reality. Cohen's (1980, p. 171) proposition also includes an important characteristic of scientific theories. To earn the status of being scientific, theoretical explanations need to go together, connect according to specific rules, and follow a unique grammar. Denzin (1970) called this set of rules, or this grammar, a deductive system. Explanations of cause and effect, by themselves, do not constitute a theory: They are merely explanations. What lends these explanations the status of theory is the manner in which the explanations are connected, derived from, or related to each other. Denzin (1970) explains it this way: "A theory must contain a set of propositions or hypotheses that combine descriptive and relational concepts. . . . Unfortunately, a set of propositions taken alone does not constitute a theory either. The set must be placed in a deductive scheme" (p. 34).

This particular feature of scientific theories (relationships among explanations or constructs) is similar to the craft of quilting. Quilting consists of sewing fabric together, usually combining large squares of material with different textures and colors to form an intricate pattern. This craft offers a very useful image for the process of theory building because it helps one see how, depending on the way the blocks of fabric are connected, entirely different images can emerge (see **Figure 4-1**).

The designs displayed in the last row of Figure 4-1 were all formed by combining the top square into blocks of four squares each (shown in the second row). The variation in shape is a result of how the original block is combined with other identical blocks. The same idea applies to scientific theories: String the data or facts together using a certain logic or set of beliefs as the starting point, and one set of explanations emerges; combine them within another logic, structure, or paradigm, and the resulting explanations might look very different. The important point to remember from this illustration is that individual blocks of fabric do not make a quilt. Similarly, a scientific theory is not developed until various explanations are weaved within a logic pattern.

Surprisingly, in neither the hard sciences nor the social sciences do scholars share a single agreed-upon view of what a theory is, nor do they care to reach consensus over a single definition (Cohen, 1980; Turner, 1986). Although for some people the term *theory*

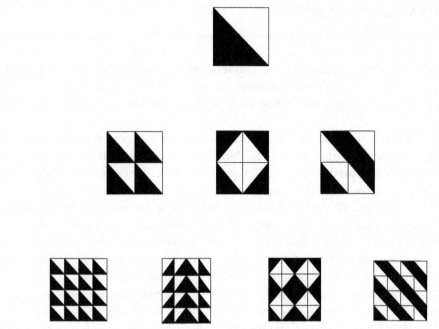

Figure 4-1 Quilt blocks.

may refer to a "set of tested empirical generalizations" or to a "unified, systematic causal explanation of a diverse range of social phenomena" (Schwandt, 2001, p. 252), others may view theory as broad "theoretical orientations or perspectives (e.g., functionalism, symbolic interactionism, behaviorism)" or, more specifically, as a single theory (e.g., critical theory) (Schwandt, 2001, p. 252).

At the same time, various types of ideas, speculations, hypotheses, models, criticisms, conceptual frameworks, and propositions, when interconnected with words (and even scholars' personal beliefs), are sometimes called theories in certain disciplinary fields (Cohen, 1980; Denzin, 1970). Therefore, despite the apparent rigor, order, logic, and systematic thinking needed in scientific theorizing, social scientists themselves use the term *theory* to mean many different things. Far from indicating that these scientists are incorrect in their use of the term, this lack of consensus reinforces the notion that theory is a complex, multidimensional phenomenon that resists attempts to be simplified, unidimensionalized, and boxed into one specific container. The beauty of theory lies precisely in its intricate complexity, much like the beauty of a kaleidoscope, a fractal image, or the inner workings of the human body.

THEORIZING AND THEORETICAL THINKING

The way that some authors attempt to simplify theoretical thinking, to reduce it to its bare bones, to skeletonize the phenomenon, and thus to distance the person from the forces involved in its creation, implementation, and refinement is perhaps merely an attempt to be didactic. In trying to help readers understand, authors have instead figuratively taken readers into an anatomy lab, made them look at a cadaver, and declared, "Here is what life looks like."

The problem is that definitions of scientific theories ignore a crucial element within the theory domain—the theorizing *process*. To think about theory is to think about explanations, descriptions, and predictions, but it is more than that. It means also considering the questions and the reasoning that lead to these explanations, descriptions, and predictions.

I define theorizing or theoretical thinking as the dynamic process of asking and answering specific types of questions. Theory may be defined also as the result, the outcome, or the outgrowth from this operation. Theorizing implies movement, dynamics, and dialogue—a volleying between questions and replies. Theory is the answer part of the equation. This conception of theory and theoretical thinking is diagrammed in **Figure 4-2**.

Within this framework, scientific theories are characterized by questions focused on causes and with explanations or answers that attempt to tell the story of why phenomena occur as they do. Theoretical questions in scientific-type thinking about health promotion, for example, ask the following questions: What influences or determines healthy behaviors among older adults? Do attitudes lead to behavior change among adolescents? Why is education level associated with certain health outcomes? Scientific theories—when they have already been proposed and tested—provide clean, decluttered answers to these questions.

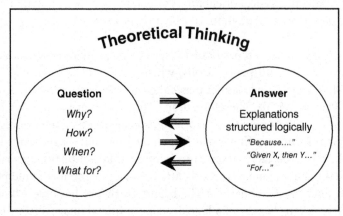

Figure 4-2   The theorizing process.

They have been carefully thought out, tentatively proposed (at first), and repeatedly tested to see whether the explanations will hold over time and across various contexts. Only after much tweaking, adjusting, and testing do these explanations gain the status of a scientific theory, and, in science, all of the tweaking, adjusting, and testing follow carefully outlined protocols. In other words, they are done in a systematic way, following principles and procedures of scientific practice (Pedhazur & Schmelkin, 1991).

Other types of theories (policy, ethics, nursing, and commonsense theories) ask different types of questions. They are not cause-and-effect theories; rather they focus on questions such as the following: What is the ultimate end of health promotion? Why should healthier lifestyles be promoted? Are the means being used to promote health healthy themselves? Which nursing interventions result in patient well-being? Is health a human right to which all human beings are naturally entitled? How can a country's public health system protect its populations against potentially dangerous illnesses? What can be expected from globalization, in terms of its effects on health promotion, on a worldwide basis?

THEORY AS PRACTICE

What Does Theory Do?

Setting aside the differences between commonsense and scientific theories, it is evident that both categories have a pivotal common element: meaning attribution. Elucidating meaning is precisely the job of theoretical thinking. It is exactly what theory—or more precisely, theorizing—does (Nealon & Giroux, 2003). Theory-type questions and their answers lend meaning, provide explanation, impose order, and organize logically the events that engulf healthcare professionals. Theorizing, in other words, leads practitioners to take the following steps:

- *Ask* certain types of questions
- *Question* the status quo
- *Seek* the most plausible and meaningful answers
- *Build* a narrative or logical structure for the questions and the answers

Theory should be viewed as a type of practice precisely because theorizing involves all of these actions. It is important to keep this point in mind: *Theory is practice.* If practice is action or doing, then theory does quite a lot more than might first be suspected. Thinking theoretically is, indeed, engaging in very practical tasks.

What Does Theory Look Like?

If one views theoretical thinking as a process of asking specific types of questions and obtaining certain kinds of answers, then scientific theories and commonsense theories become merely different manifestations—different "looks"—of the theorizing process. They appear different, but the difference lies on the surface, in the types of questions raised. The bottom-line processes of sense making, meaning attribution, explanation, and description remain the same for both (for all) types of theories.

Many scholars defend the notion that humankind's most universal strategy for making sense of reality is that of creating and telling stories. "We are storied selves," according to Nash (2004, p. 8). Because theories are one way to explain and attribute meaning to reality, theories undeniably constitute a specific type of story (Hoffmann, 2003). Edberg (2007) described the notion well:

> It could be said that a key characteristic of modern humans from prehistoric times has been the creation of tales, myths, and stories that, for example, describe an entire cosmological system, explain the creation of society, explain how men and women came to be what they are, and so on. These are all theories in the broad sense, for they present a coherent account from which more specific judgments and conclusions can be drawn. (p. 26)

When theories are compared with stories, it does not mean that theories are the product of fantasizing about make-believe worlds. Rather, theories themselves are built following certain narrative structures, certain "story-building rules" and purposes. What these stories or theories "look like" depends on whether they are scientific theories, public policy theories, nursing theories, ethics theories, commonsense theories, or conspiracy theories. Packaged in different formats, they all represent ways to provide accounts of phenomena in orderly, logical, and meaningful ways (Lemert, 1993). In this sense, theories are stories. Notice how Frank (1995), author of *The Wounded Storyteller*, described the book in which he analyzed the human experience of disease by focusing on his and others' personal stories of illness:

> This book [*The Wounded Storyteller*] is a *work of theory*, but it is equally a collection of stories and a kind of memoir. For almost a decade I have been a wounded storyteller, and I have cultivated the stories of others who are wounded, each in different ways. The "theory" in this book elaborates my story and theirs.
>
> Charles Lemert introduces his social theory textbook calling theory "a basic survival skill" (Lemert, 1993). *The Wounded Storyteller* is a survival kit, put together out of my need to make sense of my own survival, as I watch others seeking to make sense of theirs. The wounded storyteller, like Lemert's theorist, is trying to survive and help others survive in a world that does not immediately make sense. (p. xiii)

If stories are crafted and told for sense-making purposes (for survival, Frank and Lemert might say), however, they have meaning only within a given context. The biblical story of the creation of the cosmos makes no sense within the context of physics and astronomy. Theories of health promotion that emphasize individual responsibility for wellness have little relevance in refugee camps, among victims of natural disasters, or among populations afflicted by wars. To understand what theory looks like or what kind of meaning it is creating, a theory must be understood within its particular context, against the backdrop of the particular stage on which it is enacted. Edberg (2007) stated:

> [Theories] are propositions that have meaning, validity, and truth (or falsity) within a specific context, such as a historical context, a social context, or a cultural context. Within their contexts, they are commonly held to be meaningful. Thus, to understand why a particular theory is meaningful or to evaluate its validity, you need to understand the contextual ground rules, so to speak. (p. 26)

It is important to note that theories will look different, depending on the context within which one searches for them. They will have unique appearances depending on the needs they were designed to meet at the time they were created. Furthermore, they will be considered true, valid, or even useful only after considering the historical, social, professional, and cultural circumstances within which they were developed.

If that context is the natural sciences in the 20th and 21st centuries, for example, theories will look very rigid or authoritative, and some will have gained the status of universal laws (e.g., the law of gravity). In this context, the need being met is that of discovering realities existing outside of human experience—of developing factual, predictable knowledge: hard-fast, lasting, and stable rules that are efficient at prediction and control.

In contrast, if the context is the behavioral sciences within modern Western societies, theories will be numerous, varied, and much more malleable, and almost none will have achieved the status of universal explanations despite much testing. Some of these theories will even question the theorizing or sense-making processes themselves, asking whether the search for meaning is, indeed, a universal trait among humans. Within the context of behavioral sciences—lying at the intersection of biological and social sciences—the need being met by scientific theories is both to explain or gain clarity (Buchanan, 2004) regarding humans as individuals and social beings, and to predict and control human behavior.

If the context is public policy, theories will be less concerned with the aim to understand human behavior and more directed toward facilitating healthy community living and protecting individuals within specific population groups. If the context is Western ethics, theories will focus on normative aspects of human lives (what should be done, what is ethically right or wrong) and the development of guidelines for seeking out the common good. In a nursing context, theories are focused on knowing how to achieve positive patient outcomes.

Thus the outcome of the theorizing process, as well as the theorizing process itself, will assume many personas; theories wear the clothing provided by their historical and practical contexts. Much in the same way that tofu takes on the taste of the sauce in which you cook it, theories take on the form, shape, language, norms, and values of the many contexts in which they are built and applied.

THEORY VERSUS PRACTICE

In the fall of 2006, at the start of my Behavioral Foundations of Health Education class (an introductory, graduate-level health behavior theories course), I asked the students to jot down brief answers to this question: "What comes to mind when you hear the word 'theory'?" I told them that I was looking for emotions, beliefs, descriptions, or definitions that immediately surfaced when they thought about the term.

Not surprisingly, of the 14 responses I collected, none listed a single positive emotion. Half contained what I considered neutral or descriptive elements (such as "relationship," "explanation," "ideas," "hypotheses," "logical process," "concepts," "road map"). The remaining half of the class brought up negative or critical elements. Here are a few examples:

- Not factual
- Old—dating back many years and may or may not be improved or changed
- Hard to prove and understand
- Something abstract, difficult to understand
- Not useful
- Lack of concrete parameters and confusing guidelines/boundaries

My favorite response was this one: "Theory is complex, something I don't like thinking about. . . . It's a lot of thoughts with no specific answers."

A recounting of my students' beliefs is not needed, however, to illustrate the negativity that some people exhibit regarding theory. These same attitudes are sometimes apparent in textbooks. Here is an example of a preface to a well-known book on theory-driven evaluations (Chen, 1990):

> I would be more sympathetic to [the author's] use of "theory" if that term did not carry with it such a load of unwanted meanings. For example, in sociology, "theory" is often equated with the abstract essays written by sociologists who are long dead. In other fields, theory is equated with sets of integrated mathematical statements concerning highly abstract properties. (p. 9)

Could it be that the separation between theory and practice is so pronounced because scholars and practitioners have applied the wrong types of theories to their practice? In other words, is it possible that researchers or academics (the theorists) have been asking theoretical questions that are not productive for understanding why human beings do what they do? Could they perhaps be theorizing about human health behaviors by asking the wrong types of questions? Theorists and researchers have insisted on asking what causes human behavior (in the same way they would ask what causes a certain cell to replicate or what causes a planet to maintain its orbit). Should they instead be asking questions about the purpose and the meaning of human behavior (Buchanan, 2000)?

In considering whether this approach might be possible, I invoke the words of Aristotle. Theorizing or philosophizing about human knowledge, Aristotle classified human experience into three types—*theoria, poiesis*, and *praxis*. Each of these types generates a specific kind of knowledge—*episteme, techne*, and *phronesis* (practical wisdom), respectively (Buchanan, 2000, p. 54). To this day, Western thinking about what knowledge is has been influenced by Aristotle's typology; in a way, it is helpful to understand the multiple ways in which humans experience reality and learn from such experience.

For Aristotle, *episteme*-type knowledge—or the type of knowledge gained from observing "events that are constant, universal, and eternal" (Buchanan, 2000, p. 54), the type of knowledge being generated in the natural sciences—is "inadequate and inappropriate for analyzing social situations." As Buchanan (2000) explained:

> Aristotle observed that human relationships are historical, contextual, and contingent. Action in the social domain must be responsive to the novel features of each situation, to contexts in which a limitless variety of features fluctuate in salience, and to the ethical relevance of the particular persons in the specific situation at hand. . . . While the force of gravity is uniform throughout the known universe (except, possibly, in black holes), Aristotle noted that relationships in the sociohistorical domain do not display the same invariability. On the contrary, how people respond to events depends on when and where they occur, who is present, and what the individuals hope to accomplish. (p. 54)

Thus the negative feelings that theory often generates among students and healthcare practitioners may indeed be the product of approaching human behavior as resulting from fixed, universal forces (*theoria–episteme*). Negative views of theory may arise because people insist on asking the wrong questions, because they fail to admit that health behaviors lie in the domain of *praxis*-type experience (transient, fluctuating, contingent, contextual) and, therefore, lead to practical reasoning; that is, health behaviors involve *phronesis*-type knowledge, not *episteme*-type knowledge. Some current theories of health behavior, for example, provide "one size fits all" answers to questions such as "What causes people to choose a healthy lifestyle?" or "What may lead people to better manage their diets and eating habits?" Most of the answers available tend to be universal and fixed, blatantly ignoring that health behaviors are contingent on their sociocultural and socioeconomic contexts.

If this truly is the case, then why would practitioners want to use these theories that do not answer the "right here, right now" questions that they have? For example, if a nurse wonders, "How can I help Ms. Smith manage her diabetes, given the small retirement income she manages and the large family she always says 'comes first'?" then the answers provided by health behavior theories, such as "increase Ms. Smith's self-efficacy" (Bandura, 1997) and "increase her perception of the severity of diabetes" (Champion & Skinner, 2008), are totally irrelevant. In fact, if the nurse is not careful, focusing on these scientific answers can do more harm than good or become iatrogenic. Because Ms. Smith's context (low income, large family, and her place within this family network) seems to shape her health problems, intervention attempts to increase self-efficacy or perceived severity of the disease may actually exacerbate Ms. Smith's anxiety and guilt (Becker, 1993). The practitioner's intervention—if he or she is concerned about applying "one size fits all" health behavior theories to develop her educational program—may transform Ms. Smith from a "person at risk" into an "anxious person at risk," thereby worsening what has been dubbed an "epidemic of apprehension" (Becker, 1993, p. 2).

From this perspective, one might even conclude that it may, in fact, be positive for theory and practice to maintain a healthy distance from each other. Yet, I would argue that the current status of theory and practice in health care is a significant symptom of an underlying illness that has been institutionalized among the healthcare professions. To separate theory and praxis (or theoretical thinking from action) is an artifact. There is nothing more valuable, more enlightening, and more empowering than the marriage of the right type of question with the appropriate answer—to build understanding, to shape professional practice, and to sharpen professional awareness. Theoretical thinking that is relevant is intricately tied to practice. Divorcing the two becomes nonsense (no sense). It is breaking something that is a unit, a one, a whole, into pieces and expecting the pieces to survive and perform on their own—like splitting a peanut butter and jelly sandwich by pulling apart the slices of bread. Try doing this, and nothing remains: not a peanut butter and jelly sandwich, not peanut butter and bread, not bread and jelly. If split, the final product is something else, but it is not a peanut butter and jelly sandwich.

Paulo Freire—the Brazilian critical theorist and philosopher of education whom health promoters have come to know well because of his contributions related to empowerment theories (Wallerstein, Sanchez-Merki, & Dow, 1997)—deftly articulated this unity between theory and practice. For him, the relationship is the same as the one between action and reflection. He called the relationship between theory and practice a dialogical one. For Freire, individual behavior and the way people live in society constitute a constant conversation or dialogue between one's doing and thinking about what was done—the thinking about what was done, in turn, shaping what will be done next, and so forth in a continual iterative process.

Willinsky (1998), writing about theory in the context of teaching literature, argued this point quite eloquently:

> Try thinking of how we practice theory, that is, of how theory is a form of practice. After all, theory is practiced, whether by a young child facing a plate full of different foods or a teacher in front of a class on the first day. Theory takes practice. Theory shapes practice.
>
> Take this a step further and consider how this habit of naming one thing as "practice" and another as "theory" is in itself the work or practice of theory. It is a theoretical distinction. Such is the practice of theory. In this way, it seems fair to say that a theory of the world is what enables us to work with it. Or to put this another way, the world makes little sense without a theory about it. Our practices exist by virtue of our theories. (p. 244)

When relevant questions and appropriate answers are developed and applied, what is generated is theory and practice as action and reflection, or reflexive praxis: two sides of the same coin. If one wants to use metaphysical images, this unity can be thought of as being similar to a person. People consist of a physical dimension (body) and a nonphysical dimension (spirit, mind, or whatever is not solely physical). If these two dimensions of a person were separated, the result would be disastrous. Similarly, if one tried to artificially separate theory from practice and action from reflection, the result would be deficient. It is not surprising that healthcare professionals and students complain that theory is dry, irrelevant, and boring. A comparison is a person walking around, interacting with others, with no personality, emotions, hopes, dreams, or quirks. The beauty in humankind lies in the dynamic life force within people, the interaction among all of the dimensions that constitute who they are.

When theorizing is viewed as an interplay, a dance, or a constant dialogue between a specific type of question and its respective answers, when the questions asked and the answers given match, and when both emerge from action, theory/theoretical thinking and practice are one. This constant, dynamic dance/dialogue of action and reflection, theory and practice, makes the two inseparable. It also reinforces the notion that theory or theorizing is itself a type of practice. Because theory questions actions, questions the status quo (the manner in which things are done), seeks the most plausible and meaningful answers, and builds a narrative in which to frame the questions and the answers, it does indeed require practitioners to engage in quite a bit of practical work.

Viewed in this way, theory has a necessary practical dimension. Without practice (understood as everyday living), theory would not happen—it would not exist. Conversely, without theory, living would be undefined and meaningless, merely biological subsistence. Therefore, to divorce theory from practice becomes detrimental to sense making: Practice and those things that are extremely relevant to practice cannot be explained, nor can the way of doing things be improved, because they are not questioned.

SUMMARY

I would like to add one final observation to the claims that scientific theories provide practitioners with the ability to predict behaviors, and I will use an example from my own specialty of health promotion. Similar comparisons can be made with nursing and other healthcare professions. Despite widespread dissatisfaction in the field with health behavior theories' power to describe, foretell, and prevent risky behaviors, the mere notion that theories aspire to predict behavior with precision and efficiency is, to me, very scary.

Imagine this scenario: A certain theory proposes that an individual's theoretical self-esteem (TSE—defined as the regard one has for oneself in terms of the ability to think theoretically) is associated with his or her theorizing behavior. If I—the theorizing expert—knew the TSE scores of a certain group of students, I could easily predict to what extent those students would practice theorizing behaviors, or better yet, I could devise educational or marketing strategies to enhance that group's TSE and, therefore, to wheedle more frequent theorizing behavior out of them. Fortunately, there is no such thing as TSE (interestingly enough, though, there is such a thing as "web-esteem," so it may not be long until we see TSE as a bona fide theoretical construct; see Brock, 2006).

While the construct of TSE is merely a product of my imagination and predictions of ability to think theoretically are not life threatening, the ability to predict behavior is not science fiction. It is, in fact, one of the main goals of scientific theorizing. As has been learned from the natural sciences, prediction of behavior is possible. But should it be done? Buchanan, for instance, argues that if health behavior theories and health promotion methods were to become ultraefficient at predicting and changing health behaviors, human beings' autonomy would be lost:

> To me, the quest to find such power is deeply disturbing. Whoever controlled these new behavioral technologies would have the power to control your and my behavior. If effective scientific models [or theories] were ever developed, then the government, for example, would have the power to decide whether I would eat that dessert, exercise today, smoke pot, have sex outside marriage, or change any other behavior that it wanted to control. If effective scientific models were ever developed, then the very foundations of human autonomy, responsibility, dignity, and respect would be destroyed. We would have no autonomy, no moral responsibility, and no dignity because (1) scientists would have identified the causes of the behavior in question, and ipso facto, (2) they would have the power to change or eliminate that behavior. It would, in short, be a brave new world, beyond freedom and dignity. (Buchanan, 2004, p. 150)

Theorists and researchers are quick to point out that prediction is not very precise at the level of the individual; thus I really cannot do a good job of anticipating a person's behavior. Prediction works best at the level of aggregate data—when dealing with averages—and with populations or groups, not with individual persons. Even so, if one considers that public policy is usually predicated on such averages and on target groups or populations, it can still be a scary thought that people would try to predict (and, therefore, control and tweak) other people's behaviors.

To end this chapter on a positive note, consider the words of Lemert (1993):

> Theory is a basic survival skill. This may surprise those who believe it to be a special activity of experts of a certain kind. True, there are professional . . . theorists, usually academics. But this fact does not exclude my belief that . . . theory is something done necessarily, and often well, by people with no particular professional credential. When it is done well, by whomever, it can be a source of uncommon pleasure. (p. 1)

DISCUSSION QUESTIONS

1. Conduct an informal survey of your colleagues. Ask them this question: "When I say the word 'theory' [or the phrase 'health behavior theories'], what comes to mind?" Assess whether their answers carry positive, negative, or neutral connotations.
2. Engage in a discussion with your colleagues regarding (1) which types of ideas have earned the label of "theory" in nursing and (2) whether nursing is asking the appropriate theoretical questions.
3. Discuss the ethical implications of using theory to predict and control behavior.

REFERENCES

Bandura, A. (1997). *Self-efficacy: The exercise of control.* New York, NY: W. H. Freeman.

Becker, M. H. (1993). A medical sociologist looks at health promotion. *Journal of Health and Social Behavior, 34*(1), 1–6.

Brock, R. (2006, July 21). Women diminish their web-surfing skills, but the sexes are even study finds. *Chronicle of Higher Education.* Retrieved from http://business.highbeam.com/434953 /article-1G1-148314000/women-diminish-their-websurfing-skills-but-sexes-even

Buchanan, D. R. (2000). *An ethic for health promotion: Rethinking the sources of human well-being.* New York, NY: Oxford University Press.

Buchanan, D. R. (2004). Two models for defining the relationship between theory and practice in nutrition education: Is the scientific method meeting our needs? *Journal of Nutrition Education and Behavior, 36,* 146–154.

Champion, V. L., & Skinner, C. S. (2008). The health belief model. In K. Glanz, B. K. Rimer, & K. Viswanath (Eds.), *Health behavior and health education: Theory, research, and practice* (4th ed., pp. 45–65). San Francisco, CA: Jossey-Bass.

Chen, H. T. (1990). *Theory-driven evaluations.* Newbury Park, CA: Sage.

Cohen, B. P. (1980). *Developing sociological knowledge: Theory and method.* Englewood Cliffs, NJ: Prentice Hall.

Denzin, N. K. (1970). *The research act: A theoretical introduction to sociological methods.* Chicago, IL: Aldine.

DiClemente, R. J., Crosby, R. A., & Kegler, M. C. (Eds.). (2002). *Emerging theories in health promotion practice and research: Strategies for improving public health.* San Francisco, CA: Jossey-Bass.

Edberg, M. (2007). *Social and behavioral theory in public health.* Sudbury, MA: Jones and Bartlett.

Frank, A. W. (1995). *The wounded storyteller: Body, illness, and ethics.* Chicago, IL: University of Chicago Press.

Glanz, K., Rimer, B. K., & Viswanath, K. (2008). *Health behavior and health education: Theory, research, and practice* (4th ed.). San Francisco, CA: Jossey-Bass.

Hoffmann, R. (2003). Why buy that theory? *American Scientist, 91,* 9–11.

Kurtz, M. L. (2006). *The JFK assassination debates: Lone gunman versus conspiracy.* Lawrence, KA: University Press of Kansas.

Lemert, C. (1993). *Social theory: The multicultural and classic readings.* Boulder, CO: Westview Press.

Nash, R. J. (2004). *Liberating scholarly writing: The power of personal narrative.* New York, NY: Teachers College Press.

Nealon, J., & Giroux, S. S. (2003). *The theory toolbox: Critical concepts for the humanities, arts, and social sciences.* New York, NY: Rowman & Littlefield.

Pedhazur, E. J., & Schmelkin, L. P. (1991). Theories, problems, and hypotheses. In E. Pedhazur & L. P. Schmelkin (Eds.), *Measurement, design and analysis: An integrated approach* (pp. 180–210). Hillsdale, NJ: Lawrence Erlbaum Associates.

Schwandt, T. A. (2001). *Dictionary of qualitative inquiry* (2nd ed.). Thousand Oaks, CA: Sage.

Turner, J. H. (1986). *The structure of sociological theory.* Chicago, IL: Dorsey Press.

Wallerstein, N., Sanchez-Merki, V., & Dow, L. (1997). Feirian praxis in health education and community organizing: A case study of an adolescent prevention program. In M. Minkler (Ed.), *Community organizing and community building for health* (pp. 195–211). New Brunswick, NJ: Rutgers University Press.

Willinsky, J. (1998). Teaching literature is teaching in theory. *Theory Into Practice, 37*(3), 244–250.

Chapter 5

Components and Levels of Abstraction in Nursing Knowledge

Janie B. Butts

INTRODUCTION

This chapter is a to-the-point summary for graduate students and advanced practice nurses. It is not a comprehensive review of nursing knowledge development, conceptual models, theory, or empirical indicators. Rather it is an overview of the components and levels of abstraction in nursing knowledge. The backdrop is the structural holarchy of contemporary nursing knowledge described by Jacqueline Fawcett. Her internationally recognized expertise on theory, her duration and experience in studying theory, and, especially, the significance and value of her work on theory and knowledge development continue to attract many advanced practice nurses and scholars to her work.

Graduate nursing students, who are at the stage of relearning components of nursing knowledge and theory in more detail, often become confused as they attempt to interpret different authors' terminology, especially when trying to distinguish uses for different aspects of nursing knowledge and the levels of abstractness involved in thinking. Graduate nursing students, who are earning degrees in a doctor of nursing practice program or master of science in nursing program, focus on theory, at varying levels of specificity and detail, and the translation of theory to practice; likewise, so do advanced practice nurses. The American Association of Colleges of Nursing (2006) specified in Essential I, Scientific Underpinnings for Practice, in *The essentials of Doctoral Education for Advanced Nursing Practice* that scientific-based theories and concepts will be used for nursing practice and the evaluation of outcomes. Essential I is relevant to the content in the holarchy of contemporary nursing knowledge.

COMPONENTS OF NURSING KNOWLEDGE: *THE KNOWLEDGE HOLARCHY*

Nurses and others often pose the question "What do nurses *do*?" in an attempt to understand the nature of nursing and nursing practice. In reality, another question, "What do nurses *know*?", is more critical to the development of knowledge for the discipline of nursing (Rodgers, 2005, pp. 1–2). The development of nursing as a discipline and a profession in the past century has been extraordinary. It is beyond the scope of this chapter to explore the historical development of nursing knowledge, but Rodgers's discussion of the history of nursing knowledge development is an excellent source. Knowledge today is "the culmination of the integration of what is known and understood through learning and experience. Knowledge is dependent on theory and research to provide a cumulative, organized, and dynamic body of current information that can be used to answer questions, solve problems, explore phenomena, and generate new theory" (Johnson & Webber, 2005, pp. 11–12). Nursing knowledge development and practice must be in a constant state of evolution so that nurses will be equipped to fulfill the ever-changing societal needs.

Fawcett (2005a, 2005b), then later Fawcett and DeSanto-Madeya (2012), recognized nursing as a distinct discipline with a structural holarchy of contemporary nursing knowledge in which all components are functionally integrated into an order of wholeness or unity, where the largest whole makes up the scheme of nursing knowledge. Nursing knowledge is acquired by levels of abstraction, from the most abstract to the most concrete thinking, and vice versa. The holarchy described by Fawcett consists of five components that make up nursing knowledge, each of which is both a whole in itself and also one part of a larger whole (see **Figure 5-1**): (1) metaparadigm (most abstract), (2) philosophy, (3) conceptual model, (4) theory, and (5) empirical indicator (most concrete).

In formulating his own beliefs about the predicament of the human condition, Arthur Koestler (1975/1967) coined the term *holarchy* as an intended substitution for the word

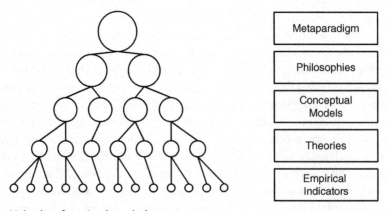

Figure 5-1   Holarchy of nursing knowledge.

hierarchy. A holarchy is a type of fractal that consists of conceptual arrangements such as the one presented in Figure 5-1. Numerous depictions of other holarchies can be found in the literature. Additionally, several creative representations of holarchies based on others' perceptions of how entities work in the world can be located on the Internet. Koestler (1975/1967) used the ancient term *holon* (originating from the pre-Socratic Greek word *holos*) in his book *The Ghost in the Machine* as a way to explain humans' predicament of having to live divided between emotion and reason and to point out how that predicament affects humans' personal and larger involvement in social and political processes and in war. As a side note, Ken Wilber (1996) later adapted Koestler's concept of holarchy and integrated his own view of it in his "chain of being" philosophy.

One can think of a holon as a node that functions independently but also interacts with other holons or nodes (wholes, or wholes within wholes) in a holarchical structure. Through their own cognitive processes, holons coordinate and include holons of a subordinate level and transmit the information necessary "to conform the superordinate level, thereby producing an evolutionary dynamic process" (Mella, 2009, p. 27). In other words, a holarchy is not just a two-directional vertical interactive connection (top-down, bottom-up) made up of successive holons that transcend and include all holons to the point of succession from the direction of the interactions. Koestler (1975/1967) and Mesarovic, Macko, and Takahara (1970) suggested that some holons also interact with other holons in their environment (how the philosophy component interacts within the holarchy is discussed later in this chapter). If individuals were viewing these interactions, they would see how holons relate to one another as the point of focus moves up, down, or across the nodes (holons) of the holarchy; these interactions change with individual eye movement and interpretation.

Two other ways of mentally viewing the nursing knowledge holarchy provided in Figure 5-1 are possible. To create these mental images, think about theory development, for instance. There are two ways that knowledge development takes places in theory: testing theory (top-down) and generating theory (bottom-up). Both of these processes are accomplished by research.

The first mental image of the holarchy focuses on *testing theory*. Testing theory is accomplished by research through deductive reasoning and thinking, from a broad generalization to a specific entity. To think deductively about the holonic interaction, imagine being on top of the holarchy, above the metaparadigm component, and looking downward. Looking at the holarchy as a whole, you would see each of the components as one unit (wholes within the whole). Then you would see the metaparadigm as the inner "ring" or core, which is the most abstract component. As your eye moved outward, the rings would progress from the most abstract, general ring (metaparadigm) to the ring with the most concrete, specific entities (empirical indicators).

Generating theory is a second mental image of the holarchy. Generating theory is accomplished by research through inductive reasoning and thinking, from a concrete specific entity to an abstract broad generalization. To think inductively about the holonic interaction, you would first see the most concrete specific entities of the outer ring (empirical indicators) of the holarchy, and moving inward you would see the most abstract inner ring (metaparadigm).

Imagining these rings by levels of abstractness clarifies one's perspective on the knowledge components of the holarchy. Any of the ways of viewing the holarchy, whether seeing it in Figure 5-1 or imagining it deductively or inductively, provides some degree of reference to help facilitate understanding of the levels of abstractness in thinking about nursing knowledge development and the ways in which to acquire and process that knowledge.

In several publications (e.g., 2005a, 2005b), Fawcett framed the components of nursing knowledge (metaparadigm, philosophy, conceptual model, theory, and empirical indicator) around the notion of the holarchy. In some of her earlier work (e.g., 1999 and previously), she used the term *hierarchy*; in later publications, she adopted the term *holarchy* as part of her framework. In many of her publications (e.g., Fawcett, 1999, 2005a, 2005b; Fawcett & Garity, 2009), Fawcett discussed the components in the holarchy of nursing knowledge in relation to how the C-T-E (conceptual–theoretical–empirical) structures are linked by means of research analysis of data (discussed briefly in the section on functions of theory in this chapter).

Metaparadigm

A *metaparadigm* is the worldview of a discipline—the view that distinguishes the focus of a discipline. A metaparadigm, which is thought to be the most abstract viewpoint of a discipline, is made up of concepts that define the discipline. The most accepted nursing metaparadigm concepts are *human beings* (also known as persons), *environment, health*, and *nursing*, initially identified by Fawcett (1978a, 1978b, 2005b) as essential units of nursing. Several theorists have presented variations of the terms and concepts for the metaparadigm. Kim (1997), for example, defined the typology of the four domains as client, client–nurse, practice, and environment. King (1984) identified the primary concepts as man, health, role, and social systems. Other theorists, such as Morse (1996), recommended that nurses concentrate on formulating and using theories that they can directly link to practice instead of using an overarching metaparadigm that is possibly too abstract to be applied to practice.

To be a discipline obliges us to have a metaparadigm, and to have a metaparadigm obliges us to call nursing a discipline. The general consensus in nursing is that nursing is a discipline with a metaparadigm. Donaldson and Crowley (1978) defined a *discipline* as "a distinct way of viewing all phenomena, which ultimately defines the limits and nature of its inquiry" (p. 113). In terms of the overall function of a metaparadigm, Fawcett (2005b) said, "Articulation of the metaparadigm brings a certain unity to a discipline" (p. 4). Being able to articulate the central focus of the nursing discipline means that nurses can communicate who they are and who they are not, what they do and what they do not do, and what they are about and what they are not about.

Philosophies

Philosophers question and search for explanations and analyze common reason in an effort to enrich our lives and to increase our understanding about the very existence and experiences of human beings. Scholars in the discipline of philosophy ask many questions, such as "Who are we?," "Where do we come from?," "Why do we exist?," and "What is the nature of our existence?" The same or similar questions are asked by nursing scholars and philosophers as they seek understanding not just of human beings from a global perspective, but also of the substance revealing the nature of our existence as a discipline. For years, nursing scholars have searched for and documented the existence and nature of phenomena that identify nursing as a discipline.

Although slight language variations can be discerned in the definitions of philosophy, all in all philosophy is the searching for and communicating of a viewpoint. Fawcett (2005b) defined philosophy as "a statement encompassing ontological claims about the phenomena of central interest to a discipline, epistemic claims about how those phenomena come to be known, and ethical claims about what the members of a discipline value" and noted that the function of a philosophy is "to communicate what the members of a discipline believe to be true in relation to the phenomena of interest to that discipline" (pp. 11–12).

Answers to empirical questions cannot explain any discipline's ontological, epistemic, and ethical philosophical questions that serve as a discipline's foundation for science, mainly because philosophy is concerned with questions of a second-order nature. Second-order questions are asked by philosophers as part of their search for the meaning and nature of the first-order acquired knowledge (Edwards, 2001). Examples of inquiry by way of second-order knowledge include "What is meant by sexual abstinence?," "What is the nature of sickness?," "What is meant by health?," and other questions concerning "What is meant by . . . ?" and "What is the nature of . . . ?"

The four philosophical areas of inquiry are *ontological, epistemology, ethics*, and *logic*. The *ontological* area (study of reality or the metaphysical) is inquiry along the lines of "What is said to exist or be?" and "If it exists, what is there to it?" In nursing, ontology is what we believe to be "true" in terms of the central interest to the discipline; it answers the question, "What is it that we believe exists?" The *epistemology* area (study of knowledge) is inquiry into the creation, dissemination, and categorization of knowledge. In nursing, this area includes questions such as "What can we know?," "How do we know what we know about the phenomena of interest?," and "In which category does the knowledge belong?" The *ethics* area (moral philosophy) is normative inquiry about what is valued by a discipline in terms of actions and practices. In nursing, we ask normative moral questions such as

"What *ought* I do as a nurse?," "How *ought* I act to be ethical in practice?," and "What *ought* we do as a profession?" The *logic* area is a *method* of inquiry or logical reasoning through which arguments are presented and evaluated.

Nursing scholars communicate and disseminate their ontological, epistemological, and ethical assertions about the discipline of nursing by developing a philosophical view about the world and human beings. Fawcett (2005a, 2005b) identified three worldviews that have materialized from the work of nursing scholars: (1) reaction worldview, (2) reciprocal interaction worldview, and (3) simultaneous action worldview. These worldviews are further explained in **Table 5-1**.

The Philosophy Connection to the Holarchy

At first glance, the philosophy component appears to fall in line (in Figure 5-1) directly under the metaparadigm and directly before the conceptual model component. However, this is not the case. Remember that a holon, such as philosophy, can interact up and down or all around its own environment with other holons. Fawcett (2005b) made the following statement about the philosophy component:

> The metaparadigm of a discipline identifies the phenomena about which ontological, epistemic, and ethical claims are made. The unique focus and content of each conceptual model then reflect certain philosophical claims. The philosophies therefore are the foundation for other formulations, including conceptual models, grand theories, and middle-range theories. (p. 22)

Conceptual Models

The terms *conceptual framework*, *conceptual system*, *paradigm*, and *disciplinary matrix* often are used interchangeably with the term *conceptual model*. Fawcett (2005b) defined a conceptual model as follows:

> A set of relatively abstract and general concepts that address the phenomena of central interest to a discipline, the propositions that broadly describe those concepts, and the propositions that state relatively abstract and general relations between two or more of the concepts. (p. 16)

The overall function of a conceptual model is to characterize relationships of phenomena in a coherent format in order to shape a distinctive frame of reference. Specifically, conceptual models assist us in communicating concept links that we believe exist and then in communicating those concepts with some degree of assurance that we understand what we are conveying to one another (Shoemaker, Tankard, & Lasorsa, 2004).

Conceptual models have practical value because they guide research and practice. A "reciprocal relationship" exists between conceptual models and nursing practice in that conceptual models provide the characterization and structure for nursing practice. In turn,

Table 5-1   Three Worldviews of Nursing

Worldview	Foundation	Perspectives
Reaction worldview	Mechanistic	Human beings are bio-psycho-social spiritual beings.
	Persistence	Human beings react to external environmental stimuli in a linear, causal manner.
	Totality	Change occurs only for survival and as a consequence of predictable and controllable antecedent conditions.
	Particulate-deterministic	Only objective phenomena that can be isolated, observed, defined, and measured are studied.
Reciprocal interaction worldview	Organismic	Human beings are holistic and parts are viewed only in the context of the whole.
	Simultaneity	Human beings are active, and interactions between human beings and their environments are reciprocal.
	Totality	Change is a function of multiple antecedent factors, is probabilistic, and may be continuous or may be only for survival.
	Change	Reality is multidimensional, content dependent, and relative.
	Persistence	
	Interactive-integrative	
Simultaneous action worldview	Organismic	Unitary human beings are unified by pattern.
	Simultaneity	Human beings are in mutual rhythmical interchange with their environments.
	Change	Human beings change continuously, unpredictably, and in the direction of more complex self-organization.
	Unitary-transformative	The phenomena of interest are personal knowledge and pattern recognition.

Modified from Fawcett, J. (2005). *Contemporary nursing knowledge: Analysis and evaluation of nursing models and theories* (2nd ed., pp. 12–13). Philadelphia, PA: F. A. Davis. Used with permission.

the outcomes of nursing practice supply evidence for theorists to determine the degree to which a conceptual model has credence (Fawcett, 1992; Kahn & Fawcett, 1995).

A unique facet of each conceptual model is that it provides an individual with the ability to interpret and characterize reality from that particular model (Fawcett, 2005b). Each discipline does not have just one reality, but rather multiple realities. The seven conceptual models of nursing recognized by Fawcett enable nurses to view the world and its functions in different ways (see **Table 5-2**). Each conceptual model of nursing gives the discipline a unique perspective of the metaparadigm concepts and provides a path for concrete theories (specifically, middle-range theories) to be generated and tested for practice.

Fawcett (1995, 2005b) has always contended that individuals cannot view the world and make observations about the world apart from a conceptual model frame of reference. Philosophers such as Karl Popper (1959) have noted that we see, hear, and process information through some determinate frame of reference, or belief and value system, painting everything we perceive and influencing how we interpret it. Fawcett (2005b) emphasized that because nurses see the world and their observations about the world through some frame of reference, choosing a credible conceptual model is central to expert practice.

Fawcett (2003) was resolute in her statement on the essentialness of conceptual models to the discipline of nursing: "Conceptual models . . . are the foundation on which claims of disciplinary status for nursing rests" (p. 229). For several years, Fawcett has communicated her concern about whether the discipline of nursing will survive given that many nursing researchers no longer use, support, or value conceptual models as integral to the viability of the discipline (Fawcett, 2003, 2008; Fawcett & Alligood, 2005; Fawcett, Newman, & McAllister, 2004). Without specific nursing conceptual models for guiding research and nursing practice, Fawcett (2003) has expressed her worry that the discipline will become extinct and nurses will regress to no more than "skilled tradespeople" (p. 229).

Nursing must have its own identity with its own conceptual models, and not borrow from other disciplines. As a discipline, it has reached a bifurcation point where a decision must be made. Without using our own conceptual models of nursing, we stand to lose nursing's identity.

Table 5-2 Conceptual Models of Nursing

Conceptual Model	Publication Dates and Revisions
Johnson's behavioral system model	1959, 1980, 1990
King's conceptual system	1968, 1971, 1981
Levine's conservation model	1969, 1991, 1996
Neuman's systems model	1982, 1995, 1996
Orem's self-care framework	1971, 1983, 1987, 2001
Rogers's science of unitary human beings	1980, 1990, 1994
Roy's adaptation model	1971, 1976, 1999

Modified from Fawcett, J. (2005). *Contemporary nursing knowledge: Analysis and evaluation of nursing models and theories* (2nd ed., pp. 1–48). Philadelphia, PA: F. A. Davis. Used with permission.

Conceptual Models Versus Theories

More than 30 years ago, Fawcett (1978b) distinguished conceptual models and theories by the level of abstraction. Since then she has built on this distinction as part of her work. Along the way, she devised a rule for making this distinction, based on a determination of the purpose of the work being examined (Fawcett, 2005b). This approach uses what can be referred to as *if–then determinations* (**Box 5-1**). Such determinations are useful for advanced practice nurses and students as they attempt to decipher the level of abstractness required for each work being examined. To answer the questions related to Determinations 1 to 3 in Box 5-1, the advanced practice nurse would examine the purpose of the work in terms of three different *if–then* conditions. Determination 4 has to do with the number of

Box 5-1 *If–Then* Determinations: Is It a Conceptual Model or a Theory?		
Determination	**If**	**Then**
Determination 1	*If* the purpose of the work is to articulate a body of distinctive knowledge for the whole of the discipline of nursing	*Then* the work is probably a conceptual model
Determination 2	*If* the purpose of the work is to further develop one aspect of a conceptual model	*Then* the work is probably a grand theory
Determination 3	*If* the purpose of the work is to describe, explain, or predict concrete and specific phenomena	*Then* the work is probably a middle-range theory
Determination 4	*If* the work requires that one must work through four steps to directly link the concepts to empirically testable hypothesis	*Then* the work is probably a conceptual model
Process Steps to Linking Step 1: Create the conceptual model. Step 2: Derive the middle-range theory. Step 3: Identify empirical indicators Step 4: Identify empirically testable hypotheses.	*If* three steps are required	*Then* the work is probably a middle-range theory

Modified from Fawcett, J. (2005). *Contemporary nursing knowledge: Analysis and evaluation of nursing models and theories* (2nd ed., pp. 1–48). Philadelphia, PA: F. A. Davis. Used with permission.

Table 5-3 Grand Theories of Nursing

Grand Theory	Publication Dates and Revisions
Newman's theory of health as expanding consciousness	1979, 1986, 1994, 1997
Parse's theory of human becoming	1981, 1987, 1992, 1994, 1996, 1997, 1998
Leininger's theory of culture care, diversity, and universality	2006

Modified from Fawcett, J. (2005). *Contemporary nursing knowledge: Analysis and evaluation of nursing models and theories* (2nd ed., pp. 1–48). Philadelphia, PA: F. A. Davis. Used with permission; and from Fawcett, J., & Garity, J. (2009). *Evaluating research for evidence-based nursing practice* (pp. 55–71). Philadelphia, PA: F. A. Davis.

steps required for one to work and think through the process of formulating concepts and translating them into empirically testable hypotheses. These steps are embedded within the components of the holarchy.

Fawcett (2005b) specified the level of abstractness of conceptual models in more detail:

> The concepts are too abstract and general for direct observation of phenomena to occur. The concepts are not restricted by anyone—individuals, groups, situations, or events. The propositions are too abstract and general for direct empirical observation to occur. The related concepts are stated in an abstract and general manner.

Fawcett and Garity (2009) mentioned an additional condition for a conceptual model to be designated as such: A conceptual model must be complete in terms of the four concepts of the metaparadigm. The three theories they listed as "grand" contain only three of four metaparadigm concepts that designate a conceptual model (see **Table 5-3**).

Distinction Between Conceptual Models and Other Models for Middle-Range Theories

Fawcett and Garity (2009) found that nursing scholars from time to time incorrectly refer to a conceptual model as a grand theory or theoretical framework, and vice versa, or refer to a schematic diagram for middle-range theories as a conceptual model. An important point to consider is that Fawcett's description of a conceptual model is not the same as a model for middle-range theory often seen in some nursing articles and in other disciplines, such as in the social sciences and philosophy of science.

Fawcett (2005b) articulated the differences between a conceptual model and a model for a middle-range theory. Unlike Fawcett's description of a conceptual model, a *model for middle-range theory* is a schematic diagram of theories, a representation of testable theories, or a graphic representation that helps one to comprehend the theory. Shoemaker and colleagues (2004) called a model a "theoretical tool" that is used to represent a theory; a theory can talk to a model, and a model can talk to a theory. Models not only suggest relationships, but they also can imply relationships in middle-range theory; nevertheless, these are the models of middle-range theories and not conceptual models.

In contrast, each conceptual model has its own distinctive language of its concepts and propositions, and the definition of each term and phrase is directly connected to the essence and meaning of the conceptual model (Fawcett, 2005b). A conceptual model is extremely abstract and represents the physical, psychological, and logical processes of the world (Neuliep, 1996).

Theories

Theorists and metatheorists define, classify, and stack theories in different ways. These differences are evident in nursing, for example. Some theorists do not try to place conceptual models and theories in echelons, whereas others do place them in echelons but in differing ways. Graduate nursing students who are at the stage of relearning theory in more detail could become confused as they try to interpret different authors' terminology, especially when trying to sort out the answers to questions such as "What is the difference between a conceptual model and a theory?," "Should theories be categorized?," "How are theories sorted?," "Which way is right?," and "Who is right?" Much of this chapter has followed Fawcett's way of distinguishing theory; refer to Box 5-1 for the *if–then* determinations that allow for differentiating a conceptual model from a theory.

Fawcett (2005b) defined a theory as "one or more relatively concrete and specific concepts that are derived from a conceptual model, the propositions that narrowly describe those concepts, and the propositions that state relatively concrete and specific relations between two or more concepts" (p. 34).

Meleis (2007, pp. 38–39) found six different ways that theory is defined, where each type is based on how it is defined:

1. Based on structure (McKay, 1969)
2. Based on practice goals (Dickoff & James, 1968)
3. Based on tentativeness (Barnum, 1998)
4. Based on research (Ellis, 1968)
5. Based on creativity in developing and connecting concepts and the use of theory in practice and research (Chinn & Kramer, 2004, 2008)
6. Based on progression from conceptual models to theory (Fawcett, 2005b)

Functions of Theory: Theory to Practice

The function of theory is closely connected to "how good" the theory is. According to Jaccard and Jacoby (2010), a good theory is one that helps us better understand the world. Fawcett and Garity (2009) note that each theory is evaluated in terms of how good it is for guiding research and practice; thus, if we are to judge whether a theory is good, we must evaluate its *utility*. Shoemaker and colleagues (2004) stated the function of theory in a concise way: Its major purpose, they say, is to "condense and store knowledge . . . and put our discoveries of the nature of the world into statements" (p. 169). To accomplish this goal, the information within the theory must be good.

Fawcett (2005b) detailed the functions of theory development as twofold: (1) *research* inquiry based on theory-testing or theory-generating research and (2) research-supported theory translated into *practice*. In an article published in 1992, she emphasized that a reciprocal relationship exists between conceptual models and nursing practice (see the Conceptual Models section in this chapter). The *conceptual–theoretical–empirical* (C-T-E) formalization for theory development has been presented by her in many publications. The C-T-E formalization is a way to analyze research by systematically testing or generating theory; it is sometimes called *theoretical substruction*, a term still used today by a few scholars and educators (Fawcett, 1999). Within the C-T-E formalization, there are two major C-T-E structures: (1) one C-T-E formalization for theory-testing research (top-down) and (2) one C-T-E formalization for theory-generating research (bottom-up). These functions of theory are noted throughout Fawcett's discussion of the C-T-E structures.

Conceptual models inform and transform practice by systematically providing evidence; in turn, the systematic use of the conceptual model provides information that is used for modifications of the conceptual model and documentation of outcomes (Fawcett, 1992, 2005b). Fawcett (1992) summed it up by saying, "Indeed, the reciprocal relationship between a conceptual model and nursing practice progresses from the abstract content of the conceptual model to the real world of clinical practice back to the conceptual model" (p. 226).

Theory by Levels of Abstractions

Fawcett (2005a, 2005b) categorized theories on the basis of their levels of abstraction and scope, with grand theory being more abstract with a broad scope, but less abstract than a conceptual model, and middle-range theory being more concrete and narrower in scope. It is important to note that Fawcett mentioned only grand theory and middle-range theory as the two categories in the theory component of the holarchy of nursing knowledge. Metatheory and practice theory were not named components of Fawcett's holarchy of nursing knowledge, but they are briefly defined in this section to familiarize advanced practice nurses with these terms and the way in which some theorists view them.

Metatheory is not a named level of abstraction of Fawcett's theory component in the holarchy of nursing knowledge, possibly because metatheory is philosophical study about theory and is not itself theory content. As described by Meleis (1997), metatheory is a theory of theories. Metatheory encompasses a philosophical stance, debate, or evaluation about theory and its methods and processes for generating knowledge (Chinn & Kramer, 2008). Metatheory involves scholars debating theory in an effort to move the discipline toward a coherent body of knowledge. A *metatheorist* "talks" theory, analyzes theory, and develops processes for theory development, whereas a *theorist* develops the actual theory and its content (Meleis, 1997). Some scholars refer to metatheory as being the highest level of abstraction of theory.

Grand theory is a named level of abstraction of Fawcett's theory component in the holarchy of nursing knowledge. This kind of abstract, broad theory consists of concepts and propositions that are less broad and abstract than a conceptual model but not as specific and concrete as middle-range theory (Fawcett, 2005b). Grand theory is sometimes referred to as macro theory, meaning that the theory is far too abstract to state relationships or hypotheses in empirical terms or to specify actions and processes for nursing practice (McKenna & Slevin, 2008). Fawcett recognized three theories in nursing as grand theories (see Table 5-3). Grand theories are derived from conceptual models and often become "the starting points for middle-range theory development" (Fawcett, 2005b, p. 19). A grand theory sometimes can be used as the "C" (conceptual) of the C-T-E structure, replacing the conceptual model in this structure (Fawcett & Garity, 2009). It should be noted here that middle-range theories also frequently originate directly from conceptual models (discussed in the next section).

Middle-range theory is a named level of abstraction of Fawcett's theory component in the holarchy of nursing knowledge. It is less abstract, is narrower in scope, and has fewer concepts and propositions than grand theory. Numerous middle-range theories have been formulated in the past 15 years because they provide elements that especially align with practice in nursing (Peterson, 2009). Robert Merton (1957/1949), a sociologist who is known for his position on middle-range theory, stated that theories of this level guide research and have specificity for practice; according to Merton, theories of the middle range are strongly supported by empirical data (indicators).

Fawcett's long-term aims have been to express (1) the importance of middle-range theories to practice; (2) how middle-range theories fit in the holarchy, specifically with the conceptual model component; (3) how middle-range theories can be tested, evaluated, and translated into practice; and (4) how middle-range theories signal the onset of a maturing discipline. In her book of contemporary nursing knowledge, Fawcett (2005b) highlighted three middle-range theories that were derived from conceptual models but noted that many middle-range theories have been derived from conceptual models of nursing (see **Table 5-4**). Two other examples are King's theory of goal attainment (1981, 1995), which is derived from King's conceptual system (1981), and Tulman and Fawcett's (2003) theory of adaptation during childbirth, which is derived from Roy's adaptation model (Roy & Andrews, 1999; Roy & Roberts, 1981).

Conceptual models guide the direction of the propositions and empirically testable hypotheses used to create or refine middle-range theories. As stated previously in this chapter, every person views the world and how it works from a frame of reference

Table 5-4 Middle-Range Theories of Nursing

Middle-Range Theory	Publication Dates and Revisions	Type
Theory of deliberative nursing process	Orlando, 1961, 1972	Predictive middle-range theory
Theory of interpersonal relations	Peplau, 1952, 1987, 1989	Descriptive middle-range theory
Theory of human caring	Watson, 1979, 1985, 1996, 2001	Explanatory middle-range theory
Theory of goal attainment	King, 1981, 1995	Derived from King's conceptual system (1981)
Theory of adaptation during childbirth	Tulman and Fawcett, 2003	Derived from Roy's adaptation model (1981, 1999)

Modified from Fawcett, J. (2005). *Contemporary nursing knowledge: Analysis and evaluation of nursing models and theories* (2nd ed., pp. 1–48). Philadelphia, PA: F. A. Davis. Used with permission; and from Fawcett, J., & Garity, J. (2009). *Evaluating research for evidence-based nursing practice* (pp. 73–88). Philadelphia, PA: F. A. Davis.

(i.e., a conceptual model). Popper (1959) maintained that everything a person observes is screened and interpreted through that person's conceptual backdrop. The implicit understanding of this view is that nurses have assumptions about the world and the way the world functions on the basis of their historical and cultural underpinnings. Those assumptions guide nurses toward their choice of a credible conceptual model of nursing for use in practice.

When theorists develop middle-range theories, they do so from a chosen conceptual model that aligns with their own assumptions about the world. Many middle-range theories come from the same conceptual model. As Fawcett (2005a) noted, "Many middle-range theories are needed to deal with all of the phenomena encompassed by any one conceptual model because each theory deals with only a limited aspect of the total reality encompassed by a conceptual model" (p. 36). Thus, when many middle-range theories have emerged from a conceptual model, there is more detail and specificity to that particular model. Because grand theories are also derived from conceptual models, many grand theories are also needed to detail and specify any one conceptual model (Fawcett, 2005b).

Middle-range theory is categorized in similar but slightly different ways. Fawcett (2005a) specified three types of middle-range theories: (1) descriptive, (2) explanatory, and (3) predictive. McKenna and Slevin (2008) defined four types of scientific theories: (1) descriptive, (2) explanatory, (3) predictive, and (4) prescriptive, and concisely designated them as "information presenting," "knowledge building," "knowledge confirming," and "knowledge utilization," respectively (p. 30). *Descriptive theory*, the most basic type of theory usually involving one concept, is "information presenting" in the sense that phenomena are classified and described. For descriptive theory, "an explanation is called for but not yet available" (McKenna & Slevin, 2008, p. 30). *Explanatory theory*, or "knowledge building," attempts to explain how two or more concepts relate to each other. *Predictive theory*, or "knowledge confirming," predicts cause and effect relationships between two or more concepts. *Prescriptive theory* is "knowledge utilization" that goes beyond the predictive cause and effect relationships. This type of theory builds on descriptive, explanatory, and predictive theory. McKenna and Slevin (2008) emphasized the strength of prescriptive theory:

> We must have considered the evidence for the cause–effect relationship. We must have considered the "expected utility" of one or some actions as opposed to others. And, we will have taken account of the context. (p. 31)

Some theorists label prescriptive theory as practice theory, which has a narrower scope than what is often labeled as middle-range theory (practice theory is discussed later in this section).

Other slight variations on types of theory exist as well. For example, Meleis (2007) defined theory by goal orientation and divided it into two major categories—descriptive and predictive. Within descriptive theory, she delineated two classifications: (1) "factor-isolating, category-formulating, or labeling theory" and (2) "explanatory" (p. 44). McEwen (2011) specified four types of theories: (1) descriptive theory as factor-isolating theory, (2) explanatory theory as factor-relating theory, (3) predictive theories or promoting or inhibiting theory as situation-relating theory, and (4) prescriptive theory as situation-producing theory.

A derivative of middle-range theory is *practice theory*, which is a very narrow theory resulting from empirical testing (Peterson, 2009). Practice theory is also known as prescriptive theory. Fawcett (2005b) does not compartmentalize practice theory or prescriptive theory apart from her middle-range theory category, but she does refer to descriptive, explanatory, and predictive theories as types of middle-range theories. Specifically, Fawcett and Garity (2009) refer to predictive theory as empirical, experimental theory for practice on the basis of the effects of actions and processes on people and situations. This definition encompasses prescriptive theory.

As Peterson (2009) has explained, labeling any theory that is very concrete and narrow in scope can present challenges. Synonyms for practice theory include *situation-specific theory* and *micro theory* (Peterson, 2009). Dickoff and James (1968), who were noted for their stance that theory exists only for the sake of practice, categorized practice theory as goal-incorporating, prescriptive, and situation-producing theory.

The concepts of practice theory (or micro theory) are precisely defined for specific populations, desired situations, or fields of practice. Numerous practice theories exist, including these five theories:

1. The praxis theory of suffering (Morse, 2001, 2005)
2. The theory of postpartum depression (Beck, 1993)

3. The theory of breastfeeding (Nelson, 2006)
4. The theory of health promotion for preterm infants (Mefford, 2004)
5. The theory of dependent care in research with parents of toddlers (Arndt & Horodynski, 2004)

Empirical Indicators

Fawcett (2005b) defined an *empirical indicator* as "a very concrete and specific real world proxy for a middle-range theory concept; an actual instrument, experimental condition, or procedure that is used to observe or measure a middle-range theory concept. The information obtained from empirical indicators is typically called data" (p. 21).

Empirical indicators provide a way for middle-range theories to be tested or generated, but there is no direct link between empirical indicators and conceptual models, philosophies, or the metaparadigm. The only way that empirical indicators are connected to theory is by way of an operational definition for each concept in the middle-range theory. Research instruments with data about concepts, nursing protocols, nursing practice quality indicators, and other outcome data used by nurses, among many other methods, can be used as empirical indicators. In turn, those empirical indicators can be used to test or generate middle-range theories.

USING THE COMPONENTS IN PRACTICE

The C-T-E system is a whole system of nursing knowledge that is implemented for conceptual model-based or theory-based scientific practice. A conceptual model, a theory (or more than one), and empirical indicators are strongly linked to form a C-T-E system for application of a conceptual model or theory to nursing practice, research, and education. Fawcett (2005b) defined the C-T-E system as "service to the society guided by knowledge that is specific to the discipline of nursing, as articulated in conceptual models of nursing and nursing theories" (p. 32). Fawcett described two functions of the C-T-E system: (1) "to provide an intellectual lens" for human beings participating in nursing, their health, and their environment, and (2) "to provide a purposeful and systematic process for practice, that is, a practice methodology" (p. 33). The C-T-E system can be implemented by nursing departments within healthcare institutions, advanced practice nurses and other nurses working in private practice, and nursing educators to guide curriculum development or to teach students this system for practice. This section provides a brief synopsis of the substantive elements of the C-T-E system for practice.

Three substantive elements must be considered if the C-T-E system is adopted and used. Referring back to the discussion of the components of nursing knowledge will help clarify this section's meaning. **Figure 5-2** provides an overview of the holarchy translated into practice.

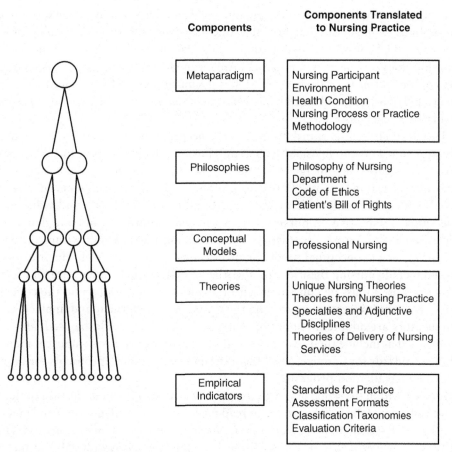

	Components	Components Translated to Nursing Practice
	Metaparadigm	Nursing Participant Environment Health Condition Nursing Process or Practice Methodology
	Philosophies	Philosophy of Nursing Department Code of Ethics Patient's Bill of Rights
	Conceptual Models	Professional Nursing
	Theories	Unique Nursing Theories Theories from Nursing Practice Specialties and Adjunctive Disciplines Theories of Delivery of Nursing Services
	Empirical Indicators	Standards for Practice Assessment Formats Classification Taxonomies Evaluation Criteria

Figure 5-2 Holarchy of nursing knowledge.

Modified from Fawcett, J. (2005). *Contemporary nursing knowledge: Analysis and evaluation of nursing models and theories* (2nd ed., p. 34). Philadelphia, PA: F. A. Davis. Used with permission.

The first element is translation of the metaparadigm of nursing into practice. The metaparadigm includes the human beings requiring nursing care, meaning the participant, family, or community; the environment of the human beings requiring care and the nursing practice environment; the health status of the participant; and the nursing practice methodology. In healthcare institutions, the mission statement sets the tone of the institution, the scope of nursing practice and its methodology, and types of service.

The second element is translation of philosophies into nursing practice. As previously discussed, the nursing philosophy is a worldview about the beliefs and values of nursing as a discipline. The institution has a philosophy of its beliefs and values about human beings, the institution's environment, health, and nursing methodology. Some of the ways in which philosophy is communicated include the American Nurses Association's *Code of Ethics for Nurses* (2001) or other codes of conduct; the patient's bill of rights for the particular institution (for hospitals, for example, the American Hospital Association has written and adopted *The Patient Care Partnership* [2008] document, which has replaced its universal Patient's Bill of Rights); and the nursing department's philosophy statement that is uniquely formulated by each institution.

The third element is translation of the conceptual model, theories, and empirical indicators into a comprehensive "formal nursing knowledge system," the C-T-E system. This step "requires the linkage to a conceptual model, one or more theories, and one or more empirical indicators" (Fawcett, 2005b, p. 34). There are numerous ways that a C-T-E system becomes evident. The conceptual model can be the individual nurse's professional perspective on nursing and/or the institution's and nursing department's adopted conceptual model or theory. The practicing nurse works within the institution's or agency's conceptual model or professional practice model. Theories that are adopted include nursing theories and theories of delivery of nursing care and services. All theories used must be consistent with the adopted philosophy and the conceptual model. Once the conceptual model and the theories are congruent and in place, empirical indicators are adopted. Numerous empirical indicators could be used, along with documents that include their own empirical indicators. Sources for empirical indicators include standards for practice, assessment designs, taxonomies, protocols for intervention, and an evaluation program.

It is not within the scope of this chapter to present an in-depth discussion of the substantive elements of the C-T-E system. To read more about the C-T-E system and guidelines using the C-T-E system for practice, research, education, or administration, refer to Chapter 2 of Fawcett's *The Structure of Contemporary Nursing Knowledge* (2005b). In that same chapter, Fawcett offers a perspective on the process elements of the C-T-E system; successful implementation of a C-T-E system; the phases of evolution during the implementation, a process called perspective transformation; strategies to facilitate perspective transformation; and levels of integration of the C-T-E system.

SUMMARY

This chapter presents a review of the holarchy of nursing knowledge that was formulated by Fawcett. The components of nursing knowledge—that is, the metaparadigm, philosophy, conceptual model, theory, and empirical indicator—were discussed. According to Fawcett, middle-range theories must be strongly linked to nursing's conceptual models if nursing is to remain a viable and bona fide discipline. As Fawcett pointed out, nursing stands to lose its identity if nursing researchers and scholars continue to abandon nursing's own conceptual models in favor of models and theories of other disciplines. Linking conceptual models of nursing, theories, and empirical indicators to the C-T-E system is necessary for the application of a conceptual model of nursing and, therefore, for the translation of the components of nursing knowledge into real-world practice.

DISCUSSION QUESTIONS

1. Examine each of the components in the holarchy of nursing knowledge. Identify one conceptual model of nursing, one grand theory of nursing, and one middle-range theory of nursing. Either search this text for the content of each one, or search in the CINAHL or Medline databases. Using the *if–then* determinations in Box 5-1 of this chapter, explain the distinguishable levels of abstraction characteristics of each one (conceptual model, grand theory, and middle-range theory).
2. Which one of the three philosophical worldviews from Table 5-1 reflects your philosophical worldview? Explore how your philosophical worldview (reaction, reciprocal interaction, or simultaneous action) interweaves with the philosophical worldview adopted by your workplace.
3. Determine which conceptual model of nursing you prefer. Then, choose a middle-range nursing theory that has been formulated or derived from your preferred conceptual model of nursing. Analyze the parts of your chosen middle-range theory that reveal the derivation characteristics from your chosen conceptual model of nursing. An example includes (but is not necessarily the model and theory that you will choose) King's theory of goal attainment (1995), which is a middle-range nursing theory derived in 1981 from King's conceptual system (1971).
4. Explore specific strategies that you or other advanced practice nurses can implement to advance the discipline of nursing. What is the critical nature of the relationship between conceptual models of nursing and middle-range nursing theories?
5. Analyze how the C-T-E structures translate into nursing practice (see Figure 5-2). Use actual examples. You may use the middle-range nursing theory and the conceptual model of nursing that you chose in Discussion Question 3. In addition, choose two or more empirical indicators that are consistent with your middle-range nursing theory and that can be translated into a testable hypothesis. Give an overview of this C-T-E structure process.

REFERENCES

American Association of Colleges of Nursing. (2006, October). *The essentials of doctoral education for advanced nursing practice.* Retrieved from http://www.aacn.nche.edu/publications/position /DNPEssentials.pdf

American Hospital Association. (2008, April 1). *The patient care partnership.* Washington, DC: Author. Retrieved from http://www.aha.org/aha/issues/Communicating-With-Patients/pt-care-partnership.html

American Nurses Association. (2001). *Code of ethics for nurses with interpretive statements.* Washington, DC: Author.

Arndt, M. J., & Horodynski, M. A. O. (2004). Theory of dependent-care in research with parents of toddlers: The NEAT project. *Nursing Science Quarterly, 17,* 345–350.

Barnum, B. J. S. (1998). *Nursing theory: Analysis, application, and evaluation* (5th ed.). Philadelphia, PA: Lippincott Williams & Wilkins.

Beck, C. T. (1993). Teetering on the edge: A substantive theory of postpartum depression. *Nursing Research, 42,* 42–48.

Chinn, P. L., & Kramer, M. K. (2004). *Integrated theory and knowledge development in nursing* (6th ed.). St. Louis, MO: Mosby.

Chinn, P. L., & Kramer, M. K. (2008). *Integrated theory and knowledge development in nursing* (7th ed.). St. Louis, MO: Mosby.

Dickoff, J., & James, P. (1968). A theory of theories: A position paper. *Nursing Research, 17*(3), 197–203.

Donaldson, S. K., & Crowley, D. M. (1978). The discipline of nursing. *Nursing Outlook, 26*(2), 113–120.

Edwards, S. D. (2001). *Philosophy of nursing: An introduction.* New York, NY: Palgrave.

Ellis, R. (1968). Characteristics of significant theories. *Nursing Research, 17*(3), 217–222.

Fawcett, J. (1978a). The relationship between theory and research: The double helix. *Advances in Nursing Science, 1*(1), 49–62.

Fawcett, J. (1978b). The "what" of theory development. In J. Fawcett, L. T. Zderad, J. G. Paterson, J. M. Rinehart, & M. E. Hardy (Eds.), *Theory development: What, why, and how?* (pp. 17–33). New York, NY: National League for Nursing [Pub. No. 15–1708].

Fawcett, J. (1992). Conceptual models and nursing practice: The reciprocal relationship. *Journal of Advanced Nursing, 17,* 224–288.

Fawcett, J. (1995). *Analysis and evaluation of conceptual models of nursing* (3rd ed.). Philadelphia, PA: F. A. Davis.

Fawcett, J. (1999). *The relationship of theory and research* (3rd ed.). Philadelphia, PA: F. A. Davis.

Fawcett, J. (2003). Guest editorial: On bed baths and conceptual models of nursing. *Journal of Advanced Nursing, 44,* 229–230.

Fawcett, J. (2005a). Middle-range nursing theories are necessary for the advancement of the discipline. *Aquichan, 5*(001), 32–43.

Fawcett, J. (2005b). *Contemporary nursing knowledge: Analysis and evaluation of nursing models and theories* (2nd ed., pp. 1–48). Philadelphia, PA: F. A. Davis.

Fawcett, J. (2008). Editor's choice: The added value of nursing conceptual model-based research. *Journal of Advanced Nursing, 61,* 583.

Fawcett, J., & Alligood, M. R. (2005). Influences on advancement of nursing knowledge. *Nursing Science Quarterly, 18,* 227–232.

Fawcett, J., & DeSanto-Madeya, S. (2012). *Contemporary nursing knowledge: Analysis and evaluation of nursing models and theories* (3rd ed., pp. 3–25). Philadelphia, PA: F. A. Davis.

Fawcett, J., & Garity, J. (2009). *Evaluating research for evidence-based nursing practice.* Philadelphia, PA: F. A. Davis.

Fawcett, J., Newman, D. M. L., & McAllister, M. (2004). Advanced practice nursing and conceptual models of nursing. *Nursing Science Quarterly, 17,* 135–138.

Jaccard, J., & Jacoby, J. (2010). *Theory construction and model-building skills: A practical guide for social scientists* (pp. 22–36). New York, NY: Guilford Press.

Johnson, B. M., & Webber, P. B. (2005). Language, meaning, and structure. *An introduction to theory and reasoning in nursing* (2nd ed., pp. 9–29). New York, NY: Lippincott Williams & Wilkins.

Kahn, S., & Fawcett, J. (1995). Continuing the dialogue: A response to Draper's critique of Fawcett's "Conceptual models and nursing practice: The reciprocal relationship." *Journal of Advanced Nursing, 22,* 188–192.

Kim, H. S. (1997). Terminology in structuring and development nursing knowledge. In I. M. King & J. Fawcett (Eds.), *The language of nursing theory and metatheory* (pp. 27–36). Indianapolis, IN: Sigma Theta Tau International Honor Society of Nursing.

King, I. M. (1981). *A theory for nursing: Systems, concepts, process.* New York, NY: Wiley.

King, I. M. (1984). Philosophy of nursing education: A national survey. *Western Journal of Nursing Research, 6,* 387–406.

King, I. M. (1995). The theory of goal attainment. In M. A. Frey & C. L. Sieloff (Eds.), *Advancing King's systems framework and theory of nursing* (pp. 23–32). Thousand Oaks, CA: Sage.

Koestler, A. (1975/1967). *The ghost in the machine.* New York, NY: Random House.

McEwen, M. (2011). Overview of theory in nursing. In M. McEwen & E. M. Wills (Eds.), *Theoretical basis for nursing* (3rd ed., pp. 21–45). Philadelphia, PA: Wolters Kluwer/Lippincott Williams & Wilkins.

McKay, R. (1969). Theories, models and systems for nursing. *Nursing Research, 18*(5), 393–399.

McKenna, H. P., & Slevin, O. D. (2008). *Nursing models, theories and practice* (pp. 1–61). Oxford, UK: Blackwell.

Mefford, L. C. (2004). A theory of health promotion for preterm infants based on Levine's conservation model of nursing. *Nursing Science Quarterly, 17,* 260–266.

Meleis, A. I. (1997). Theoretical nursing: Definitions and interpretations. In I. M. King & J. Fawcett (Eds.), *The language of nursing theory and metatheory* (pp. 41–50). Indianapolis, IN: Sigma Theta Tau International Honor Society of Nursing.

Meleis, A. I. (2007). *Theoretical nursing: Development and progress* (4th ed.). Philadelphia, PA: Lippincott Williams & Wilkins.

Mella, P. (2009). *The holonic revolution: Holons, holarchies and holonic networks: The ghost in the production machine.* Pavia, Italy: Pavia University Press.

Merton, R. K. (1957/1949). *Social theory and social structure* (revised ed.). New York, NY: Free Press.

Mesarovic, M., Macko, D., & Takahara, Y. (1970). *Theory of hierarchical, multi-level systems.* New York, NY: Academic Press.

Morse, J. M. (1996). Nursing scholarship: Sense and sensibility. *Nursing Inquiry, 3,* 74–82.

Morse, J. M. (2001). Toward a praxis theory of suffering. *Advances in Nursing Science, 24*(1), 47–59.

Morse, J. M. (2005). Creating a qualitatively-derived theory of suffering. In U. Zeitler (Ed.), *Clinical practice and development in nursing* (pp. 83–91). Aarhus, Denmark: Center for Innovation in Nurse Training.

Nelson, A. M. (2006). Toward a situation-specific theory of breastfeeding. *Research and Theory for Nursing Practice, 20*(1), 9–27.

Neuliep, J. W. (1996). *Human communication theory: Applications and case studies.* Boston, MA: Pearson/Allyn & Bacon.

Peterson, S. J. (2009). Introduction to the nature of nursing knowledge. In S. J. Peterson & T. W. Bredow (Eds.), *Middle range theories: Application to nursing research* (2nd ed., pp. 3–45). New York, NY: Lippincott Williams & Wilkins.

Popper, K. (1959). *The logic of scientific discovery.* New York, NY: Basic Books.

Rodgers, B. L. (2005). *Developing nursing knowledge: Philosophical traditions and influences.* Philadelphia, PA: Lippincott Williams & Wilkins.

Roy, C., & Andrews, H. A. (1999). *The Roy adaptation model* (2nd ed.). Stamford, CT: Appleton & Lange.

Roy, C., & Roberts, S. L. (1981). *Theory construction in nursing: An adaptation model.* Englewood Cliffs, NJ: Prentice Hall.

Shoemaker, P. J., Tankard, J. W., & Lasorsa, D. L. (2004). *How to build social science theories.* Thousand Oaks, CA: Sage.

Tulman, L., & Fawcett, J. (2003). *Women's health during and after pregnancy: A theory-based study of adaptation to change.* New York, NY: Springer.

Wilber, K. (1996). *A brief history of everything.* Boston, MA: Shambhala Books/Random House.

III

Interdisciplinary Philosophies and Theories

Chapter 6

Complexity Science and Complex Adaptive Systems

Joan C. Engebretson
Joanne V. Hickey

INTRODUCTION

Complexity science (CS) is an emerging paradigm that is being integrated into the healthcare literature as a new approach from which to view clinical care and healthcare organizations (HCOs). Grounded in physics and mathematics, it offers a fresh approach for studying regularities that differ from traditional science. Unlike traditional science that incorporates laws of science, CS is based on the notion that complexity emerges from simple rules (Phelan, 2001).

The theoretical concepts of complexity have been broadened into a paradigm of science concerned with the interconnection between individual units or agents (Kauffman, 1995; Waldrop, 1992). CS has expanded recently to include the ability to analyze huge amounts of data through computers. Thus, it has expanded the view of scientific research beyond purely linear reductionism. CS has been applied to fields such as weather forecasting, economics, and the neurosciences as well as social and organizational behavior. The term *complex adaptive system* (CAS) refers to a special application of complexity that bears some similarity to systems theory. As such, this framework will likely have an inherent resonance with nurses. The idea of nested systems from the individual patient, family, and community—as well as the healthcare unit, organization, and healthcare system—is familiar to most nurses. CASs have recently been applied to health care in relation to physiology and medicine. Additionally, complexity frameworks have been applied to local healthcare systems (Anderson, Issel, & McDaniel, 2003; Crabtree, Miller, & Strange, 2001) and organizations.

Biomedical scientific frameworks of mechanism and reductionism, which have produced excellent medical advances, have not always been a good fit for nursing. This lack of fit

Table 6-1 Complexity Science Terminology

Complexity science: The science based in physics and mathematics that uses basic principles such as simple rules or functions to explain the relationship between variables, and that allows for variations and emergent behaviors that are not fully predictable. Computer modeling using these rules/functions has accommodated large amounts of data that allow for the study of phenomena on intermediate levels in dynamic systems.

Nonlinear dynamics: The mathematics used to understand complex deterministic systems with complex behavior.

Complexity theories or concepts: The basic principles or concepts from complexity science and complex adaptive systems that are *applied,* often metaphorically, to other biological and social systems.

Complex adaptive systems (CASs): The application of complexity theories and systems perspectives to living, dynamic systems in biology and other systems.

Complex responsive processes (CRPs): The application of complexity to organizations in which a CAS is not completely applicable based on organizational structure and the ways in which people learn and form mental models in structured organizations. Currently, new mathematical models are being applied to science at all levels and the language has begun to penetrate other areas.

---

has led to a long-standing problem for nursing professionals when they try to ground practice, research, and scholarship in reductive scientific approaches. In reality, many nursing activities could be better understood through a complex, dynamic systems framework. Therefore, it is important for nurses to understand this movement and become familiar with its basic concepts and principles (see **Table 6-1** for definitions). A word of caution is offered; the vocabulary that supports CS is often confusing, and the concepts sometimes seem to be inconsistent.

The purpose of this chapter is threefold: (1) to introduce the reader to the roots, common terminology, and basic concepts of CS and math, which serve as a foundation for understanding their application to nursing, health care, and HCOs; (2) to explore the CAS, a special form of complexity particularly relevant for nurses; and (3) to discuss the implications of CS for practice and health care.

INTRODUCTION TO COMPLEXITY SCIENCE

CS is not a single theory but rather an emerging field of science that is engaging scholars and scientists in a new paradigm of interdisciplinary study. Complexity, CS, and the CAS are being described in a number of fields, including physics, mathematics, biology, economics, and the biological and social sciences. CS is attracting a diverse group of scholars and scientists across disciplines to view phenomena of interest through a new lens. Many scholars have identified it as a new paradigm in science. A prominent physicist has stated recently that complexity is a technical scientific revolution that will change the focus of research in all scientific disciplines, including human biology and medicine (Baranger, 2009).

For the past century, science has been focused largely on an analytical/reductionist paradigm of breaking things down into smaller units and isolating the parts from their contexts in an effort to understand how these parts operate in nature. The reductionist approach has been very successful in many ways and has engendered tremendous progress in health-related fields. Nevertheless, this approach is not sufficient to understand nature, especially living entities that are dynamic and adaptive. This limitation has been a concern in the nursing profession, which is oriented to a more holistic approach.

Several scientists from the physical and biological sciences have postulated that CS will be the preeminent science of the 21st century (Baranger, 2009). Robert Laughlin, Nobel laureate and physicist, has been quoted as stating that science has shifted from the *age of reductionism* to the *age of emergentism* (as cited in Kelso & Engstrom, 2006). This trend represents a fundamental shift away from breaking things down into the smallest parts and toward supplementing this approach with understanding of the behavior of the whole.

This paradigm shift is echoed by Sturmberg and Martin's (2009) speculation that the unilateral focus on reductionist thinking has resulted in some of the problems that we now face in health care. These authors call for the application of complexity systems thinking to address the social dimensions of health care. Their call is not to abandon the reductionist view, but rather to embrace both the holistic and reductionist perspectives to gain a new and more complete understanding of the world. This shift toward examining the whole, as well as appreciating the component parts and their relationship, combines the two views as a "both/and" perspective rather than an "either/or" approach in CS.

While CS is not a unified theory, its constructs have been applied to health care, and many of the general principles and concepts have an inherent resonance with nursing. The perspective of seeing the whole, which is perceived as more than the sum of its parts, is fundamental to nursing theory; therefore, this perspective is an important opportunity for nurses to understand the CS movement and become familiar with its key concepts and principles. As noted previously, the vocabulary that supports CS is often confusing, and the concepts are defined inconsistently.

CS has been applied to a number of fields such as computing, economics, and earth sciences. Aspects such as agent-based modeling and computer simulations have recently been applied to health care in relation to physiology and medicine. Complexity frameworks have also been applied to local healthcare systems, social behavior, and organizations. These latter applications have significant relevance to nursing because many nursing theorists have a systems theory orientation. While notable debate has ensued about the relationship between complexity and systems theory, especially in relation to some of the more recent advancements proposed by Richardson (2005), many authors point out that CS has many of the same elements of systems theory, which is a theory very familiar to nursing. The systems orientation situates patients, families, and organizations within hierarchies of systems. With these systems orientations and theoretical frameworks, the biomedical scientific framework of mechanism and reductionism has resulted in a less precise fit for nursing than was previously thought. The lack of fit has produced a long-standing problem for nursing researchers who try to ground practice, research, and scholarship in reductive scientific mechanisms. It is apparent that many nursing activities could be understood better through complex dynamic systems frameworks.

BACKGROUND

It may be helpful to differentiate between CS as the application of mathematical and physics science to large data sets and the use of computer modeling. CASs are special cases of complexity in which some of the basic constructs are used and generally thought of more as complexity theory or a conceptual framework. CS is grounded in theoretical mathematics and physics and is concerned with the interconnection between agents (Kauffman, 1995; Waldrop, 1992). Agents are units or components of the system; they may consist of individual people, birds in a flock, bees in a hive, or a component of a human system such as genes or neurons. An example is the heart and circulatory system, both of which act as agents within a body.

Many of the complexity concepts come from chaos theory, quantum mechanics, and nonlinear mathematics. It is the interconnection between or among these agents that is the focus of CS. *Chaos theory* signifies a different concept from the common usage of the term chaos. In a chaotic system that conforms to chaos theory, behaviors may appear to be chaotic, random, or incoherent when analyzed in a linear fashion; in contrast, when analyzed using nonlinear approaches, the system exhibits dynamic *patterned* variation. For this reason, chaos theory is described as patterned complexity rather than being equivalent to the common usage of the terms chaos and random incoherence.

CS provides language, metaphors, conceptual frameworks, models, and theories that can be applied to health care. A *metaphor* is a figure of speech in which a word or phrase literally denotes one kind of object or idea in place of another to suggest a likeness or analogy between them. Metaphors are useful in describing complicated concepts because they provide a good conceptual analogy, allowing us to communicate and think about abstract concepts. For example, the metaphor of a machine is used to convey the idea of parts that can be identified and understood. This metaphor has been successfully applied to understanding the mechanisms of how things behave or operate.

The use of metaphors in CS also can help communicate abstract information. These metaphors shape our thinking and perspective by connecting an idea to a known concrete entity. In one sense, then, all scientific thinking is metaphorical because the metaphors influence which questions we ask and how we understand phenomena. The machine metaphor has been the predominant metaphor shaping our thinking about physiology and guiding medical research. Indeed, a large amount of medical research is devoted to understanding the mechanisms, whether they are at the genetic, biochemical, structural, or physiological levels. For example, clinical practice and research trials are predicated on understanding the mechanism of a disease or disorder, developing an intervention to repair function, or interrupting a disease process. The expected outcome is better function or a reduction in signs or symptoms of the disease. This linear process approach is a dominating factor in terms of the way we think about clinical research and patient care, with the outcomes being based on efficacy and efficiency.

The machine metaphor not only has been used to make sense of physiological functions of the body, but it has also been applied to social organizations. Although useful, this metaphor has limitations for understanding individual behavior and organizations. CS, by comparison, provides a different metaphor that looks at living systems as complex, adaptive, self-organizing systems. CS is concerned with the relationship among the units, components, or agents rather than just the components themselves. This perspective sheds light on how individuals and organizations behave and how change happens (Zimmerman, Lindberg, & Plsek, 1998). Physicists have identified laws of quantum mechanics on the micro (atomic and subatomic) and cosmic levels, which have been metaphorically applied at the intermediate levels (i.e., the behavior between the atomic and cosmic levels). Currently, new mathematical models are being applied to science at all levels, and the language has begun to penetrate other areas, including health care. Adding this perspective of understanding is most relevant to health care and to the profession of nursing.

Many healthcare disciplines are beginning to acknowledge the limitations of using only reductive approaches and the machine metaphor (Plsek & Greenhalgh, 2001; Sturmberg & Martin, 2009). Consider an example from the field of genetics. Researchers who identified human genes inspired new questions about how these genes are activated. Genetic researchers have become aware of the importance of understanding the gene and its molecular aspects (micro level) as well as the context, the environment, and the ecosystem of behavior (macro level) influencing gene behaviors. Elucidation of both levels is necessary for understanding how genes behave in a human organism related to expressions of health and disease. As noted previously, scholars are not suggesting that CS wholly replace analytical reductive science; rather, CS embraces both the reductive and the complexity perspectives (Lindberg, Nash, & Lindberg, 2008). Using this approach in nursing allows us to begin to address the complex challenges of patient behaviors, work environments, and care environments.

THE SCIENTIFIC ROOTS OF COMPLEXITY SCIENCE

A brief introduction to the mathematical and scientific roots of CS grounds the understanding of the concepts, which are applicable to other systems such as individuals, groups, and organizations. The following descriptions of nonlinearity are adapted from Liebovitz's

(1998) explanations of fractals and chaos, with the concepts being simplified here for the life sciences. Another scientific application of CS lies in coordination dynamics where mathematics is applied to reconcile the polarized world of contradictory pairs for the purpose of understanding the poles and the world between them.

Nonlinear Mathematics

Nonlinear mathematics provides a language to explain complex dynamic changes over time and three-dimensional space (four dimensions); it focuses on the interactions among variables, rather than the variables themselves. Some of the major concepts are presented in this section, although a full discussion of the mathematical and science concepts is beyond the scope of this chapter. Nonlinear approaches can be applied when the data do not follow a normal distribution pattern or when additional data do not fall close to the norm. Given that these concepts apply to the mathematical functions and patterns, one must be careful when applying them directly to other observed phenomena. **Table 6-2** lists some nonlinear dynamics concepts.

Focus on Simple Rules

These mathematical functions refer to the rule that describes relationships. For example, in the common equation $1 + 1 = 2$, a linear approach deductively examines the dependent variable as 2 and then focuses on the two independent variables of 1. In contrast, the nonlinear approach focuses on the plus ($+$) symbol, which is the rule or mathematical function that explains the relationship between the variables.

Coupling

Coupling examines the strength of the relationship between functional units. Additionally, the whole may be greater than the sum of the parts.

Table 6-2 Nonlinear Dynamics Concepts

- Nonlinearity
- Focus on simple rules
- Coupling
- Deterministic
- Sensitivity to initial conditions
- Fractals and self-similarity
- Scaling
- Emergence

Deterministic Systems

In a *deterministic system*, system behavior is not random, but rather has coherence or a pattern. A small number of equations and the understanding of their variables from the past can be used to compute values in the short term. Computer modeling may be used to make these explanatory predictions. The simple rules/functions specify how these variables change over time and space, at least in the short run.

Sensitivity to Initial Conditions and Perturbations

An *initial condition* is the starting point of a dynamic system, and a small difference in starting values can result in significantly different trajectories. To understand this concept, picture a plot on a graph where a minuscule difference in the starting point could alter the angle of the trajectory so that it points in a different direction if you tracked it over time. These perturbations can disrupt a system or create new emergent behaviors.

Fractals and Self-Similarity

A *fractal* is a geometrical pattern or structure that is self-similar and repeating. Similar patterns are repeated on different scales or resolutions. The similarity may be apparent, but when used strictly in mathematics and science, it is also mathematically similar so that the scales are proportional (i.e., self-similar). A common classic example from the discovery of fractal geometry is provided by Mandelbrot (1967, 1982). He described the coastline of England as a fractal because as it is observed from closer points of view (i.e., by changing the scale of magnification), the patterns appear to be repeated in a self-similar pattern. If you were to use binoculars and take repeatedly closer looks (different scales of resolution) at the entire coastline, you would likely see similar patterns, albeit on an even smaller scale. In CS, one finds self-similar mathematical patterns.

Scaling

The different resolutions of measurement are referred to as *scaling*. Perhaps more familiar examples of fractals would be the body's networks of blood vessels or the branches of a tree, in which the patterns are repeated on different scales; in other words, patterns are repeated at increasingly finer and finer resolution. In CS, new information is apparent at finer resolutions. As the object is viewed under continually closer resolutions, the object appears more complex rather than exactly the same. Liebovitz (1998) distinguished non-fractal objects from fractal objects when he stated, "As a non-fractal object is magnified, no new features are revealed. As a fractal object is magnified, ever finer features are revealed. The shapes of the smaller features are kind of like the shapes of the larger features" (p. 4).

Emergence and Coordination Dynamics

The unpredictability of a complex system that allows for new and unexpected behavior that is generated by the system itself is called *emergence*. Another scientific application of complexity lies in *coordination dynamics*—the study of patterns of coordinated behavior in living things.

In addressing coordination dynamics, Kelso and Engstrom (2006) noted, "It is a set of context dependent laws or rules that describe, explain, and predict how patterns of coordination form, adapt, persist and change in natural systems" (p. 90). These dynamics exist between two points or between complementary pairs. In their book *The Complementary Nature*, Kelso and Engstrom explored many of the contraries or oppositional pairs that are ubiquitous in the way humans make sense of the world. Coordination dynamics are a way to begin to understand these dichotomies, dualities, and polar opposites.

Complementary Pairs

By definition, complementary pairs are opposed; they actually are coexistent, linked, and often mutually dependent. Kelso and Engstrom (2006) recommended that these dichotomized pairs be written with the tilde symbol (~)—for example, mind~body, random~determined, objective~subjective, local~global, stability~instability, and qualitative~quantitative. In approaching complementary pairs, it is important to understand not only both poles of the pairs, but also the dynamics that occur between them. A scientific example is the wave~particle theory of light. The dynamics of waves and particles, as well as the interaction between them, are needed to describe light comprehensively.

Coordination dynamics offers a way to address the whole~part phenomena. Using coordination dynamics harkens back to the appeal to think in terms of "both/and" rather than "either/or" or "black/white." Likewise, the study of living things can be studied by reductive/analytical~emergent approaches. One key feature of coordination dynamics is control parameters, which can be either endogenous or exogenous. Control parameters can cause the system to adapt and change; conversely, they can be stabilizing to the system. Thus, the control parameters may be described as stabilizing~destabilizing/transformative. Life is replete with ambiguities and paradoxes.

COMPLEX ADAPTIVE SYSTEMS

The term *complex adaptive system* (CAS) refers to special cases of complex systems. CASs have been studied for more than 40 years, beginning at the Santa Fe Institute, where interdisciplinary researchers investigated the application of CS in physical, biological, computational, and social sciences. Other groups across the world also have engaged in the application of CS and CASs to real-world problems. The control within a CAS is decentralized and dispersed. Coherent behavior in the system arises from competition and cooperation among the agents (Waldrop, 1992). A CAS is a collection of individual agents with freedom to act in ways that are not always totally predictable and whose actions are interconnected so that the action of one part changes the context for other agents (Wilson, Holt, & Greenhalgh, 2001).

A CAS is a network consisting of many agents that follow simple rules, are in constant dynamic interaction with one another, and can generate complex structures. The CAS has the capacity to adapt and become a good fit within a changing environment. This ability to adapt allows the organism or organization to continually modify itself relative to a changing environment by changing the rules of interaction among component agents. The process of adaptation occurs through learning new rules or behaviors and accumulating new experiences. In this process, the organism/organization evolves through a process of self-organization, which, in turn, allows for creativity and lacks complete predictability. A cardinal aspect of a CAS is that small actions or inputs may have large effects; conversely, large inputs may have small effects.

A CAS has a high degree of adaptive capacity and is characterized by self-similarity, complexity, emergence, and self-organization. The concept of CASs has been used to describe a flock of birds, a school of fish, a hive of bees, a human body, a family, and a community in which each level is considered a system that is different from, and more than, the sum of its parts of components. Each of these CASs is embedded in larger contexts. Moreover, CAS concepts have been applied to human physiology, such as cellular networks, neural networks, and body systems such as the cardiovascular system. It is clear that the application of a CAS perspective is broad and wide, and relevant to health care and nursing.

Components of Complex Adaptive Systems

A CAS is composed of agents that interact within the system. These agents also may be considered a CAS embedded in a larger CAS. For example, an individual in a family is a CAS as well as an agent in the family. These agents act within the system according to patterned behavior. That behavior may self-organize at the CAS level, leading to new emergent behavior. The components of these networks are agents and patterns.

Agents

Agents are units or components of the system, which, as previously mentioned, can be individuals, birds in a flock, bees in a hive, or a component of a human system such as genes or neurons. These agents interact in a particular way, and their interactions and the patterns of interaction are the focus of CS, rather than understanding the agent in isolation. The interaction enables the system to function in a way that could not be understood from the examination of only the components.

Each agent also may be a CAS and, in turn, is also part of a larger CAS. For example, a nurse in a clinic is a CAS as well as an agent in the CAS of the clinic. The nurse coevolves with the unit as the system emerges from the patterns of interactions. In this way, the nurse also contributes to and is affected by the organization of the unit.

Control of a CAS is highly dispersed and decentralized, and the overall behavior of the system is the result of multiple decisions by individual agents (Waldrop, 1992). The agents, as well as the system, are adaptive. Agents have fuzzy boundaries and simultaneously may be members of several systems. Examples include the immune system, a financial market, and a hospital unit.

Patterns

Patterns are formed by agents acting from a set of internalized rules. In a biochemical system, these patterns can be a series of chemical reactions; in an organization, they comprise the behavior of individuals or groups. Patterns and behaviors are the focus of understanding the CAS. Again, the emphasis is the relationships among the agents, rather than the agents themselves. Agents within a CAS have patterns of behavior that evolve. They absorb their past history and experiences, as well as respond to endogenous and exogenous changes. The CAS can develop rules that shape the interaction of the agents. Such systems are capable of emergent patterns that may be incorporated into the CAS's future behavior.

Characteristics of Complex Adaptive Systems

The following characteristics are part of the CAS. Many of these constructs are similar to some of the features of the mathematical and science disciplines (see **Table 6-3** for a summary of CAS characteristics). Here, however, they are applied in a more conceptual or theoretical framework, which allows them to be applied to clinical situations, thereby demonstrating both a patient and an organizational focus.

Connectivity

Agents or components of a system are connected to other components both within the system and within larger systems.

Complex Adaptive Systems Are Dynamic and Adaptive

A key characteristic of a CAS is that it is *dynamic*; that is, the system can adapt to changes in both its internal and external environments. The organism or organization demonstrates transformations of behavior through multiple modes of behavior. According to general systems theory, a system that loses its ability to maintain its equilibrium may cease to exist. Lindberg and colleagues (2008) note that nurses, physicians, and other healthcare

Table 6-3   Complex Adaptive Systems Concepts

Components
- Agents
- Patterns

Characteristics
- Connectivity
- CASs are dynamic and adaptive
- Simple rules allow CASs to function
- Emergence is a property of a CAS
- CASs are self-organizing
- Control is distributed rather than centralized
- Diversity maximizes self-organization
- CASs are deterministic
- CASs are exemplified by embeddedness (i.e., a CAS may be nested within a larger CAS)
- Coordination dynamics occur within a CAS
- CASs are sensitive to initial conditions
- Coevolution occurs with a CAS
- CASs are robust and adaptable

professionals often have an orientation toward homeostasis and strive to maintain the status quo both in physiology and in organizations. A healthy system often features processes that keep the system in a balanced or dynamic state of equilibrium so that the system can adapt to both internal and external stimuli. Complexity exists in the dynamic balance between stability and instability.

Goldberger (1996) provided a physiological illustration of this balance through a discussion of heart rate, rhythm, and cardiac output. At one extreme is a patient who is stable, but whose electrocardiographic tracing strip reflects heart failure with minimum variability. This lack of variability indicates a system that is unable to respond or adapt to changes or demands on the system. This is a most unhealthy, nonadaptive state. Conversely, fibrillation, in which the heart demonstrates chaotic, highly irregular, and unpatterned rhythms, is both dysfunctional and life threatening. These examples stand in contrast to a healthy cardiac system, which operates within the range of complexity so that there are continual alterations in the heart rate in response to small and large stimuli. Thus, the heart is capable of adapting to its changing environment by adjusting output.

Simple Rules Support Complex Adaptive Systems

It is posited in CS that a CAS operates by an adherence to a few *simple rules* that allow the system to function. These rules are not overly specific, written, or overt; rather, they are part of the function of the components of the system. A frequently cited example is used to illustrate some of the rules that allow a flock of birds to fly in a group. The following rules have been suggested by computer modeling: (1) Maintain a minimum specific distance from other birds; (2) match velocity with other birds in the flock; and (3) move toward the center of the mass of birds in the neighborhood. Imagine what it would take to give specific instructions to each bird, depending on the bird's location within the flock.

A different set of rules operate in a bee hive, where residents of the hive have different specific roles and each bee (the agent) adapts to certain external and internal environmental stimuli based on simple rules. When agents follow these rules, a form of collective behavior, a structure or a process that is more complex than the rules that produced it, emerges (Paley, 2007). These simple rules guide the CAS and allow it to act as a system. For example, an application of simple rules allows social insects such as bees to form a collective unit that enables them to behave like a single organism or system (Kauffman, 1995; Waldrop, 1992). Scientists and mathematicians have begun to discover some of these rules and are seeking to construct mathematical models to understand the behavior of the CAS—namely, its ability to behave as a single organism with multiple agents.

Emergence Is a Property of Complex Adaptive Systems

Emergence has been compared to novelty, flexibility, and the creative advancement of a system (Capra, 2002). Novel or new structures, patterns, properties, or processes can emerge during the process of self-organization in a CAS. Examples of emergence include the ways in which termites and ants build large complex structures that appear to have had an architect, designer, or structural engineer guiding the process. The human brain may operate in a similar fashion, as individual neurons (i.e., agents) operate locally and in networks through some simple patterns of reciprocal activation. In both cases, the collective structure or activity cannot be deduced from individual behaviors. These emergent behaviors can be innovative and creative. It is also a possibility that some emergent patterns will not be sustainable or adaptive over the long run.

Complex Adaptive Systems Are Self-Organizing

A cardinal property of a CAS is that it is *self-organizing*. Most CASs operate on a stability~instability dynamic. Self-organization requires appropriate conditions, often described as far from equilibrium or on the edge of chaos. This terminology indicates a zone that is closer to the instability pole where change can occur. Given its ability to exhibit emergent collective behavior, the CAS can self-organize into novel or new patterns. In this way, it moves away from a simple equilibrium or stable state and activates the nonlinearity inherent in the system. This evolution may lead to a new pattern and change the dynamics of the system. The important concept here is that these activities, behaviors, or patterns come from the CAS without the imposition of a central grand plan or control, or an externally imposed plan.

Control Is Distributed Rather Than Centralized

A characteristic of self-organization in a CAS is *distributed control*. This term implies that the agents or components do not act through a central agent or blueprint within or outside of the system. There is no central control that is responsible for the behavior or structures that emerge; rather, the CAS is a network of disparate agents exhibiting coherence and the ability to change without central direction or a single intelligent executive function. The commonality in the examples of emergence is that the activity or structure is produced by local interactions, without any central command center. This principle is often referred to as *distributed control* (Lindberg et al., 2008), previously addressed.

Unexpected complex results from the decentralized local interaction of agents often appear to mimic more centralized organized and planned activities that are evident in a growing number of disciplines (Paley, 2007). For example, the brain has approximately 100 billion individual neurons—agents interacting with one another through hormonal and other mediators, which are themselves often localized (Holt, 2004). The individual neurons have no cognitive capacity, but nonlinear interactions between them may generate higher-level cognitive functions. Distributed control is an important characteristic of self-organization. Nevertheless, the self-organization is not always independent of the environment because often it is the environment to which the CAS adapts.

Complex Adaptive Systems Have Diversity

Diversity has been identified as a characteristic that maximizes self-organization. The greater the diversity of the components or patterns, the more robust and adaptable the system can be. Having diversity allows for the use of multiple resources to respond to external stimuli and internal adaptations (Lindberg et al., 2008). Diversity in a system provides for novelty and is a source of the capability for adaption. It is a key to innovation and long-term viability in both individuals and organizations. In addition, diversity has been demonstrated to be an essential ingredient in healthy ecosystems (Wilson, 1992). When the ecosystem is unhealthy and the environment is ruined, civilizations can collapse.

Complex Adaptive Systems Are Deterministic

CASs tend to have patterns that follow or are *determined by* earlier ones. This stands in contrast to stochastic or random systems, in which there is no predictability or coherent pattern from previous states. The CAS operates by applying simple rules, and often these patterns continue and are predictable in the short run. The tendency toward determinism can be cause for confusion because this characteristic coexists with emergence and self-organization. Even in complex emergence, there is generally a pattern that is not totally chaotic, but rather demonstrates a self-similar pattern.

Complex Adaptive Systems Are Exemplified by Embeddedness

Similar to the hierarchy of systems in systems theory, CASs exist in an ecological nest of *embeddedness*. Similar to systems theory, one can locate the level of the system as the focal system, with those systems within it being considered subsystems. This system is embedded then in larger systems, which form its context. It is important to locate the level that one is addressing to discuss it. Complexity scientists often refer to the concept of embeddedness as levels that represent (1) an external level as the context, (2) the middle level as the focus of the interactions among the agents, and (3) the inner level as the agents and behaviors within the focal system. All actions and dynamics influence and are influenced by all three levels, with each level influencing all of the others. The degree of cohesion between the three levels depends on each nested system's behaviors. When one of the nested systems experiences a change or perturbation, the entire system is affected. An example of how changes in a system can alter the network of embedded systems can be seen with fluctuations in the stock markets. In 2008, when the U.S. stock market experienced a crisis, stock markets around the world experienced the effects.

Coordination Dynamics Occur Within Complex Adaptive Systems

Coordination dynamics are context dependent and operate according to a three-part process of interaction between parts: (1) within a focal (or part of a) system, such as the firing of neurons within the brain; (2) between different parts of the same system, such as between the heart and the lungs; and (3) between other systems, the person, and the environment (Kelso & Engstrom, 2006). A significant amount of this interaction is related to self-organization. These coordinating elements interact with one another, as well as their surroundings, and they organize themselves into dynamic patterns.

Complex Adaptive Systems Are Sensitive to Initial Conditions

Given these dynamics, one can see how initial conditions could have a great impact on outcomes. Even a small perturbation in the system has the capacity to greatly alter the future structures, patterns, and processes. Lorenz (1993), a leading figure in chaos theory, noted that a small change in the initial condition of a system might trigger a chain of events that could lead to large-scale alterations of outcomes. The metaphor of the *butterfly effect* has become very popular. As small an input as a butterfly flapping its wings in Brazil can, at a critical point, alter the weather system so that a tornado occurs in Kansas. This highly sensitive nature of the CAS underscores the difficulty of making long-term predictions. Indeed, a condition in a certain time or space may significantly affect the dynamics of the system under certain conditions, but not others. Thus small inputs may have large effects, and large effects may have simple causes. For example, a person may be exposed to multiple viruses many times yet never become sick; in contrast, at a different time and place, just a minimum exposure may result in sickness.

Coevolution Occurs With Complex Adaptive Systems

When the environment includes other CASs, a process of reciprocal adaptive dynamics often occurs. In this case, two systems are simultaneously changing and self-organizing, a process termed *coevolution*. Many scientists cite coevolution and the adaptive changes that organisms and the universe have made as an explanation for evolution (Kauffman, 1995). An example might be the way in which a parasite and its host coevolve to form a single system, with each party benefiting from and adapting to the other, but evolving to a different system than either one independently (Lindberg et al., 2008).

Robustness and Adaptability

Robust systems are able to continue to function and adapt to changes within the system as well as changes in the environment. A robust system can respond to external and internal changes while still maintaining the integrity and function of the system. Some of this adaptability is related to the coordination of stability with disruption/transformation.

COMPLEX ADAPTIVE SYSTEMS, COMPLEX RESPONSIVE PROCESSES, AND ORGANIZATIONS

Several authors have applied CAS concepts to organizations (Plsek, 1997), while others have made a distinction between CASs and complex responsive processes (CRPs; Stacey, 2001) in applying complexity to systems. CAS is the term more widely used in the United States when dealing with HCOs. The following sections provide brief discussions of organizations from both perspectives.

Organizations as Complex Adaptive Systems

Plsek (as cited by the Institute of Medicine [IOM], 2001), in reference to organizational systems, defined a CAS as a system of individual agents who are interconnected, yet have freedom to act in novel and unpredictable ways. One agent's action changes the context for other agents, which illustrates how control is dispersed throughout the interaction among agents.

Applying complexity to organizational structure was advocated by Plsek (2001). He illustrated his advocacy for complexity first with an example of the mechanistic approach, and he then contrasted it with an example of complex, self-organizing behaviors. A good surgical team operates via a mechanistic approach, such that their actions are predictable and ordered. This is seen as the only viable approach because an "either/or" perspective fears any approach that is not ordered. Thus the choice in the operating room is strict control—an ordered mechanistic approach that has both benefits and limitations. Plsek contrasts that example with a unit that is more complex and that self-organizes and emerges with creativity. In this area, new and novel behaviors occur. It is important to note that this emergent behavior can manifest as either innovation or error. Plsek advocated for an application of CAS concepts to describe a middle zone of complexity in which a CAS can act within a range of adaptability from highly ordered to an area of emergence, with the ability to adapt to different conditions.

Plsek (2001) criticized traditional management theory because of its emphasis on ways to establish order and control through the actions of a few people at the top of the organizational hierarchy. Jordan and colleagues (2009) described order and structure, as well as innovation, spontaneously coming about through self-organization. Emergent properties can be produced from self-organization of agents at lower levels, which then leads to patterns and order at higher levels, which in turn can reinforce existing patterns or create systems change. Plsek (1997) described the perspective of viewing the organization through the lens of a CAS, which would avoid the limitations associated with overcontrolled hierarchical organizations. By expressing general direction and a few basic principles, CAS leaders could allow enough flexibility for the adaptability and creativity of the organization to emerge.

It was contended that the organization could be able to achieve a balance by integrating a planned, ordered approach with a more flexible approach. Plsek used the metaphors of clockware (planned, rational, repeatable, standardized, and measured) and swarmware (exploring new possibilities, trials, freedom, autonomy, and intuition) to describe this process. By working at the edge of knowledge and experience or near the edge of chaos, maximum flexibility and innovation can be realized. Operating from this edge of chaos allows creativity to emerge, but at the same time, creates a need to balance the tension fostered by simultaneously maintaining the status quo and allowing creative change. In advocating for this blending of approaches, Plsek emphasized a need for interaction among agents to work through the tensions of perspectives as well as allowing new ideas to emerge.

Plsek (2001) described how a few simple rules can be demonstrated in organizations that allow for both functional order and creativity, citing the Internet as a prime example. He highlighted the many successful high-tech firms that have fewer rules, structures, and policies than their less successful competitors. Plsek identified three types of simple rules that can apply to organizations: (1) rules that point to a general direction such that management provides the general direction or goals for the organization; (2) prohibitions or regulatory and boundary-setting rules, which restrain and maintain standards and order; and (3) recourses, incentives, and permission-providing rules, which allow for innovation and rewards.

Lanham and colleagues (2009) also used the concept of CASs in an analysis of four studies dealing with primary care. These researchers found that the CAS was a useful and comprehensive theory to explore emergence of systems-level properties arising over time from local interactions among agents. They determined that practice-level quality is viewed best in holistic ways as systems issues rather than individual components. Thus, making an effort to improve the relationships among the members, rather than focusing on the individual components, allows for more effective strategies for improvement.

Organizations and Complex Responsive Processes

Organizational theorist Ralph Stacey (2001) applied complexity thinking to organizations and coined a new term, *complex responsive process* (CRP). Stacey objected to the systems approach, which he contended placed the organization and individuals at different explanatory levels. Instead, he focused on learning and knowledge creation. His premise is that organizational knowledge can be found in the relationships and conversations between people within an organization. The individual mind and the social world are the same process; thus knowledge is in perpetual construction. The potential for both continuity and change exist within these everyday conversations. Therefore, change comes from the interaction between or among individual people. The complexity concepts of self-organization, emergence, and nonlinear patterns of behavior are applied in this model as well.

Complex Responsive Processes and Relationship-Centered Care

CRP approaches have been promoted by Suchman (2006) as part of *relationship-centered care* (RCC) and through *complex responsive processes of relating* (CRPRs). RCC is based on a Pew–Fetzer task force effort to advance humanism in medicine in order to combat the objectivist and reductive approach of science-based practice. RCC went a step further by advocating the notion of patient-centered care and the biopsychosocial model. RCC is founded on four principles:

1. Relationships in health care include the personhood of the participant.
2. Affect and emotions are important components of these relationships.
3. Healthcare relationships occur in the context of reciprocal influence.
4. Genuine relationships in health care are morally valuable, and the patient–clinician relationship is central, but relationships of clinicians with one another, with the community, and within themselves are important as well (Beach, Inui, & The Relationship-Centered Care Research Network, 2006, p. 53).

Drawing on Stacey's work on CRP, Suchman (2006) used a process of CRPR to examine pieces of meaning and relating in each relationship encounter. These patterns reflect role structures, dominance hierarchies, and behavioral norms, as well as vocabulary, concepts, and knowledge (particular and specific). The self-organization of patterns in social process is ubiquitous. Self-organization at this level requires the simultaneous action of order~disorder and constraint~freedom. CRPR allows one to determine how these patterns are created and maintained. Suchman has applied this approach to patient–provider encounters, as well as to interprofessional relationships. These applications, which are often of a reciprocal nature, could have significant relevance to the relationships between nurses and patients.

IMPLICATIONS FOR PRACTICE

Practice as Complex Adaptive Systems

The IOM (2001) noted that complexity in the practice setting is a leading variable in the "significant unpredictability and variation in clinical outcomes." One can think of practice from the perspective of various sizes of systems. Microsystems, mesosystems, and macrosystems are all CASs that are related and connected through relationships (Roussel, 2014). It is through the connections within these systems that providers interact with patients, that providers interact with other providers, and so forth. The clinical microsystem, for example, is the frontline unit of care that interacts with the patient, and those interactions affect outcomes. High-performance clinical microsystems foster a positive culture of open and respectful interaction focused on the patient's and the provider's mutual goal of optimal patient outcomes (Batelden, Nelson, Edwards, Godfrey, & Mohr, 2003). Clinical microsystems are dynamic and sensitive to small changes such as the attitude of one of its members, which can have a major influence on group dynamics and patient outcomes.

Any number of CAS microsystem interactions can be cited as examples, but one of great current interest is the interaction that occurs during a transition in care. What happens when several clinical microsystems interact—as they do during transitions of care—in increasingly rapid cycles? Care transition is defined as hospital discharge of the patient or movement of the patient from one healthcare setting to another (Geary & Schumacher, 2012). Many of these transitions occur in the context of increasingly fragmented care. One of the strengths of using a CAS approach to clinical situations is that CAS concepts can be integrated with other models and theories to expand understanding. One useful model is Meleis's (2010) middle-range transition theory. As Geary and Schumacher (2012) point out, combining CAS concepts from CS with transition theory provides a powerful new lens through which to view care transitions and ultimately a means to improve transition outcomes within the current context of limited continuity and consistency in care.

Viewing Healthcare Organizations Through the Lens of Complexity

It is generally accepted that HCOs are examples of a high order of complexity systems because these organizations typically contain systems embedded within other systems. From a macrosystems perspective, each HCO is part of a larger entity. An individual healthcare facility could be part of a larger healthcare system that includes a number of other facilities. The individual facility or system is, in turn, part of the local and national healthcare system that provides for the comprehensive healthcare needs of the nation across care settings and services. From a microsystems perspective, the HCO is composed of a number of traditional administrative and service lines, all of which are divided into smaller units that provide a variety of focused services to specific populations.

In examining an organization such as an acute care facility, the number of different units within larger units is striking. For example, major units on the organizational chart may include nursing administration, nursing/patient care units, food services, pharmacy, rehabilitation services, diagnostics (laboratory and radiology), business management, and environmental services. Each of these major units, in turn, has subunits. For example, patient care units may be organized around body systems, such as cardiovascular surgery, orthopedics, or neurology. Nurses who work within these units become highly specialized in the care of the target population. These nurses tend to develop expert knowledge related to the care of this population and create a culture that addresses and supports the special problems and needs of the population of interest. Such a unit is also part of the system of nursing services, with the unit and nursing service interacting. Additionally, each unit interacts with other nursing units and departments such as rehabilitation, radiology, and food services.

The overall purpose of HCOs is to deliver high-quality, comprehensive care that is coordinated, integrated, and cost-effective. In *Crossing the Quality Chasm: A New Health System for the 21st Century* (IOM, 2001), six recommendations to improve the current healthcare system are outlined: Health care should be safe, effective, patient centered, timely, efficient, and equitable. In preparing its report, the IOM committee was guided by the belief that care must be delivered by systems that have been designed carefully and consciously. The committee noted the following:

> Such systems must be designed to serve the needs of patients, and to ensure that they are fully informed, retain control and participate in care delivery whenever possible, and receive care that is respectful of their values and preferences. Such systems must facilitate the application of scientific knowledge to practice, and provide clinicians with the tools and supports necessary to deliver evidence-based care consistently and safely. (IOM, 2001, pp. 7–8)

When describing systems in the report, reference is made to all systems that affect healthcare delivery, such as regulatory, insurance, and HCOs; here, the focus is limited to HCOs, though we fully recognize that other systems interact with and influence HCOs and healthcare delivery. All systems must have at least two core values that include to serve the needs of patients and to allow patients to retain control over and fully participate in their own health care. Viewing HCOs through the lens of CS provides a dynamic framework for examining HCOs as CASs.

Healthcare Organizations as Complex Adaptive Systems

CASs are special cases of complex systems. No format or guideline exists to help one determine precisely what qualifies as a simple system or a complex system, although individual and collective wisdom are thought to make the distinction. In complex systems, unpredictability and paradox are ever present, and some things will inevitably remain unknowable (Plsek & Greenhalgh, 2001). This section addresses some key issues related to the framing and understanding of HCOs in terms of contemporary and highly complex organizations. They include new models of HCOs, leadership, and research.

New Models of Healthcare Organizations

Models of organizational development and change based on linearity, vertical organization, hierarchal decision making, and controlled change strategies are outmoded and do not work within contemporary HCOs. New models are needed to understand the dynamic fast-paced volatility of healthcare delivery changes that influence HCOs.

New mental models must replace outdated ones, and CS offers a new paradigm. CS is as much a vehicle for change as it is for creating a lens to understand organizations and change (Norman, 2009). As defined by cognitive scientists, a *mental model* is a concept that refers to deeply held or ingrained assumptions or generalizations about external reality, which can take the form of patterns or images that, in turn, frame and focus how we understand the world (Werhane, 1999). Individuals construct mental models based on knowledge and experience gained in the past. These mental models are used then to understand the present, allowing the individual to make decisions and to act (Rouse & Morris, 1986). Two important points about mental models are noteworthy. First, mental models are socially learned and, therefore, incomplete. Second, because they are socially learned, they are open to change (Chen, Mills, & Werhane, 2008). Mental models shape the way we see the world, and they can change over time.

The past is populated with mental models that primarily represent only linear thinking. In fact, the complexity of modern-day HCOs and healthcare delivery makes simple linear thinking obsolete. To manage the escalating complexity in HCOs and healthcare delivery, healthcare professionals must abandon the unitary approach of linear models, accept unpredictability, respect and make use of autonomy and creativity, and respond flexibly to emerging patterns and opportunities (Plsek & Greenhalgh, 2001). This transformation requires incorporating a complexity perspective to better understand the dynamics of these organizations. As previously emphasized, a "both/and" perspective rather than an "either/or" assumption is appropriate.

New Models of Leadership

Leadership styles change in a culture of complexity. An understanding of the organization as a CAS allows its leaders to accommodate their leadership style by engaging the natural dynamics of groups to self-organize to new situations and changes in both the ecosystem and the internal system. One such model applied in a CAS milieu is sometimes referred to as an *emergent model of leadership.* In CAS networks, leaders are open, responsive catalysts; they are collaborative co-participants who are connected and adaptable and who acknowledge paradoxes. These leaders value people and are engaged, continuously emerging, and able to shift as processes unfold. They decrease the burden imposed by rules, help others, and are good listeners.

By contrast, in many traditional hierarchical linear-oriented systems, leaders value position and structure; they are controlling, in charge, autonomous, self-preserving, and disengaged; they hold and value formal positions, set rules, make decisions, and repeat the past. This system bears little resemblance to a CAS, in which there are a few simple rules and the self-organizing dynamics are understood, thereby allowing for emergent adaptive behavior.

Leaders who embrace complexity and the CAS perspective view their roles differently. With a vision that allows the system to evolve, they support and encourage emergence and self-organization, rather than being controlling and dictatorial. Creativity is stimulated and encouraged. Key stakeholders are supported as they work to find solutions to problems affecting them. The vertical authority gradient of the top-down hierarchy is flattened, and new collegial partnerships based on respect, trust, and values replace autocratic leadership.

To facilitate the creation of such leaders in this new age of CS, major changes must occur in how leadership is perceived and prepared through formal educational processes and mentorships. This effort will also require a receptive organizational environment with a new vision of an organizational culture.

New Models for Research

Viewing HCOs from a reductionist perspective and using the machine as a metaphor to understand dynamic and adaptive systems have clear limitations. The randomized controlled trial (RCT), often described as the gold standard of research design, comes from the tradition of reductionism and, therefore, is not sufficient for the nonlinear and dynamic nature of the CAS. This is not to say that RCTs and other research designs based on a reductionist foundation are not useful; rather, the key point is that envisioning these designs as the *only* approach to understanding is knowledge limiting. It is important for researchers to apply the appropriate model and methodology to investigations and be open to expanding paradigms and methods.

Researchers McDaniel, Lanham, and Anderson (2009) emphasize that because HCOs are CASs, the phenomena of interest tend to be dynamic and unfold in unpredictable ways, and these unfolding events are often unique. Current research designs and methodologies fail to capture either the dynamic nature of the area of interest or the unpredictable unique occurrences. McDaniel and colleagues (2009) note that the traditional classification of research as either qualitative or quantitative is distracting and often not helpful in this setting because both approaches begin with a question, build or test models, and aim to understand or explain the phenomena of interest. Neither category alone is a perfect match for CASs, although the use of mixed-methods models in conjunction with new methodologies will more likely capture the richness of CASs and lead to better understandings. Using qualitative-quantitative research embraces a "both/and" approach rather than an "either/or" philosophy.

One emerging approach is *action research*, in which researchers incorporate action perspectives to change organizational patterns by actively engaging stakeholders in the change process (Koch & Kralik, 2006). For example, researchers are also using other techniques such as *positive deviance* to discover a unit within an organization that has significantly better outcomes or better approaches to problems with similar resources and constraints and in which others hold the view that the unit or area is exceptional. A positive deviance approach can be used as a model for change in other areas of the organization. Another approach, *appreciative inquiry*, is used by researchers to discover and then amplify what works "well" within an organization and to discover the direction that the organizational team chooses to take based on what has transpired in the past. When this strategy is employed, a culture of positive innovation can flourish.

The state of the science of CAS research is developing as well. Bar-Yam (2000) developed techniques to study nonlinear dynamics in complex systems. McDaniel and Driebe (2001) applied CAS theory to the analysis of HCOs. Agar (2004) combined ethnographic approaches with agent-based modeling to understand social systems. Non-reductionist strategies also have been frequently applied to understand large-scale systems such as hurricanes (Sornette, 2006).

Maguire, McKelvey, Mirabeau, and Oztas (2006) conducted a survey of CS and organizational studies. The 2009 issues of the *Journal of Evaluation in Clinical Practice* include a collection of articles about CS, and an ongoing section appears in subsequent issues. The interest in HCOs and CASs is growing, and new research methodologies are emerging to support this interest.

Recently, complexity has been applied to clinical research. Understanding the human as a complex system has led to new approaches in clinical research. Systems biology, which examines the network structures and dynamics with regard to regulatory circuits, is exploring the system's robustness in regard to adaptation to external forces, internal stability, and graceful degradation, which allows for a gradual aging process (Kitano, 2002). Complexity has been applied to multiple organ dysfunction syndrome (Seely & Christou, 2000) and sepsis (Mann, Engebretson, & Batchinsky, 2013). Research techniques that track multiple points of physiological data using computers to analyze very large data sets are now available. One example of computational analysis of large data is analyses of fractal dynamics and presence of loss of complexity. Research in complexity is generally conducted with interdisciplinary teams, representing clinical, biological, mathematical, and computational expertise.

APPLICATION TO HEALTH CARE AND NURSING

Application to Clinical Care

With the advent of computers and the corresponding ability to manage large amounts of data quickly, interdisciplinary teams have begun to apply complexity concepts to physiology and the management of patient care. West (2008), a physicist, advocated a medical application of a complexity approach, using it to program life-support equipment to a more appropriate variability in healthy people. For example, he suggested that the patterns of respirations should be studied and that the finer variability be programmed into respirators, rather than relying on a mechanically regular pulsation. Use of the complexity concept in this way addresses the adaptive pattern that can be predicted in the short run. This kind of agent-based modeling simulates the operations of complex physiological behavior in an attempt to re-create and predict the appearance of complex phenomena.

A key notion in CS is that simple behavioral rules generate complex behavior. This principle facilitates developing supportive interventions to mimic that pattern. The pattern can be drawn from theory or from actual empirical data of an individual patient. In another application, a team of researchers in the Veterans Administration used detailed monitoring of heart rate variability in trauma victims to identify early changes in the autonomic nervous system, thereby allowing for earlier intervention than was possible with the existing technology (Salinas, 2010). This is also applied in some intensive care units where panels of biomarkers are fed into computers that can generate patterns that might indicate a loss of complexity, thus allowing for earlier detection of changes in the patient's condition. Other researchers have advocated for the use of complex systems modeling as a means to obtain a better understanding of the obesity epidemic (Hammond, 2009).

Application to Nursing

CS and its application to nursing, health care, and HCOs is emerging as a new paradigm capturing the interest of scholars across a number of diverse disciplines (see **Box 6-1**). The use of computers has assisted researchers in refining CS, which in turn, has inspired a new paradigm in scientific thinking. This paradigm shift has influenced the way people interpret the world.

SUMMARY

The concepts of complexity are pervading many areas of study and have multiple applications to health care. A paradigm based on CS is congruent with the holistic paradigm familiar to nursing. The ability to apply the science as well as the associated change in thinking about physiology, human beings, groups, and organizations has significant implications for the

---

Box 6-1 CS Application to Health Care

In this chapter, advanced practice nurses (APNs) are introduced to an important paradigm through which to view clinical practice and care environments in new ways. Clinically, nurses need to be aware of a new spectrum of thought that can capture the details and complexities of human physiology. Adoption of this paradigm will enable the APN to provide more individualized patient-centered care to augment the adaptive capacity of the human body. Because new research findings based on CS are becoming available, it is important for APNs to understand the terminology and conceptual framework so that they can apply this new knowledge to patient care. In addition, this paradigm shift will spawn numerous applications of emergent technologies in patient care.

The complexity paradigm has major implications for health care through its application to organizations and work environments. As organizations struggle to be more responsive to internal and external issues, the ability to be flexible, adaptive, and innovative becomes essential for survival. Many organizations are beginning to apply CS at all levels within the organization. Nurses at all levels must understand this important framework of CASs if they are to maximize their ability to function both individually and as part of teams to sustain a dynamic and relevant organization poised for innovation and change in response to the ever more complex healthcare environment.

---

discipline of nursing. In keeping with the holistic approach, it is important to remember that the complexity perspective is complementary to the reductionist model. Together, they offer a more complete and holistic view of the world. For further reading on CS and CASs, see **Table 6-4**.

Table 6-4   Sources for Further Reading

General References of Interest
Kauffman, S. (1995). *At home in the universe: The search for laws of self-organization*. New York, NY: Oxford University Press.
Kelso, J. A. S., & Engstrom, D. A. (2006). *The complementary nature*. Cambridge, MA: MIT Press.
Stacey, R. (2001). *Complex responsive processes in organizations*. New York, NY: Routledge.
Waldrop, M. M. (1992). *Complexity: The emerging science at the edge of order and chaos*. New York, NY: Simon & Schuster.
Zimmerman, B., Lindberg, C., & Plsek, P. (1998). *Edgeware: Lessons from complexity science for health care leaders*. Bordentown, NJ: Plexus Press.

Specific to Nursing
Lindberg, C., Nash, S., & Lindberg, C. (2008). *On the edge: Nursing in the age of complexity*. Bordentown, NJ: Plexus Press.

Website
Plexus Institute: http://www.plexusinstitute.org

DISCUSSION QUESTIONS

1. How does more diversity in the nursing profession relate to CASs?
2. How could some of the agent-based modeling concepts be applied to patient-centered care?
3. How could local units in a hospital or clinic setting apply concepts of self-organization to become more adaptive to situational demands?
4. How could the APN apply the concepts of a CAS to individual patient care?
5. Reflect on a professional or personal experience when a seemingly small incident had a much larger impact than expected. What did you learn from this experience?

REFERENCES

Agar, M. H. (2004). We have met the other and we're not all nonlinear: Ethnography as a nonlinear dynamic system. *Complexity, 10*(2), 16–24.

Anderson, R. A., Issel, L. M., & McDaniel, R. R. (2003). Nursing homes as complex adaptive systems: Relationship between management practice and resident outcomes. *Nursing Research, 52*(1), 12–21.

Baranger, M. (2009). *Chaos, complexity and entropy: A physics talk for non-physicists* (Unpublished manuscript). Massachusetts Institute of Technology, Boston, MA.

Bar-Yam, Y. (Ed.). (2000). *Unifying themes in complex systems: Proceedings of the International Conference on Complex Systems.* Cambridge, MA: Perseus Books.

Batelden, P. B., Nelson, E. C., Edwards, W. H., Godfrey, M., & Mohr, J. J. (2003). Microsystems in health care: Part 9. Developing small clinical units to attain peak performance. *Joint Commission Journal on Quality and Patient Safety, 11,* 575–585.

Beach, M. C., Inui, T., & The Relationship-Centered Care Research Network. (2006). Relationship centered care: A constructive reframing. *Journal of General Internal Medicine, 21,* S3–S8.

Capra, F. (2002). *The hidden connections.* New York, NY: Doubleday.

Chen, D. T., Mills, A. E., & Werhane, P. H. (2008). Tools for tomorrow's health care system: A systems-informed mental model, moral imagination, and physicians' professionalism. *Academic Medicine, 83*(8), 723–732.

Crabtree, B. F., Miller, W. L., & Strange, K. C. (2001). Understanding practice from the ground up. *Journal of Family Practice, 50*(10), 881–887.

Geary, C. R., & Schumacher, K. L. (2012). Care transitions: Integrating transition theory and complexity science concepts. *Advances in Nursing Science, 35*(3), 236–248.

Goldberger, A. (1996). Non-linear dynamics for clinicians: Chaos theory, fractals and complexity at the bedside. *Lancet, 347,* 1312–1314.

Hammond, R. A. (2009). Complex systems modeling for obesity research. *Preventing Chronic Disease: Public Health Research, Practice and Policy, 6*(3), 1–10.

Holt, T. (2004). *Complexity for clinicians.* Oxford, UK: Radcliffe Medical Press.

Institute of Medicine. (2001). *Crossing the quality chasm: A new health system for the 21st century.* Washington, DC: National Academy Press.

Jordan, M. E., Lanham, H. J., Crabtree, B. F., Nutting, P. A., Miller, W. L., Strange, K. C., & McDaniel, R. R. (2009). The role of conversation in health care interventions: Enabling sensemaking and

learning. *Implementation Science, 4*(15). Open access BioMed Central. Retrieved from http://www
.implementationscience.com/content/4/1/15

Kauffman, S. (1995). *At home in the universe: The search for laws of self-organization.* New York,
NY: Oxford University Press.

Kelso, J. A. S., & Engstrom, D. A. (2006). *The complementary nature.* Cambridge, MA: MIT Press.

Kitano, H. (2002). Systems biology: A brief overview. *Science, 295*(560), 1162–1664.

Koch, T., & Kralik, D. (2006). *Participatory action research in health care.* Malden, MA: Blackwell.

Lanham, H. J., McDaniel, R. R., Crabtree, B. R., Miller, W. L., Strange, K. C., Tallia, A. F., & Nutting,
P. A. (2009). How improving practice relationships among clinicians and nonclinicians can improve
quality in primary care. *The Joint Commission Journal on Quality and Patient Safety, 35*(9), 457–466.

Liebovitz, L. S. (1998). *Fractals and chaos simplified for the life sciences.* New York, NY: Oxford
University Press.

Lindberg, C., Nash, S., & Lindberg, C. (2008). *On the edge: Nursing in the age of complexity.*
Bordentown, NJ: Plexus Press.

Lorenz, E. N. (1993). *The essence of chaos.* Seattle, WA: University of Washington Press.

Maguire, S., McKelvey, B., Mirabeau, L., & Oztas, N. (2006). Complexity science and organization
studies. In S. R. Clegg, C. Hardy, T. B. Lawrence, & W. R. Nord (Eds.), *The Sage handbook of
organization studies* (2nd ed., pp. 165–214). London, UK: Sage.

Mandelbrot, B. B. (1967). How long is the coast of Britain? *Science, 156,* 636–638.

Mandelbrot, B. B. (1982). *The fractal geometry of nature.* San Francisco, CA: W. H. Freeman.

Mann, E., Engebretson, J., & Batchinsky, A. (2013). A complex systems view of sepsis: Implications
for nursing. *Dimensions of Critical Care Nursing, 32*(1), 12–17.

McDaniel, R. R., & Driebe, D. J. (2001). Complexity science and health care management. In J. D. Blaire,
M. D. Fottler, & G. T. Savage (Eds.), *Advances in health care management* (Vol. 2, pp. 11–36). Stamford,
CT: JAI Press.

McDaniel, R. R., Lanham, H. J., & Anderson, R. A. (2009). Implications of complex adaptive systems
theory for the design of research on health care organizations. *Health Care Management Review,*
14(2), 191–199.

Meleis, A. (2010). *Transitions theory: Middle range and situation specific theories in nursing research
and practice.* New York, NY: Springer.

Norman, C. D. (2009). Health promotion as a systems science and practice. *Journal of Evaluation
in Clinical Practice, 15*(5), 868–872.

Paley, J. (2007). Complex adaptive systems and nursing. *Nursing Inquiry, 14*(30), 233–242.

Phelan, S. E. (2001). What is complexity science, really? *Emergence, 3*(1), 120–136.

Plsek, P. E. (1997). *Creativity, innovation, and quality.* New York, NY: McGraw-Hill.

Plsek, P. E. (2001). Redesigning health care with insights from the science of complex adaptive systems. In Institute of Medicine, Committee on Quality of Health Care in America (Ed.), *Crossing
the quality chasm: A new health system for the 21st century* (pp. 322–335). Washington, DC:
National Academy of Sciences.

Plsek, P. E., & Greenhalgh, T. (2001). The challenge of complexity in health care. *British Medical
Journal, 323,* 625–628.

Richardson, K. A. (2005). Systems theory and complexity: Part 3. *Emergence: Complexity & Organization, 7*(2), 104–114.

Rouse, W. B., & Morris, N. M. (1986). On looking into the black box: Prospects and limits in the search for mental models. *Psychological Bulletin, 100,* 349–363.

Roussel, L. A. (2014). The nature of the evidence: Microsystems, macrosystems, and mesosystems. In H. R. Hall & L. A. Roussel (Eds.), *Evidence-based practice: An integrative approach to research, administration, and practice* (pp. 171–184). Burlington, MA: Jones & Bartlett Learning.

Salinas, J. (2010). *Analysis, classification, and complexity of physiologic signals to support medical decision support: Why is my computer smarter than me????* Presentation at University of Texas–Houston School of Nursing, February 2, 2010.

Seely, A. J. E., & Christou, N. V. (2000). Multiple organ dysfunction syndrome: Exploring the paradigm of complex nonlinear systems. *Critical Care Medicine, 28*(7), 2193–2200.

Sornette, D. (2006). *Critical phenomena in natural sciences: Chaos, fractals, self-organization and disorder: Concepts and tools* (2nd ed.). Berlin, Germany: Springer-Verlag.

Stacey, R. (2001). *Complex responsive processes in organizations.* New York, NY: Routledge.

Sturmberg, J. P., & Martin, C. M. (2009). Complexity and health: Yesterday's traditions, tomorrow's future. *Journal of Evaluation in Clinical Practice, 15*(5), 543–548.

Suchman, A. (2006). A new theoretical foundation for relationship-centered care: Complex responsive process of relating. *Journal of General Internal Medicine, 21,* 40–44.

Waldrop, M. M. (1992). *Complexity: The emerging science at the edge of order and chaos.* New York, NY: Simon & Schuster.

Werhane, P. H. (1999). *Moral imagination and management decision making* (pp. 11–12). New York, NY: Oxford University Press.

West, B. (2008). A physicist looks at physiology. In C. Lindberg, S. Nash, & C. Lindberg (Eds.), *On the edge: Nursing in the age of complexity* (pp. 97–123). Bordentown, NJ: Plexus Press.

Wilson, E. O. (1992). *The diversity of life.* Cambridge, MA: Belknap Press.

Wilson, T., Holt, T., & Greenhalgh, T. (2001). Complexity science: Complexity and clinical care. *British Medical Journal, 323,* 685–688.

Zimmerman, B., Lindberg, C., & Plsek, P. (1998). *Edgeware: Lessons from complexity science for health care leaders.* Bordentown, NJ: Plexus Press.

Chapter 7

Critical Theory and Emancipatory Knowing

Peggy L. Chin

INTRODUCTION

This chapter provides an overview of emancipatory knowing and the critical philosophy and theory upon which emancipatory knowing is founded. Emphasis is placed on the importance of critical perspectives for best practices in nursing. The chapter provides specific guidelines for developing and evaluating nursing practice based on critical approaches.

Emancipatory knowing in nursing is a term that refers to a pattern of knowing that has conceptual roots in critical social theory and practice. Critical social theory is a general perspective that uncovers social, historical, and ideological forces and structures that limit human potential and that produce injustice and inequity in society. Emancipatory knowing in nursing is defined by Chinn and Kramer (2015) as "the human capacity to be aware of and critically reflect on the social, cultural, and political status quo, and to figure out how and why it came to be that way." In short, emancipatory knowing is a central, critical, and necessary pattern of knowing that underpins the development of all nursing knowledge and that shapes all nursing practices that flow from nursing's disciplinary knowledge. The recent collection of original works by leading nurse scholars in the area of emancipatory nursing identifies emancipatory nursing as a type of nursing practice that is grounded in awareness of social and political factors that create injustices in health and well-being and that takes action to address these social structures in order to improve health and well-being of all people (Kagan, Smith, & Chinn, 2014).

The critical philosophical perspective of emancipatory nursing frames social problems as circumstances that are unjustly created by humans. Furthermore, it posits that humans can change these circumstances. All too often, however, the social order is taken for granted and assumed to just be "the way things are." In fact, social structures have developed over generations and are well entrenched. Thus, they typically have been thought not to be open to challenge, even when the structure sustains serious injustices and harm.

Politics is the process of exercising one's values and desires in a social situation. Critical perspectives view all human activities as political, in the sense that what humans do and say inevitably affects others. When human actions harm or disadvantage others, or limit human potential in any way, those actions are inherently wrong and need to be changed so that no member of the society is harmed or disadvantaged.

Despite the persistent assumption that nurses shy away from political matters, the fact remains that nursing practice, by definition, is inherently and deeply political. Put simply, a fundamental goal of nursing is to bring about maximum health and well-being for every individual, family, and community. This goal is intentionally aimed at establishing an explicit value in a social community. To accomplish this goal, nurses must remain constantly vigilant in identifying circumstances that impede its achievement. The more deeply nurses probe to identify and address the underlying causes or circumstances that create barriers to maximum health and well-being, the closer they come to identifying social, cultural, and political barriers that limit the potential for maximum health (Kagan, Smith, Cowling, & Chinn, 2009).

Consider, for example, a relatively simple low-tech nursing activity—setting up and conducting a clinic to provide health screening, monitoring, and supervision for elders served by a community senior center. Such a clinic is assumed to contribute to the health and well-being of the people to be served and to promote their achievement of optimal health. Typically, establishing such a clinic represents an effort to change something about the kinds of services the people can access and to provide a social network of support that was not available in the community previously. To get the clinic set up and functioning, myriad community-based arrangements are required, including the very political activities involved in working with various agencies and individuals to gain their cooperation in making the clinic a reality. Once the clinic is functioning, each individual who comes to the clinic brings with him or her huge packages of personal and social circumstances that nurses must take into account if their practice is to actually achieve the goal of improving the health of the individual and the community.

The package of individual circumstance that individuals bring with them to the clinic is, in turn, wrapped in a complex network of social factors that influence the effectiveness of nursing care. For example, if patients have trouble understanding their condition and the things they need to do to take care of themselves, the nurse is drawn to consider various things that might be contributing to this challenge—for example, media messages, family and cultural belief systems, overriding economic concerns, and unspoken fears based on misperceptions. Each possible barrier is not simply an individual's problem; it has roots in social relations and circumstances, and effective nursing approaches must address those underlying roots.

This chapter begins with an overview of the fundamental patterns of knowing in nursing. It then provides a brief explanation of the underlying philosophy and theory on which emancipatory knowing is based, with a particular emphasis on how the philosophy and theory are made visible in advanced nursing practice. Next, the chapter outlines criteria for assessing and developing advanced nursing practice from an emancipatory perspective. The final sections of the chapter offer an explanation of the necessity of emancipatory knowing approaches to achieve the essential competencies required for advanced nursing practice.

NURSING'S PATTERNS OF KNOWING

Barbara Carper (1978) conducted a philosophical analysis of early nursing literature and identified four fundamental patterns of knowing in nursing: (1) empirics, the science of nursing; (2) ethics, the component of moral knowledge in nursing; (3) the component of personal knowing in nursing; and (4) aesthetics, the art of nursing. Carper's analysis opened the way for a broad, comprehensive, and holistic view of nursing knowledge and nursing practice beyond the confines of empirics or science alone.

However, as nurse scholars and practitioners began to delve further into the broader fundamental understandings that form a foundation for nursing, it became increasingly clear that there is yet another pattern of knowing that has long been a foundation for nursing practice. This realm of knowing, first identified in the literature by White (1995), was identified as sociopolitical knowing. Later, Chinn and Kramer (2007) developed a conceptualization of emancipatory knowing that embraced White's conceptualization but expanded it to emphasize the nature of this pattern of knowing as expressed in nursing. In addition, Chinn and Kramer used the term *emancipatory* to emphasize the driving force underpinning this pattern of knowing—the universal human longing for liberation from those circumstances that limit human potential. The contributing authors in *Philosophies and Practices of Emancipatory Nursing: Social Justice as Praxis* (Kagan et al., 2014) provide a comprehensive collection of works advancing emancipatory nursing as a distinct and essential approach to practice that leads to fundamental changes in social and political structures in which health and well-being are embedded.

All patterns of knowing in nursing have both a *knowing* dimension and a *being/doing* dimension. The knowing (epistemological) dimension addresses how we come to know or understand things and what is required to admit something as knowledge. In all disciplines, methods and standards for conducting those methods exist so that the members of the discipline can agree on what is valid knowledge and what is not (meaning those things that are considered myths, falsehoods, or misconceptions). In nursing, practitioners rely on fundamental knowledge that has been verified as valid and reliable in related disciplines, as well as knowledge that has been verified within nurses' own discipline related to phenomena identified as central to processes of achieving maximum health. For example, in nursing,

Mishel (1990, 1997) developed knowledge of uncertainty from her practice observations and research focusing on people's experiences of illness.

The being/doing (ontological) dimension addresses how what nurses know is manifested in who they are and what they do. This is the very practical dimension of nursing that brings knowledge and practice together as one. Nurses have a long history of sensing that knowledge (theory) and practice need to be fully integrated. Unfortunately, theory and practice have often seemed to dodge integration because nursing theory development and academic research have tended to be a dominant focus in discussions of nursing knowledge. Recognizing the crucial doing (ontological) dimension of knowing and knowledge development is a major step toward a more complete integration of theory and practice.

For example, consider what it means to know and understand Mishel's theory of uncertainty. One can read all that has been written about this theory, including the reports of the research studies that were conducted to develop aspects of the theory. Nurses would probably think about what all this might mean for their practice. Understanding the theory might shift their perceptions of who they are and how they respond when working with someone who is struggling to cope with a difficult illness experience. As nurses experience this shift in practice, they become more aware of things about the experience that are as yet poorly understood; in response, they may seek new evidence, or knowledge, concerning this experience. This scenario is a circle of knowing and doing—a close connection between practice and theory that is not often acknowledged but that often enters into daily nursing. This kind of connection is increasingly being recognized and promoted by recent movements toward evidence-based practice, practice-based evidence, and translational research.

PHILOSOPHICAL AND THEORETICAL FOUNDATIONS OF EMANCIPATORY KNOWING IN NURSING

Emancipatory knowing and the approaches to practice that flow from this pattern of knowing are grounded in several fundamental assumptions:

- *There is no ahistorical, value-neutral knowledge.* All knowledge is constructed by humans and is saturated with value-laden and culturally situated perceptions. That which is taken as "true" or "real" is shaped by humans and can shift over time and over different contexts.
- *Research is a political activity.* Even the act of forming a research question is grounded in human values, intentions, and vested interests. The choice of research focus and the results that flow from this activity shape human actions and interactions.
- *Power relations inform knowledge development.* Those who conduct knowledge development activities have the privileges of a certain kind of academic experience and the economic privilege that is required for this experience. Their social position in society carries with it a privileged lens that shapes all knowledge development activities.

- *Language is constructed to carry power meanings.* Modern English discourse is saturated with militaristic, adversarial, and confrontational metaphors and expressions. Most of this language is not even recognized as carrying power meanings, but these meanings do, in fact, shape our perceptions and attitudes.
- *Social oppressions are not natural or fixed.* Social structures are constructed by humans and can be changed. In fact, social structures evolve and change over time, shaped by emerging contexts and circumstances. People can let change happen, but it is in their best interest to help shape the course of change in a direction of creating justice for all.

These fundamental assumptions are shared by a number of philosophers and theorists who are generally recognized as advocating a critical social perspective (Kagan et al., 2009). The ideas of two significant philosophers who have formed the foundation for nursing's emancipatory critical perspective—Jürgen Habermas and Paulo Freire—are summarized in the following sections.

Habermas's Critical Social Philosophy

Habermas's (1973, 1979, 1981) critical social philosophy is concerned with everyday life and the practices that sustain people on a daily basis. A very pragmatic philosophy, it is one of the first philosophical approaches to recognize that understanding the world requires a number of different approaches. These traits make this line of thought particularly appealing from a nursing perspective. After all, nursing deals with the most ordinary, and yet deeply significant, realities of life—illness, death, activities of daily living, and human relationships. In addition, nursing is grounded in the recognition that daily human experience is complex and requires many different approaches in order to be understood in ways that support effective nursing practice.

Habermas's works are massive and complex and cover immense philosophical, political, and theoretical territory. The brief discussion presented here touches on central ideas that form the foundation for the concept of emancipatory knowing. This philosopher's ideas are centrally concerned with the public sphere and the communicative action that sustains public life. Communicative competence is a unique human capacity that has evolved over time to create social and political structures that are necessary for social coexistence. However, forces that create dominance and advantage for some, and disadvantage and injustice for others, have suppressed capacity for communicative competence. Habermas's philosophy and theory are intended to provide a framework for emancipation from such social forces of injustice.

Habermas described three human interests that are fundamental to everyday life: technical, practical, and emancipatory. Each interest demands its own method and involves a particular kind of knowledge that makes human survival possible.

Technical interest involves the human interest and capacity to work with and create tools and systems that make it possible to carry out daily activities of living. It is rooted in the human interest in predicting and controlling the environment. Technical interest requires empirical methods that measure things, predict outcomes based on statistical significance, and calculate probabilities of natural phenomena. A significant portion of nursing and health care involves our technical interest—for example, drugs and interventions to treat illness, knowledge and use of nutrition for maintaining health, and knowledge and use of physical activity as it relates to health and well-being.

Practical interest is concerned with what Habermas termed *communicative* functions of life—the ways that people seek to get along with one another and to understand themselves within the context in which they live. Practical interest is vital to survival, to getting along with others, and to forming meaningful connections with acquaintances, friends, and family. Practical interest requires interpretive/philosophical methods that provide interpretive insight into the illusive yet vital human experiences of interacting with one another. The significant aspects of nursing that involve our caring relationships with individuals, families, and communities—the art of nursing—all involve professionals' practical interest.

Emancipatory interest is the human capacity to recognize that something in the social milieu is wrong, unjust, or failing, and subsequently the human impulse to make things right. Emancipatory interest also involves the capacity to recognize self-deception and the ideologies that shape human perception of the world. This feat requires the use of critical methods to probe for underlying patterns that arise from ideologies, often shaping circumstances of inequality and injustice. Critical methods seek understanding of social structures and interactions that create and sustain unjust circumstances within the status quo. Nursing concerns for promoting health and well-being for individuals and communities require our emancipatory interest.

Freire's Theory of Human Liberation

Paulo Freire's theory of human liberation was developed from his experience of instituting an unorthodox form of literacy education among sugarcane workers in Brazil during a time when literacy was required to vote. His approach to education is described in his classic book *Pedagogy of the Oppressed* (Freire, 1970), which remains the foundational work for all critical approaches in education, as well as in other disciplines.

Freire explained the conditions that sustain privilege for some and disadvantage for others and outlined specific propositions that point these parties in the direction toward liberation and freedom. Along the way, Freire identified certain traits that tend to dominate the life space of those who are privileged, who are called *the oppressor* in his early works:

- The dominant group is powerful and unified.
- Those who are privileged fail to recognize others as human, meaning that those who are not part of the dominant group are assumed to be "others" and are subject to manipulation and control.

- Those who are privileged have a consciousness and ethic of self-interest, and they use their power and privilege to sustain their own interests.
- The dominant group prescribes and defines reality for all, often in subtle ways, so that the status quo ends up being viewed by all as "the way things are" (hegemony).
- The dominant group exploits and manipulates others without apology.

By contrast, those who are disadvantaged (termed *the oppressed* in Freire's early works) exhibit traits that complement the traits of the dominant group and that serve to help sustain the circumstances of their disadvantage:

- The oppressed are powerless and divided. Their lack of unity contributes to their powerlessness, which in turn sustains the privilege enjoyed by the dominant group.
- Because they are not granted the rights and responsibilities of full humanity, the oppressed are prevented from being authentic; they are barred from realizing their full human potential.
- Those who are disadvantaged think and behave according to the prescribed norms of the dominant group and assume that those norms are natural or fixed.
- Those who are disadvantaged deny the self; instead, they internalize the consciousness of the oppressor.
- Those who are disadvantaged are exploited and manipulated, and because they deny the self, they do not typically recognize their own exploitation.

These complementary characteristics of the dominant and disadvantaged groups exist not by individual will or intention, but rather because of systematic conditions inherent in the social structure that sustain injustice. Even those who are privileged often do not recognize their own self-interest and the actions that sustain exploitation of others.

Within an unjust social system, those with power and privilege can seem generous when they demonstrate even small, insignificant acts of generosity, which, in fact, do little or nothing to change the injustice of the system. Educational opportunities are distributed unequally, with those who are relatively oppressed being denied access to adequate education. Specifically, oppressed groups are not taught their own history; as a consequence, they are not able to see their circumstance in its historical context, and they do not understand the roots of the divisiveness that exists in their own group. People who are disadvantaged tend to avoid forming associations with members of their own group; they do not join organizations with others of their own group, but instead they invest time and energy into becoming involved in the activities of those who are privileged.

Individuals in the oppressed group are vulnerable to being used as tokens because they believe the illusion that pleasing or serving the oppressor will eventually garner more power and privilege for those who are relatively disadvantaged. When members of the oppressed group do achieve some relative status (usually by token acts of generosity), they tend to become the oppressors of those who are now subordinate to them.

Furthermore, systematically embedded conditions make action toward liberation very difficult in these circumstances. The relative power of those who are privileged conveys the illusion that they are right, that their perspective is good and to be desired. Related to the internalization of this notion that those who are privileged are right, disadvantaged groups tend to see themselves as incapable of taking risks and sometimes even as deserving of their present situation. It is also a frightening prospect to challenge the status quo and to seek freedom because examples exist of the dangers that come to those who act. For example, when individuals do begin to act in a manner seeking liberation from disadvantage, they are often subjected to danger, ridicule, firing from a job, or other feared outcomes. The message to the oppressed is clear: It is safer to not "rock the boat."

What is required for liberation, for moving toward freedom from the constraints of disadvantage, is actually quite simple yet very difficult to do. First, disadvantaged groups must become aware of their situation, of the limits of the context in which they exist. This process, which has been termed *consciousness raising* in feminist and other activist groups, involves coming to realize one's own consciousness and becoming aware of the actual circumstances of one's own situation. Beyond the basic consciousness of the limits of the situation, liberation requires *consciousness of actions* that are feasible but have not yet been tried or tested—the untested feasibilities.

To take action requires unity with others who are also disadvantaged; it is not possible to take action alone (see **Box 7-1**). Together, groups of people begin to test the feasibility of possible actions. Most important, it is essential for the steps toward liberation to be fully and consciously grounded in love for self *and* for those who are privileged—the oppressor. It is this grounding in love, for both self and the oppressor, that makes it possible for people to move toward liberation without becoming, in turn, the oppressors of those subordinate to them (Freire, 1970).

IMPLICATIONS OF THE PHILOSOPHY AND THEORY FOR PRACTICE

If you are a reader who has typically thought of philosophy and theory as unrelated to practice, ideally the discussion so far has conveyed a sense of how vitally important one's own philosophy and theoretical perspective are in shaping the nature of one's practice. Because an emancipatory approach is so dramatically different from the traditional approaches to both theory and practice, it requires a more complete explanation than other individual-focused perspectives on which practice and theory are based. Once an emancipatory perspective is brought to bear on an individual's practice, several shifts become possible. The shifts include, but are not limited to, viewing the problems that people bring to health care as intrinsically linked to social and political processes, recognizing the need for action

Box 7-1   Application of Freire's Theory of Liberation

Jane and her best friend Sue have worked together on a surgical unit for more than 10 years. To celebrate their long and close working relationship, they plan an overnight getaway at a spa, where they can be pampered with great meals (cooked by someone else!), saunas, massages, pedicures, and manicures. When they arrive at the spa late in the afternoon on Friday, they begin with massages and some relaxing time in the sauna. They then enjoy an exquisitely prepared dinner. Over dinner, Jane shares with Sue that she has enrolled in a doctor of nursing practice (DNP) program to become an advanced practice nurse. Sue is shocked; usually Jane tells her about something like this long before it actually happens. The news that Jane has already decided, and has enrolled, throws her off balance. Sue gathers her composure and offers a toast to Jane's new adventure, and they continue to enjoy their good time together.

When Sue arrives home, she becomes aware of her growing resentment that Jane has made this decision. She decides to talk to Jane about it when they take their break on Monday. When Sue brings up the subject, she explains that she wishes Jane had told her about what she was doing. Sue says, "Jane, you know I can't afford to go into the DNP program, and I wish you well, but I wish you had told me you were thinking about this. But, most of all, I hope that this change in your life won't interfere with our friendship." Jane brushes off the comment and assures her that they will remain close friends.

Sue and Jane do remain close for a while, but gradually Jane begins to be critical of everything that Sue and other staff nurses are doing, and they begin to see Jane as having a chip on her shoulder and acting in a "holier than thou" manner. Eventually Jane moves on to a private practice, but occasionally she comes back to the unit to see her patients. She is cordial, but she makes demands on the staff nurses as if she had never been part of their life. The staff nurses, in turn, resist following Jane's orders and try to avoid her as much as possible. When one of them does cooperate with Jane, the others tend to view their staff nurse colleague as "sucking up" to Jane, and resentment builds among the staff nurses.

Based on Freire's theory of liberation, consider the following questions related to this situation:

1. What, theoretically, is going on here?
2. What needs to happen for this situation to change?
3. What is the most important factor for real change to occur?
4. How would you feel if you were one of the staff nurses hearing this theoretical explanation?
5. If you were Jane, how would you feel if someone explained this situation to you in terms of Freire's theory?

to change social circumstances, and recognizing the potential for every person to become an agent for change. The following sections detail the various ways in which an emancipatory perspective shapes the reality of nursing practice.

Emancipatory Nursing Practice

Joyce Fontana (2004) conducted an analysis of the foundations of critical/emancipatory scholarship and the various published works in nursing that were conducted using critical approaches. She identified seven traits that characterize critical work in nursing: (1) critique, (2) context, (3) politics, (4) emancipatory intent, (5) democratic structure, (6) dialectic analysis, and (7) reflexivity. These seven traits are explained in the following subsections in relation to nursing practice. Fontana focused on critical research, but critical methods do not draw a firm line of distinction between research and practice. Because critical emancipatory approaches require participation by those who are disadvantaged and aim to achieve change in their lives, a research project is also *practice*.

Drawing on Fontana's conceptualization, the sections that follow describe the features of emancipatory practice in relation to nursing. Examples are drawn from the Nurse Manifest projects, which were designed to explore the circumstances of practice that limit nurses' ability to practice nursing as they themselves wish to practice (Jacobs, Fontana, Kehoe, Matarese, & Chinn, 2005; Jarrin, 2006; *Nurse Manifest Research Study Report*, 2002). Examples are also drawn from a project in which a nurse engaged adolescent girls in examining the experience of menarche, which illustrates an emancipatory approach in practice (Hagedorn, 1995).

Critique

Assuming that people have a desire to be free of constraints that limit them, critique is central to critical methods in emancipatory nursing practice. From a critical perspective, this activity involves much more than simply taking stock of a situation to figure out what is wrong (as in problem solving). Rather, critique requires an analysis that exposes the political and social structures that sustain patterns of injustice and imbalance (Fontana, 2004). In practice, it typically requires a group of people who first examine their experiences of a situation on an individual basis and then, working as a group, begin to identify the common dynamics of each of their unique experiences. Given the assumption that all humans have an emancipatory interest, as soon as people recognize the conditions of their experience that constrain their human potential, they shift to figuring out how to eliminate these barriers and change the situation.

For example, in the project reported by Hagedorn (1995), adolescent girls shared stories of their own menarche. When they did so, they began to realize that—contrary to their preconceived assumption—they were not alone in their experience. Their critique of their experiences led them to examine the social and political forces that shaped their experience, including the roles of culture, the influence of the for-profit corporate entities that sell menstrual care products, and the lack of appropriate education for girls related to menarche.

Context

Emancipatory methods are fully situated in the circumstances of daily life. As a consequence, the people who are directly affected by the conditions of disadvantage and injustice play central roles as active participants (not subjects), whether it is a research project or a clinical project (Fontana, 2004). Allies who are relatively advantaged, or at least not seriously disadvantaged in the situation, can join with those who are directly experiencing injustice or limitations, but allies are always present only to facilitate, encourage, and support those who are the central actors in the situation (Chinn & Kramer, 2015).

The process of taking the project to the people and their context was demonstrated in powerful ways in Freire's (1970) early work, which, as mentioned, focused on teaching Brazilian sugarcane workers to read. Freire and his fellow teachers went into the villages and spent time simply experiencing the conditions of the lives of the workers. Through this effort, they developed a stance of complete love and respect for the people and a fuller understanding of their lives. Rather than announcing at the outset that they were there to teach the people to read, the teachers began by inviting small groups of workers to examine photos and drawings of ordinary life experiences in the village and simply asked the question, "What is going on in this picture?" Freire called the pictures "codifications"—things that illustrated the ordinariness of daily life.

As people began to discuss what was going on, they recognized dynamics of their situation that were not right and needed to change. Their recognitions did not necessarily differ from what the teachers might have identified, but their personal, inner recognition brought with it a realization of their own authentic consciousness—not a consciousness based on what someone else told them to think or see.

Politics

Critical approaches, in contrast to most mainstream approaches to research and practice, acknowledge up-front the value basis of the work. Philosophically, critical science is based on the assumption that all research and all human actions are political in the sense that they enact values in the world and, by doing so, affect the world and others who inhabit that world. However, most scientists, scholars, and practitioners do not overtly acknowledge their value stance or their political intentions, and they may not be consciously aware of this aspect of their work. In contrast, those who work from a critical perspective make explicit their fundamental intent to expose injustice and discrimination and their plan to initiate steps to correct these conditions.

For example, in the various Nurse Manifest projects, the facilitators of each project conveyed to potential nurse participants their concern for the contexts in which nurses are practicing—the strained economy, the shortage of nurses, the demands placed on nurses to work long hours, and so forth—and their hope that the project would lead to new ideas about how to change those situations. The groups began their discussion based on a simple question concerning their experience of practicing nursing: "What is it like to practice nursing today?" (Jarrin, 2006).

Emancipatory Intent

Closely related to politics is the emancipatory intent that is explicit in any critical approach. This intent shapes an emancipatory approach from the outset, requiring that the people who are most directly affected by a situation of injustice be central. Their perceptions and voices must dominate any discourse and must be fully respected. This intent is fully disclosed at the outset, but with the clear understanding that the facilitators or caregivers do not come with preconceived ideas about what is required to make the situation better for those who are involved. Rather, people are assured that any ideas or solutions or actions that might come from their discussion will be their ideas, and that the role of any ally or facilitator will be to support their exploration of what is feasible as they test the various options for action that might be considered.

The actions that arose from the Nurse Manifest projects were typically not large or earth-shattering, but they were significant in a very practical sense. The outcomes included (but were not limited to) significant shifts in awareness among the participating nurses concerning the historical and political contexts of their work, awareness of the importance of working together and supporting one another, increased respect for nurses and nursing, renewed determination to gain control over their own priorities, and working toward finding nursing's own voice in the healthcare system (Jarrin, 2006).

Likewise, in the project in which adolescent females explored their experience of menarche, the immediate outcome was an educational video that the young women made themselves, which both reported the findings of their discussions and fact-finding projects and sought to educate younger women about the experience of menarche. Their primary conclusion was that menarche education should not be provided by the corporations that sell menstrual care products, but rather should be designed and conducted by "peers"—adolescent girls who best understand the challenges of the experience and can best convey to younger girls what to expect and how to manage their menstruation once it starts (Hagedorn, 1995).

Democratic Structure

All who participate in an emancipatory project are equal agents; the processes used are collegial, with every participant learning from others and also teaching others. There is no one voice of authority. Instead, all aspects of the project are negotiated among equals, and leadership shifts based on the needs of the group and the particular capabilities of each participant. Given that this approach is not the way in which most people are accustomed to working together, accomplishing a democratic structure that places everyone on equal footing requires conscious effort and willingness by each participant to own responsibility for the process itself and to turn the critical lens inward to better shape the democratic ideal.

In the Nurse Manifest projects, groups used variations of the processes described in *Peace and Power* (Chinn, 2013a, 2016). When groups convene for discussion using this process, each person has equal opportunity to speak. A discussion begins with everyone checking in to share their intentions for the discussion; it ends with each person speaking to share critical reflections on the discussion and ideas for what that individual hopes will happen next. During the discussion, a process of "rotating chair" is used, in which the person who is speaking recognizes the next person to speak (instead of a single "chair" calling on people to speak). Jacobs and her colleagues (2005) described the role of the researcher or leader in a group using this process, illustrating how a leader can shape a genuinely democratic process without imposing the leader's own will on the group:

> The role of the researchers was to engage the participants in the initial identification of codifications, to respectfully hear the views of all participants, pose questions, and suggest possibilities to assist in discovering background awareness of the dialectical relations between two or more dimensions of reality. (p. 10)

The experience of participating in a group that functions in this manner is itself an experience of empowerment and change, and adapting this approach to group interactions was the major recommendation of the Jacobs report (Jacobs et al., 2005).

Dialectic Analysis

Emancipatory approaches focus on understanding the many contradictory elements of any social structure, but particularly the contradictions between the ideal and the real. A critical approach assumes that the totality of the world involves contradiction, or seemingly opposing sides that in actuality constitute the whole—day and night, front and back, general and specific, abstract and concrete, thought and action, subjective and objective, global and local. Each component of a contradiction must be understood if one is to understand the whole.

In the Nurse Manifest projects, nurses realized that they already knew the ideal but that they had lost sight of what might be possible because of their immersion in the realities of daily nursing. Exploring the ideal brought into better focus the situation of their real-world practice and engendered new realizations of ways in which the ideal could be feasible. The simple yet challenging personal project of gaining a sense of respect for other nurses and finding ways to support one another gradually became viewed as actually possible. Through this process, participants come to see themselves as active agents, rather than passive objects subject to others' dominance (Jacobs et al., 2005).

Reflexivity

Reflexivity means the nurse and the group examine not only *what* they are doing, but also *how* they are doing what they are doing. The central question that focuses this kind of reflective commitment is, "Do I know what I do, and do I do what I know?" Given the democratic nature of this approach, each individual engages in this kind of personal reflection, and the group members also discuss and share individual insights with one another concerning the activities of the group.

In groups that use the processes outlined in *Peace and Power* (Chinn, 2013b), critical reflections shared at the end of each gathering serve to bring this ideal into reality. This exercise becomes one of the most valuable aspects of working together to create change. Everyone in the group respects each member's reflections on how the group is functioning and how well their shared intentions and values are expressed in their actions. Each shared perspective reveals insights for everyone about the struggle of overcoming the tendencies associated with the dominant power structure and the challenges of creating social and political change.

Emancipatory Knowing and the Essentials of Advanced Nursing Practice

Emancipatory knowing, and the approaches that flow from this pattern of knowing, are essential for anyone who is a nurse, whether one is practicing as a staff nurse, nurse manager, administrator, educator, researcher, or advanced practice nurse in a specialty area. Most of the nursing literature that describes emancipatory approaches focuses on research methods (see, for example, Fontana, 2004; Jarrin, 2006; Kagan et al., 2009; Kagan et al., 2014) or nursing education (see, for example, Anthony & Landeen, 2009; Falk-Rafael, Anderson, Chinn, & Rubotzky, 2004; Falk-Rafael, Chinn, Anderson, Laschinger, & Rubotzky, 2003).

Emancipatory knowing lies at the heart of nursing practice, even though it is not typically acknowledged explicitly. Bringing forth awareness of this vital component of knowing and action provides a bridge to actualize the ideals of nursing practice, particularly the ideals of advanced nursing practice. To illustrate, consider the *Essentials of Doctoral Education for Advanced Nursing Practice* (2006), which the American Association of Colleges of Nursing formulated as a guide for the development of advanced nursing practice roles. The first seven of the *Essentials* address competencies for advanced nursing practice in all specialties:

1. Scientific underpinnings for practice
2. Organizational and systems leadership for quality improvement and systems thinking
3. Clinical scholarship and analytical methods for evidence-based practice
4. Information systems/technology and patient care technology for the improvement and transformation of health care
5. Healthcare policy for advocacy in health care
6. Interprofessional collaboration for improving patient and population health outcomes
7. Clinical prevention and population health for improving the nation's health

The following subsections outline ways in which an emancipatory approach can vitally strengthen each of these essential competencies.

Essential I: Scientific Underpinnings for Practice

An emancipatory lens is essential in determining adequate scientific underpinnings for practice. This determination requires questioning the value and worth of what is taken to be a scientific underpinning. An *emancipatory critique* goes deeper than simply determining the methodological strengths and weaknesses of research reports and begins to ask questions such as the following:

- What ideology does this report reflect?
- Which biases and implied assumptions shaped the design and outcomes of this study?
- Who benefits if these findings are used as a basis for practice?
- Does this report adequately account for the social and political context of the people for whom I provide care?

These questions are not only posed by individual nurses, but they are also used as a basis for discussion among members of the team evaluating scientific worth.

Essential II: Organizational and Systems Leadership for Quality Improvement and Systems Thinking

Emancipatory knowing and the approaches that flow from this pattern of knowing are, by definition, *systems thinking*. This pattern of knowing demands not simply a local systems approach, but a global, social, and political systems approach. The emancipatory processes described in *Peace and Power* (Chinn, 2013b, 2016) provide a kind of leadership that moves organizations and systems to seek quality improvement constantly on a level that goes beyond something that can be easily measured. When teams of individuals who are providing care come together in small, meaningful discussions to examine not only what they are doing but also how they are doing it, each person becomes invested in the processes required to improve the care that is provided, as well as the conditions of their own experience in the workplace.

This kind of emancipatory leadership is facilitative rather than prescriptive and supportive rather than demanding. During work with nurses involved in daily nursing care roles, it becomes clear that nurses deeply yearn to create conditions in which they can provide the highest quality of care. Leadership that facilitates the impulse to bring this ideal into reality is, indeed, transformative.

Essential III: Clinical Scholarship and Analytical Methods for Evidence-Based Practice

Clinical scholarship that is founded in an emancipatory approach brings together scholarship and practice in ways that are not possible with research approaches that lack this perspective. Emancipatory approaches do not prescribe a method; rather, any research method can be employed as a component of an emancipatory project.

For example, the adolescent women who explored their experience of menarche used their group discussion as a basis for undertaking a qualitative analysis of the common elements of their unique experience. From this discussion, however, they grew curious about the larger social, historical, and cultural forces that had shaped their experience. Once they realized that the corporations that sell menstrual care products also produced all of the educational materials they had been given about menarche, they gathered evidence of the corporate motives (profit) that shaped the approaches and content that were presented in these materials. The young women's findings led them to engage in a more critical appraisal of the educational materials that are produced by these companies. For example, the adolescents sought evidence of the nature of the menarche experience in cultures other than their own and discovered that this event in a young woman's life was treated as a sacred event in Native American cultures, leading to their realization of the mutability of their own Eurocentric experiences. They interviewed their mothers and grandmothers to gain a sense of the generational roots of their own experiences. They conducted a survey of all schools in their district to determine if there was variability between and among schools in how menarche education was conducted. They accomplished all of this research and produced the video documenting their experience in the course of one semester (Hagedorn, 1995).

In addition to the diversity of methods that can be employed, the example of the adolescent women's project illustrates the kinds of questions that arise from an emancipatory perspective, which tend to broaden and deepen the exploration of what might be considered evidence for practice. Emancipatory scholarship demands asking questions such as, Who will benefit if we base our practice on this evidence?, Who will be disadvantaged?, and Which ideology (or stereotype) does this evidence sustain?

Essential IV: Information Systems/Technology and Patient Care Technology for the Improvement and Transformation of Health Care

Several critical questions that an emancipatory lens focuses on technology are vital in determining the worth and desirability of technological tools:

- Is this technology appropriate for the people we serve and in the context in which we work?
- What are the underlying motivations in adopting and using this technology?
- Who actually benefits from this technology?
- Does this technology actually improve and transform care, or does it serve other interests, such as profit or aggrandizement for some at the expense of others?

Essential V: Healthcare Policy for Advocacy in Health Care

The policy initiatives that emerge from a grassroots level, which by definition is inherent in emancipatory approaches, are those that best serve the interests of the people. Allies and advocates are essential in the policy-making process, of course. Rather than imposing policy on groups of people, emancipatory approaches take the discussion to the people, and allies and advocates follow the will of the people. When examining policy initiatives, the questions posed from an emancipatory perspective can guide both grassroots activists and allies/advocates in selecting and refining the ideals they seek through policy:

- Who benefits?
- Who is disadvantaged?
- Which social values does this policy reflect?
- From which motives does this policy arise?
- Is this policy good for the health of all members of our community?

Essential VI: Interprofessional Collaboration for Improving Patient and Population Health Outcomes

Emancipatory approaches demand the involvement of all who are party to a situation. Therefore, all members of a healthcare team or provider unit, as well as people served in the community, must collaborate in any project that arises from an emancipatory perspective. The initial commitment, and then the subsequent effort required to make this happen, are immense—but the benefits are immeasurable. When every voice is heard, when people have a meaningful role to play in a situation, and when people are given the opportunity to understand a situation from the outset, the chances of achieving good cooperation and collaboration in providing high-quality care are significantly increased.

Essential VII: Clinical Prevention and Population Health for Improving the Nation's Health

Because emancipatory thinking is an upstream approach, by definition it leads to prevention and population health. A parable-like story is often used to illustrate upstream thinking: A small group of people were walking along a river, and they saw a child being swept downstream, desperately struggling to get out of the current and reach the shore. One of the walkers dove into the river and pulled the child to shore. Before long, another child came along being swept by the current, then another, and another. Finally, one of the walkers said, "I am going to walk upstream and find out who is throwing these children into the water and stop what they are doing." Emancipatory approaches ask the fundamental question, What is happening upstream to create the patterns of injustice, discrimination, and disadvantage?

This approach seeks to understand patterns within a social and political structure that are much less obvious than children being swept down a river. An emancipatory lens also brings the patterns into focus as a social construction that can be changed. Understanding the social structures that create and sustain such patterns is essential to change what is happening and, in turn, is key to successful prevention efforts aimed at improving population health.

SUMMARY

Clearly, the challenges inherent in modern-day nursing and health care are immense. Emancipatory perspectives provide a lens that may seem to make the challenge more complex and more difficult, in that this approach shifts to a more global, deeper probing of the issues and problems than is required from other perspectives. Even so, given the assumption that the challenges are created and sustained within a social and political structure, the most effective approaches for addressing the challenges must lie within the realm of the social and political. Emancipatory knowledge, and the approaches that flow from it, provides a means to move in this direction and, in turn, to better meet the needs of those who receive nursing care.

DISCUSSION QUESTIONS

1. Think about a recent situation in nursing that you recognized as needing to change in some way and share your reflections with others in your group.
2. Did you take action to change the situation in Question 1? If not, why not? If so, consider the following:
   a. Who did you connect with in some way to create change?
   b. What were the barriers that you faced in making the change?
   c. What facilitated getting something done?
   d. Looking back, what would you do differently next time around?
3. Identify an object, painting, or picture that represents to you the current practice of nursing. Identify another object, painting, or picture that represents to you what the practice of nursing should or could be at its best. Share what each of these representations means with others in your group and identify common ground that you all have related to nursing as it is and nursing as it could be.
4. Identify a situation in nursing that you encounter frequently, preferably one that you experience as frustrating or unsatisfying. Write a brief account of a recent experience you had with this type of situation. After you have written this account, think about what tends to go through your mind as the situation unfolds and what you think needs to happen differently the next time. Imagine the situation occurring but with the changes you imagine in effect; if possible, try to enact the situation as you imagine it might be. Share your experience with others in your group and invite them to help you imagine a different kind of experience in this situation.
5. Think about the relationships you experience (or have experienced in the past) with your coworkers. Write a brief synopsis of these relationships and then do the following:
   a. Identify the groups (or individuals) who are the most advantaged or privileged in the work environment.
   b. Identify the groups (or individuals) who are the most disadvantaged. You might identify more than two layers of relative advantage.

c. Describe the traits of those who are advantaged and disadvantaged in light of Freire's theory of liberation.

d. Write a brief action plan, based on Freire's theory, describing what could happen to change the work situation.

e. Discuss your insights with your group, and invite their suggestions about how to change this kind of situation.

REFERENCES

American Association of Colleges of Nursing. (2006). *Essentials of doctoral education for advanced nursing practice*. Retrieved from http://www.aacn.nche.edu/publications/position/DNPEssentials.pdf

Anthony, S. E., & Landeen, J. (2009). Evolution of Canadian nursing curricula: A critical retrospective analysis of power and caring. *International Journal of Nursing Education Scholarship, 6*(1), 1–14.

Carper, B. A. (1978). Fundamental patterns of knowing in nursing. *Advances in Nursing Science, 1*(1), 13–23.

Chinn, P. L. (2013a, 2016). Peace and power: Group process for empowerment, cooperation, growth and solidarity. Retrieved May 16, 2016, from http://peaceandpowerblog.wordpress.com

Chinn, P. L. (2013b). *Peace and power: New directions for building community* (8th ed.). Burlington, MA: Jones & Bartlett Learning.

Chinn, P. L., & Kramer, M. (2007). *Integrated theory and knowledge development in nursing* (7th ed.). St. Louis, MO: Mosby.

Chinn, P. L., & Kramer, M. (2015). *Integrated knowledge development in nursing* (8th ed.). St. Louis, MO: Mosby.

Falk-Rafael, A. R., Anderson, M. A., Chinn, P. L., & Rubotzky, A. M. (2004). Peace and power as a critical feminist framework for nursing education. In M. H. Oermann & K. T. Heinrich (Eds.), *Annual review of nursing education* (Vol. 2, pp. 217–235). New York, NY: Springer.

Falk-Rafael, A. R., Chinn, P. L., Anderson, M. A., Laschinger, H., & Rubotzky, A. M. (2003). The effectiveness of feminist pedagogy in empowering a community of learners. *Journal of Nursing Education, 42*(12), 1–9.

Fontana, J. S. (2004). A methodology for critical science in nursing. *Advances in Nursing Science, 27*(2), 93–101.

Freire, P. (1970). *Pedagogy of the oppressed* (M. B. Ramos, Trans.). New York, NY: Seabury Press.

Habermas, J. (1973). *Theory and practice* (J. Viertel, Trans.). Boston, MA: Beacon Press.

Habermas, J. (1979). *Communication and the evolution of society* (T. McCarthy, Trans.). Boston, MA: Beacon Press.

Habermas, J. (1981). *Theory of communicative action* (T. McCarthy, Trans.). Boston, MA: Beacon Press.

Hagedorn, S. (1995). The politics of caring: The role of activism in primary care. *Advances in Nursing Science, 17*(4), 1–11.

Jacobs, B. B., Fontana, J. S., Kehoe, M. H., Matarese, C., & Chinn, P. L. (2005). An emancipatory study of contemporary nursing practice. *Nursing Outlook, 53*, 6–14.

Jarrin, O. F. (2006). Results from the Nurse Manifest 2003 study: Nurses' perspectives on nursing. *Advances in Nursing Science, 29*(2), E74–E85.

Kagan, P. N., Smith, M. C., & Chinn, P. L. (2014). *Philosophies and practices of emancipatory nursing: Social justice as praxis*. New York, NY: Routledge.

Kagan, P. N., Smith, M. C., Cowling, W. R., & Chinn, P. L. (2009). A nursing manifesto: An emancipatory call for knowledge development, conscience, and praxis. *Nursing Philosophy, 11,* 67–84.

Mishel, M. H. (1990). Reconceptualization of the uncertainty in illness theory. *Image: The Journal of Nursing Scholarship, 22,* 256.

Mishel, M. H. (1997). Uncertainty in acute illness. In J. J. Fitzpatrick & J. S. Norbeck (Eds.), *Annual review of nursing research* (Vol. 15, pp. 57–80). New York, NY: Springer.

Nurse Manifest 2002 research study report. (2002). Retrieved from http://www.nursemanifest.com /research_reports/2002_study/2002_study.htm

White, J. (1995). Patterns of knowing: Review, critique, and update. *Advances in Nursing Science, 17*(4), 73–86.

Chapter 8

Feminist Ethics: Some Applicable Thoughts for Advanced Practice Nurses

Rosemarie Tong

INTRODUCTION

Feminist approaches to ethics provide professionals in the field of nursing with nontraditional ways to examine moral issues critically, apply moral principles judiciously, and call forth human emotions appropriately. Myriad in number, these moral perspectives fall into two basic groups: *care-focused approaches* and *power-focused approaches* (Code, Mullett, & Overall, 1988; Gilligan, 1982; Jaggar, 1992; Noddings, 1984; Ruddick, 1989; Sherwin, 1992). Care-focused feminists are particularly attentive to the moral dramas that play out in the private realm. As they see it, a feminine style of moral reasoning that works to weave and maintain good human relationships is just as valid as a masculine style of moral reasoning that aims to establish just and fair universal laws. Care-focused feminists claim that individuals should try to meet others' genuine needs simply because everyone is subject to the same vicissitudes of human carnality and the inevitability of human mortality. In contrast to care-focused feminists, power-focused feminists are more intent on understanding the moral implications of power relationships, asking questions about why women usually have less social standing, economic wealth, and political clout than men have. The latter feminists are generally very active politically, seeking ways to develop strategies and policies to eliminate or at least ameliorate discrimination against women and other groups of people who experience unfair and systematic subordination.

Importantly, both care-focused and power-focused feminists agree with feminist thinker Alison Jaggar (1992), who suggested that any approach to ethics that calls itself feminist must meet the following criteria: (1) view men and women as having fundamentally dissimilar life situations; (2) provide ways to undermine the "systematic subordination of women"; (3) offer methods for dealing with issues that arise in the private sphere, but particularly in domestic life; and (4) "take the moral experience of all women seriously, though not, of course, uncritically" (p. 364). Interestingly, neither care-focused nor power-focused feminists maintain that gender oppression is necessarily the worst form of human oppression. On the contrary, they assert that oppression rooted in race, class, age, nationality, health status, and so forth can be equally pernicious. Even so, gender oppression has a universality that other forms of oppression may lack. Women everywhere, to some extent or another, have less power, authority, and autonomy than men do. Because this state of affairs stubbornly persists, feminists ally with one another in an attempt to transform familial relationships, political structures, economic policies, social norms, and cultural attitudes. They insist that women—no less than men—are full human persons and, as such, deserve the same respect and standing that men have. This chapter examines several feminist perspectives in the hope that nurses may find them of use in their lives and work.

CARE-FOCUSED FEMINIST APPROACHES TO ETHICS

Care-focused feminists spend considerable time explaining the differences between an *ethics of justice* (rights) and an *ethics of care* (responsibilities and relationships). They also devote energy to developing paradigms for appropriately caring relationships. Importantly, most care-focused feminists believe that women's caregiving skills are far more developed than are men's. For example, in the United States, 91.7% of registered nurses are women (U.S. Department of Labor & U.S. Bureau of Labor Statistics, 2008). The fact that most men avoid fields of work such as nursing is a worrisome state of affairs that care-focused feminists seek to address. For men generally to dismiss care work as "women's work" is, in some ways, for men to devalue this essential human labor as beneath them. Indeed, one study revealed that some men would prefer not to work at all than to do "women's work" (Williams, 2000, p. 309).

Probably the most well-known thinker who has promulgated a care-focused feminist approach to ethics is moral psychologist Carol Gilligan (1982). She argued that because women have traditionally focused on meeting the needs of children, elderly family members, and people with illnesses or disabilities, they have developed a language of care that helps create and maintain a thick web of loving (or at least friendly) human relationships. In contrast, because men have traditionally thrust themselves into the marketplace and the civic arena, they have developed a language of justice that shapes and maintains contractual agreements between supposedly rational and free adults eager to specify and protect their respective rights. Gilligan also maintained that scales that measure moral development privilege the ethical language of justice over the ethical language of care. For example, Lawrence Kohlberg's widely used six-stage moral development scale relegates care considerations to the lower stages of moral development and justice considerations to the higher stages of moral development (as cited in Tong, 1993, p. 82).

Thinking about Kohlberg's ladder of moral development, Gilligan asked why women rarely get past stage 3, whereas men usually get to stage 4 or even 5. Hypothesizing that Kohlberg's scale is constructed in ways that favor men, Gilligan watched Kohlbergian researchers at work. She noted that they usually asked their research subjects to resolve hypothetical moral dilemmas. The case of Heinz, a husband whose wife's life depends on his stealing an expensive drug for her, was typical of these dilemmas. Heinz's wife desperately needs a drug, but he cannot afford to purchase it. The moral question is: "Should Heinz steal the drug under these circumstances?"

When Jake and Amy, two 11-year-old children, were asked this question by Kohlbergian researchers, they gave very different answers. Jake approached the question as a math problem. He said Heinz should steal the drug because the right to life trumps the right to property. In contrast to Jake, Amy did not view Heinz's dilemma as a conflict between competing rights. Instead, she viewed it as a relationship issue: how Heinz's theft of the drug might affect him and his wife in the long run. Commented Amy:

> If he stole the drug, he might save the wife then, but if he did, he might have to go to jail, and then his wife might get sicker again, and he couldn't get more of the drug, and it might not be good. So, they should really just talk it out and find some other way to make the money. (Cited in Tong, 1993, p. 83)

Importantly, the Kohlbergian researchers gave a higher test score to Jake than to Amy. If one thinks about it, though, Amy's answer was probably the better one, all things considered. Certainly, it opened up the possibility of discussing what might really be morally wrong with Heinz's situation—namely, a pharmaceutical industry that overprices drugs, the lack of affordable healthcare insurance, or the absence of a welfare safety net for people like Heinz and his wife.

Gilligan contrasted Jake's and Amy's differing responses not to negate Jake's style of moral reasoning, but rather to affirm Amy's style of moral reasoning and to set the stage for more deeply understanding it. As the result of several empirical studies, including interviews with 29 relatively diverse women who were deciding whether to have an abortion, Gilligan concluded that women's *ontologies* and *epistemologies*, as well as *ethics*, typically diverge from men's. Focusing on the different roles of intimacy and self-individuation in men's and women's lives, Gilligan observed that the importance of individuality and autonomy for men often leads them to center discussions of morality on issues of justice, fairness, rules, and rights. In contrast, the importance of family and friends for women prompts them to center discussions of morality on people's wants, needs, interests, and aspirations. Gilligan also claimed that for women—much more than for men—moral development means learning how to integrate other-directed demands with self-centered concerns.

During the process of their moral development, women supposedly move between three levels of moral reasoning: an overemphasis on self (Level 1), an overemphasis on others (Level 2), and a proper emphasis on self in relation to others (Level 3). Although a woman's moral development is always in process, as a woman morally matures, an increasing number of her decisions will exhibit Level 3 characteristics (as cited in Tong, 1993, p. 85).

Comparing Gilligan's and Kohlberg's diverging accounts of moral development, it is easy to understand why Gilligan thought Kohlberg's account reflected men's moral development rather than everyone's moral development. She claimed that a "formal logic of fairness" informs Kohlberg's mode of reasoning and style of discourse; his scale interprets moral phenomena in terms of a set of rights and rules. In contrast, a "psychological logic of relationships" informs Gilligan's mode of reasoning and style of discourse; her scale interprets moral phenomena in terms of a set of responsibilities and connections. To be sure, Gilligan's scale is no more a scale of human moral development than is Kohlberg's. Rather than denying this fact, however, Gilligan asked nurses to reflect on the different ways in which men and women describe their distinctive moral journeys, viewing them as alternative ways to achieve the ultimate goal of a morality that requires both rights (justice) and responsibilities (care) (as cited in Tong, 1993, p. 87).

Like Gilligan, Nel Noddings, a philosopher of education (as cited in Tong, 1998, pp. 132–135), suggested that ethics is about creating and maintaining caring relationships. She claimed that traditional Western ethics is so fixated on "principles and propositions" and values such as "justification, fairness, and justice" that it fails to recognize the importance of "human caring and the memory of caring and being cared for" (as cited in Tong, 1993, p. 108). Convinced that traditional ethics had gone wrong by emphasizing justice and deemphasizing care, Noddings proposed to set it right by injecting "eros, the feminine spirit" into "logos, the masculine spirit." Although women are just as capable of rational moral reasoning as men are, in Noddings's estimation, most women still prefer to consult their "feelings, needs, impressions, and . . . sense of personal ideal" when they make moral decisions (p. 109).

According to Noddings, sentiments of sympathy and empathy are innate in all human beings, but they need to be cultivated if they are to guide everyday moral decisions. Noddings identified two sorts of human caring: *natural caring* and *ethical caring*. As she saw it, caring comes easily to us when we are young. We want to help others because they matter to us and we want their love and approval at all costs. Later, said Noddings, it becomes more difficult for us to help others because our own self-interest begins to dominate. We want our own way, even if getting it separates us from others. To the extent that this happens, said Noddings, we need to remember how others have cared for us. Noddings claimed that it is through this process of "remembrance" that ethical caring—the kind of caring that expresses itself as "I *must* care"—comes into existence. This form of caring is more deliberate and less spontaneous than what Noddings termed natural caring (as cited in Tong, 1993, p. 112). It comes into being when our feelings are dormant, distant, or otherwise temporarily diminished.

Importantly, Noddings did not think that ethical caring should replace caring. Rather, she suggested that our "oughts" should build on our "wants." Commented Noddings, "An ethics built on caring strives to maintain the caring attitude and is thus dependent upon, and not superior to, natural caring" (p. 112). When we engage in ethical caring, we are not denying, negating, or renouncing ourselves in an effort to affirm, posit, or accept others. Rather, we are acting to fulfill our "fundamental and natural desire to be and to remain related" (p. 112).

In an attempt to further elucidate why care is fundamentally about connection, Noddings wrote a book about evil (1989). In it, she argued that for women, an evil event is a bad event—something that harms someone. By comparison, for men, an evil event is a rule-breaking event—a violation of God's commandments or the state's laws. Noddings wanted to replace the father's idea of evil as sin, guilt, impurity, and fault with the mother's experience of evil as "that which harms or threatens harm" (as cited in Tong, 1993, p. 113). Noddings insisted that evil is not about disobeying authority figures. Rather, it is about experiencing, in a wide variety of ways, the kind of pain, separation, and helplessness we all experience shortly after being born. In Noddings's estimation, this new conception of evil, and its concomitant stress on relationships, may make it easier for us to resist evil throughout our lives, but especially as we grow older (p. 113).

Noddings used Doris Lessing's novel *The Diary of a Good Neighbor* (1983) to better articulate women's understanding of evil. In the novel, Jane, a middle-aged, well-heeled novelist and magazine editor, tries to alleviate the suffering of Maudie, a skinny, unkempt, lower-class, 90-year-old woman. A cadre of nurses and nurse's aides (all women) assist Jane in her work. In contrast to a male physician who views Maudie as a "case," the women view Maudie as a unique individual who needs their help as she suffers through the infirmities of old age. They do not find abstract meaning in Maudie's suffering because her pain serves no healing purpose. Nor do they speak of God's will, as if Maudie's suffering were the price she must pay for her past transgressions. On the contrary, they simply work "to relieve her pain, alleviate her loneliness, and preserve—as nearly as they can—her autonomy" (as cited in Tong, 1993, p. 114).

Using the story of Maudie as a specific example of evil, Noddings proceeded to construct a phenomenology of evil. As she sees it, evil is not an abstract phenomenon, but rather a concrete reality that takes at least one of the three following forms:

1. Inflicting pain (unless it can be *demonstrated* that doing so will or is at least likely to spare the victim greater pain in the future)
2. a. Inducing the pain of separation
   b. Neglecting relation so that the pain of separation follows or those separated are thereby dehumanized
3. a. Deliberately or carelessly causing helplessness
   b. Creating elaborate systems of mystification that contribute to the fear of helplessness or to its actual maintenance (Cited in Tong, 1993, p. 122)

These actions, said Noddings, are evil, as many people in the nursing profession know all too well. No higher or better good can ever justify causing another person unnecessary pain or rendering another person separate or helpless (p. 122). Ethics is about overcoming pain, separation, and helplessness—a task that requires human beings to relate to one another as people whose goodness requires a sense of community.

To read *Women and Evil* together with *Caring* is to realize that Noddings espoused a relational ethics that is built on a relational ontology. According to Noddings, most individual dilemmas are, in fact, *relational* dramas that require dialogue, not monologue. Seeking to make her point more concretely, Noddings claimed that patients, for example, should not make healthcare decisions ordinarily—particularly end-of-life decisions— unilaterally. Rather, they should make these decisions in consultation with their families and friends. Noddings suggested that the process of someone dying can be an opportunity for family members to draw closer to one another, although she also realized that some families ruin this opportunity as they play out old rivalries and engage in power struggles. Under such strained and stressful conditions, patients who are competent must determine whether their own needs outweigh those of their families and friends. There are some things one person is not entitled to ask another person to do. Dying is one; not dying is another. Relationships are important, but so is the individual. In other words, any viable relational ethics must resist the tendency to make the relationship something individuals must serve no matter what. A self that is disconnected from others may be a solipsistic atom, but a self that is totally welded to others is no longer a self.

Although nurses may find an ethics of care valuable in their workplace, it is not a flawless ethics. A nurse can care or be expected to care too much. The phenomenon of nurse burnout attests to this fact. Sometimes caring is taken to its limits in the nursing profession. Commented Allethaire Cullen (1995):

> The *nursing system* itself contributes to burnout by presenting as "normal" the kinds of situations most people would find uncomfortable and frightening. How many people, for example, would feel comfortable holding babies born addicted to drugs or children who have died? Nurses do these things routinely as part of their role and care to patients. Few people in other professions are directly responsible for another person's life, yet nurses shoulder this responsibility daily. (p. 25)

In expressing concern about the dangers of caring too much, Gilligan's critics echoed Elizabeth Cady Stanton's 19th-century warning that, given society's tendency to take advantage of women, it is vital that women make self-development, rather than other-directed self-sacrifice, their first priority. Even so, it is important not to overemphasize the problems associated with caring too much. Whatever weaknesses an ethics of care may have, the world would be a worse place were women—and especially women in the caring professions— suddenly to stop meeting the physical and psychological needs of those who depend on them. Care is worth rescuing from the power structures that misshape it. If it is to be rescued, however, we need to recognize the differences between what feminist Sheila Mullett (1988) termed *distortions of caring* on the one hand and *undistorted caring* on the other hand.

According to Mullett, a person cannot truly care for someone if he or she is economically, socially, or psychologically coerced to do so. In other words, genuine or fully authentic caring cannot occur under conditions characterized by unfairness, domination, and subordination. Only under conditions of equality and freedom can women in the caring professions, for example, tend to patients' needs without being diminished, disempowered, or disregarded. Absent such ideal conditions, women in the caring professions must care cautiously, asking themselves whether the kind of caring in which they are engaged is:

- Care that fulfills the one caring
- Care that calls upon the unique and particular individuality of the one caring
- Care that is not produced by a person in a role because of gender, with one gender engaging in nurturing behavior and the other engaging in instrumental behavior
- Care that is reciprocated with caring, and not merely with the satisfaction of seeing the ones cared for flourishing and pursuing other projects
- Care that takes place within the framework of consciousness-raising practice and conversation (Cited in Tong, 1993, p. 103)

Care can be freely given only when the person caring is not taken for granted (p. 104).

Reasoning much like Gilligan and Noddings, so-called maternal thinkers have used the mother–child relationship as a springboard for discussing the necessary and sufficient conditions for truly moral human relationships. Specifically, feminist Sara Ruddick argued that from the work mothers do for their children emerges a distinct mode of moral reasoning best termed *maternal thinking* (as cited in Tong, 1993, pp. 136–137). To meet the three fundamental goals of maternal practice—namely, the preservation, growth, and social acceptability of children—mothers or persons who engage in motherly behavior must cultivate a multitude of very specific virtues, the most important of which is the metavirtue of attentive love. This metavirtue, which is at once cognitive and affective, enables mothers to really know their children. Realizing what is bad as well as good about their children, "good" mothers try to help their children eliminate their vices and weaknesses, slowly replacing them with virtues and strengths.

Concerned that men of goodwill might feel that, by virtue of their XY chromosome, they cannot think maternally, Ruddick noted that all human beings are capable of thinking in terms of preserving one another, helping one another grow, and making one another socially acceptable. To survive as a human species and to thrive as individual human beings, we all need to think maternally. Ruddick hypothesized that because women were largely excluded from the public realm until relatively recently, maternal thinking has not made its way into the public realm's power-wielding central offices. Instead, a very nonmaternal kind of thinking has dominated the public realm—the kind of thinking that leads to ecological disorder, social injustice, and even war.

People who do not think like mothers, said Ruddick, do not see like mothers. They do not make a connection, for example, between war as an idea and war as a reality. For them, war is about winning, defending one's way of life, and establishing one's position of power. For a maternal thinker, war is about conceivably destroying the child one has spent years preserving, nurturing, and training: a unique human person who cannot be replaced. In summary, for a maternal thinker, war is about killing—about canceling out the "product(s)" of maternal practice, and such a realization catapults maternal thinkers in the direction of peace activities (as cited in Tong, 1993, pp. 382–383).

Building on Ruddick's work, feminist philosopher Virginia Held (1993) noted that just because a maternal ethics exceeds the "moral minimum" of taking everyone's rights seriously, that does not mean it is free to dispense with this "moral minimum." Mothering persons must be fair, as well as compassionate, rational, and emotional, and able to make generalizations about human relationships as well as to articulate their specific features. A maternal thinker who says that no two human relationships are ever alike invites moral chaos. Like principles, relationships can be qualified as good, better, or best (bad, worse, or worst), and that which is subject to *qualification* is also subject to *evaluation*. In the same way that we can ask what makes a principle good or bad, so we can ask what makes a relationship good or bad.

Held (1993) stressed that both men and women can be mothering persons. Inviting girls but not boys to do caregiving work, she noted, produces boys with personalities "in which the inclination toward combat is overdeveloped and the capacity to feel for others is stunted" (p. 146). Because bellicose, unfeeling boys usually mature into bellicose, unfeeling men in positions of power, Held claimed that human survival may depend on society's ability to get men as well as women to care for children and, by parity of reasoning, for other vulnerable people (p. 146).

Despite the fact that Held believed that both men and women can mother, she nonetheless suggested that there could be a *qualitative* difference between female mothering and male mothering. The fact that women bear children as well as rear children could signal that "women are responsible for the existence of new persons in ways far more fundamental than are men" (p. 146). Women need men to begin a pregnancy, but they do not need men to end a pregnancy. Through abortion or suicide, women can say a definite "no" to life.

Even if rearing a child to adulthood is overall more taxing and demanding than the process of pregnancy and giving birth, Held asserted that the birthing act should not be discounted as if it had no special effect on subsequent parent–child relationships. In suggesting that biological experiences may influence "the attitudes of the mother and father toward the 'worth' or 'value' of a particular child" (p. 147), Held sought to explore the relationship between the kind of feelings women and men have for their children on the one hand and the kind of obligations they have to them on the other hand. If ethicists assume that natural male tendencies play a role in determining men's moral rights and responsibilities, then they should likewise make the same assumption about natural female tendencies:

> Traditional moral theories often suppose it is legitimate for individuals to maximize self-interest, or satisfy their preferences, within certain constraints based on the equal rights of others. If it can be shown that the tendency to want to pursue individual self-interest is a stronger tendency among men than among women, this would certainly be relevant to an evaluation of such a theory. And if it could be shown that a tendency to value children and a desire to foster the developing capabilities of the particular others for whom we care is a stronger tendency among women than among men, this too would be relevant in evaluating moral theories. (Cited in Tong, 1993, p. 147)

Held joined Gilligan and Noddings in their condemnation of the biblical character Abraham, who was willing to kill his son, Isaac, to honor God's command. Women who birth children—who preserve, nurture, and train them—are not likely to believe that obeying a command, including one from God, is more sacred than preserving the very lives of their children. To be sure, from the standpoint of traditional ethics, a mother's refusal to subordinate the concrete life of her child to the abstract commands of duty or higher law may indicate her underdevelopment as a moral agent. Yet, in an age where a blindness to interconnection has led to the destruction of the environment and a perilous buildup of the war arsenal, it can be argued reasonably that a focus on connections rather than rights may constitute a higher and better morality than does traditional ethics (Tong, 1993, pp. 145–148).

As a result of her awareness of how socioeconomic as well as physical and psychological conditions affect women's (and men's) ability to care, Eva Kittay (1998), another proponent of care ethics, focused on dependency workers—people who take care of people (most often for pay) but who view their job as more than a mere job—as the paradigm for caregivers. Nurses and other paid careworkers fall into this class of workers in a marked way. Kittay used Sasha, the woman who cared for her severely developmentally disabled daughter for more than 25 years, as her prime example of a dependency worker. In describing how Sasha's "labor of love" enabled her to succeed as a scholar and teacher, Kittay made the general point that we need to understand how people are interrelated. Without careworkers, domestic laborers, public health workers, and the like, human beings could not survive. Yet we often take our support systems for granted, paying meager salaries to the people (mostly women) who tend to our wounds, clean our bodies, and remove our dirt. Worse, we often view our caregivers as somehow less equal—less deserving of respect—than those who rule over us on Wall Street or in the White House.

It was this thought that pushed Kittay to use the mother–child paradigm to articulate the bottom-line rationale of her ethics of care. She thought of her mother, who used to sit down to dinner after serving her and her father, pointedly asserting: "After all, *I'm* also a mother's child" (Kittay, 1998, p. 25). In this statement—"I, too, deserve to eat"—is contained the fundamental source of human equality, according to Kittay. We are all equal because we are all the product of some mother's labor. We are the same not in our independence, but rather in our dependence.

POWER-FOCUSED FEMINIST APPROACHES TO ETHICS

Although power-focused feminist approaches to ethics appreciate the value of care, they are interested primarily in analyzing practices, policies, systems, structures, ideologies, and attitudes that contribute to the oppression of women and other groups that suffer equal or even worse forms of damaging subordination (Card, 1999). The ultimate goal of power-focused feminist ethicists is to transform a world burdened by covert and overt forms of sexism, racism, classism, ableism, heterosexism, ethnocentrism, and colonialism into a world in which all people are treated equally. In a transformed world, caregiving tasks would be equally distributed, and caregivers would receive as much care as they give.

Power-focused feminist approaches to bioethics can generally be divided into two groups: (1) those that emphasize the ways in which political, economic, and social forces systematically cause gender oppression and other forms of human oppression; and (2) those that stress the ways in which ideology, identity issues, and cultural forces account for women's (and other marginalized groups') second-class status. Liberal feminists belong to the first group, whereas radical, multicultural, global, and third-wave feminists are members of the second group.

Liberal Power-Focused Feminists

Liberal feminists have their historical roots in Mary Wollstonecraft's (1988) *A Vindication of the Rights of Woman*, John Stuart Mill's (1970) "The Subjection of Women," and the women's suffrage movement of the 19th century. Among the organizations with which contemporary liberal feminists are most aligned is the National Organization for Women (NOW). Liberal feminists maintain that the primary cause of women's remaining subordination to men is a set of lingering social norms and formal laws that have made it hard for women to succeed in the public world. When a woman chooses to be a nurse today, for example, this decision is not made because she cannot be a physician. Rather, it is because she wants to be a nurse, not a physician. One hundred years ago, a woman would not have had such a choice. The doors of medical schools would have been closed to her.

Although many people think that liberal feminism is passé and that the ethical issues that preoccupied them have been resolved, the fact of the matter is that as of 2010, the Bill of (Women's) Rights, which was first articulated by NOW in 1967, had yet to be fully implemented. Furthermore, U.S. women's reproductive rights are still not secure (the right to have an abortion remains under siege), and the Equal Rights Amendment has yet to pass. If the goal of liberal feminism is to push women full force into the public world and catapult them into its higher orbits, then its work is far from done.

Radical Power-Focused Feminists

Pointing to what they perceive as the central weakness of liberal feminism—the view that "I can be a man, too"—*radical feminists* claim that women's fundamental strength rests in their differences from men. Radical feminists do not think it is in women's best interest to become part of a system that devalues, among other things, caregiving practices and occupations. On the contrary, they think women should reject this system because its values—power, dominance, hierarchy, and competition—breed injustice. Not only must patriarchy's legal, political, educational, and economic structures be overturned, in radical feminists' estimation, so too must its sexual and reproductive practices and institutions be challenged.

Although all radical feminists focus on issues related to gender, sex, and reproduction, they do so in different ways depending on whether they are *radical-libertarian feminists* (the chapter author's terminology) on the one hand or *radical-cultural feminists* (also the chapter author's terminology) on the other hand. With respect to gender-related inequities, radical-libertarian feminists think that both men and women suffer when women are required to exhibit feminine characteristics only (e.g., "interdependence, community, connection, sharing, emotion, body, trust, absence of hierarchy, nature, immanence, process, joy, peace and life" [as cited in Tong, 1993, p. 163]) and men are required to exhibit masculine characteristics only (e.g., "independence, autonomy, intellect, will, wariness, hierarchy, domination, culture, transcendence, product, asceticism, war and death" [p. 163]). As radical-libertarian feminists see it, this enforced divide between the feminine and the masculine deforms both women and men, rendering both sexes deficient. Thus it is vital for society to permit both men and women to be androgynous—to exhibit a full range of masculine and feminine qualities. Men should be permitted to explore their feminine dimensions and women their masculine ones. No person should be forbidden the sense of wholeness that comes from combining his or her masculine and feminine dimensions. Such a view would enable more men to feel at home in the caring professions, and the terms *male nurse* and *female physician* would cease to exist.

Disagreeing with radical-libertarian feminists that a turn to androgyny would be a liberating strategy for women, radical-cultural feminists argue against this move. Some anti-androgynists maintain that the problem is not femininity in and of itself, but rather the low value that patriarchy assigns to feminine qualities and the high value that it assigns to masculine qualities. They claim that if society learned to value the feminine side of human existence as much as the masculine side of human existence, women's oppression would end. Other anti-androgynists disagree. They claim that femininity, as it is commonly understood, is a problem because it was constructed by men to achieve patriarchal purposes. To be liberated, they say, women must give new gynocentric meanings to femininity. According to this view, femininity should no longer be understood as those traits that deviate from masculinity and those traits that equip women to serve men's needs and desires. Rather, femininity should be reinterpreted as an authentically female way of being designed to support, delight, and satisfy women.

Radical feminist thought is as diverse on issues related to reproduction as it is on matters related to gender. Radical-libertarian feminists claim biological motherhood drains women both physically and psychologically. Women should be free, they say, to use both the old reproduction-controlling technologies of contraception, sterilization, and abortion and the new reproduction-assisting technologies of in vitro fertilization, egg donation, and surrogate motherhood on their own terms—to prevent or terminate unwanted pregnancies or, alternatively, to initiate pregnancies that require third-party intervention. Women should be able to have children when they want to, how they want to (in their own womb or that of another woman), and with whom they want to (a man, a woman, or alone through reproductive cloning). Some radical-libertarian feminists take this position even further, however. They look forward to the day when *ectogenesis* (extracorporeal gestation in an artificial placenta) entirely replaces the natural process of pregnancy and women no longer have to experience the physical discomforts that accompany gestation and/or the birthing process.

Objecting to radical-libertarian feminists' celebration of assisted reproduction, radical-cultural feminists caution that technology is not necessarily women's friend. According to these theorists, technology is breaking the links between conceiving, gestating, birthing, and rearing a child. Women had best keep an eye on technology lest it push them into the kind of dystopia Margaret Atwood imagines in *The Handmaid's Tale* (1985). In Atwood's novel, some women serve men as sexual toys; other women clean their homes. Still other women called handmaidens breed their children, and another group of women rear their children. Following a birth, the central character, Offred—a handmaiden whose name literally means "to be of Fred"—recalls better times and speaks in her mind to her mother, who had been a feminist leader: "Can you hear me? You wanted a woman's culture. Well, now there is one. It isn't what you meant, but it exists. Be thankful for small mercies" (as cited in Tong, 2009, p. 81).

Multicultural, Global, and Third-Wave Power-Focused Feminist Ethics

Multicultural and *global feminists* add new thoughts to those of liberal and radical feminism. They believe that women need to focus on the ways in which race, ethnicity, nationality, sexual identity, gender identity, age, religion, educational level, profession or occupation, marital status, health, and so forth contribute to some women being more powerful, free, and well-off than other women. Being a nurse in the United States, for example, is far different from being a nurse's aide in the United States or being a nurse in the Philippines or Kenya.

Audre Lorde (1992), bell hooks (1990), and Patricia Hill Collins (2008) were among the first multicultural feminists who stressed the ways in which some women are multiply jeopardized. The way for a marginalized woman to liberate herself from thoughts that she is deviant or inferior, said Lorde, is for her to "integrate all the parts of who [she is], openly, allowing power from particular sources of [her] living to flow back and forth freely through all [her] different selves, without the restrictions of externally imposed definition" (as cited in Tong, 2009, p. 539). Women must fight the enemy without—the political, economic, legal, and social systems and structures that keep women oppressed—but they also must fight the enemy within.

Global feminists are particularly attuned to the ways in which women in the so-called "First World" countries (i.e., heavily industrialized and market-based countries located primarily in the Northern Hemisphere) often unknowingly take advantage of women living and working in "Third World" countries (i.e., economically developing countries located primarily in the Southern Hemisphere). According to these feminists, relatively wealthy women in the upscale urban homes should think twice before buying inexpensive goods produced by poor women in global sweatshops. To be sure, purchasing such goods may be morally justifiable in the short run so that the women who make them now can survive; yet in the long run, this short-term remedy may actually prevent Third World women from organizing the kind of protests necessary to effect major social change.

Truth be told, reliance on immigrant women to do low-paid care work seems to be the order of the day. First World countries increasingly view Third World countries as a source of female caregivers willing to work for next to nothing. For example, in the United Kingdom, 35% of the nurses who work in the eldercare environment are immigrants. In London, more than 60% of the people who do eldercare work are immigrants (Cangiano, Shutes, Spencer, & Leeson, 2009, p. 182). These immigrant workers are nearly exclusively women, and they come mostly from Zimbabwe, Poland, Nigeria, the Philippines, and India. Their employers like their work ethic and their "warmth, respect, empathy, trust and patience in the care relationship" (p. 184). They also like the fact that they are willing to work for wages that native-born eldercare workers find outrageously low.

As in the United Kingdom, there is an exceptionally high demand for immigrant careworkers in Taiwan. Since the early 1980s, significant numbers of immigrant women without legal papers have worked in Taiwanese households (Lan, 2002, p. 188), thereby enabling Taiwanese women to remain in the paid workforce. Comments Pei-Chan Lan, "The filial duty of serving aging parents is transferred first from the son to the daughter-in-law (a gender transfer); later, it is outsourced to migrant careworkers (a market transfer)" (p. 188). As a result of citizens' increasing demand for inexpensive eldercare workers for their aged relatives, the Taiwanese government decided to legalize large numbers of immigrant careworkers. Specifically, in 1992, Taiwan started to grant work permits to domestic care-takers who agreed to care for severely ill or disabled people, children younger than the age of 12 years, or elders older than the age of 70 years (p. 171). Moreover, the country's leaders began to describe the importation of eldercare workers from the Philippines and Indonesia in particular "as a solution to the growing demand for paid care work among both nuclear households and the aging population" (p. 172).

Interestingly, Taiwanese female employers sometimes bond with their Filipina employees. They ally with them against husbands who are often viewed as tyrannical or extensively demanding. For the most part, however, no such bond is created and the Filipina employee may suffer accordingly. She may be abused verbally or discriminated against on account of her race, for example. Not having any real way to defend herself against mistreatment, the Filipina employee, like other immigrant eldercare workers, may do what she is told to do and leave it at that. The fact that she has legal documents does not mean she can quit and secure another job that pays well enough to support herself and her family back home.

If it is easy to take advantage of immigrant eldercare workers with proper legal documents, it is far easier to intimidate, harass, or bully immigrant eldercare workers without legal documents. Fearing deportation, undocumented eldercare workers are a particularly vulnerable group of careworkers. One rich New York businesswoman described her ideal careworker as a person who "basically [did] not have a life" of her own and who had nowhere to turn for help (Chang, 2006, pp. 43–45). The words of this wealthy woman are, of course, disconcerting. They clearly reduce the ideal careworker to a mere means—that is, a thing or instrument to serve one's own interests with no concern for the interests of the person one is using.

Although multicultural and global feminism are still alive and very well (Howard & Allen, 2000), these perspectives have been joined by yet another form of feminism: *third-wave feminism*. Contradiction, including self-contradiction, is expected and even willingly welcomed by third-wave feminists. So, too, is conflict. Two leading third-wave feminists, Leslie Heywood and Jennifer Drake (1997), commented:

> Even as different strains of feminism and activism sometimes directly contradict each other, they are all part of our third-wave lives, our thinking, and our praxes: we are products of all the contradictory definitions of and differences within feminism, beasts of such a hybrid kind that perhaps we need a different name altogether. (p. 3)

Heywood and Drake's suggestion that feminism may be passé is perhaps troubling, but it is understandable.

Being a feminist in a society where a growing number of people can literally choose their gender or racial/ethnic classification is different from being a feminist in a society where one's identity is more of a given and is difficult, if not impossible, to escape. Moreover, engaging in feminist action is extraordinarily challenging in a global context. According to third-wave feminist Chilla Bulbeck (1997), women in the First World have a lot of learning to do about women in the Third World. She stressed that the term *Third World* is "double valenced" (p. 35); that is, the Third World can be understood either negatively as a backward, poor, and bad place to live, or positively as "a subversive, immense repressed voice about to burst into centre stage of the globe" (p. 35).

Yet, however great the positive potential of the Third World is in Bulbeck's estimation, it still works against the women who live in it. Most Third World women are disadvantaged, as are women in the Fourth World (1997, p. 34), the world in which indigenous people in settler societies live—for example, the world of Native American women in the United States. Also disadvantaged are women in the Fifth World (O'Keefe & Chinouya, 2004), the world of migrants and immigrants who have left their native lands either because they wanted to or because they had to—for example, immigrant African women in the United Kingdom. Thus third-wave feminists realize just how elusive the concept of some sort of universal sisterhood is.

In addition to being open to women's different social, economic, political, and cultural differences, third-wave feminists are open to women's sexual differences. In the 1970s, feminists debated whether sex between heterosexuals and lesbians always needed to be egalitarian, feeling, and gentle, or whether it could sometimes be mechanical, rough, and violent. Even more specifically, they wondered about the appropriateness of women working in the sex industry as porn models, call girls, lap dancers, exotic dancers, and prostitutes. Were these women the victims of sexual objectification and dire economic conditions, or were they instead cagey entrepreneurs who realized they could make far more money selling their sexual services than working as waitresses at local diners? Although some second-wave feminists were willing to applaud women who used their sexuality in ways that served their self-reported interests, the general consensus of most second-wave feminists was that the dangers of sex were greater than its pleasures and that women had best steer clear of violent sex and commercialization of their bodies.

In contrast to most second-wave feminists, third-wave feminists are less prescriptive about what counts as good sex for women. They are also more comfortable with women who enhance their bodies to meet cultural expectations about what counts as beautiful. If a woman wants to wear makeup, have cosmetic surgery, and wear sexually provocative clothes, then, as far as many third-wave feminists are concerned, she should feel free to do so, provided she feels empowered by her actions and not somehow demeaned, diminished, or otherwise objectified by them. Unlike most second-wave feminists, third-wave feminists think that a woman can be both a feminist and a star in porn flicks. The apparent contradiction in the term *feminist porn queen* does not seem to bother third-wave feminists. Likewise, these feminists are very comfortable living in a transgendered world, in which people can change their sex or present themselves in a way that resists gender categorization.

Third-wave feminists are shaping a new kind of feminism that is not as interested in getting women to want what women should want as it is in responding to what women say they want and not judging whether their wants are authentic or inauthentic. Indeed, third-wave feminists describe the context in which they do feminism as one of "lived messiness" (Heywood & Drake, 1997, p. 8). Theorist Rebecca Walker has speculated that because many third-wave feminists grew up "transgender, bisexual, interracial, and knowing and loving people who are racist, sexist, and otherwise afflicted" (Walker, 1995, p. xxxiii), they are not as judgmental as second-wave feminists were. She stressed that because "the lines between Us and Them are often blurred," third-wave feminists seek to create identities that "accommodate ambiguity" and "multiple positionalities" (p. xxxiv).

Clearly, the openness of third-wave feminists is generally appealing and, in many instances, particularly liberating. When Walker (1995) said her third-wave feminist goal is to "debunk the stereotypes that there is one lifestyle or manifestation of feminist empowerment" (p. xxxiii) and instead offered "self-possession, self-determination, and an endless array of non-dichotomous possibilities" (p. xxxiv) to women, most young nurses would likely second her views. Yet just because third-wave feminists are able to deal with difference in admirable ways, it does not mean that third-wave feminism is flawless.

Whereas the challenge for second-wave feminists was to see and use women's differences productively to overcome the idea that all women are necessarily the same or some sort of victims, the challenge for third-wave feminists is to recognize that to have feminism, one has to believe that women constitute a distinct social group (Ferguson, 1989, p. 352) and that just because some women feel empowered does not mean all women feel this way. Thus it is troubling when second-wave feminism is dismissed as unalloyed victim feminism and third-wave feminism is celebrated as unalloyed power feminism.

In the hands of third-wave feminists such as Heywood and Drake, as well as Walker, power feminism seems inviting enough. Conversely, in the hands of other thinkers, sometimes described as third-wave *postfeminists*, power feminism gets very mean-spirited. Specifically, third-wave postfeminists such as Katie Roiphe (1993), Camille Paglia (1992), and Rene Denfeld (1995) insisted that nowadays women are free to be whomever they want to be and to do whatever they want to do. Women's only possible enemy is themselves, they implied. Forgetting how much their power is connected to their advantaged position, Roiphe, Paglia, and Denfeld have failed to recognize the vulnerability and victimization of disadvantaged women in the United States and elsewhere. For every nurse who loves her job, there is another one who hates it; and for every nurse who heads a team, there is another one who knows better than to disagree with a physician, an administrator, or even a demanding patient. This is not the time for women to reject the label feminist; far from it, it is the time for women, especially women in the caring professions, to embrace it more enthusiastically lest women's progress reach a dead end as it has in the past. Think about all the women who are leaving their careers because they cannot handle both career and family responsibilities; more specifically, think of all the nurses who are leaving nursing because their workplaces are anything but female-friendly, paradoxical as that claim may seem.

All women, but especially women in the caring professions, should rally around the feminist flag to call attention to their caregiving powers. This statement is not intended to dismiss the important roles played by men in the nursing professions and men who proudly call themselves feminist. Rather, the intention is to agree with feminist theorist Christine di Stephano, who claimed, "Gender is basic in ways that we have to fully understand" and "functions as 'a difference that makes a difference,'" even as it can no longer claim the legitimating mantle of the difference (di Stephano, 1990, p. 70). If any group of people—including men—can figure out what this difference is, it is nurses; nursing is almost an intractably gendered field, and we would all do well to understand why this is so.

REFERENCES

Atwood, M. (1985). *The handmaid's tale.* Toronto, Canada: McClelland & Stewart.

Bulbeck, C. (1997). *Re-orienting Western feminisms: Women's diversity in a postcolonial world.* New York, NY: Cambridge University Press.

Cangiano, A., Shutes, I., Spencer, S., & Leeson, G. (2009). *Migrant care workers in ageing societies: Research findings in the United Kingdom.* Oxford, UK: COMPAS: ESRC Centre on Migration, Policy, and Society, University of Oxford.

Card, C. (1999). *On feminist ethics and politics.* Lawrence, KS: University Press of Kansas.

Chang, G. (2006). Disposable domestics: Immigrant women workers in the global economy. In M. K. Zimmerman, J. S. Litt, & C. E. Bose (Eds.), *Global dimensions of gender and carework* (pp. 39–47). Stanford, CA: Stanford Social Sciences.

Code, L., Mullett, S., & Overall, C. (Eds.). (1988). *Feminist perspectives: Philosophical essays on method and morals.* Toronto, Canada: University of Toronto Press.

Cullen, A. (1995). Burnout: Why do we blame the nurse? *American Journal of Nursing, 95*(11), 22–28.

Denfeld, R. (1995). *The new Victorians: A young woman's challenges to the old feminist order.* New York, NY: Routledge.

di Stephano, C. (1990). Dilemmas of difference. In L. J. Nicholson (Ed.), *Feminism/postmodernism* (pp. 63–82). New York, NY: Routledge.

Ferguson, A. (1989). Sex and work: Women as a new revolutionary class. In R. S. Gottlieb (Ed.), *An anthology of Western Marxism: From Lukacs and Gramsci to socialist-feminism* (pp. 348–372). Oxford, UK: Oxford University Press.

Gilligan, C. (1982). *In a different voice.* Cambridge, MA: University Harvard Press.

Held, V. (1993). *Feminist morality: Transforming culture, society, and politics.* Chicago, IL: University of Chicago Press.

Heywood, L., & Drake, J. (Eds.). (1997). *Third wave agenda: Being feminist, doing feminism.* Minneapolis, MN: University of Minnesota Press.

Hill Collins, P. (2008). *Black feminist thought: Knowledge, consciousness, and the politics of empowerment.* New York, NY: Routledge Classics.

hooks, b. (1990). *Yearning: race, gender, and cultural politics.* Boston, MA: South End Press.

Howard, J. A., & Allen, C. (2000). *Feminisms at a millennium.* Chicago, IL: University of Chicago Press.

Jaggar, A. M. (1992). Feminist ethics. In L. Becker & C. Becker (Eds.), *Encyclopedia of ethics* (pp. 363–364). New York, NY: Garland.

Kittay, E. F. (1998). *Love's labor: Essays on women, equality, and dependency.* New York, NY: Routledge.

Lan, P. C. (2002). Among women: Migrant domestics and their Taiwanese employers across generations. In B. Ehrenreich & A. R. Hochschild (Eds.), *Global woman: Nannies, maids, and sex workers in the new economy* (pp. 169–189). New York, NY: Metropolitan Books.

Lessing, D. (as J. Somers, pseudonym). (1983). *The diary of a good neighbor.* New York, NY: Alfred A. Knopf.

Lorde, A. (1992). Age, race, class, and sex and women redefining difference. In M. L. Anderson & P. H. Collins (Eds.), *Race, class, and gender* (2nd ed., pp. 503–509). Belmont, CA: Wadsworth.

Mill, J. S. (1970). The subjection of women [1869 orig pub by Mills]. In A. S. Rossi (Ed.), *Essays on sex equality* (pp. 123–243). Chicago, IL: University of Chicago Press.

Mullet, S. (1988). Shifting perspectives: A new approach to ethics. In L. Code, S. Mullett, & C. Overall (Eds.), *Feminist perspectives: Philosophy essays on methods and morals* (pp. 109–126). Toronto, Canada: University of Toronto Press.

Noddings, N. (1984). *Caring: A feminine approach to ethics and moral education.* Berkeley, CA: University of California Press.

Noddings, N. (1989). *Women and evil.* Berkeley, CA: University of California Press.

O'Keefe, E., & Chinouya, M. (2004). Global migrants, gendered tradition, and human rights: Africans and HIV in the United Kingdom. In R. Tong, S. Dodd, & A. Donchin (Eds.), *Linking visions: Feminist bioethics, human rights, and the developing world* (pp. 217–234). Lanham, MD: Rowman & Littlefield.

Paglia, C. (1992). *Sex, art, and American culture: Essays.* New York, NY: Random House.

Roiphe, K. (1993). *The morning after: Sex, fear, and feminism on campus.* New York, NY: Little, Brown.

Ruddick, S. (1989). *Maternal thinking: Towards a politics of peace.* Boston, MA: Beacon Press.

Sherwin, S. (1992). *No longer patient: Feminist ethics and health care.* Philadelphia, PA: Temple University Press.

Tong, R. (1993). *Feminine and feminist ethics.* Belmont, CA: Wadsworth.

Tong, R. (1998). The ethics of care: A feminist virtue of care for healthcare practitioners. *Journal of Medicine and Philosophy, 23*(2), 131–152.

Tong, R. (2009). *Feminist thought: A more comprehensive introduction* (3rd ed.). Boulder, CO: Westview Press.

U.S. Department of Labor & U.S. Bureau of Labor Statistics. (2008). Women in the labor force: A databook. *Report, 1011,* 31.

Walker, R. (1995). *To be real: Telling the truth and changing the face of feminism.* New York, NY: Anchor Books.

Williams, C. L. (2000). The glass escalator: Hidden advantages for men in the "female" professions. In M. S. Kimmel & A. Aronson (Eds.), *The gendered society reader* (pp. 294–310). New York, NY: Oxford University Press.

Wollstonecraft, M. A. (1988) [C. H. Polston, Ed.]. *A vindication of the rights of woman.* New York, NY: W. W. Norton.

Chapter 9

Theories and Methods in Ethics

Karen L. Rich

INTRODUCTION

The first purpose of this chapter is to analyze the theoretical nature of ethics—that is, to provide a framework to answer the question, "Do ethical theories really exist?" The reader should be an active participant in answering this question. To conduct this analysis, the nature of philosophy, ethics, science, and theory are each explored. The second purpose of the chapter is to discuss several important approaches to ethics. In the literature, these approaches often are referred to as *theories* of ethics. Before reading further, visit **Box 9-1** to begin an analysis of theory in the field of ethics.

PHILOSOPHICAL INQUIRY

Philosophy, translated literally, means the love of wisdom. One of the oldest scholarly disciplines, it retains at its roots an effort to understand the abstract questions about the nature of *knowledge* and *being* and a search for *truth*. The discipline remains esoteric, but it has evolved over the years to include formal systems and principles such as those used in the practice of logic.

Philosophical inquiry can be grouped into content areas, which may differ slightly among philosophers. Three main content areas or types of inquiry in philosophy are (1) *epistemology*, the study of knowledge; (2) *ontology* (metaphysics), the study of the nature of being; and (3) *axiology*, the study of values. Ethics is concerned with axiological inquiry. Philosophy provides a method of studying and, consequently, knowing something about the nature of knowledge, reality, and existence, and what is highly desirable, good, or useful.

Billington (2003) divided philosophy into two areas of focus—one that asks questions of "Why?" and one that asks questions of "How?" or "What?" The *why* questions relate to epistemology, metaphysics, and logic; the *how* and *what* questions focus on decisions

---

Box 9-1   Ethics-Focused Inquiry

In *Essentials of Doctoral Education for Advanced Nursing Practice* (American Association of Colleges of Nursing [AACN], 2006), it is stated that doctor of nursing practice programs prepare graduates to "integrate nursing science with knowledge from" other sciences and disciplines "as the basis for the highest level of nursing practice" (p. 9). Advanced practice nurses (APNs) need to be able to think critically about, question, and analyze epistemological, ontological, and empirical matters. Probing the following questions and considering possible answers is an exercise in preparing to integrate knowledge into practice. *Ethics* can be defined simply as the study of ideal ways of being and behavior. With this in mind and before reading this chapter, reflect on and use your current knowledge to answer the following questions:

1. Is ethics a science? What does one have to know to answer this question?
2. As a field of study, is ethics suitable for theory development and use? Why or why not?
3. Which methods of inquiry or research do you believe are appropriate for ethics?

---

about behavior, priorities, and relationships. According to Billington, ethics belongs in the second category of focus.

Durant (1933) included five fields of study and discourse within the discipline of philosophy: (1) logic, (2) esthetics, (3) ethics, (4) politics, and (5) metaphysics. The first four of these fields constitute a study of the *ideal*, which is described as the study of ideal "method in thought and research," "form or beauty," "conduct," and "social organization," respectively (p. 3). According to Durant, metaphysics does not fit the same pattern as other forms of philosophy. Specifically, it does not focus on trying to accommodate the real with the ideal. Instead, metaphysics is a study of ultimate reality. Included in metaphysics is a study of the nature of mind (philosophical psychology), matter (ontology), and knowledge (epistemology).

No matter how ethics is classified, whether as a primary field of philosophy or as a field subsumed within another field, ethics is always considered to be a subdivision of philosophy. Because it is a branch of philosophy, ethics resides in the tier of the most abstract approaches to studying and understanding the nature of human beings and reality. Ethics means different things to different people. When the term is narrowly defined according to its historical use, ethics is the study of ideal human behavior and ideal ways of being. The approaches to ethics and the meanings of related concepts have varied over time among philosophers and ethicists. For example, Aristotle believed that ideal behaviors are those practices that lead to the end goal of *eudemonia*, which is synonymous with a special or high level of happiness or human well-being, whereas the 18th-century philosopher and ethicist Immanuel Kant (1785/2012) believed that ideal behavior entails acting in accordance with one's duty. Human well-being, according to Kant, is having the freedom to exercise self-determination (autonomy), being respected, and having the capability to think rationally.

As a field of study, ethics is a systematic approach to understanding, analyzing, and distinguishing matters of right and wrong, good and bad, and admirable and deplorable and how these matters relate to the well-being of and the relationship among sentient beings. Ethics is an active process rather than a static condition. Therefore, some ethicists prefer to use the phrase *doing ethics* to describe work in this field. When people are doing ethics, they need to support their beliefs and assertions with sound reasoning. In other words, even if people believe that ethics can be done subjectively, they must be able to justify their positions through logical, rational arguments.

As contrasted with ethics, *morals* are specific beliefs, behaviors, and ways of being derived from doing ethics. As a practical matter, these terms are often used interchangeably.

SCIENCE: THE DAUGHTER OF PHILOSOPHY

Philosophy has been practiced since ancient times, when Plato declared that philosophers would be kings in ideal republics. Lovers of wisdom provided much of the means of humans' intellectual progress for hundreds of years. Eventually, it was philosophy that inevitably gave birth to science (Magee, 2001) as people sought more certainty to explain their external environment and human nature. As people moved out of the Middle (Dark) Ages and into the Age of Enlightenment, those in the Western world began to feel confident that human nature and the material world could be explained, predicted, and controlled.

After Newton, science reigned as the authoritative definer of the universe, and philosophy defined itself in relation to science—predominantly supportive, occasionally critical and provocative, sometimes independent and concerned with different areas, but ultimately not in a position to gainsay the cosmological discoveries and conclusions of empirical science, which now increasingly ruled the Western worldview (Tarnas, 1991, p. 280).

Russell (1945) called philosophy an intermediate discipline between theology and science. Philosophy has commonalities with both: Like theology, philosophy is speculative and provides no definitive answers; like science, philosophy is based on reason rather than on dogma and tradition. Russell contended that the most interesting questions of speculative minds reside in what he called the "no man's land" of philosophy. Science cannot answer these questions, and theologians no longer hold the authority that they did in past centuries.

Philosophy can enrich the lives of people because it is focused on this no man's land of questions that have confounded humans for ages. As Lund (2003) articulates, "Philosophizing is thinking hard about life's most fundamental questions" (p. 2). Thinking hard, using reason, and evaluating arguments about the fundamental questions of life liberate one from dogma and small-minded customs. Although many philosophers have religious beliefs, good philosophizing does not resort to the use of religion to support philosophical positions (Magee, 2001). Instead, good philosophy is an attempt to "see how far reason will take us" (p. 7). In **Box 9-2**, the reader is asked to consider some of the questions related to the ideas proposed in this paragraph.

Although both philosophers and scientists search for truth using rational thought processes, the answers to the questions of philosophical inquiry are neither well defined

---

Box 9-2   How Do We Know What We Know?

In *Essentials of Doctoral Education for Advanced Nursing Practice* (AACN, 2006), it is stated that "the [APN] scholar applies knowledge to solve a problem via the scholarship of application (referred to as the scholarship of practice in nursing)" (p. 11). But how do nurse scholars know what they know? Reflect on the following questions posed by Magee (2001, p. 7). How would you answer them?

1. Can we ever really know, in the sense of being sure of, anything? If so, what?
2. Even if we do know, how will we be able to be sure that we know? In other words, can we ever know that we know?

Now compare and contrast your answers to these questions as they relate to moral knowledge and scientific knowledge. Consider the following quote in your process of answering these philosophical questions:

> It is a conclusion which—like all other philosophical conclusions—we shall require good reasons for believing. We shall not be willing just to accept it on spec, or on faith, or because we have an intuition to that effect: we shall want to know why we should believe it to be true. (Magee, 2001, p. 8)

---

nor unequivocal. Scientists, however, use experiments in an attempt to elucidate them. Of course, there is no experiment that can answer some of society's most fundamental ethical questions, such as "What is the meaning of good?" and "How beneficent are people or nurses required to be?"

Philosophy is used to address problems that are prescientific or nonscientific, problems such as the determination of good and evil (Durant, 1933). Science begins with a hypothesis that is tested with the scientific method; if the scientist is successful, doing science ends with a practical achievement. Philosophy, by comparison, "is a hypothetical interpretation of the unknown (as in metaphysics), or of the inexactly known (as in ethics or political philosophy)" (p. 2). Durant used a military metaphor to compare philosophy and science. In a siege of truth, philosophy occupies the most forward trench, whereas science represents the captured land. However, philosophy "leaves the fruits of victory to her daughters the sciences" (p. 2).

Science should be conducted impartially and objectively; it is focused on fact finding. Philosophy, although conducted with rational thinking, is value laden and is used to interpret and synthesize ideal possibilities, meanings, and the significance of experience. Science breaks the whole into parts, and then philosophy puts the parts together again in a form that is better than the original whole. According to Durant:

> Science tells us how to heal and how to kill; it reduces the death rate in retail and then kills us wholesale in war; but only wisdom—desire coordinated in the light of all experience—can tell us when to heal and when to kill. (p. 2)

METHODS AND OUTCOMES OF INQUIRY

Scientists generally use the scientific method to conduct *scientific inquiry*. Some of the characteristics of scientific inquiry are objectivity, generalizability, reproducibility, and being able to achieve outcomes of practical importance. In his classic book *A Primer in Theory Construction*, Reynolds (1971) listed five characteristics that a scientific body of knowledge should provide: (1) typology, (2) predictions, (3) explanations, (4) understanding about causes (i.e., independent variables' effects on dependent variables), and (5) control.

Often the outcomes of philosophy as compared to science provide knowledge and satisfaction for its own sake rather than for its practical benefits (Lund, 2003). In referring to medical ethics, Sulmasy and Sugarman (2001) stated that it is not always clear whether work done in the field of ethics by disciplines such as nursing, medicine, sociology, economics, law, and others is scholarly work. Three accepted scholarly methods of ethical inquiry or thinking that relate to ethics exist: *normative ethics*, *meta-ethics*, and *descriptive ethics* (Frankena, 1973). Sulmasy and Sugarman contended that "normative ethics [inquiry] is at the core of scholarship in ethics" (p. 4).

Normative Ethics

Normative ethics is an attempt to decide or prescribe values, behaviors, and ways of being that are right or wrong, good or bad, and admirable or deplorable. When using the method of normative ethics, inquiries are made about how humans should behave, what ought to be done in certain situations, or which type of character one should have or how one should be. Outcomes of normative ethics are the prescriptions derived from asking normative questions. These prescriptions include accepted moral norms, standards, and codes.

One such accepted moral standard is the *common morality* (Beauchamp & Childress, 2009). The common morality consists of normative beliefs and behaviors about which the members of society generally agree and that are familiar to most human beings. For example, the belief that robbing a bank is wrong is part of the common morality in the United States. In contrast, because of the many and varying positions about the rightness or wrongness of abortion, accepting abortion as a moral act is not a part of our common morality. A normative belief in the nursing profession is that nurses ought to be compassionate; that is, nurses should work to relieve suffering. This claim is supported by the *Code of Ethics for Nurses With Interpretive Statements* (American Nurses Association, 2015) and *The ICN Code of Ethics for Nurses* (International Council of Nurses, 2006).

Meta-ethics

The focus of meta-ethics, which means "about ethics," is not an inquiry about what ought to be done or which behaviors should be prescribed. Rather, meta-ethics is concerned with understanding the language of morality through an analysis of the meaning of ethically related concepts and theories, such as the meaning of good, happiness, and virtuous character. For example, a nurse who is engaging actively in a meta-ethical analysis might try to determine the meaning of a good nurse–patient relationship.

Descriptive Ethics

Of the three methods of inquiry, descriptive ethics comes closest to a scientific method of inquiry as opposed to philosophical ethical inquiry. This approach is used when researchers or ethicists want to describe what people think about morality or how people actually behave (i.e., their morals). Professional moral values and behaviors can be described empirically through nursing research using traditional descriptive research methodology. An example of descriptive ethics is the outcome of research that identifies nurses' attitudes regarding telling patients the truth about their terminal illnesses.

The Fact/Value Distinction

In conducting ethical inquiry, one should be aware of the "fact/value" distinction to avoid the pitfall in moral reasoning called the "is/ought" gap. During the 18th century, the philosopher David Hume (1711–1776) made an important point about good moral reasoning, when he argued that there is a distinction between facts (for example, scientific or descriptive findings) and values (normative beliefs) when moral reasoning is considered. Not being sensitive to the fact/value distinction can leave one with an is/ought gap. A skeptic, Hume suggested that people should not acknowledge a fact of what is and then believe they can legitimately prove the rightness or wrongness of a value judgment based on that fact. In other words, one logically cannot take a fact of what is and then extrapolate an ethical judgment of what ought to be.

If Hume's argument is accepted as valid, people should refrain from making the following assumption: (1) I see Sara practicing hard paternalism with her terminally ill cancer patient; (2) many bioethicists caution that a hard form of paternalism is unethical; therefore, (3) Sara ought not practice paternalism because it is unethical (a value statement). According to people who believe in the truth of the "fact/value" distinction, it is a fact that Sara is acting paternalistically toward her cancer patient, and it is a fact that many bioethicists believe that paternalism is unethical. However, the two facts in this example do not prove the moral nature of Sara's act of paternalism. The conclusion that Sara's act of paternalism is unethical is only a feeling that places a certain value on a particular act. Although Hume's fact/value distinction requirement for doing ethics precludes being able to prove the rightness or wrongness of value statements, it does not minimize the need for people to support their moral positions (value judgments) with valid arguments. Nevertheless, accepting Hume's argument does mean that identifying the truth in value statements is an interminable endeavor.

PERSPECTIVES ON THEORY

The meaning and purposes of theory have been described and analyzed differently among myriad people both within and outside of nursing. Different perspectives about theory are discussed briefly in this section. Rather than providing a definitive conclusion about whether theories of ethics exist, and if they exist, the type of theory into which moral theory can be classified, readers are encouraged to draw their own conclusions about these points. It is important to note that most ethicists and other writers do refer to theories of ethics or moral theory when discussing ethics; however, most ethicists do not typically analyze the theoretical nature per se of ethical approaches.

Reynolds (1971) referred to "scientific theory" (p. 10) in his primer. He proposed that three primary forms of theories exist: (1) set-of-laws, (2) axiomatic, and (3) causal process. The first form is composed of theories that can be classified as scientific laws; the second includes sets of definitions, existence statements, and relational statements; and the third form is composed of sets of definitions, existence statements, and causal statements. Axiomatic theories are rare in social and human phenomena. Plane geometry is a good example of an axiomatic theory. Reynolds acknowledged that the following are sometimes considered to be other forms of theory: "(1) vague conceptualizations or descriptions of events or things, (2) prescriptions about what are desirable social behaviors or arrangements, or (3) any untested hypothesis or idea" (p. 11). Nevertheless, he avoided a discussion of these latter forms of theory in his classic theory primer.

Some nurse authors and theorists distinguish nursing philosophies from nursing theories (McEwen, 2007; Tomey & Alligood, 2006). The structural holarchy of contemporary nursing (Fawcett, 2005) is depicted visually with a figure that lists the following elements in top to bottom order, although no assumption should be made that these elements exist linearly: metaparadigm, philosophies, conceptual models, theories, and empirical indicators. Fawcett defined theory as "one or more relatively concrete and specific concepts that are derived from a conceptual model, the propositions that narrowly describe those concepts, and the propositions that state relatively concrete and specific relations between two or more of the concepts" (p. 18).

Meleis (2005) defined theory as "an organized, coherent, and systematic articulation of a set of statements related to significant questions in a discipline that are communicated in a meaningful whole" (p. 12). These statements are used to describe, explain, predict, or prescribe "events, situations, conditions, or relationships" (p. 12). According to Meleis, a theory should contain concepts related to a discipline's phenomena of interest.

The philosophers Dickoff and James (1968) argued that theory for the practice discipline of nursing should be of the highest level—a type of theory that these authors called *situation producing*. They outlined the following characteristics of situation-producing theory: (1) it is invented for a purpose; (2) it includes specific goal content aimed at the outcome of some activity; (3) it is prescriptive in nature; and (4) it contains a survey list of aspects of related activity. Beckstrand (1978, 1980) specifically criticized Dickoff and James's conception of situation-producing theory as being too personal in nature, as well as being unnecessary for nursing. Although the term *evidence-based practice* was not in vogue when she wrote her articles, Beckstrand contended that when nurses use situation-producing theory, they essentially decide on their own goals for patient care without subjecting the goals to consensus or examining evidence for and against the goals. Beckstrand's other criticism is discussed later in this section.

Wiedenbach (1970), who wrote and worked with Dickoff and James, also developed a philosophy-based practice theory for nurses that she classified as prescriptive. Wiedenbach defined theory as follows:

> Theory is an abstract phenomenon. It develops within the mind but derives from reality and influences action. It is the outgrowth of an intellectual process set in motion by observations. From them, ideas are generated. Then, by means of the intellect, the ideas—we'll call them concepts—may be consciously brought into meaningful relationship with one another for such purposes as to identify or isolate factors, to characterize or classify them, to predict effect from cause, or to prescribe a course of action by which to obtain desired results. (p. 1057)

Wiedenbach (1970) asserted that nurses use theory to guide practice, which can be interpreted as a personal use, and to improve nursing practice, which can be interpreted as a use for the common good of the profession. According to Wiedenbach, each nurse must identify (theorize about) what underlies his or her practice. To meet this challenge, the nurse must answer three questions: (1) "What needs to be accomplished?", (2) "How will it be accomplished?", and (3) "In which context will it be done?" When these questions are answered, the nurse has the information needed to identify a prescriptive theory for practice. The three essential characteristics of the prescriptive theory are (1) the nurse's professional commitment (purpose), (2) the prescription for achieving the nurse's purpose, and (3) the realities that affect the process and, ultimately, the outcomes of the nurse's actions. In regard to the first characteristic, nurses need to specify their beliefs. Wiedenbach's prescriptive form of practice theory is subject to the same criticism that Beckstrand (1980) used in evaluating Dickoff and James's situation-producing theory—namely, that it might be viewed as too subjective.

In 1978, Beckstrand asserted that while much buzz focused on developing a practice theory for nursing, such as the situation-producing theory suggested by Dickoff and James (1968), the profession does not really need a practice theory at all. She argued that nurses have access to scientific and ethical theories and that all other knowledge needed by nurses is reducible to these two fields. Science is needed "to describe, to explain, and to predict natural and social phenomena" and "the purpose of ethical or normative theory is to describe and to predict what actions and characteristics will lead to the realization of morality and goodness" (Beckstrand, 1978, p. 606). Nursing practice is focused on changing entities so that more good can be achieved. Beckstrand distinguished ethical theory useful to nursing as being of the normative type. She discussed important ethical knowledge in terms of moral obligations and moral values. Also essential to justify the goals of nursing practice is knowledge about theories of nonmoral value, which can be evaluated in terms of utility or being intrinsic, extrinsic, contributory, or instrumental. Ultimately, Beckstrand concluded that scientific theory and ethical theory (including nonmoral value theory) are sufficient to guide nursing practice without the development of additional practice theories.

According to Vaughn (2010), "moral theories are meant to explain what makes an action right or a person good" (p. 43). Thus Vaughn's position indicates that moral theory is of the explanatory type, but he added that moral theory also "must be filled out with details about how to apply them in real life and the kinds of cases to which they are relevant" (p. 31). This means that moral theory is prescriptive as well as explanatory. He divided moral theories into those that focus on right action and those that focus on good or bad character. To identify the best theory for determining what is right and good, three criteria were proposed: "consistency with our considered moral judgments, consistency with the facts of the moral life, and resourcefulness in moral problem solving" (p. 44).

Vaughn (2010) called morality a "normative, or evaluative, enterprise" (p. 5) that can be distinguished from nonmoral norms, which also are applied in everyday life. Moral norms are different because they possess the following characteristics: (1) *normative dominance*—accepting the practice of allowing moral norms to dominate or override non-moral norms; (2) *universality*—recognizing that certain moral norms should be applicable across all comparable situations; (3) *impartiality*—the notion that all individuals' interests should be considered equally (note: this characteristic has been debated among ethicists depending on preferred theories, such as in feminist ethics and communitarianism); and (4) *reasonableness*—norms having sound support in good moral reasoning.

The ethicists Beauchamp and Childress have been highly influential in the development of the field of bioethics. Beauchamp and Childress (2009) proposed that the following characteristics may be used to describe ethical or moral theory: "(1) abstract moral reflection and argument, (2) systematic presentation of the basic components of ethics, (3) an integrated body of moral principles, and (4) a systematic justification of moral principles" (p. 333). Major moral theories include a hypothesis that offers a moral framework. These authors distinguish two conceptions of ethical theory, which are separated temporally. The task of ethical theory in the older conception (late 18th to early 20th century) "is to locate and justify general norms as a system" (p. 334). In the more recent conception, which is less well formed, ethical theory is tasked with reflecting "critically on actual and proposed moral norms and practices" (p. 334).

Beauchamp and Childress (2009) have outlined eight conditions against which ethical theories can be evaluated: (1) clarity (clearness), (2) coherence (no conceptual inconsistencies or contradictory statements), (3) comprehensiveness (accounts for a sizable number of justified moral norms or judgments), (4) simplicity (narrows morality to only a few basic

---

Box 9-3   Evaluation of Theory for Ethics

Formulate answers to these questions before reading the final section of the chapter. After reading the final section, revisit these questions and continue to refine your judgments. Supplementary information may be needed to accomplish this activity, especially additional readings about specific moral theories or approaches.

1. Do ethical or moral theories exist? Support your answer.
2. Which type of classification best fits the purpose of ethical theories or approaches (for example, prescription, explanation, prediction, or control)? Support your answer.
3. How do ethical theories or approaches differ from nursing theories? Compare and contrast.

---

norms), (5) explanatory power (helps people understand morality), (6) justificatory power (provides new grounds for beliefs or a justified criticism of defective beliefs), (7) output power (produces new moral judgments), and (8) practicability (requirements of the theory are not too demanding to make it unfeasible to use). It is not expected that all ethical theories will be able to fulfill all eight of these conditions.

The next section of this chapter covers specific approaches to ethics that most ethicists call theories. Before reading this section, review **Box 9-3** and begin to formulate your positions about theory as it relates to ethics.

THEORETICAL APPROACHES TO ETHICS

Assuming that ethical or moral theories exist, they generally are considered to be normative in nature. Normative ethical theories function as moral guides to answer the questions, "What should I do or not do?" and "How should I be?" A moral theory can provide individuals with guidance in moral thinking and reasoning, as well as offering justification for moral actions.

The descriptions of the theories in this section are not all inclusive, nor do they necessarily include all variations of the theories that are discussed. Theories of ethics overlap and often are quite abstract and difficult to study. Therefore, the theories discussed in this chapter, because of their brief presentation, provide a somewhat oversimplified view. The goal was to include enough discussion to illustrate the major concepts important to the content of each theory. Readers are encouraged to seek more information about each theory, consider related concepts, and construct propositional statements that are reasonable given what is included in discussions of the theories in ethics literature.

Rule-Based Theories

Natural Law Theory

Most modern versions of natural law theory have their basis in the philosophy of St. Thomas Aquinas (ca. 1225–1274). People who adhere to natural law theory believe that the rightness of actions is self-evident because morality is determined by inherent human nature, not by customs and preferences. According to this theory, the law of reason is incorporated within the order of nature (usually thought to be implanted by God), and this law provides the rules or commands for human actions. Consequently, natural law theory is often associated with rule-based Judeo-Christian ethics. Natural law theory is the basis of religious prohibitions against acts that some people consider to be unnatural, such as homosexuality, the use of birth control, and fertility procedures.

Rights Theory

Since the time of Thomas Hobbes (1588–1679), the concepts of individualism and liberalism have been associated with a rights-based theory of ethics (Beauchamp & Childress, 2009). "Rights are *justified claims* that individuals and groups can make on other individuals or on society" (p. 350). Decisions about allowing or disallowing rights come from a society's normative framework. In the United States, legal rights stem from the Constitution and federal, state, and local legal systems. Moral rights are less well defined. For example, in the United States, groups continue to argue about whether health care is a right or a privilege. Libertarians believe in market justice; that is, they believe that people should earn and pay for the benefits that they receive. In contrast, communitarians believe that health care for all citizens contributes to the common good of the community.

Disagreements also exist about whether moral rights are always absolute or whether they sometimes are *prima facie* claims that must give way to other rights. To exercise one's rights ethically, it is generally accepted that a person should not violate the rights of other people. An example of an absolute right is the right to choose one's religion, whereas a *prima facie* right is the right to autonomy. Sometimes one's autonomy must be overruled when, for instance, it might cause an infringement on another person's right to health.

Deontology

Deontology, literally "the study of duty," is an approach to ethics that focuses on duties and rules. The most influential philosopher associated with the deontological way of thinking was Immanuel Kant (1724–1804). Kant (1785/2012) defined a person as a rational, self-legislating (autonomous) being with the ability to know universal, objective moral laws and the freedom to decide to act morally, which means to act according to one's duty. Kantian deontology prescribes that each rational being is ethically bound or obligated to act first and foremost from a sense of duty. When deciding how to act, the consequences of one's actions are considered to be irrelevant.

According to Kant, only dutiful actions have moral worth. Even when individuals do not want to act from a motivation of duty, Kant believed they are required ethically to do so. In fact, having one's actions motivated by duty is superior to acting from a motivation of love. Because rational choice is within one's control, whereas one has only tenuous control over personal emotions, only reason—and not emotion—is sufficient to lead a person to moral actions. In Kantian deontology, the only intrinsically good thing is a goodwill that motivates dutiful actions.

Kant believed that people are ends in themselves and should be treated accordingly. Each autonomous, self-directed person has dignity and is due respect. An individual should never act in ways that involve using other people as a means to his or her personal ends. In fact, according to Kant, when people use others as a means to ends, even if they believe they are using persons to reach ethical goals, the dignity of the used persons is harmed. An example would be a failure to obtain full, informed consent from a research participant even though the researcher steadfastly believes the research will be beneficial to the participant.

Kant identified rules to guide people in thinking about their obligations. In doing so, he drew a distinction between two types of duties or obligations: the *hypothetical imperative* and the *categorical imperative*. Hypothetical imperatives are optional duties or rules that people ought to observe or follow if certain ends are to be achieved. Such statements are sometimes called *if–then* imperatives, which means they involve conditional or optional actions—for instance, "If I want to eat tonight, then I should go to the grocery store today."

However, where moral actions are concerned, Kant believed duties and laws are absolute and unconditional. He proposed that people ought to follow a universal, unconditional framework of maxims, or rules, as a guide to know the rightness of actions and one's moral duties. According to Kant, these absolute and unconditional duties constitute categorical imperatives. When deciding about matters of ethics and acting according to a categorical imperative, one needs to ask the question, "If I perform this action, could I will that it should become a universal law for everyone to act in the same way?" No action can ever be judged as right, according to Kant, if it is not reasonable that the action could become a binding, ethical law for all people. For example, Kant's ethics imposes the categorical imperative that one should never tell a lie because a person cannot rationally wish that all people should be able to pick and choose when they have permission not to be truthful. Another example of a categorical imperative is that suicide is never acceptable. A person, when committing suicide, cannot rationally wish that all people should feel free to commit suicide or the world would become chaotic.

Kantianism is valued highly in Western medicine because of the focus on individual rights, autonomy, and informed consent. In the U.S. healthcare system and in Western bioethics, the choices of rational individuals generally are respected. In public health, however, practitioners often must balance the rights of individuals against the rights of populations and communities. Sometimes navigating this delicate balance can be controversial or generate dilemmas, such as considering appropriate actions that may breach confidentiality when a person with a stigmatizing communicable disease may jeopardize the health of other people. This situation results in a need to balance the need to respect the autonomy and protect the confidentiality of one person against the need to protect the safety of other persons.

Consequentialism

Consequentialists, as distinguished from deontologists, do consider consequences to be an important indication of the moral value of one's actions. *Utilitarianism* is the most well-known consequentialist theory of ethics. Under utilitarianism, actions are judged by their utility; that is, they are evaluated according to the usefulness of their consequences. When people use the theory of utilitarianism as the basis for ethical behavior, they attempt to promote the greatest good (happiness or pleasure) and to inflict the least amount of harm (suffering or pain) that is possible in a situation. In other words, utilitarians believe that it is useful to society to achieve the greatest good for the greatest number of people who may be affected by a rule or action. People who use a utilitarian approach to ethics place great emphasis on what is best for collective groups, not individual people, although each individual's happiness is worthy of equal consideration as compared to every other individual in a group.

The British philosopher Jeremy Bentham (1748–1832) was an early promoter of the principle of utilitarianism. During Bentham's life, British society functioned according to aristocratic privilege. Poor people were mistreated by people in the upper classes and were given no choice other than to work long hours in deplorable conditions. Bentham tried to develop a theory that could be used to achieve a fair distribution of pleasure among all British citizens. He went so far as to develop a systematic decision-making method that relied on mathematical calculations. Bentham's method was designed to determine ways to allocate pleasure and to diminish pain by using the measures of intensity and duration. His approach to utilitarianism has been criticized, however, because Bentham equated all types of pleasure as being equal.

Another Englishman, John Stuart Mill (1806–1873), challenged Bentham's views when he pointed out that particular experiences of pleasure and happiness clearly do have different qualities and that different situations do not necessarily produce equal consequences. For example, Mill stated that the higher intellectual pleasures may be differentiated from lower physical pleasures. The higher pleasures, such as enjoying a work of art or a scholarly book, are considered to be better because only human beings, not other animals, possess the mental faculties to enjoy this higher level of happiness.

According to Mill, happiness is measured by quality and not quantity (duration or intensity). In making these distinctions between higher and lower levels of happiness, Mill's philosophy focuses more on ethics than does Bentham's philosophy, which was devised as a means to change social or political policy. Mill believed that communities usually agree about what is good and about those things that best promote the happiness of the most people. An example of an application of Mill's utilitarianism is mandatory vaccination laws, under which individual liberties are limited so that the larger society is protected from diseases. The consequence is that people generally are happier because they are free of diseases. Because of the emphasis on population-focused care, utilitarianism is one of the most widely used ethical approaches in public health practice.

People using Mill's form of utilitarian theory often can defer to widely supported traditions to guide them in deciding which rules and behaviors will probably produce the best consequences for the most people, such as the maxim, "Stealing is wrong." Through experience, humans generally have identified many behaviors that will produce the most happiness or unhappiness for society as a whole.

Communitarianism

According to Wildes (2000), "All communities have some organizing vision about the meaning of life and how one ought to conduct a good life" (p. 129). Communitarian ethics is based on the position that "everything fundamental in ethics derives from communal values, the common good, social goals, traditional practices, and cooperative virtues" (Beauchamp & Childress, 2001, p. 362). Communitarian ethics is relevant to moral relationships in any community.

The notion that communitarian ethics is based on the model of friendships and relationships that existed in the ancient Greek city-states described by Aristotle was popularized in modern times by the philosopher and ethicist Alasdair MacIntyre (1984) in his book *After Virtue*. In general societal ethics and in bioethics, the valuing and consideration of community relationships have come to mean different things to different people, however (Beauchamp & Childress, 2001). Communitarian ethics is distinguished as an ethical approach in that the epicenter of communitarian ethics is the community, rather than any one individual (Wildes, 2000). The value of discussing and articulating an approach to communitarian ethics lies in the benefit that can be gained from illuminating and appreciating the relationships and interconnections between people that are often overlooked in everyday life.

According to this philosophy, although personal moral goals, such as the pursuit of personal well-being, are significant, the importance of forming strong communities and identifying the moral goals of communities must not be neglected if both individuals and communities are to flourish. An important distinction that legitimately can be drawn between communitarian and other popular ethical approaches, such as rule-based ethics, lies in communitarian ethicists' proposal that it is natural for humans to favor the people with whom they live and have frequent interactions. Kantian deontologists base their ethics on an impartial stance toward the persons who experience the effects of their morally related actions. However, using a communitarian ethic and valuing partiality as a way of relating to other people do not necessarily exclude caring about people who are personally unknown to moral agents. Although it is often easier for people to care about and have compassion for people who are relationally closest to them, it is not unrealistic to believe that people can develop empathy or compassion toward people who are personally unknown to them. Such behavior and expectations are an integral part of Christian and Buddhist philosophies, for example. Accepting the notion that humans usually are more partial to those people

Table 9-1 Theoretical Approaches to Ethics

Theory	Concepts
Natural Law	Self-evident; nature; natural; inherent
Rights	Justified claim; individualism; liberalism; absolute right; *prima facie* right
Deontology	Categorical imperative; duty; ends and means; goodwill
Utilitarianism	Happiness; consequence; greatest good; utility
Communitarianism	Common good; flourishing; traditional practices; cooperative virtues

with whom they are most closely related, while at the same time believing that it is possible to expand the scope of their empathy and compassion to unknown others, broadens the sphere of morality in communitarian ethics.

The education of communities often occurs through role modeling (Wildes, 2000). Members of communities learn about what is and is not accepted as moral through personal and group interactions and dialogue within their communities. Nurses share narratives about the lives of exemplars, such as Florence Nightingale and Lillian Wald, to illustrate moral living. By her efforts to improve social justice and health protection through environmental measures and her efforts to elevate the character of nurses, Nightingale exhibited moral concern for her local society, the nursing profession, and people remote from her local associations, such as the population of soldiers affected by the Crimean War. Likewise, Lillian Wald was an excellent role model for members of communities because of her efforts to improve social justice through her work at the Henry Street Settlement. When learning from the examples of Nightingale and Wald, communitarian-minded nurses are in an excellent position to educate the public and other nurses and healthcare professionals about why they, in many ways, should assume the role of being their brothers' and sisters' keepers. (For a summary of the theories discussed in this section, see **Table 9-1**.)

SUMMARY

Rather than providing in-depth information about a variety of theories of ethics, this chapter seeks to raise awareness about the philosophy of ethics and the ways in which related theories are constructed and classified. Doing ethics is a significant part of advanced nursing practice, as is using appropriate theory in practice. Being moral and acting in moral ways is not accidental. Aristotle believed that morality (for him, virtue) can be taught and must be ingrained through habit. With Aristotle's position in mind, readers are reminded to learn more about ethics and consciously develop moral habits grounded in reasonable moral theories.

DISCUSSION QUESTIONS

1. Choose one ethical theory discussed in this chapter. Define the related concepts outlined in Table 9-1. Examine literature about the theory, and identify and define other concepts used in the theory.
2. Use the concepts that you defined for Question 1 and develop proposition statements specific to the ethical theory.
3. Compare your chosen theory to Beauchamp and Childress's and Vaughn's criteria discussed in this chapter. What are your conclusions?
4. Analyze your chosen theory using Fawcett's criteria.
5. Do you agree with Beckstrand's argument that all knowledge in nursing is reducible to theories in the fields of science and ethics? Support your position.

REFERENCES

American Association of Colleges of Nursing. (2006). *Essentials of doctoral education for advanced nursing practice*. Washington, DC: Author.

American Nurses Association. (2015). *Code of ethics for nurses with interpretive statements*. Silver Springs, MD: Author.

Beauchamp, T. L., & Childress, J. F. (2001). *Principles of biomedical ethics* (5th ed.). New York, NY: Oxford University Press.

Beauchamp, T. L., & Childress, J. F. (2009). *Principles of biomedical ethics* (6th ed.). New York, NY: Oxford University Press.

Beckstrand, J. (1978). The notion of a practice theory and the relationship of scientific and ethical knowledge to practice. *Research in Nursing and Health, 1,* 131–136. Reproduced in L. H. Nicoll (1997), *Perspectives on nursing theory* (3rd ed., pp. 605–613). Philadelphia, PA: Lippincott.

Beckstrand, J. (1980). A critique of several conceptions of practice theory in nursing. *Research in Nursing and Health, 3,* 69–70. Reproduced in L. H. Nicoll (1997), *Perspectives on nursing theory* (3rd ed., pp. 620–631). Philadelphia, PA: Lippincott.

Billington, R. (2003). *Living philosophy: An introduction to moral thought* (3rd ed.). New York, NY: Routledge, Taylor & Francis.

Dickoff, J., & James, P. (1968). A theory of theories: A position paper. *American Journal of Nursing, 17*(3), 197–203.

Durant, W. (1933). *The story of philosophy*. New York, NY: Simon & Schuster.

Fawcett, J. (2005). *Contemporary nursing knowledge* (2nd ed.). Philadelphia, PA: F. A. Davis.

Frankena, W. K. (1973). *Ethics* (2nd ed.). Retrieved from http://www.ditext.com/frankena/e1.html

International Council of Nurses. (2006). *The ICN code of ethics for nurses*. Geneva, Switzerland: Author.

Kant, Immanuel. (Trans. M. Gregor). (1785/2012). *The groundwork of the metaphysics of morals*. Cambridge, MD: Cambridge University Press.

Lund, D. H. (2003). *Making sense of it all*. Upper Saddle River, NJ: Prentice Hall.

MacIntyre, A. (1984). *After virtue: A study of moral theory* (2nd ed.). Notre Dame, IN: University of Notre Dame Press.

Magee, B. (2001). *The story of philosophy.* New York, NY: Dorling Kindersley.

McEwen, M. (2007). Theory development: Structuring conceptual relationships in nursing. In M. McEwen & E. M. Wills (Eds.), *Theoretical basis for nursing* (2nd ed., pp. 73–94). Philadelphia, PA: Lippincott Williams & Wilkins.

Meleis, A. I. (2005). *Theoretical development and progress* (3rd ed. rev. reprint). Philadelphia, PA: Lippincott Williams & Wilkins.

Reynolds, P. D. (1971). *A primer in theory construction.* Indianapolis, IN: Bobbs-Merrill Educational.

Russell, B. (1945). *The history of Western philosophy.* New York, NY: Simon & Schuster.

Sulmasy, D. P., & Sugarman, J. (2001). The many methods of medical ethics (or, thirteen ways of looking at a blackbird). In J. Sugarman & D. P. Sulmasy (Eds.), *Methods in medical ethics* (pp. 3–18). Washington, DC: Georgetown University Press.

Tarnas, R. (1991). *The passion of the Western mind.* New York, NY: Ballantine.

Tomey, A. M., & Alligood, M. R. (Eds.). (2006). *Nursing theorists and their work* (6th ed.). St. Louis, MO: Mosby Elsevier.

Vaughn, L. (2010). *Bioethics: Principles, issues and cases.* New York, NY: Oxford University Press.

Wiedenbach, E. (1970). Nurses' wisdom in nursing theory. *American Journal of Nursing, 70*(3), 1057–1062.

Wildes, K. M. (2000). *Moral acquaintances: Methodology in bioethics.* Notre Dame, IN: University of Notre Dame Press.

Chapter 10

Educational and Learning Theories

Margaret M. Braungart
Richard G. Braungart

INTRODUCTION

To learn is to gain knowledge, understanding, or skills through experience. Learning is fundamental to human development. It may be formal or informal, direct or indirect, or consciously or unconsciously acquired. From a psychological perspective, learning involves a relatively permanent change in an individual's thinking, emotions, attitudes, or behavior. A lifelong process, the key to learning is experience. The more we know about learning through research, the more we realize learning is complex, involving biological, emotional, cognitive, and social-cultural dimensions. Much of an individual's identity is based on what he or she has learned through family, schools, and culture, while growing up during a particular era in history. Not only are people challenged to learn new information and skills throughout their lives, but they may also need to unlearn or relearn behaviors, emotions, and attitudes—challenges that are especially evident in the healthcare field.

Nurses spend a significant amount of their time and energy involved with learning and teaching, whether acquiring new information as part of their professional and continuing education or instructing others in health care. Advanced practice nurses, in particular, are concerned with teaching and learning in numerous ways. In part, this focus reflects their leadership roles in healthcare education, administration, and planning. For example, how can a nursing instructor motivate a classroom of diverse students to learn when many are juggling the demands of education with the burdens of work and family? How can nurses in management and policy-making positions address the need to change staff behavior regarding ethical breaches, medical mistakes, infection control, and workplace conflicts?

And how might nurses construct and implement an effective hospital or community education campaign to improve health behaviors? These examples from nursing and health care suggest three fundamental questions about learning:

1. What are effective ways to learn new information or change attitudes and behaviors in health care?
2. How can people be motivated to learn, and which kinds of experiences facilitate learning?
3. What are effective ways to teach so that information and skills will be remembered rather than forgotten and will transfer correctly outside the immediate learning situation?

This chapter examines learning from an educational, psychological, and research-based perspective by reviewing the basic principles of learning theories and suggesting how they can be applied to advanced nursing practice. Learning theory is defined and discussed in relation to nursing, and the most widely used learning theories are described and illustrated with examples from health care. Neuropsychology research on the underlying physiological dynamics of learning is mentioned briefly as well. The perspectives on learning are then pulled together into a general model of learning, followed by a discussion of how nurses can decide which theories and principles to use and how the three fundamental questions about learning pertain to nursing practice.

LEARNING THEORY

Learning theory in education is rooted in the field of psychology. Psychology is the scientific study of mental processes and behavior and represents a research-based approach to understanding human behavior. Educational psychology is a specialty area devoted to the study of learning, teaching, and assessment (Ormrod, 2014; Woolfolk, 2012). Reflecting different schools of psychology, the principal learning theories were formulated during the first half of the 20th century in the attempt to describe, explain, and predict how learning occurs. Learning theories are useful for understanding how people gain knowledge and skills, as well as how emotions, attitudes, and behaviors are acquired and can be changed. These theories are highly applicable and provide the foundation for educational practices, counseling, advertising, workplace management, and rehabilitation.

To help nurses understand the various dimensions and dynamics of learning, the chapter summarizes four learning theories that are widely recognized in psychology and education: (1) behaviorist theory, (2) cognitive theory, (3) psychodynamic theory, and (4) humanistic theory. Behaviorist and cognitive theories were prominent in education during the first half of the 20th century; by the 21st century, however, cognitive theory had begun to dominate academic research and practice in psychology and education. Nonetheless, principles of behaviorist theory continue to be useful in education, the workplace, counseling, health care, and other areas in society. While not always considered learning theories per se, psychodynamic and humanistic theories are included and discussed in this chapter because they highlight emotional learning and emphasize the importance of the teacher–learner relationship (Hilgard & Bower, 1966). Illness and health care are often highly charged experiences. Consequently, nurses conducting health education and endeavoring to achieve behavior change should not ignore the role of emotions in the learning process.

Each of the four theories discussed here reflects a different perspective on learning and comprises a distinct set of constructs and principles. The theories include information regarding the kinds of experiences that motivate learning and how to maximize the likelihood that learning will be remembered and can be transferred to a variety of settings. The theories differ in terms of whether the learner is viewed as more passive or active, whether the focus of the theory is on external environmental influences or on internal processes within the learner, and whether the principal route to learning is through behavior, thinking processes, or emotions and feelings. These days, learning theory cannot be fully discussed without including information from neuropsychology research, which helps educators sort out conflicting claims of learning theories. Principles of learning can be applied to nursing, patient, staff, and community education, as well as to changing attitudes and behavior in a variety of circumstances. Healthcare research data reveal that using learning theories to design professional education and intervention programs enhances their success (Clark, Mitchell, & Rand, 2009; Ferguson & Day, 2005; Leinster, 2009; Sargeant, 2009).

This chapter is organized as follows. An overview of each learning theory is presented, including its origins, basic constructs, and principles. Focus is given to each theory's perspective on motivation, practice, retention, and transfer, as well as to which kinds of teaching approaches and experiences aid or hinder learning. Criticisms of the theories are also offered. The theories and principles selected for discussion are considered useful to advanced practice nurses. Behaviorist and cognitive theories are emphasized, and psychodynamic and humanistic theories are viewed as supplementing and strengthening nursing education and professionalism. For organizational clarity, each theory is presented as a unit. In practice, the theories are often used in combination. To help nurses make decisions about how to use learning theories, a general model of learning is offered, and the three fundamental questions raised earlier about learning and teaching are addressed in relation to nursing practice. Learning theories provide a toolbox of approaches from which nurses can select the appropriate option to address problems related to nursing and health education or to modify attitudes and behavior in a variety of settings.

BEHAVIORIST LEARNING THEORY

According to behaviorist theory (also referred to as behaviorism), since there is no way to know accurately what is going on within a person's mind, the focus should be on only what is directly observable. What is observable in any learning situation are the stimulus conditions (S) in the environment and the behavior (movements, acts, actions) that is exhibited in response (R) to stimulus conditions (Kazdin, 2013). In this model, learning is relatively simple; it is based on the associations people make between *stimuli* and *responses* (termed the *S–R model of learning* or *association learning*), and the belief that life is largely a matter of habit that requires little thinking. For example, people learn their health habits, such as their responses to foods, their physical exercise patterns, and their reactions to stress. For better or worse, much behavior is learned in the family through socialization and is passed from generation to generation.

According to behaviorists, what is learned can be unlearned by modifying stimulus conditions in the environment or changing the response to stimuli. The route to learning, then, goes through behavior and action—the learning is in the doing—rather than through inner processes such as thinking and feeling. Changes in thinking and feeling, in fact, may come about by first changing behavior; thoughts and emotions then follow. For instance, if nurses who lack self-confidence are given responsibilities where they can perform well, their self-confidence may improve over time. Thus the route to personal change proceeds through behavior and practice.

Behaviorist principles are useful for breaking bad habits, designing practice sessions for sports and rehabilitation, and working with people who are more comfortable engaging in actions than reflecting on thoughts and emotions. Behaviorism provides the foundation for behavior modification programs, behavioral medicine, commercial advertising, and some therapies. The principles of the behaviorist model of learning can be applied to animals as well as people.

To promote learning, behaviorists change the stimulus–response (S–R) associations the learner makes in the environment and may follow a learner's response with some kind of reinforcement. To learn, of course, people must be motivated to make a response. Motivation is based on drive reduction—that is, having a drive that needs to be alleviated or satisfied. Primary drives are unlearned, such as the drive for food, warmth, sleep, sex, and avoidance of pain. In contrast, secondary drives are learned, such as the drive for financial security, popularity, or achievement. Culture plays an important role in learning secondary drives. It is difficult to encourage people to learn if there is no drive to be reduced, such as when people are satisfied, complacent, and satiated, or when another drive overpowers the drive to learn.

According to behaviorist learning theory, the process of learning proceeds as follows. Once a primary connection is made between the stimulus and the response, learning can be said to have occurred, which is somewhat of an "all or nothing" experience (e.g., not being able to ride a bike, then suddenly being able to steer and ride the bike; not being able to insert an intravenous [IV] line after many tries, then suddenly inserting it correctly). Most initial learning needs to be strengthened with practice. According to behaviorists, memory and retention are helped by repeating S–R connections, although there is a point at which practice becomes redundant and a waste of time. In its early stage, learning tends to be generalized to similar objects, situations, and stimuli. With additional and varied experiences, however, learners begin to make more sophisticated distinctions, called *discrimination learning*. In a sense, advanced practice nursing education is an exercise in discrimination learning.

The goal of most learning is to be able to transfer what is learned to other settings, such as teaching self-care to patients in the hospital—learning that is intended to be transferred to the home and workplace once patients have been discharged from the hospital. Transfer of learning is enhanced when the stimulus conditions and responses in the practice session and in the transfer situation are similar. Thus, working with patients in a hospital or rehabilitation center is necessary, but it may not be sufficient for the transfer of patients' learning outside the institution.

In the behaviorist model, the learner is relatively passive. The teacher or instructor plays a significant role in influencing learning through astute observation of S–R conditions and learners' reactions. Teachers are also responsible for the selection of motivating and well-chosen experiences to maximize learning, retention, and transfer. Likewise, the effectiveness of teaching depends on identifying appropriate stimulus conditions, reinforcement, practice, and feedback to ensure learning.

Two behaviorist perspectives on how learning occurs have had a significant impact on education and promoting behavior change: (1) classical conditioning and (2) operant conditioning. Conditioning is a powerful tool of learning, largely because little, if any, thinking is required in the learning process.

Classical Conditioning

Classical conditioning, sometimes referred to as respondent conditioning or Pavlovian conditioning, is a simple model of learning identified by Russian physiologist Ivan Pavlov in the late 19th century. Pavlov's classical experiment demonstrated how organisms become conditioned or learn their responses to stimuli. Simple conditioning works as follows. Take a naturally occurring S–R connection that did not have to be learned (an unconditioned stimulus–unconditioned response connection). In Pavlov's experiment, hungry dogs salivate when presented with food; in this case, food is the unconditioned stimulus (UCS) and salivation is the unconditioned response (UCR).

Pavlov then decided to introduce a neutral stimulus (NS) into the experiment; an NS is an arbitrary stimulus that has no natural connection to the UCS–UCR association. In one experiment, he used a bell as the NS. Initially, when Pavlov rang the bell, it did not signal anything in particular to the dog. To demonstrate how simple learning occurs, he decided to condition the dog to salivate at the sound of the bell. As Pavlov presented food (UCS) to the dog, he rang the bell (NS), and the dog salivated (UCR); the salivation occurred in response to the presentation of the food at this time. Pavlov then repeated the UCS–NS–UCR sequence. After several repeated trials, he rang the bell but did not present food, and the dog salivated. The dog's reaction demonstrated that learning had occurred—the bell had become the conditioned stimulus (CS) and salivation the conditioned response (CR). In other words, the former NS, which initially had no meaning to the dog, had been learned as a signal for food, and the dog responded by salivating (CS–CR). Pavlov later conditioned the dog to respond to a light as a signal, demonstrating how diverse neutral stimuli can become associated with responses.

A pervasive example of classical conditioning in health care in the United States occurs with prescription drug advertising. (Only the United States and New Zealand currently permit direct-to-consumer prescription drug advertising.) Each pharmaceutical company attempts to condition potential customers to prefer its drug to competitors' drugs to treat the same medical condition. In the ads, a company's drug is the NS, which is then paired with a naturally occurring association, such as images of patients' happiness about relief from pain, their comfort and attractiveness in being able to perform normal functions, or their ability to remain active and independent. The drug's brand name is repeated a number of times so that it becomes associated with images of relief, attractiveness, or independence, and consumers are urged to ask their doctor about the brand-name drug. To see how this association changes depending on the target audience, compare ads for a particular prescription drug in commercial trade magazines with ads for the same drug in medical journals. In medical journals, prescription drugs are often associated with images of physician power, authority, or even magical healing abilities.

Classical conditioning has been used to demonstrate how emotions such as fear can be learned. In fear conditioning, an NS is paired with an aversive stimulus (e.g., pain, loud noise, shock, traumatic experience) until the NS alone comes to elicit the fear response (freezing, stress reaction, agitation, and anxiety). Behaviorists have shown that fear can be taught (conditioned) in animals and in people, which represents one explanation for how anxiety, phobias, and delayed-stress syndrome may be learned. As an illustration, people may learn to genuinely fear hospitals if they have several unfortunate or painful (physical or emotional) experiences with hospitals as a patient or a visitor.

What has been learned can be unlearned, according to the behaviorists. Indeed, over the years behaviorists have shown how principles of conditioning can be used to extinguish negative emotions (fears, anxieties, rage) and break bad habits (unhealthy behaviors) simply by changing S–R connections and practicing the new response. Note that in classical conditioning, rewards are not needed.

A first step in this type of effort is to carefully assess the stimulus conditions or cues in the environment that automatically trigger the undesirable response. Some of the following procedures may be used to extinguish problematic emotions or unhealthy habits:

• Introduce the fear- or anxiety-producing stimulus (e.g., fear of heights, dark spaces, or a certain animal; anxiety about public speaking or social situations) at a low level so the client does not respond negatively. Gradually increase the strength of the fearful or anxious stimulus presented until the client can be in its presence without being afraid or agitated. For instance, someone with a fear of dogs might be shown pictures of dogs first, be given a cute toy dog, then view a live dog at a distance, slowly moving the dog closer until the client pets the dog. This conditioning technique, which is termed *systematic desensitization*, may take several sessions and is useful for extinguishing many fears, phobias, and anxieties. Clients are sometimes taught relaxation techniques so they can remain relatively calm (not anxious) in the presence of a fearful or threatening stimulus.

- Rechain events (S–R connections) by identifying the stimuli or cues that trigger unwanted behavior and then constructing a new chain of responses that does not include the unwanted behavior in response to the cues. This approach is useful for dieters, procrastinators, and persons with anger management issues, among others. To illustrate, procrastinating students often engage in a host of distracting tasks once they arrive home. Studying is postponed until late at night when they are tired. As part of their retraining, students realize the S–R chain starts when they enter the door at home, and their first task in rechaining events is to study for at least an hour before performing other tasks. Practicing this sequence of events for several weeks can help students' procrastination decrease and their studying behavior improve at home.

- Interfere with an S–R association, which can be accomplished in two ways. First, one can create new stimulus conditions. People who abuse alcohol, for example, may need to change friends and avoid stimulus environments (e.g., bars, cocktail parties, restaurants serving alcohol) that increase the likelihood of substance abuse. Second, one can substitute a healthy response for the unhealthy response to existing cues. If individuals with an alcohol problem need to be in situations where people are drinking alcohol, they could change their response to the stimulus situation by drinking sparkling water or juice in a cocktail glass. Building a new S–R association takes time; practice is required to form new habits. This technique may be useful for dieters, smokers, and persons struggling with substance abuse, anger management, or worry and anxiety.

- "Fatiguing the response" involves performing the unwanted behavior repeatedly until the client has a negative reaction and manifests a different response. For instance, chain smokers may be told to stand in a corner and smoke cigarette after cigarette. As the smoke blows back in their face, they become disgusted or feel ill and demand to stop. When this behavior is practiced over several days, the once pleasurable cigarettes become associated with an unpleasant physical reaction. There are risks with this technique, however, and it does not apply well to many problem behaviors.

It takes much longer and is more difficult to unlearn or extinguish a response than it is to learn the response. Moreover, although a response may appear to be extinguished, it can return at any time (termed *spontaneous recovery*), especially under similar stimulus conditions when the response was often performed in the past. If the response resurfaces, it may recover at full strength. For example, people who have smoked cigarettes and quit can easily experience spontaneous recovery. They may not have had a cigarette for months or years, yet at a party accept and smoke one. Their smoking habit then may return at full strength. The problem of spontaneous recovery needs to be given serious attention in any health program to change behavior, such as substance abuse, weight loss, or nutrition.

Operant Conditioning

Operant conditioning is another widely recognized behaviorist approach. Popularized by B. F. Skinner (1974), operant conditioning gives less attention to stimulus conditions and more attention to a response and what happens to an individual after he or she responds. According to operant conditioning principles, behavior is most effectively influenced or changed by following an individual's response with some kind of reinforcement. A *reinforcement* is defined as a stimulus that increases the probability that a response will occur again under similar stimulus conditions.

According to operant conditioning principles, learning can be enhanced and behaviors increased or decreased simply by applying reinforcement on a proper schedule. Often working with animals such as rats and pigeons, Skinner formulated a well-organized way to understand how desirable and undesirable responses are learned, and how to change behaviors using scheduled reinforcement. Operant conditioning principles lie at the heart of behavioral modification programs in institutions, as well as instructional technologies where learners teach themselves by using teaching machines or computer programs.

Four types of reinforcement can be applied after a response is made to either increase or decrease the likelihood of the response being performed in the future: (1) positive reinforcement—applying a pleasant stimulus; (2) negative reinforcement—removal of an unpleasant stimulus; (3) nonreinforcement—not applying any kind of pleasant or unpleasant stimulus; and (4) punishment—applying an unpleasant stimulus. Of these four types of reinforcement, positive reinforcement is the most powerful way to promote learning.

Increasing a Response

To increase a response, apply (1) positive reinforcement or (2) negative reinforcement.

Positive reinforcement entails providing a pleasant stimulus or reward after a response is made, which increases the likelihood that the response will be performed in future similar situations. Keep in mind that both desirable and undesirable behaviors may be strengthened with positive reinforcement. For instance, acknowledging a staff member's cooperative behavior increases the likelihood that he or she will continue to act in cooperative ways. Operant conditioning also helps us understand why people engage in unhealthy, annoying, or damaging behaviors. For example, smokers, attention-getters, and angry people are receiving some kind of positive reinforcement for their behavior, which explains why they keep making the same unwanted responses. To change behavior, identify what is positively reinforcing to the person, make sure not to reinforce the undesirable behavior, and then positively reinforce the person's desirable responses. As an example, if a principal goal of patient care is to help patients be independent, then individuals should not be rewarded when they complain or act in a dependent manner; instead, every attempt should be made to recognize and reward them when they strive for independence. For some patients, the more active they become, the less they are concerned with pain, and the experience of pain appears to lessen. This approach may not work with all patients, however.

Negative reinforcement involves removing an unpleasant stimulus, which acts to increase a response in similar situations. Two types of negative reinforcement are distinguished: escape conditioning and avoidance conditioning. The difference between the two relates to their timing.

Escape conditioning occurs when an unpleasant stimulus is applied (e.g., a clinical instructor chastises a student) and the person (student) makes a response (cracks a joke) that stops the unpleasant stimulus from being applied (the instructor ceases chastising and laughs at the joke). In this case, the student has escaped the unpleasant stimulus (being chastised). Consequently, humor is the response that is likely to be increased the next time the student is in a difficult situation.

Avoidance conditioning occurs when aversive stimuli are anticipated but not yet applied. In particular, when people want to avoid an unpleasant situation (e.g., a test or a job interview), they may say they are sick. If they continue to claim they are sick to avoid difficult situations, they may actually become ill when they feel threatened or anxious. Sick behavior is the response that has been increased through avoidance conditioning.

Decreasing a Response

To decrease a response, apply (1) nonreinforcement or (2) punishment.

Nonreinforcement involves ignoring behavior (not applying any kind of reinforcement), which acts to lessen the frequency of a response. Attention-getting behaviors, temper tantrums, and attempts to upset people emotionally may be reduced when no reinforcement is given. Ignoring desirable behavior may also result in its decline. In a healthcare setting, if nurse managers preoccupy themselves with problem behaviors and fail to reward those nurses who are performing well, the frequency of this desirable behavior may decrease.

Punishment involves applying an unpleasant or aversive stimulus, which serves to reduce the likelihood of a behavior. Punishment is used only as a last resort if nonreinforcement and other techniques do not work. Physical punishment should not be employed for obvious reasons. Verbal confrontation, removing disruptive individuals from situations where they can get attention, and imposing penalties (e.g., fines, being grounded, "three strikes and you're out") are some examples of unpleasant stimuli that might be used. If punishment is utilized, keep the focus on the behavior that needs to be changed and avoid personal disparagement (i.e., punish the behavior, not the person).

Punishment is risky, with behaviorists finding that punishment may not weaken responses or decrease behavior in the long run (Hilgard & Bower, 1966; Kazdin, 2013). This tactic also arouses emotions that may work against learning what needs to be learned and may well create a negative attitude toward the punisher. Even so, there are situations when it becomes necessary to apply an unpleasant stimulus to decrease a response. An illustration is the punishment administered by hospital committees and state boards that deal with unethical, irresponsible, and harmful behavior by health professionals. The behavior may be punished by putting professionals on probation or even suspending their license to practice. Dealing with frequent medication errors and blatant disregard for infection control are other behaviors where nonreinforcement hardly seems a viable option.

How and when to use positive reinforcement, and which kind to use, are important considerations in operant conditioning. First, in initial learning, it is necessary to reinforce the learner after each response (continuous reinforcement); once the response is established, one must then move to intermittent reinforcement (sufficient to keep the response functioning). Second, the reinforcement has to be of value to the particular learner, and unhealthy rewards (e.g., sweet or fattening foods, large amounts of money, risky pleasures) should not be used. Third, administrators need to know that rewarding the group is not as effective in maintaining positive behavior as rewarding the individual. Saying "Good job—I am very proud of all of you" has less impact than acknowledging each staff member because rewards are more effective if they are personal and directed individually.

There are many criticisms of behaviorist learning theory. Foremost is the ethical concern about who is to decide what the desirable behavior should be. Should it be docile patients who give the staff little trouble, or passive students who do not take issue with or criticize others? Second, the emphasis on rewards and gains may foster materialism and manipulation. Should students be given tangible rewards for studying, or should they study to develop a genuine love of learning? Third, research indicates behaviors learned through classical and operant conditioning techniques may fade away quickly once the individual moves to a different setting—perhaps the same kind of environment and irrational reinforcement system that got the person in trouble in the first place. Finally, when working with people in the classroom or in the healthcare setting, it seems unrealistic to ignore learners' inner processing, such as their thoughts, emotions, motivations, and interpretations.

COGNITIVE LEARNING THEORY

Cognitive learning theory focuses on the perceptions, thinking, reasoning, memory, developmental changes, and processing of information that transpire within the learner (Matlin, 2013; Sawyer, 2006). Taking issue with the behaviorists, researchers advocating this perspective undertook a series of cognitive experiments that demonstrated a number of factors related to learning, such as reward is not necessary to learn, and thinking and reasoning develop in stages over the course of childhood and adolescence. Researchers also documented that learning is an active process in which learners perceive, interpret, and respond to the environment in their own ways, with social factors having a strong influence on each learner's construction of reality.

The introduction of several important subtheories has contributed to the advancement of cognitive theory over more than a century, with cognitive theory currently influencing much of educational practice. Cognitive theory is useful for appreciating the different ways that individuals approach and respond to any learning situation, recognizing the complexity of learning, and prompting instructors to take their cues from learners to be effective.

According to the basic principles of cognitive theory, the way individuals approach any learning situation reflects their level of cognitive development, their past experiences, the way they perceive and process information, and the way they think about themselves and respond to instruction. Attention is the key to learning, with each learner incorporating, organizing, and interpreting new information in relation to what he or she already knows. Learners have an awareness of how they acquire knowledge and think—a capacity termed *metacognition*. The ability to alter his or her thoughts, beliefs, and behavior rests on the learner discovering some kind of insight that causes him or her to reorganize these perceptions and thoughts. Thus a change in one's perception and thinking may lead to behavior change.

In cognitive theory, motivation is based on the learner's goals and expectations, which create disequilibrium and a tension to act. People without goals or with low expectations for themselves are not motivated to act. Conversely, people whose goals and expectations are too high may be at risk for disappointment and becoming discouraged about education and learning. Research suggests that having realistic goals (goals that stretch accomplishment but are achievable for the person) and taking responsibility for one's actions (internal locus of control) result in better academic performance, compared to having unrealistic goals (too high or too low) and blaming outside forces for one's success or failure (external locus of control).

In using cognitive theory, the educator's job is to assess readiness to learn; provide a variety of meaningful, developmentally appropriate experiences; and allow individuals to discover what they learn for themselves. Teachers and other students may provide feedback to correct faulty conceptions. Thus, according to this view, education is a social experience that benefits from human interactions. Sharing different perceptions and ways of thinking enhances learning and fosters an appreciation for the rich diversity in human thought.

When operating from a cognitive perspective, instructors need to be organized, with clear goals and expectations and a well-structured approach to presenting information. It may be helpful to provide a framework for understanding (advance organizers) to prepare learners for maneuvering through information on their road to discovery and insight.

Creativity and original thought contribute to the excitement of learning and are encouraged. Creativity is engendered by a novel and insightful reorganization of information and experience. Practice for the sake of practice—such as using boring repetition, requiring rote memory, and demanding that thinking conform to instructor expectations and remain "inside the box"—is not helpful. Instead, offering diverse experiences linked to learning is a more beneficial kind of practice.

Memory and retention are facilitated by the organization and meaningfulness of the educational material, along with proper pacing and time to reflect on the information. Recognition must be given to the various ways that individuals approach and respond to what is to be learned. Because learning is subject to social and personal influences within a cognitive framework, it is important to determine how information has been perceived, interpreted, and stored. It may be helpful to offer techniques that aid memory and transfer (Matlin, 2013).

When a cognitive theoretical approach is used, it is essential to give feedback to learners so they can make adjustments in how they process information. The transfer of learning to future situations is not likely to be total, however, since every experience and situation where learning is to be performed will have its own set of differences and anomalies. Thus, the emphasis is on fortifying learners' abilities to solve problems by providing a variety of experiences, encouraging flexibility in thinking and creativity, and promoting feelings of competence or self-efficacy. Such training prepares learners to adjust to new cognitive patterns and changing situations—and it explains why clinical experiences need to be carefully selected and structured for nursing students. Having students rotate through different kinds of healthcare facilities broadens their clinical education.

The remainder of this section profiles some useful concepts and principles from the leading subtheories within cognitive theory.

Gestalt Theory

Gestalt theory was formulated in the early 20th century around the same time that the behaviorists were gaining influence in psychology. This theory stresses the importance of sensory perception, attention, and the unique ways in which people may organize information and experiences. Gestalt means *configuration*; thus gestalt experiments demonstrate how people can encounter the same event yet perceive, interpret, and respond to it differently (Hilgard & Bower, 1966; Murray, 1995). According to gestalt theorists, people feel a tension to try to make sense out of confusing reality and to structure events in personal and sometimes idiosyncratic ways.

Some useful principles from gestalt theory are highlighted here, with examples from health care being used to illustrate each principle:

• Given the wealth of stimuli at any one time, people pay attention (orient) to some information while screening out (habituate to) other information. For example, patients may not attend to the health information a nurse presents because they are focused on their personal worries, other people in the room, or various other distractions.

- Perception strives for simplicity, equilibrium, and regularity. When patient education is conducted, patients and their families endeavor to make the information easy to understand, to remain balanced or be comfortable with the information, and want to relate the information to something familiar. Imagine what it is like for someone from a non-Western culture to be sick or injured in a U.S. hospital and how stressful it is to strive for simplicity, equilibrium, and regularity in such an unfamiliar environment! Young children or older patients hospitalized for the first time may have reactions similar to a foreigner.

- Perception is selective in terms of what is screened out and what is attended to; thus, perceptions and interpretations may be distorted or at odds with those of other individuals in the same situation. Patients and their doctors may selectively pay attention and interpret information in their own ways, which can be a source of misunderstanding. As an illustration, well-meaning doctors may tell patients they have a 95% probability of surviving their disease or operation, yet some patients may then stay awake all night worrying that they have a 5% chance of dying.

- Perception is influenced by structure and directed toward organization and closure—"the whole is greater than the sum of the parts." For example, when a diagnosis is unclear, patients may go to great lengths to find information (e.g., from books, the Internet, journals, friends) that can suggest a diagnosis for their condition. The diagnosis may not be accurate, but patients may organize their symptoms into an identifiable pattern and find comfort in having some kind of answer to bring closure to their tension. Clearly, certain people have a much greater need for perceptual structure and meaning than others do.

- The patterns that people select and perceive in events are strongly influenced by their background, past experiences, needs, aspirations, and emotional attachments. Patients with the same disease may view their illness and react quite differently because of differences in their culture, age, religion, and gender. Anne Fadiman's book *The Spirit Catches You and You Fall Down* (1997), which illustrates the perplexing dilemmas of a Hmong family caught up in the California healthcare system, exemplifies these differences in perspective.

With regard to teaching, while gestalt theorists believe that discovery learning encourages retention, creativity, and problem solving, they stress that the way the material is presented and framed/structured can make all the difference in learning. The goal of learning is understanding, not rote memory and drill. There is a long-standing debate about association or behaviorist learning versus discovery learning and which is the most effective. Recent efforts have been made to acknowledge the value of each theory and to identify ways of using them together (Hee & Anderson, 2013; Shanks, 2010).

Presenting material in various ways—appealing to multiple senses, employing different methods and techniques—acknowledges the diverse ways that information and experiences are subjectively perceived and organized by each learner. Looking at the same problem in different ways encourages flexibility in thinking and creativity in problem solving. Presenting an issue in incomplete form invites learners' involvement as they strive for insight, originality, and meaning. Relearning or retraining involves motivating a structural reorganization into a new configuration.

Gestalt theory remains the backbone of cognitive theory and has spawned many ideas in education about how to teach and learn. The importance of structuring perception using well-known gestalt principles is reflected also in medical and drug advertising. In health care, gestalt theory has been applied to addressing addictive and self-medicating behaviors (Brownell, 2012).

Cognitive Development Theory

Cognitive development theory focuses on changes and advancements in perception and thought that occur from infancy through old age. Demonstrating that children's reasoning progresses sequentially through a series of stages from early childhood through adolescence, Jean Piaget's work represented a significant breakthrough in how to understand and work with children (Piaget & Inhelder, 1969). By observing, asking questions, and listening to children try to solve problems, Piaget identified four stages of cognitive development:

1. In the *sensorimotor* stage, infants learn to coordinate sensory information with motor activity.
2. Once they begin to be able to represent mentally what is not present, children move to the second or *preoperational* stage, where the use of symbols and language advances rapidly. At this stage, the child remains egocentric (only able to perceive the world from his or her own perspective and deal with one dimension at a time).
3. The third stage, called *concrete operations*, occurs around school age as children become able to grasp more than one dimension and deal with relationships among objects, such as "greater than" and "less than," and manipulate concepts and numbers.
4. As children become adolescents, they are able to begin to think abstractly, termed the *formal operations* stage.

While Piaget initially attached approximate ages to the four stages, he subsequently decided that it was the sequence of development that was important. Indeed, research has shown that some adults may never reach formal operations and can reason in only concrete terms; a few adults may function at a preoperational stage.

Piaget described two central processes involved in learning. The first is *assimilation*, in which information is incorporated and made to fit the existing cognitive framework or schema. The second process is *accommodation*, where the information taken in actually changes the schema. Given the limitations of young children's perception and reasoning, their efforts to understand the world around them are often geared toward assimilating information and interpreting it in their own way. Accordingly, young children may think the moon or a mountain follows them around. School-age children do not deal well with abstractions such as literary criticism, philosophy, and ideas about universal morality. Adults, too, engage in assimilation and accommodation, sometimes evident when confronting prejudice, bias, and religious or political beliefs.

Cognitive development theory seriously challenged the behaviorists' view of learning and had significant implications for understanding and teaching children. Comparing children to little scientists, Piaget advocated active discovery learning, claiming that perception rather than language was the key to learning. Another cognitive development theorist, Lev Vygotsky (1986), agreed that teaching must be in keeping with the child's level of understanding but suggested that language was most critical to learning and that social interaction facilitates learning. Vygotsky advocated that teachers exercise a stronger role in guiding children's learning than Piaget recommended. According to Vygotsky, adults give meaning and provide understanding to children's actions. Of course, some children may respond better to discovery learning, whereas other children may benefit from social interaction and guidance. Both Piaget and Vygotsky's views of learning continue to have a significant impact on education.

Piaget's theory goes no further than adolescence in describing cognitive development, leaving the question, what about cognitive development in adults? Research in psychology, gerontology, and education needs to be considered for those in health care working with young, middle-aged, and older adults. First, research indicates it may not be until late adolescence and early adulthood—if ever—that abstract thinking functions well. Teenagers have been characterized as engaging in black-and-white thinking, and they may behave in risky experimental ways without giving forethought to the possible consequences of their actions (Adelson, 1986). Second, adult cognitive processing may advance beyond the characteristics of formal operations to become more adept at synthesizing experiences, integrating information, and dealing with contradictions (Kramer, 1983). For this reason, adult learners require special consideration in education. They need to be treated with respect; they learn more effectively if allowed to discuss learning with others (cooperative and collaborative learning) and bring their own experiences to bear in a learning situation. Adults like independence and taking an active role in determining what and how they learn (Tennant, 2006).

Cognitive change in older adulthood is the subject of considerable research in gerontology and aging. Relative to health care, some older adults are burdened with cognitive deficits that may come with disease, medications, depression, or lack of interest in dealing with life's challenges. Other older adults may progress to an advanced stage of cognitive development where they demonstrate excellent judgment, a sophisticated perspective based on their years of experience, and a desire to give to others (Hooyman & Kiyak, 2007). In general, reaction time slows down and sensory declines occur with age. Thus, nurses attempting to educate older patients need to slow the pace of instruction and gear it to the patient's best sensory functioning. Relating new information to what is familiar to older persons may be helpful. As Sparks and Nussbaum (2008) urged, healthcare providers need to communicate at appropriate levels and meaningfully with older adults caught up in a healthcare system that demands high levels of literacy. Motivation can be a problem for older adults for a host of reasons, so it may be necessary to work to get their attention and involvement to solve problems.

Information-Processing Theory

Information-processing theory provides another cognitive perspective on learning and teaching. Explicit attention is given to how information is encountered, taken in, stored, and remembered. Information-processing theory is especially useful in trying to understand what is going on within each learner, discovering how to structure a learning situation to facilitate retention, and learning why distortions and errors occur in faulty learning or behavior (Bjork, 2013; Sternberg, 2006). The stages in processing information and learning are described next and illustrated with examples from health care:

- *Attention stage:* This is the initial crucial stage when learners decide whether to pay attention to the relevant information to be learned. If individuals are habituating to the information being presented and orienting to something else, then the intended learning will not occur. For example, it is generally a waste of everyone's time to try to educate patients when distractions are present (e.g., noisy setting, hallways and rooms bustling with human activity, people talking, television turned on, or patients feeling tired, nauseated, or worried).
- *Sensory memory stage:* The information is taken in and quickly processed by the senses. For example, patients and students generally have preferred sensory modes for encountering and remembering information. For some persons, the preferred mode is visual; for others, it is auditory; for still others, the mode of touching and manipulating is effective. When dealing with a group of learners, it is helpful to present pertinent health information in several different modes. Of course, sensory deficits must be factored in when deciding how to present and structure information.
- *Short-term* or *working memory stage:* Information is transferred from sensory memory to short-term memory, where it is encoded. Encoding is the form in which sensory information is transferred, such as the various ways people may briefly remember a telephone number—visualizing the numbers, remembering the numbers as a rhythm,

or repeating the numbers vocally. Information lasts only seconds or less in short-term memory and then is either discarded and forgotten or transferred to long-term memory. Researchers found it is helpful to try to reduce the *cognitive load* in the working memory stage in order to aid the incorporation of material into long-term memory (Sweller, Ayres, & Kalyuga, 2011). Make it easy to learn in a variety of ways. As an example, teaching at too rapid a pace and presenting too many ideas in quick succession work against memory and retention. Unfortunately, physicians, instructors, health educators, and those charged with obtaining informed consent ("consenting the patient") may be more concerned with getting through all the information in a restricted time period than with making sure that information is fully processed, understood, and remembered.

- *Long-term memory stage:* Information is organized by the learner for storage. Efficient learners may already have effective ways to structure and retain information. If they do not, instructors and health educators may provide learning strategies to aid effective storage, such as mnemonic devices, heuristics, rehearsal techniques, and memorable metaphors, among others (see Matlin, 2013).

- *Information retrieval stage:* The final stage involves retrieving information that is to be used—a feat that, as any student knows, can be problematic. It is not uncommon for nursing students to know the necessary information yet be unable to reproduce it when called on to do so on a test or in class. Older people, who generally have stored considerable information, may face issues of recognition versus recall. They may recognize something and know "they know it," but be unable to recall it. For instance, they may know they take a medication for arthritis and be able to describe exactly what the pills look like, but they cannot recall the name of the drug when asked. In the converse situation, someone really does not know the information but is able to provide a correct answer or guess correctly. The issue of competence versus performance is at the crux of any learning situation.

Information-processing theory encourages both students and teachers to organize information and make it meaningful so that the information can be remembered. Instructors need to be aware that what happens right before or right after information has been given may interfere with accurate storage and retrieval. Also, it is not sufficient merely to teach information; time must be provided for learners to demonstrate mastery of the information. Both students and patients may want to appear intelligent and agreeable, so they may say they understand information when, in fact, they do not. Instructors must check whether the information is accurately retained and can be performed. Feedback may need to be given to correct faulty learning, and the learner must demonstrate at a later time that the information was retained and can be performed correctly.

Information-processing theory is especially useful when teaching patients self-care, cautions about their medications, and behaviors to avoid so that they can heal properly. It is also useful when teaching students skills such as performing cardiopulmonary resuscitation, inserting IVs, providing information for informed consent, and performing a host of other professional skills.

Social Learning Theory

Social learning theory was developed largely by psychologist Albert Bandura (1977, 2001) over several decades and remains widely used today. Bandura (1977) observed that people do not need to have direct experience to learn; much of learning is based on observing others and what happens to them after they behave in particular ways. Initially, his theory reflected a behaviorist perspective on learning in that Bandura demonstrated the power of role models on learning and behavior. Role models are persons in positions where their behaviors are likely to be both observed and copied; examples are parents, teachers, and those in authority.

Observers are attuned also to whether the role model is rewarded for behavior, which Bandura termed *vicarious reinforcement*. Role model behavior that is positively reinforced is likely to be copied. Yet, in a disturbing finding, role models who engaged in undesirable behavior but who were perceived to be rewarded were more likely to be copied than role models who behaved properly and were rewarded. No wonder organizational behavior can deteriorate quickly when executives and administrators behave in devious or destructive ways yet are perceived to be rewarded for their actions. The predictions are that such results will prove damaging, with the unethical behavior being copied by others throughout the organization.

Principles of social learning theory have been widely adopted in health care. For example, they are evident in mentoring programs where inexperienced health professionals work closely with experienced members of their profession as a way to teach clinical skills and performance in the workplace.

In the next stage of theory development, Bandura (1977) became more interested in the role of the learner and shifted toward a cognitive perspective. As Bandura noted, the learner exercises a strong degree of control (self-regulation) over what is learned and how it is perceived, interpreted, and stored. Just because a role model is viewed as being rewarded does not mean the behavior will be copied. Much depends on the learner's internal processes. Accordingly, Bandura identified four processes or phases within the learner:

1. In the *attentional* phase, the learner decides whether to pay attention to a role model. High-status, attractive, compelling role models and role models who have similar characteristics as the learner are more likely to be copied.
2. In the *retention* phase, the learner engages in storage and retrieval of what was observed.

3. In the *reproduction* phase, the learner copies the role model's behavior. Rehearsal and feedback are important at this stage.
4. In the *motivational* phase, the learner may or may not be motivated to perform the role model's behavior. In deciding whether to copy a behavior, the motivational phase is very important. It is strongly affected by the likelihood of positive reinforcement or punishment, the learning situation, and the learner's evaluation of subsequent situations where the behavior might be performed.

In his more recent work on social learning theory, termed *social cognitive theory*, Bandura (2001) includes sociocultural factors in his model and conceptualizes the individual as an agent exerting considerable control over the learning process. Reflecting the interaction among the environment, the person, and behavior, the emphasis is on the learner's role in mediating and filtering social and cultural influences through the self-system to produce behavior. Personal selection, intentionality, self-regulation, self-efficacy, and self-evaluation come into play and affect both learning and performance. Bandura found self-efficacy to be especially salient in this respect. Self-efficacy has a strong cultural component, such as what stereotypes communicate about competence (e.g., men versus women, youth versus adult, employed versus unemployed). Thus one goal of behavior change and wellness in health care is to promote feelings of self-efficacy in clients trying to break bad habits or cope with their illness and a shifting sense of self. More explicit attention is given to the impact of social factors on learning in several additional cognitive theories, summarized next.

Social Constructionism, Social Constructivism, and Social Cognition Theories

Social constructionism, social constructivism, and social cognition theories are a series of theories from the fields of sociology, psychology, and education that highlight the importance of social influences on learning and behavior. All three theories reflect the idea that knowledge is socially constructed. *Social constructionism* emphasizes the impact of the social context on molding a shared reality. *Social constructivism* stresses the individual's structuring of learning based on culture and social interaction. *Social cognition theory* focuses on how individuals try to make sense of the social world (Fiske & Taylor, 2013; Matlin, 2013). While there are some differences between these three social theories, the emphasis in this chapter is on the general contribution of socially oriented theories to understanding learning and utilizing the information when charged with teaching others.

Individuals give organization and meaning to what they learn, with this process being strongly affected by social influences. In keeping with their cultural background and group affiliations, learners may misperceive, misrepresent, and distort information as they attend to it, incorporate it, store it, or retrieve it. More specifically, social factors such as gender, class, ethnicity, religion, and group memberships can affect what information is attended to and what is ignored, or what is and is not learned. Feelings of self-worth, competence, and efficacy can be critical in remembering and in performance. Given the diverse social backgrounds of people encountered by health professionals, social constructionism, social constructivism, and social cognition theories can help explain some of the widely varying—even irrational—attitudes and behavior exhibited in healthcare settings.

While cognitive theory is widely heralded in psychology and education, it is challenging for instructors to try to determine what is going on in the minds of learners. Also, many of the terms and concepts associated with this theory are not easily operationalized and measured for research purposes.

Another criticism of cognitive theory is that not much attention has been given to the role of emotions in learning until recently. First, a clue about the importance of emotions in learning has been provided by neuropsychological studies based on brain imaging of subjects as they engage in various activities. Researchers found that along with thinking and reasoning, emotional areas of the brain become activated as subjects perform various tasks, including making moral judgments (Benjamin, de Belle, Etnyre, & Polk, 2008; Greene, Sommerville, Nystrom, Darley, & Cohen, 2001). Second, cognitive psychologists have recognized the importance of self-regulation not only in learning and studying (Bjork, 2013), but also in being able to control emotions from early childhood throughout life (Baumeister & Vohs, 2007).

A third area incorporating emotions into cognitive functioning is *emotional intelligence*, which some have argued is more important in successful lives than cognitive intelligence. Emotional intelligence includes attributes such as being self-motivated, managing personal feelings, and making wise judgments, as well as being able to read other people's feelings and working effectively in interpersonal relationships (Goleman, 1995; Mayer, Roberts, & Barsade, 2008). Emotional intelligence has been applied to health care; for example, it has been used to reduce stress and violence in the workplace (Littlejohn, 2012) and as a predictor of professional well-being and satisfaction (Zeidner & Hadar, 2014). Izard (2009) incorporated emotions into cognitive theory because of their impact on motivation, perception, and cognitive processes in affecting behavior outcomes. For example, emotional schemas can lead to psychopathology when learning has fostered connections among emotional feelings and maladaptive cognitions and actions. Although emotions are accorded some consideration by cognitive theorists, a more explicit focus is given to the effects of emotions on learning and behavior in psychodynamic and humanistic theories, which are discussed next.

PSYCHODYNAMIC LEARNING THEORY

Psychodynamic theory evolved from Sigmund Freud's (1995/1938) theory of personality development, which is primarily directed toward understanding and treating dysfunctional behavior in light of childhood and past experiences, emotional conflicts, and motivational forces. Psychoanalysis is a method of treatment in which the patient freely describes his or her history, relationships, and anxieties, which the therapist then helps the patient interpret. The goal is for the patient to gain insights about the self and work through problematic emotional issues.

Mainly applied to personality pathology and abnormal behavior, psychodynamic theory had a profound impact on psychiatry and psychology in the early to mid-20th century. Subsequently, the psychodynamic perspective lost favor, both as a personality theory and as an approach to therapy. From a practical standpoint, however, some of the concepts from psychodynamic theory contribute to a fuller understanding of learning and teaching (Hilgard & Bower, 1966) and are especially useful to those working in health care and the caring professions (Bower, 2005; O'Loughlin, 2013). This theory may be helpful for identifying barriers to learning and healthy behavior, promoting more positive attitudes, and recognizing some of the destructive dynamics in teacher–student and other power relationships. In health care, psychodynamic theory is especially useful for appreciating the role of emotions and motivation in patients, staff, and self and for becoming attuned to interpersonal and intrapersonal conflicts that may hinder productivity and functioning in any setting.

Largely a theory of motivation, psychodynamic theory highlights not only conscious aspects of behavior, but also unconscious motivations. It gives less emphasis to thoughts and thinking than to emotions, tensions, and conflict as driving forces in people's behavior. According to this theory, individuals are motivated to seek pleasure and to avoid pain, an idea termed the *pleasure principle*—a simple generalization that explains a lot of behavior in health care. Personality is conceptualized as having three basic components that motivate actions: the *id* (primitive drives that seek immediate gratification); the *superego* (internalized social values, norms, and standards); and the *ego* (the mediator between the id and the superego, which is grounded in reality). Some of Freud's followers emphasized the importance of healthy ego development, which helps individuals function realistically in an environment full of conflicts, contradictions, and challenges to the self.

As Freud conceived it, personality develops from infancy through adolescence in stages, with each stage involving a psychosexual conflict. Difficulties in adulthood are attributed to problems rooted in one or more childhood stages. Erik Erikson (1968), another psychodynamic personality theorist, later modified and expanded Freud's developmental model. According to Erikson, personality develops in eight stages throughout life, with each stage revolving around a specific psychosocial crisis to be resolved: (1) trust versus mistrust, (2) autonomy versus shame and doubt, (3) initiative versus guilt, (4) industry versus inferiority, (5) identity versus identity diffusion, (6) intimacy versus isolation, (7) generativity versus stagnation, and (8) integrity versus despair.

Research generally has supported Erikson's personality theory (Steinberg & Morris, 2001). The implication is that both teaching and caring relationships should be geared to enhancing personal and social development at every stage of life. Problems in learning or behavior are traced to difficulties in resolving issues during previous stages of development. For instance, growing up in an irresponsible family may result in offspring having problems with the very first crisis of trust versus mistrust. As adults, they may need to work through the issue of trust that is getting in the way of their optimal functioning.

Although not a learning theory per se, psychodynamic theory has some useful applications that can bring an interesting perspective to the dynamics of learning. It can be particularly helpful in understanding why someone may be having difficulty acquiring information or acting in healthy ways. According to psychodynamic theory, learners are motivated to do what is pleasurable and to avoid what is painful, which has several ramifications for healthcare educators. While learning need not be made a miserable experience, students must nevertheless be able to delay gratification and perhaps struggle to learn difficult material on their own.

Students with healthy ego development are more likely to work independently to truly understand what they are supposed to learn, whereas students motivated largely by id impulses may procrastinate, fail to show up for class or turn in assignments on time, and engage in a host of behaviors that ultimately set them up for failure. They may or may not be aware of their own dynamics. If they are not aware, they need to be encouraged to become cognizant of the consequences of their actions and to work for healthier ego development so they can function more effectively.

Equally important, some students with an overdeveloped superego may approach learning by demonstrating heightened anxiety, obsessing over grades, being unhappy over the challenges they need to meet, and becoming angry when they do not receive the grade they think they deserve. Clearly, they are not enjoying learning—and this negative attitude may endure throughout life. From an analytical perspective, the root of people's difficulties with learning can be traced to previous failures and past experiences with parents and other authorities. This insight suggests that problems with learning may have more to do with emotional conflicts than with cognitive abilities.

Memory and retention are, of course, central goals of learning, but according to the psychodynamic view, memory can be faulty or even inaccessible. In addition, memory lapses and mistakes can be significant and may represent unconscious conflicts and motivations (motivated forgetting). Why, for instance, is it difficult to remember a certain patient's name, or why does a particular nurse continue to make medication errors?

Anxiety can be another reason for difficulties in either learning or recalling information. To many students and for numerous reasons, education can be an anxiety-producing process. Even so, anxiety is not necessarily detrimental because it may spur people to do a conscientious job or perform better, and life will always supply stressful and anxiety-producing situations that must be overcome. It is the ego's job to manage anxiety. As a consequence, it is crucial that the ego be able to differentiate objective anxiety that is realistic from anxiety that is unrealistic (not probable, overblown, or perhaps highly probable but ignored). When events are stressful, the ego may protect itself by employing defense mechanisms. In the short run, these defense mechanisms may help the self come to grips with a difficult situation. If they are overused or continued too long, however, the same coping strategies may become dysfunctional.

Because both education and health care can be stressful, it is worth reviewing some of the commonly employed ways of defending the self against threat. Examples from health care illustrate each mechanism in the following list:

- *Denial:* ignoring or refusing to acknowledge a threat (patients who refuse to believe their diagnosis and ignore treatment)
- *Rationalization:* excusing or explaining away a threat (staff members who make medical mistakes, which they excuse as caused by circumstances rather than their error)
- *Regression:* returning to a less mature stage as a way of coping with threat (administrators whose ideas are voted down and who then sulk and act like angry children)
- *Repression:* burying unacceptable impulses and thoughts from conscious awareness (nurses who claim they never met a patient they did not like)
- *Displacement:* rather than directing anger at the source of a threat, taking out aggressions on others as a way to release tension and anxiety (receptionists who snap at patients and give them a hard time for no good reason)
- *Projection:* perceiving one's own unacknowledged unacceptable characteristics or desires in others (staff members who gossip about lots of people having sexual affairs or consistently viewing others as devious)
- *Intellectualization:* minimizing anxiety by responding to threat in a detached, abstract, cold manner (physicians who act like technicians or absorbed scientists and fail to establish any rapport with patients)
- *Compensation:* making up for weaknesses by excelling in other areas (staff members who are refused admittance to medical school and subsequently become successful health professionals)

Two of these defense mechanisms, in particular, are endemic in health care and will be briefly discussed here: denial and intellectualization.

Denial is prevalent in professional education and health care and is a way of dealing with bad news that may seem overwhelming. Students may be in a state of denial about how poorly they are doing in a course, for example. Denial is the first stage in Elisabeth Kübler-Ross's (1969) stages of death and dying. This defense mechanism is understandable as a way to cope with a serious threat initially, but if continued it may keep students from addressing the need to study and find help, or it may hinder patients from seeking treatment for themselves or their children.

Intellectualization can be an occupational hazard in medicine. Using this mechanism, healthcare professionals protect themselves by being emotionally detached rather than genuinely engaging with patients needing support. Films such as *The Doctor* (also a book) and *Wit* (also a play) have dramatized the issue of intellectualization in medicine and its impact on patients.

Psychodynamic theory offers an insightful perspective on power relationships (teacher–student, doctor–nurse, nurse–patient). *Transference* is a term from psychodynamic theory describing the situation in which students, patients, or those in a dependent position project their feelings, conflicts, and reactions onto authority figures—often reacting to the authority figure as they would their parents. The reaction may result in hostility and rebellion or in heightened reliance and over-identification with the authority. There is a significant responsibility for those in authority not to exploit or manipulate a transference relationship. At the same time, a student or patient may remind a health professional of a person from his or her past, creating a *countertransference* reaction, in which the person in authority reacts to certain students or patients as if they were someone other than who they really are. This reaction could be either highly favorable or highly unfavorable. The problem is that the relationship becomes distorted and plagued with bias, which makes communication, learning, and treatment problematic.

Knowledge of psychodynamic theory in education and health care reminds teachers and those in authority to pay close attention to their own and others' emotions, anxieties, and conscious and unconscious motivations so that they can function in a safe, realistic manner. The goal is to promote the emotional development of patients, staff, colleagues, and self by recognizing the irrational aspects of human behavior. The psychodynamic approach has been found to be helpful in attempting to understand human trauma, patient and family noncompliance, palliative care, student anxieties, and some of the emotional undercurrents involved in caregiving and long-term care. As an example, Ferns's (2006) nursing study indicated that psychodynamic theory was useful in trying to comprehend and control bullying and abusive behavior by nurse managers, as well as the failure of nurses to report mistakes, highly unethical behavior, and incidents of violence.

Psychodynamic theory has been criticized vehemently for decades. Much of the theory rests on murky constructs and symbolism that is subject to interpretation, and some of Freud's concepts have been proven wrong or are outdated. In addition, this theory is criticized for being speculative and difficult to operationalize and measure. The data are based on descriptive anecdotal case studies of patients with emotional and behavioral problems. As a result, the findings may not be generalizable and are considered less meaningful than the conclusions reached in more rigorous, quantitative, large-sample studies (Bower, 2005). As a therapy modality, psychoanalysis may require years of expensive counseling and has not been demonstrated to be as effective as other therapies. Nevertheless, some aspects of psychodynamic theory add an important dimension to understanding the complexity and emotional nature of learning and the challenges in attempting to change behavior.

HUMANISTIC LEARNING THEORY

Humanistic learning theory in psychology was developed during the mid-20th century, partially in reaction to the dominance of behaviorism and cognitive theory. The humanists argued that these two theories ignored or dismissed the role of emotions in learning and were more concerned with methodology, experimentation, and survey research findings than with people as unique individuals and human beings. Moreover, they criticized the psychodynamic approach for its negative focus on psychological pathology and dysfunction and its ready adoption of an emotionally detached medical model of treatment (Schneider, Bugental, & Pierson, 2001; Snowman & McCowan, 2012).

To the humanists, the purpose of psychology in general, and of education and therapy in particular, is to foster the growth, self-development, and creativity of each individual. Unfortunately, achieving positive self-development is made difficult in a highly technological, materialistic, bureaucratic society that devalues humanity and the human experience. Under the humanist framework, education is criticized for promoting conformity rather than creativity and for sapping enthusiasm for learning with boring curricula, formal lectures, and rote exercises. Moreover, individuals who are viewed as different are seen as being stigmatized by society, such as people with mental health problems, disabilities, or a host of characteristics that relegate entire groups of people to lesser status in the human community. Criticism is also directed at medicine for its hierarchical professional "know it all" approach, which dehumanizes patients and treats people who seek help for their suffering in routine, mechanistic ways that do little to heal the person or the spirit.

Humanistic theory, in contrast, emphasizes a person-centered approach and stresses the importance of feelings over thoughts. The subjective human experience of each individual is seen as being of value, and human relationships depend on being spontaneous, authentic, and empathetic. The goal is to help individuals express their inner creativity, reach their human potential, and strive for personal growth. Motivation is derived from a person's needs, feelings about the self, and desire for positive self-development. Learning is facilitated by allowing people freedom and choices, by supporting their expressiveness and efforts at creative problem solving, and by making learning enjoyable. To achieve these goals, teachers, therapists, and health professionals need to engage in a collaborative relationship with students and patients based on authentic behavior, honest dialogue, and genuine therapeutic listening. When learners are encouraged to make wise choices and are free to pursue creative interests, the retention and transfer of information are more likely than in an authoritarian approach to education. Education, therapy, and healing all need to take place within a nurturing context.

Humanistic theory was given considerable impetus by the work of Abraham Maslow (1954, 1987), whose hierarchy of needs concept of motivation engendered widespread attention and had significant implications for education and health care. According to Maslow, individuals are motivated to act on the basis of their needs, where the lowest-level needs must be met before higher-order needs are pursued. A student who is financially distressed, hungry, and tired is not likely to be oriented toward pursuing competitive academic achievement at school. A fearful, anxiety-ridden patient who is worried about money, his or her job, and family may not be concerned with learning about his or her disease and self-care. Maslow's hierarchy is conceptualized as moving from lowest- to highest-level needs:

- *Physiological needs:* meeting basic survival needs of food, warmth, sleep, and thirst
- *Safety needs:* meeting the need for security, protection, and freedom from fear
- *Belonging and love needs:* meeting the need to give and receive affection
- *Esteem needs:* meeting the need to be perceived as competent; to have confidence and independence; and to have status, appreciation, and recognition
- *Self-actualization needs:* meeting the need to fulfill one's potential as a creative human being

Although Maslow's model has intuitive appeal, Pfeffer (1985) concluded that this theory is not well supported by research. For one thing, the ranking of Maslow's hierarchy of needs does not appear to hold up under scrutiny. For example, creative people may not meet lower-level needs such as warmth and safety, yet they nonetheless manage to self-actualize.

Another important construct in humanistic theory is self-concept. Educator and therapist Carl Rogers (1961, 1994) argued that what people want most is "unconditional positive self-regard"—that is, to be loved for who they are as persons rather than for what they have or can do. Individuals who are threatening, judgmental, or coercive undermine people's self-concept and desire to learn. Rogers maintained that instructors and counselors should act as facilitators by using a person-centered approach with their patients and students. With this strategy, they spend more time listening than talking and convey the idea that they genuinely value and respect each learner as a person. Teachers also need to attend to learners' interests and recognize the importance of communicating and interacting in an honest and authentic manner. A teacher–student relationship based on mutual trust and enjoyment of learning lies at the heart of meaningful education according to humanistic theory.

The humanistic approach to learning fits well with an emphasis on holistic health, wellness, complementary medicine, and health promotion. Creative openness—a hallmark of humanistic theory—furthers healing through activities such as visualization, art, music, therapeutic listening, and communication. Humanists are not afraid to borrow from Buddhism, Chinese medicine, or alternative medical practices to soothe a sick or suffering person's mind, body, and spirit. Being in touch with one's sense of self and emotions, valuing empathetic understanding, and enjoying patients and families are especially critical for anyone in the healing professions. To the humanists, knowing is different from feeling, and feelings may well be more crucial than cold, hard facts. Humanistic principles are fundamental to self-help groups, wellness programs, hospice, and palliative care. In the spirit of humanism, health professionals need to be accepting and encouraging to those who are diagnosed with mental illness, are homeless, or have HIV/AIDS or other dreaded diseases.

While humanistic psychology does not enjoy as prominent a place in the theoretical armamentarium as it once did, its principles have had a clear impact on education and counseling, particularly in regard to its view of the student and patient as central to the mission of learning and therapeutic change. However, the constructs and principles in humanistic psychology are not easily measured and quantified, and the research conducted in this area is considered weak methodologically. Humanistic psychology has been criticized also for fostering narcissism and self-centeredness in learners, with critics charging that it does not prepare students to appreciate the benefits of constructive criticism. In addition, humanists have tended to dismiss the value of expert guidance, memorization, facts, practice, and drill in education, despite research indicating that these activities have their place in learning and can further knowledge, skill acquisition, and performance (Gage & Berliner, 1992).

More popular today than humanistic psychology is positive psychology (Lopez, Pedrotti, & Snyder, 2014), which is less oriented to learning than to topics such as health and well-being, happiness and life satisfaction, positive emotions, and optimism. Positive psychology also has been targeted by a growing number of critics, however (Ehrenreich, 2009).

NEUROPSYCHOLOGY AND LEARNING

Neuropsychology is a branch of psychology concerned with the scientific study of the brain in relation to mental processes and behavior. A relatively new and flourishing area of investigation, it has attracted scientists from a variety of fields, such as physiology, neurology, psychology, cognitive science, and medicine, among other disciplines (Benjamin et al., 2008; Kolb & Whishaw, 2015; Sousa, 2012). Although not a learning theory per se, the findings of neuropsychology are providing an accumulating body of knowledge about underlying brain structures and activity that come into play in attention, perception, information processing, making decisions, and taking action.

Basic research is fundamental to neuropsychology, derived from a variety of sources, including animal studies, work with neurologically impaired patients and people with physical and mental disabilities, and laboratory experiments with healthy subjects engaged in specific tasks. The rapid development of the field of neuropsychology has been greatly aided by advancements in brain imaging technology. Methodological tools include electrical recording (electroencephalography and event-related potential technique), standardized neuropsychological tests, surgery, paper and pencil tests, and computer software.

Neuropsychology research results pertain to a variety of topics and are found scattered among a number of disciplines and scientific journals.

An important contribution of neuropsychology research has been its documentation of the significant role of emotions in learning, information processing, memory, and recall. Emotions range from positive to negative (*valence*) and vary in intensity (*arousal*). In general, emotion has been found to modulate attention, learning, memory, and the brain's executive function (Warren, Miller, & Heller, 2008). As an illustration, in classical conditioning studies of fear, a number of brain structures pertaining to emotions have been identified, including the amygdala, hippocampus, and medial prefrontal cortex. Moreover, fear conditioning does not occur without an intact amygdala (Atkins & Reuter-Lorenz, 2008). As another illustration, arousing events—whether negative or positive—are remembered better than neutral events, with the amygdala exercising a prominent role in memory storage.

Today, the study of memory is one of the largest areas of research in neuropsychology. For example, emotional areas of the brain are clearly involved in memory storage and retrieval. Moreover, by mapping the circuitry activated in doing memory tasks, researchers have identified several independent memory systems. As an illustration, Polk (2008) reported that working memory relies on different neural structures than long-term memory and sensory memory. Atkins and Reuter-Lorenz (2008) described two types of memory: (1) *implicit memory* (procedural memory or how to do tasks), which is mostly not accessible to conscious awareness, and (2) *explicit memory* (long-term memory and semantic memory), which is accessible to conscious awareness and verbal report. Studies also indicate that the depth of processing (i.e., how well the material is processed) is more important in learning and memory than the amount of repetition, rehearsal, or practice (Simon, 2008). These findings suggest that memory is more complex than is often conceptualized. In the healthcare realm, when nurses expect students, patients, or family members to remember, they may need to employ different strategies for procedural memory than for long-term memory tasks. No one should be rushed through memory processing if the goal is to have information accurately remembered.

Another area of interest in memory research is aging and changes in memory and central nervous system functioning, which affect both communications with older people and their performance. The sensory declines and expected slowdowns in processing that come with age decrease reaction time along with all facets of information processing, retrieval, and performance. Lustig and Flegal (2008) noted that older adults have more difficulty with executive processes and screening out distractions and irrelevant information, although many develop effective strategies to compensate for this difficulty. Anyone working with older adults needs to be attuned to the many physiological changes that accompany aging and may affect attention, learning, memory, and performance.

Motor learning and skill acquisition is another research interest in neuropsychology. This is an important area in medicine and health care, where patients may need to learn self-care skills, providers may need to learn caregiving skills, patients may need to relearn motor skills because of injury or disease, and health professionals must acquire the skills necessary to manipulate medical instruments and equipment. Although skill learning has been studied for decades, identifying the underlying neural basis of skill learning is a relatively new endeavor—and one made possible thanks largely to the introduction of new technologies and methodologies (Bo, Langan, & Seidler, 2008). Information gained from mapping connections between brain and motor skill acquisition is expected to lead to better treatments and teaching strategies. For example, motor learning is not an entirely mechanical process; cognition and emotions are involved, especially in the early stages of learning or relearning. Eventually, however, the skills become more automatic. While practice is essential in learning motor skills, a number of issues and considerations surrounding the amount, type, frequency, variation, and spacing of practice sessions must be resolved to ensure effective learning.

Neuropsychological research has provided concrete evidence supporting a number of constructs and principles proposed as part of the various learning theories. In general, research has confirmed the validity of Piaget's concepts of constructivism, assimilation, and accommodation. The information-processing model of learning appears accurate, and Freud's notions of conscious and unconscious forces motivating learning and behavior have been supported by neuropsychology research as well. The humanists' emphasis on the importance of emotions in learning has been verified with evidence, as have many cognitive theory principles. Moreover, not only do brain structures affect learning, but learning, experience, and practice also change brain structures—a concept termed *plasticity* (Reber, 2008). The brain turns out to be much more flexible than once conceptualized, which has important implications for relearning.

The contributions of neuropsychology research suggest some of the following generalizations about learning. Learning is an active process that entails attention and perception, transforming information into preferred modes for encoding, short-term memory, and storage. The dynamics of assimilation and accommodation account for how new information is incorporated into existing structures. Emotions color all aspects of learning, and learning can occur without awareness or thought. Because brain processing is different for each learner, gaining the learner's attention, controlling the pace of learning, and identifying the specific mechanisms that enhance or inhibit learning are important challenges for any instructor. What is clear is that the learner exerts considerable control over whether learning occurs, what is learned, whether it is accurately learned, and whether learning acquired in one setting transfers to other settings.

Neuropsychology research is diverse, fragmented, scattered, and relatively new, and thus it is subject to some criticism relative to learning. First, the subjects used in neuropsychological studies typically are animals, people with disabilities and injuries, and convenience samples of volunteers willing to participate in research. The question then becomes, do the research results generalize to most people? Second, neuropsychology experiments and laboratory studies often involve contrived and relatively simple tasks, which raises concerns about validity and suggests caution when translating findings into the real world of classrooms, health education, or any place where teaching and learning occur on a regular basis. Third, the emphasis on biological mechanisms of learning is considered reductionistic; it oversimplifies learning and ignores the complexity of learning in diverse social environments. Moreover, the humanists caution that the individuality and humanity of learners is buried by science, while infatuation with the latest expensive technology can be a distraction from the actual worth and applicability of the project and its findings.

USING LEARNING THEORIES IN ADVANCED NURSING PRACTICE

The learning theories discussed in this chapter have implications that extend beyond classroom instruction. Indeed, they may be particularly useful to advanced practice nurses in their leadership roles in education, management, or organizational and lifestyle change.

Taken together, the theories share common features that suggest some general advice about learning. Most theories indicate that learning is an active process, in which individuals have the ultimate control over what is learned and how well it is learned. Self-concept, feelings of self-efficacy, and the ability to self-regulate may need to be buttressed to improve knowledge acquisition or the confidence to change feelings, thoughts, and behaviors. Neuropsychology research documents that emotions are intertwined with learning, memory, decision making, and behavior and, therefore, must be considered in any learning situation. Social science research demonstrates that a significant amount of learning is affected by environmental influences and filtered through each learner's personal lens, which can distort perceptions, information processing, and interpretations. In addition, learning is a social experience, with many adults and some children acquiring information more effectively through social interaction.

In pulling together the learning theories, the following general model for learning is proposed (also see **Box 10-1**):

Learning experiences → learner processing → learning outcomes

A multidimensional approach to learning more accurately represents the complexity involved in learning, where the following three dimensions exist:

1. *External learning experiences:* environment or situation, stimuli, structure and configuration of teaching materials and approach, role models, and social influences
2. *Internal processing within the learner:* perceptions and cognitions; emotions and feelings; conscious and unconscious motivations; past experiences and cognitive and emotional developmental stage and schema; notions of self-efficacy, self-regulation, and self-concept; personality development and ego strength
3. *External outcomes and observable results of learning:* responses, behavior, actions, performance, transfer, feedback, and problem solving

Box 10-1 General Learning Model		
External Learning Experiences $\rightarrow$	**Internal Learner Processing** $\rightarrow$	**External Learning Outcomes** $\rightarrow$
Environment	Attention	Responses
Situations	Perceptions	Behavior
Stimuli	Thoughts	Actions
Teaching materials	Memory (retention)	Performance
Teaching approach	Emotions	Choices
Role mobdels	Motivation	Transfer
Social influences	Cognitive development	Feedback
Culture	Schema	Problem solving
Social interaction	Personality development	
	Ego development	
	Self-efficacy	
	Self-regulation	
	Self-concept	
	Transference	

What becomes evident is that the learning theories work together, with each theory proving helpful in dealing with specific considerations and problems encountered when attempting to instruct others; break bad habits; or improve studying, behavior, and performance. In addressing the three fundamental questions raised in the beginning of the chapter, the following subsections cover some of the principal issues about learning in relation to nursing practice.

1. What Are Effective Ways to Learn New Information or Change Attitudes and Behavior in Health Care?

Research for nearly a century in education and psychology suggests that there is no "one size fits all" approach to learning. The question then becomes, how are advanced practice nurses supposed to decide which theories to utilize in their practice? Part of the decision-making process involves considering the situation, assessing the learner(s), and using the theories in combination to influence learning outcomes. Decisions about how to change behavior (unlearning–relearning) must also be addressed. Multiple applications of the learning theories to situations and people are described in the following section (also see **Box 10-2**).

Box 10-2 Applications of Learning Theories to Situations and People	
Learning Theory	**Applications to Situations and People**
Behaviorist learning theory	Situations in which it works well: • Simple behaviors, skill learning, and nonverbal tasks • Breaking unhealthy habits • Organizational behavior and workplace performance • Medical advertising and public health campaigns People for whom it works well: • People who are not cognitively oriented • People who like to learn by doing and action • People who need clear structure, guidance, and rewards
Cognitive learning theory	Situations in which it works well: • Acquiring knowledge, complex learning, and understanding • Memory processing, problem solving, and creativity • Understanding distortions, misperceptions, and bias People for whom it works well: • People who are verbal and cognitively oriented • People who like challenges, problem solving, and creativity • Some people learn best by discovery, others by guidance • Some children and many adults learn well through social interaction • Consider the individual's stage in life and cognitive processing
Psychodynamic learning theory	Situations in which it works well: • Conflict situations: interpersonal and intrapersonal conflicts • Understanding conscious and unconscious motivation • Dealing with ego development and personality development People for whom it works well: • People exhibiting problems with learning or relationships • People overly motivated by the id or the superego • People who need to be in better touch with reality • Power relationships: transference and countertransference
Humanistic learning theory	Situations in which it works well: • Correcting situations that dehumanize and depersonalize • Palliative care, wellness, and emotional healing People for whom it works well: • People who are creative, self-directed, or seeking fulfillment • People with negative self-concepts or unhealthy needs • People stigmatized by society

- *Consider the situation.* One theoretical approach may be preferable to others in certain situations. For example, behaviorist theory is useful when dealing with simple behaviors, such as increasing study time, changing unhealthy habits, and promoting better organization and responsiveness in the workplace. Yet when knowledge acquisition is at stake (e.g., nursing education, patient education, or staff education), cognitive theory is essential in recognizing the control that the learner has over what is learned. Instruction must be given appropriately and in keeping with learners' developmental level, and teachers must remain attuned to the many considerations related to processing and retention within learners (e.g., pacing, organization, allowing time for reflection). Psychodynamic theory is helpful when learning and behavioral problems become evident and in promoting healthy ego development to cope more realistically with life's challenges. Humanistic theory reminds instructors of their role as facilitators in being respectful, encouraging, and supportive of learners.

- *Consider the learner(s).* People may learn more effectively with certain approaches than with others. Some patients, students, and staff members prefer to discover for themselves, whereas others do better with guidance and find that social interaction aids their learning. Individuals who are not cognitively oriented and need structure may learn better using behaviorist principles, whereas people who are self-motivated and verbal might learn more effectively using cognitive principles. Those who lack confidence can gain from a humanistic approach, as long as they do not need much structure and are self-directed. Students and staff members who encounter barriers to learning and do not function effectively might benefit from a psychodynamic approach where they can talk about their problems and, in the process, become more aware of their motivations, defensive behaviors, and consequences of their actions.

- *Consider how to use learning theories in combination to enhance learning outcomes.* Whether the goal is knowledge acquisition or behavior change, utilizing multiple learning theories can be more effective in influencing learning outcomes than relying on a single learning theory. For example, cognitive-behavioral therapy has been formalized as an approach to changing behavior. Reflecting a combination of behaviorist and cognitive principles, the emphasis with this approach is on assessing the effects of thoughts and feelings on behavior, changing responses through conditioning and reinforcement techniques, and practicing responses until an effective one has been discovered (Dobson & Dobson, 2009). Work is also being done to combine theories, utilizing the most effective concepts from each theory. Integrating association learning from behaviorist theory with discovery learning from cognitive theory is one example (Shanks, 2010). However, nurses may achieve better outcomes by carefully assessing a learning situation themselves and developing a plan by thoughtfully selecting learning principles to apply to a specific situation and person(s). Try the plan, evaluate it, and, if it does not work, formulate another plan and evaluate it. Being comfortable and flexible in employing learning theories requires understanding, application, practice, and assessment—a perspective that is in keeping with an evidence-based approach to nursing, medicine, and health care. Assessment of students, patients, or staff is critical at the learning outcomes stage, where nurses might employ before–after measures of performance, qualitative and quantitative methods, and/or indicators of learner and instructor accountability.

Advanced practice nurses spend a significant amount of their professional time concerned with changing behavior—for example, with patients and community residents who may have learned little or incorrect health information, with those needing to alter their lifestyles, or in the scenario of unhealthy organizational behavior. Thus, it may be helpful to review how learning theories can be used to replace old habits with new ways of thinking and behaving.

The simplest way to modify behavior is to have individuals alter their responses to stimulus situations; over time and with practice, attitudes and behaviors may change. As the behaviorists suggest, there are several ways to effect such a change: (1) Change the environment or situation in ways that will elicit desirable responses; (2) if the environment cannot be changed, substitute a healthier response to the environmental conditions; and (3) change responses to the situation by not reinforcing undesirable behaviors while positively reinforcing desirable behaviors. It can be helpful also for role models to demonstrate what is expected, such as through mentoring programs, visits to well-run healthcare facilities and offices, or meeting with people who successfully accomplished behavioral or organizational changes.

Another option is to work to change perceptions, thoughts, emotions, and attitudes within learners in the hope that behavior change will follow. Reflecting cognitive, psychodynamic, and humanistic theories, this aim may be accomplished by helping learners become more aware of unrealistic motivations, expectations, and goals, as well as negative thoughts, misperceptions, and damaging feelings (perhaps by journaling, keeping a diary or log, or videotaping). The next step is to encourage learners to formulate more realistic goals and motivations and then develop a plan (means) to change their perceptions and achieve their goals. Learners may need to work on what they tell themselves internally about what is contributing to dysfunctional attitudes and behavior. Both the psychodynamic and humanistic perspectives emphasize the need to achieve a balance between personal drive and desire relative to social pressures. The focus then becomes identifying and making mature choices, and practicing healthy responses to develop a better sense of self to cope with difficulties more effectively. Feedback and evaluation are critical along the way. Opportunities to discuss such changes with others may be helpful to some learners (e.g., self-help groups, group study sessions).

In keeping with the general model of learning, working on both external and internal dynamics of learning may be the wisest approach.

2. How Can People Be Motivated to Learn, and Which Kinds of Experiences Facilitate Learning?

Motivation can be the chief obstacle to acquiring knowledge or changing behavior. People may not be motivated for a host of reasons: They do not have a drive to learn, their equilibrium has not been disturbed and they are complacent, they lack self-discipline and cannot defer gratification for the long-term gain, or they lack self-confidence (self-efficacy) in their abilities. Students, patients, and staff may go through the motions of seeming to appear that they are learning when they have actually not learned, so it is important to evaluate what they have learned and to provide appropriate feedback. People must learn how to learn.

This feedback can consist of a simple check with patients to ask them to repeat instructions or have them perform self-care several times until they feel comfortable. It may also help to assess learners' goals and expectations, although behaviorists and psychoanalysts might warn that what people identify as their goals may be less reliable than what their actions and nonverbal behavior indicate. Other factors to assess are feelings of self-efficacy and self-concept. Carl Rogers (1961) noted that it may be easier for people with low self-esteem to confirm a negative self-concept than to think of themselves in positive ways. Teaching is much like coaching, in that encouragement can help some people pull through low periods and buttress their motivation. To be successful, however, such encouragement must be genuine rather than merely saying the right things without demonstrable emotional warmth, rapport, or care.

Given the need to promote active learning, an instructor's main job is to provide experiences that excite learners' motivation. However, the experiences must be at an appropriate level and sufficiently diverse to encompass the numerous ways that learners have of perceiving, interpreting, and responding to information. Since emotions are involved in learning, it is sensible to make learning pleasurable (psychodynamic), enjoyable (humanistic), rewarding (behaviorist), and meaningful (cognitive). Both cognitive theory and neuropsychology research indicate that processing information intensively (through reflection, relating to what is familiar, discussion, and criticism) is likely to lead to better retention and transfer. Learners need time to mull over experiences and opportunities to act on their newly learned information. Providing experiences where learners can discover by doing or engaging in hands-on action is recommended as an aspect of several theories. A Chinese proverb says, "I hear and I forget; I see and I remember; I do and I understand."

As an illustration, as compared to simply reviewing statistics, students may gain a fuller understanding (cognitively and emotionally) of poverty and the impact of low income on patient health by trying to fill out an application for Medicaid or going to a grocery store to see if they could buy healthy food for a family of four with the amount of money allotted for food stamps. Other recommendations are to employ gestalt and cognitive principles in structuring experiences to excite learner motivation and to invite learners' involvement by disturbing their equilibrium. Some suggestions are to create dissonance with contradictory information, set up an experience where learners will want to bring closure, or give learners a problem to solve on their own before presenting information. What is learned initially must be assessed at a later time to make sure it has been learned accurately and can be transferred to situations where it needs to be performed. Therefore, one-shot learning experiences are not likely to be effective; feedback and follow-ups are essential.

3. What Are Effective Ways to Teach So That Information and Skills Will Be Remembered Rather Than Forgotten and Will Transfer Correctly Outside the Immediate Learning Situation?

In applying the learning theories' lessons regarding retention and transfer, a planned approach to teaching is suggested. Readers may want to formulate their own list of advice points about teaching for retention and transfer utilizing learning theories, but the following suggestions are a start:

- *Prepare to teach.* Observe learners to determine their level of cognitive development, identify what they respond to and what is familiar to them, and perhaps get to know learners at a personal level by listening while they describe themselves and their goals for learning. Also, determine readiness to learn by assessing learner motivations, attention (including distractions in the environment), and possible barriers to learning such as fatigue, anxiety, preoccupation with other thoughts, or being in pain, nauseated, or ill—all of which affect attention and concentration.
- *Present information.* Help individuals prepare their schema and framework for learning by providing advance organizers to inform them about the goals of the educational session and topics to be covered. Seek reactions from learners to find out what is familiar to them; this information can then be used to relate the substantive material to be presented. Pose a question, contradiction, or problem for learners to solve to heighten their interest and involvement, and prod learners' motivation. Ideally, the material needs to be presented in ways that respect cognitive load and activate different sensory modes, in keeping with learners' metacognition and ways of processing information. It can be helpful to break complex material into units or understandable chunks to make it easier to process and store—perhaps offering some memory techniques to aid retention. Pacing and time for reflection encourage deep processing and retention.
- *Construct a way for learners to act on the information.* Some suggestions are for learners to ask questions, participate in small discussion groups, and perform an exercise to apply the information. Learners may need time for chance discovery, reflection, and creative application, and they may also need to practice the information over time. The information may need to be repeated in different ways to increase the likelihood that it

will be remembered and transferred. It is helpful if the material presented in a learning session can be practiced in settings similar to those in which it is likely to be transferred.

• *Evaluate the effectiveness of learning.* Learning can be assessed through tests, short quizzes, oral discussion, projects, and problem-solving opportunities. Learners must feel free to ask for clarification and help, and instructors need to be attuned to barriers to learning and information transfer, such as weak motivation, problems with self-efficacy and self-regulation, or faulty processing and possible rewards for not learning.

• *Provide remediation as soon as possible for weak or inaccurate learning.* Teachers may want to utilize computer technology for self-teaching and correction or have students or patients teach one another as practice (the best way to learn is to teach). In addition, some socially oriented students might benefit by working with others to remediate their learning. Perhaps some learners may not understand initially the value of acquiring certain information and, therefore, need a clearer rationale for learning, or perhaps they may benefit from having a direct experience that demonstrates the value of learning. Other students may need positive reinforcement. When difficulties in learning arise, it is essential to uncover what is inhibiting learners' processing and performance. Psycho-dynamic and humanistic learning theories can be helpful when remediation is an issue. Serious problems may require referral to formal counseling and therapy (see Box 10-2).

SUMMARY

As this review of educational and learning theories demonstrates, learning is a multidimensional process that involves external learning experiences, the internal processing within each learner, and the resulting learning outcomes as evidenced by behavior, actions, and performance. Learning theories provide a toolbox of approaches that advanced practice nurses can apply to educational activities, organizational management, medically related lifestyle and behavior change, and health communications. Research studies confirm that utilizing learning theories to formulate educational experiences in health care enhances advanced nursing practice.

Learning theories and theories in social psychology provide the rationale for successful continuing education programs to foster interprofessional collaboration and communication in preventing medical errors and ensuring patient safety (Sargeant, 2009). Graduate-level nursing programs increase in effectiveness when students are able to transfer theories and methods from classroom information about quality of care and patient safety to the wider healthcare setting (Jones, Mayer, & Mandelkehr, 2009). Equally important, when these precepts are applied to clinical education programs, students benefit by being actively engaged with patient care and receiving timely feedback (Leinster, 2009). By implementing educational and learning theories in their work, advanced practice nurses can be at the forefront of improved health care for patients, students, staff, and the human community.

DISCUSSION QUESTIONS

1. Which learning theories and principles do you think are the most useful to advanced practice nurses, and why?

2. Based on the learning theories discussed in this chapter, make a list of suggestions to help nurses do an effective job with patient education. You do not need to identify which theories you are using, but your suggestions should clearly reflect important learning principles.

3. Applying the learning theories discussed in this chapter, develop a step-by-step program to decrease the frequency of medical mistakes in hospitals, and cite the learning theories or principles that back up each step of your program. (Alternatively, choose a different application, such as decreasing workplace conflict, improving communication between physicians and nurses, reducing medication errors, or some other organizational problem confronting health care.)

4. Devise a step-by-step program for altering the lifestyles of patients who have serious health problems because of an unhealthy habit or habits (e.g., smoking, obesity, substance abuse, high stress levels, or some other unhealthy habit). Decide which specific habit or habits you want to address in your program, and then describe your program. Anchor the rationale for each step in learning theories and principles, and indicate which learning principles apply to each step.

5. As an alternative to Question 4, develop a step-by-step program to change a specific health behavior of your choice (e.g., smoking, obesity, healthier nutrition for people with diabetes, lack of exercise for cardiac patients, or some other health problem). In your program, address the elements of the three fundamental questions discussed at the beginning of this chapter—effective ways to change health behaviors, ways to motivate program participants, experiences that might encourage learning, and teaching so that information and skills will be remembered and transferred outside of the classroom.

6. Using your own experience and knowledge, explain how a multidimensional approach employing learning theories is superior to a unidimensional approach in resolving health problems.

7. How has neuropsychology research improved our understanding of the general model of learning described near the end of the chapter?

8. As mentioned at the beginning of the chapter, knowledge of the role of emotions in learning and behavior is crucial in the highly charged field of health care. How can information from each of the four learning theories and neuropsychology research help advanced practice nurses include considerations related to emotions in patient education, nursing education, and organizational behavior?

REFERENCES

Adelson, J. (1986). *Inventing adolescence: The political psychology of everyday schooling.* New Brunswick, NJ: Transaction Books.

Atkins, A. S., & Reuter-Lorenz, P. A. (2008). Learning and memory for emotional events. In A. S. Benjamin, J. S. de Belle, B. Etnyre, & T. A. Polk (Eds.), *Human learning: Biology, brain, and neuroscience* (pp. 125–135). Boston, MA: Elsevier.

Bandura, A. (1977). *Social learning theory.* Englewood Cliffs, NJ: Prentice Hall.

Bandura, A. (2001). Social cognitive theory: An agentic perspective. *Annual Review of Psychology, 52,* 1–26.

Baumeister, R. F., & Vohs, K. D. (Eds.). (2007). *Handbook of self-regulation: Research, theory, and application.* New York, NY: Guilford Press.

Benjamin, A. S., de Belle, J. S., Etnyre, B., & Polk, T. A. (Eds.). (2008). *Human learning: Biology, brain, and neuroscience.* Boston, MA: Elsevier.

Bjork, R. A. (2013). Self-regulated learning: Beliefs, techniques, and illusions. *Annual Review of Psychology, 64,* 417–444.

Bo, J., Langan, J., & Seidler, R. D. (2008). Cognitive neuroscience of skill acquisition. In A. S. Benjamin, J. S. de Belle, B. Etnyre, & T. A. Polk (Eds.), *Human learning: Biology, brain, and neuroscience* (pp. 101–123). Boston, MA: Elsevier.

Bower, M. (Ed.). (2005). *Psychoanalytic theory for social work practice: Thinking under fire.* New York, NY: Routledge.

Brownell, P. (2012). *Gestalt therapy for addictive and self-medicating behaviors.* New York, NY: Springer.

Clark, N. M., Mitchell, H. E., & Rand, C. S. (2009). Effectiveness of educational and behavioral asthma interventions. *Pediatrics, 123,* S185–S192.

Dobson, D., & Dobson, K. S. (2009). *Evidence-based practice of cognitive-behavioral therapy.* New York, NY: Guilford Press.

Ehrenreich, B. (2009). *Bright-sided: How relentless promotion of positive thinking has undermined America.* New York, NY: Metropolitan Books.

Erikson, E. (1968). *Identity: Youth and crisis.* New York, NY: W. W. Norton.

Fadiman, A. (1997). *The spirit catches you and you fall down: A Hmong child, her American doctors, and the collision of two cultures.* New York, NY: Farrar, Straus and Giroux.

Ferguson, L., & Day, R. A. (2005). Evidence-based nursing education: Myth or reality? *Journal of Nursing Education, 44,* 107–115.

Ferns, T. (2006). Under-reporting of violent incidents against nursing staff. *Nursing Standard, 20,* 41–45.

Fiske, S. T., & Taylor, S. E. (2013). *Social cognition: From brains to behavior.* Thousand Oaks, CA: Sage.

Freud, S. (1995/1938). *The basic writings of Sigmund Freud* (Modern Library Series, A. A. Brill, Trans.). New York, NY: Random House.

Gage, N. L., & Berliner, D. C. (1992). *Educational psychology* (5th ed.). Boston, MA: Houghton Mifflin.

Goleman, D. (1995). *Emotional intelligence.* New York, NY: Bantam Books.

Greene, J. D., Sommerville, R. B., Nystrom, L. E., Darley, J. M., & Cohen, J. D. (2001). An fMRI investigation of emotional engagement in moral judgment. *Science, 293,* 2105–2108.

Hee, S. L., & Anderson, J. R. (2013). Student learning: What has instruction got to do with it? *Annual Review of Psychology, 64*, 445–469.

Hilgard, E. R., & Bower, G. H. (1966). *Theories of learning* (3rd ed.). New York, NY: Appleton-Century-Crofts.

Hooyman, N., & Kiyak, H. A. (2007). *Social gerontology: A multidisciplinary perspective* (8th ed.). Boston, MA: Allyn & Bacon.

Izard, C. E. (2009). Emotion theory and research: Highlights, unanswered questions, and emerging issues. *Annual Review of Psychology, 60*, 1–25.

Jones, C. B., Mayer, C., & Mandelkehr, L. K. (2009). Innovations at the intersection of academia and practice: Facilitating graduate nursing students' learning about quality improvement and patient safety. *Quality Management in Health Care, 18*(3), 158–164.

Kazdin, A. E. (2013). *Behavior modification in applied settings*. Long Grove, IL: Waveland Press.

Kolb, B., & Whishaw, I. Q. (2015). *Fundamentals of human neuropsychology* (7th ed.). New York, NY: Worth.

Kramer, D. A. (1983). Post-formal operations? A need for further conceptualization. *Human Development, 26*, 91–105.

Kübler-Ross, E. (1969). *On death and dying*. New York, NY: Scribner.

Leinster, S. (2009). Learning in the clinical environment. *Medical Teacher, 31*(2), 79–81.

Littlejohn, P. (2012). The missing link: Using emotional intelligence to reduce workplace stress and workplace violence in our nursing and other health care professions. *Journal of Professional Nursing, 28*, 360–368.

Lopez, S. J., Pedrotti, J. T., & Snyder, C. R. (2014). *Positive psychology: The scientific and practical explorations of human strength* (3rd ed.). Thousand Oaks, CA: Sage.

Lustig, C., & Flegal, K. (2008). Age differences in memory: Demands on cognitive control and association processes. In A. S. Benjamin, J. S. de Belle, B. Etnyre, & T. A. Polk (Eds.), *Human learning: Biology, brain, and neuroscience* (pp. 137–149). Boston, MA: Elsevier.

Maslow, A. (1954). *Motivation and personality*. New York, NY: Harper & Row.

Maslow, A. (1987). *Motivation and personality* (3rd ed.). New York, NY: Harper & Row.

Matlin, M. W. (2013). *Cognition* (8th ed.). Hoboken, NJ: Wiley.

Mayer, J. D., Roberts, R. D., & Barsade, S. G. (2008). Human abilities: Emotional intelligence. *Annual Review of Psychology, 59*, 507–536.

Murray, D. J. (1995). *Gestalt psychology and the cognitive revolution*. New York, NY: Harvester Wheatsheaf.

O'Loughlin, M. (Ed.). (2013). *Psychodynamic perspectives on working with children, families, and schools*. New York, NY: Jason Aronson.

Ormrod, J. E. (2014). *Educational psychology: Developing learners* (8th ed.). Boston, MA: Pearson.

Pfeffer, J. (1985). Organizations and organizational theory. In G. Lindzey & E. Aronson (Eds.), *Handbook of social psychology: Vol. 1. Theory and method* (3rd ed., pp. 379–440). New York, NY: Random House.

Piaget, J., & Inhelder, B. (1969). *The psychology of the child* (H. Weaver, Trans.). New York, NY: Basic Books.

Polk, T. (2008). Introduction: Cognitive neuroscience of learning and memory. In A. S. Benjamin, J. S. de Belle, B. Etnyre, & T. A. Polk (Eds.), *Human learning: Biology, brain, and neuroscience* (pp. 75–76). Boston, MA: Elsevier.

Reber, P. J. (2008). Cognitive neuroscience of declarative and nondeclarative memory. In A. S. Benjamin, J. S. de Belle, B. Etnyre, & T. A. Polk (Eds.), *Human learning: Biology, brain, and neuroscience* (pp. 113–123). Boston, MA: Elsevier.

Rogers, C. (1961). *On becoming a person*. Boston, MA: Houghton Mifflin.

Rogers, C. (1994). *Freedom to learn* (3rd ed.). New York, NY: Merrill Press.

Sargeant, J. (2009). Theories to aid understanding and implementation of interprofessional education. *Journal of Continuing Education in Health Professions, 29*(3), 178–184.

Sawyer, R. K. (Ed.). (2006). *The Cambridge handbook of the learning sciences*. New York, NY: Cambridge University Press.

Schneider, K. J., Bugental, J. F. T., & Pierson, J. F. (Eds.). (2001). *The handbook of humanistic psychology: Leading edges in theory, research, and practice*. Thousand Oaks, CA: Sage.

Shanks, D. R. (2010). Learning: From association to cognition. *Annual Review of Psychology, 61*, 273–301.

Simon, D. A. (2008). Scheduling and learning. In A. S. Benjamin, J. S. de Belle, B. Etnyre, & T. A. Polk (Eds.), *Human learning: Biology, brain, and neuroscience* (pp. 61–72). Boston, MA: Elsevier.

Skinner, B. F. (1974). *About behaviorism*. New York, NY: Vintage Books.

Snowman, J., & McCowan, R. (2012). *Psychology applied to teaching* (13th ed.). Belmont, CA: Wadsworth, Cengage Learning.

Snyder, C. R., & Lopez, S. J. (Eds.). (2002). *Handbook of positive psychology*. New York, NY: Oxford University Press.

Sousa, D. A. (2012). *How the brain learns* (4th ed.). Thousand Oaks, CA: Corwin/Sage.

Sparks, L., & Nussbaum, J. F. (2008). Health literacy and cancer communication with older adults. *Patient Education and Counseling, 71*(3), 345–350.

Steinberg, L., & Morris, A. S. (2001). Adolescent development. *Annual Review of Psychology, 52*, 83–110.

Sternberg, R. J. (2006). *Cognitive psychology* (4th ed.). Belmont, CA: Thomson/Wadsworth.

Sweller, J., Ayres, P., & Kalyuga, S. (2011). *Cognitive load theory: Explorations in the learning sciences, instructional systems and performance technologies*. New York, NY: Springer-Verlag.

Tennant, M. (2006). *Psychology and adult learning* (3rd ed.). New York, NY: Routledge.

Vygotsky, L. S. (1986). *Thought and language*. Cambridge, MA: MIT Press.

Warren, S. L., Miller, G. A., & Heller, W. (2008). Emotional facilitation and disruption of memory. In A. S. Benjamin, J. S. de Belle, B. Etnyre, & T. A. Polk (Eds.), *Human learning: Biology, brain, and neuroscience* (pp. 45–59). Boston, MA: Elsevier.

Woolfolk, A. E. (2012). *Educational psychology* (12th ed.). Boston, MA: Pearson.

Zeidner, M., & Hadar, D. (2014). Some individual difference predictors of professional well-being and satisfaction of health professionals. *Personality and Individual Differences, 65*, 91–95.

Chapter 11

Health Behavior Theories

Karen Glanz
Lora E. Burke
Barbara K. Rimer

INTRODUCTION

This chapter focuses on contemporary theoretical bases for health behavior change for disease prevention and management and their applications to advanced nursing practice. It first introduces key concepts related to the application of theory in understanding and improving health behaviors. It then describes several current theoretical models that can be helpful in planning and conducting patient and family education and behavioral interventions. Finally, it highlights important issues and constructs that cut across theories.

Health behavior is central to disease prevention and management. Nurses' roles in health behavior change, including patient education and health promotion, are pivotal because of nurses' centrality in health care and their credibility as patient educators. With the focus of the Patient Protection and Affordable Care Act on achieving the Triple Aim (improving the patient experience of care, improving the health of populations, and reducing the per capita cost of health care), the role of nurses in the adoption of and adherence to healthy behaviors is more important than ever before. Contemporary evidence-based recommendations advise including intensive behavioral counseling for adult patients with known behavioral risk factors for chronic disease, noting that such counseling can be provided by physicians or other clinicians, such as nurses and trained community health workers. Also, some behaviors can be improved through brief, low-intensity counseling delivered by nurses and other health professionals. Further, nonclinical community sites, such as work sites, churches, and community centers, are becoming increasingly important as locations for health behavior interventions, especially with the growing and widespread prevalence of obesity and diabetes. Nurses may play leadership roles in these settings, as well.

THE EVOLUTION OF HEALTH BEHAVIOR THEORY

The earliest known applications of health behavior theory to population health problems occurred while social psychologists working in the U.S. Public Health Service were trying to understand how to increase participation in programs designed to prevent and detect disease (Hochbaum, 1958). Theories of health behavior reflect an amalgamation of approaches, methods, and strategies from social and health sciences. They draw on the theoretical perspectives, research, and practice tools of such diverse disciplines as psychology, sociology, anthropology, communications, nursing, economics, and marketing (Glanz, Rimer, & Viswanath, 2015). Health behavior and its close relative, health education/promotion, are also dependent on epidemiology, statistics, and medicine.

Many kinds of professionals contribute to and conduct health behavior and health education research and programs. Interdisciplinary collaborations among professionals drawn from different disciplines, each of whom is concerned with the behavioral and social intervention process and its application to health issues, ensure the best blend of perspectives. For example, nurses bring to health behavior and health education their unique expertise in working with individual patients and patients' families to facilitate learning, adjustment, and behavior change, and to improve quality of life. Psychology contributes a rich legacy of more than 100 years of research and practice on individual differences, motivation, learning, persuasion, and attitude and behavior change (Matarazzo et al., 1984), as well as the perspectives of organizational and community psychology. Other health, education, and human services professionals contribute their special expertise to health behavior theory and practice, as well.

TRENDS IN THE USE OF THEORIES AND MODELS

Theories that gain recognition in a discipline shape the field, help define the scope of practice, and influence the education and socialization of its professionals. No single theory or conceptual framework dominates research or practice in contemporary health behavior and health education, although a relatively small number of theories and models are used most often in this realm.

Over the past two decades, the authors of this chapter have reviewed a sample of publications on four different occasions to identify the most often used theories (Glanz, Rimer, & Viswanath, 2008; Glanz et al., 2015; Painter, Borba, Hynes, Mays, & Glanz, 2008). From these reviews, certain theories and models clearly emerged as the most popular and widely used choices. The first three, and by far the most dominant, are social cognitive theory (SCT), the transtheoretical model/stages of change, and the health belief model (HBM). The other leading theories and models are the theory of reasoned action (TRA) and theory of planned behavior (TPB), ecological models/social ecology, stress and coping, community organization, diffusion of innovations, social support and social networks, and patient–provider communication. The three most popular theories and models, along with the representational approach (RA, a recent adaptation that blends psychological and educational theories), are described in more detail later in this chapter.

In a review of theory use in published research between 2000 and 2005, we found that the most often used theories were the transtheoretical model, SCT, and the HBM (Painter et al., 2008). Overall, the same theories dominated as did in 1999 and 2000. As in previous reviews, this review revealed dozens of theories and models that were used, though only a few of them were used in multiple publications and by several authors. Some are minor variations of another theory. Several key constructs cut across the most often cited models for understanding behavior and behavior change: the importance of the individual's view of the world, multiple levels of influence, behavior change as a process, motivation versus intention, intention versus action, and changing behavior versus maintaining behavior change (Glanz & Oldenburg, 2001).

A recently published compendium of behavior change theories, using clearly defined inclusion criteria, provides summaries of 83 different theories and models (Michie, West, Campbell, Brown, & Gainforth, 2014). As these reviews primarily assessed individual outcomes of behavior change interventions, we also examined reviews of strategies for implementation and dissemination in health and mental health services (Powell et al., 2012; Tabak, Khoong, Chambers, & Brownson, 2012) and a review of social ecological contextual levels of health promotion interventions across a 20-year period (Golden & Earp, 2012).

It should be emphasized that there are *many* available theories and models—for example, the (acknowledged) selective review of 83 theories in Michie et al.'s book (2014); the 68 distinct strategies identified by Powell et al. (2012); and the 61 models included in Tabak et al.'s (2012) dissemination and implementation research review. These theories and models are not mutually exclusive. As Tabak and colleagues (2012) have stated, "There is substantial overlap between models, as the included constructs are often similar." Review authors have used different coding schemes to classify the theories in their reviews. A novel approach taken by Michie et al. (2014) to examine the interconnectedness of the 83 theories summarized in their book was to use network analysis methods to examine contributions, links, and patterns among the theories they described.

Our synthesis of the various reviews, and the Michie et al. network analysis (2014), leads to the conclusion that indeed, *only a small number of theories and models have been widely used and/or informed numerous other theories*. In fact, those theories are the same ones that were identified in the last three editions of this book: the HBM, SCT (and social learning theory, its predecessor), TPB (and TRA, its predecessor), social support, diffusion of innovations, and the social ecological model.

Along with the published observations about which theories are being used, concerns have been raised about how the theories are used (or not used) in research and practice. In the most recent review of theory use, we classified articles that employed health behavior theory along a continuum:

1. *Informed by theory:* A theoretical framework was identified, but there was no or limited application of the theory in specific study components and measures.
2. *Applied theory:* A theoretical framework was specified and several of the constructs were applied in components of the study.
3. *Tested theory:* A theoretical framework was specified and more than half of the theoretical constructs were measured and explicitly tested, or two or more theories were compared to one another in a study.
4. *Building/creating theory:* New or revised/expanded theory was developed using constructs specified, measured, and analyzed in a study.

Of all the theories used in the sample of articles ($n = 69$ articles using 139 theories), 69.1% used theory to inform a study, 17.9% of theories were applied theories, 3.6% were tested, and 9.4% involved building/creating theory (Painter et al., 2008). These findings should encourage researchers and practitioners to strive for more thorough application and testing of health behavior theories to advance science and move the field forward.

Health behavior is concerned with the development and application of knowledge, as well as with approaches to solving health and social problems—in other words, how to effect change (Glanz et al., 2008). Considerable scholarly and practitioner efforts have been devoted to developing techniques that change behaviors. Now, more attention is being paid to sustaining change and not just facilitating initial change. Although these efforts grew out of a desire to produce a better world, techniques that push people to change were experienced by many as manipulative, reducing their freedom of choice and sustaining a balance of power in favor of the change agent (Kipnis, 1994).

A paradigm shift has occurred recently, and many of the behavioral techniques used today (e.g., social support, empowerment, problem solving, and personal growth) are based on reducing obstacles to change and promoting informed decision making, rather than on pushing people to change. Thus, efforts respect individual autonomy while informing individuals of the benefits of change.

Advanced practice nurses employ these techniques frequently in caring for patients and their families. This is particularly the case with nurses who provide care to individuals with chronic disorders. They know that merely providing information to patients or telling patients that they need to take their medication, stop smoking, or be more active will not lead to behavior change. Instead, these nurses recognize that their practice should be guided by behavior change theories, and that teaching should be delivered in sessions that are based on mutual collaboration and accompanied by counseling strategies to enlist the individual or patient to consider making changes or adopting a new treatment regimen.

These nurse–patient interactions are guided by several of the strategies that are part of the theories discussed in this chapter. Nurses use elements of SCT in counseling patients about medication adherence (Berg, Dunbar-Jacob, & Sereika, 1997; Burkhart, Rayens, Oakley, Abshire, & Zhang, 2007; Ruppar, Cooper, Mehr, Delgado, & Dunbar-Jacob, 2016) and counseling patients with coronary heart disease about reducing risk factors (DeBusk et al., 1994; Haskell et al., 1994; Jorstad et al., 2013; Saffi, Polanczyk, & Rabelo-Silva, 2014). Self-efficacy, derived from SCT, has guided nurse-delivered interventions to improve dietary adherence (Burke, Dunbar-Jacob, Orchard, & Sereika, 2005) as well as medication adherence (Bartlett, Lukk, Butz, Lampros-Klein, & Rand, 2002; Berg, Dunbar-Jacob, & Rohay, 1995; Burke et al., 2005; Cook, McCabe, Emiliozzi, & Pointer, 2009; McKenzie & Chang, 2015). The expanded HBM (Burns, 1992) has been used extensively to guide pre-conception counseling among teens with type 1 diabetes (Charron-Prochownik et al., 2001), while another nurse researcher applied the TPB in her examination of the mediating role of condom self-efficacy between the parent–adolescent relationship and the intention to use condoms (Cha, Kim, & Doswell, 2007). Others have used the transtheoretical theory of behavior change to guide medication adherence among adults taking antidepressants. Finally, a newly derived model, the RA to patient education, was applied by a group of researchers in four studies: a study of pain management among cancer patients (Ward et al., 2008), a study of symptom management among women with ovarian cancer (Donovan et al., 2007), a study of communication about end-of-life care for patients undergoing cardiac surgery (Song, Kirchhoff, Douglas, Ward, & Hammes, 2005), and a study to improve symptom management and quality of life among women who had survived breast cancer (Donovan et al., 2007; Heidrich et al., 2009). Several of these examples will be described in further detail following the discussion of each of these theories.

THE HEALTH BELIEF MODEL

The HBM was one of the first theories of health behavior, and it remains one of the most widely recognized in the field today. This model was developed in the 1950s by a group of U.S. Public Health Service social psychologists who wanted to explain why so few people were participating in programs to prevent and detect disease. For example, the Public Health Service was sending mobile X-ray units out to neighborhoods to offer free chest X-rays as screening for tuberculosis (Hochbaum, 1958). Despite the fact that this service was offered without charge and was available in a variety of convenient locations, the program had limited success. Fortunately, these researchers asked the question, "Why?"

To find an answer, social psychologists examined what was encouraging or discouraging people from participating in the program. They theorized that people's beliefs about whether they were susceptible to disease and their perceptions of the benefits of trying to avoid disease influenced their readiness to act (Glanz & Rimer, 2005).

In ensuing years, researchers expanded upon this theory, eventually concluding that six main constructs influence people's decisions about whether to take action to prevent, screen for, and control illness. They argued that people are ready to act if they meet the following criteria:

1. Believe they are susceptible to the condition (*perceived susceptibility*)
2. Believe the condition has serious consequences (*perceived severity*)
3. Believe taking action would reduce their susceptibility to the condition or its severity (*perceived benefits*)
4. Believe the costs of taking action (*perceived barriers*) are outweighed by the benefits
5. Are exposed to factors that prompt action (e.g., a television ad or a reminder from one's physician to get a mammogram; *cue to action*)
6. Are confident in their ability to successfully perform an action (*self-efficacy*)

Because health motivation is its central focus, the HBM is a good fit for addressing problem behaviors that evoke health concerns (e.g., cancer screening, influenza vaccinations, high-risk sexual behavior and the possibility of contracting human immunodeficiency virus [HIV]). Together, the six constructs of this model provide a useful framework for designing both short-term and long-term behavior change strategies. When applying the HBM to planning health programs, practitioners should ground their efforts in an understanding of how susceptible the patient, his or her family, or the target population feels to the health problem; whether they believe it is serious; and whether they believe action can reduce the threat at an acceptable cost. Changing these factors is rarely as simple as it may appear, however.

Consider high blood pressure screening campaigns, which often identify people who are at high risk for heart disease and stroke who say they have not yet experienced any symptoms. Patient education to promote adherence to medications for hypertension also can encounter this obstacle. Because patients do not feel sick, they may not follow instructions to take prescribed medicine or lose weight. The HBM can be useful for developing strategies to deal with noncompliance in such situations. According to this model, asymptomatic people may not follow a prescribed treatment regimen unless they accept that, even though they may not be experiencing any symptoms, they do actually have hypertension (perceived susceptibility). They must understand that hypertension can lead to heart attacks and strokes (perceived severity). They must believe that taking prescribed medication or following a recommended weight-loss program will reduce the risks (perceived benefits) without negative side effects or excessive difficulty (perceived barriers). Print materials, reminder letters, or pill calendars might encourage people to consistently follow their doctors' recommendations (cues to action). For those who have, in the past, struggled with losing weight or maintaining weight loss, a behavioral contract might help establish achievable, short-term goals to build confidence (self-efficacy).

Examples of Application of the Health Belief Model

Charron-Prochownik and colleagues (2001) have developed an extensive research program based on the extended health belief model (EHBM) and have used this framework to develop a program of preconception counseling for teenagers with type 1 diabetes. One study examined the significant correlates of the variables based on the constructs of this model in relation to an intention to perform or actual performance of behaviors that would prevent an unplanned pregnancy, as well as metabolic control of the diabetes. The findings revealed that most of the 80 teenage participants perceived themselves to be moderately susceptible to severe reproductive problems, but they had little knowledge of diabetes and pregnancy and had moderate self-esteem. The participants' perception was that preconception counseling would be beneficial, and they did not envision major barriers to obtaining this type of assistance. The findings also revealed that these same participants did not use effective birth control methods all the time. The correlational analyses demonstrated that there were several significant associations among the individual variables; for example, self-efficacy was significantly associated with other constructs, including self-esteem, social support, and stress. The takeaway message of this study was that female adolescents with type 1 diabetes had limited knowledge of reproduction-related complications of diabetes and the role that preconception counseling can play in preventing complications; moreover, while participants believed that preconception counseling was beneficial, many engaged in unsafe sexual practices.

A later step in this research was the validation of the theory-based instrument to assess preconception planning behavior of adolescents with type 1 diabetes. The reproductive health attitudes and behavior (RHAB) instrument drew upon the constructs of the EHBM, the TRA, and SCT because each theory contributes unique constructs in describing the decision-making processes used by adolescents with diabetes. Overall, the RHAB had good psychometric properties for a newly developed instrument (Charron-Prochownik, Hannan, Sereika, Becker, & Rodgers-Fischl, 2006).

The third phase in this program of research involved the translation of findings from the earlier work into an educational program for teenage girls with diabetes. Charron-Prochownik and colleagues (Charron-Prochownik, Ferons-Hannan, Sereika, & Becker, 2008; Charron-Prochownik, Hannan, et al., 2006; Charron-Prochownik et al., 2001; Charron-Prochownik et al., 2013; Charron-Prochownik, Wang, Sereika, Kim, & Janz, 2006; Fischl et al., 2010) developed an extensive research program based on the EHBM and have used this framework throughout their research program. This program focuses on prevention of unplanned pregnancy, efforts to raise awareness of potential reproductive health complications related to diabetes, and ways to avoid problems. The preconception counseling educational program was developed into a video computer-based and written program (Charron-Prochownik & Downs, 2009) that is distributed currently by the American Diabetes Association (Charron-Prochownik & Downs, 2016). This program of research, from beginning to translation, is based on the EHBM, offering an excellent illustration of how a theoretical framework can guide a body of work.

THE THEORY OF REASONED ACTION, THE THEORY OF PLANNED BEHAVIOR, AND THE INTEGRATED BEHAVIORAL MODEL

People's health decisions often are influenced by how they view the actions they are considering, and by whether they believe important people, such as family members or peers, would approve or disapprove of their behavior. The TPB, which evolved from its predecessor, the TRA, focuses on the relationships between behavior and beliefs, attitudes, subjective norms, and intentions (Montano & Kasprzyk, 2015). The concept of perceived behavioral control—which incorporates beliefs about whether one can control his or her performance of a behavior (i.e., individuals may feel motivated if they believe they can do it)—received added attention in TPB. A central assumption of TPB is that behavioral intentions are the most important determinants of behavior (Ajzen, 1991).

TPB has been applied widely to help understand and explain many types of behavior. Both TRA and TPB have been used successfully to predict and explain a wide range of health behaviors and intentions, including smoking, alcohol abuse, health services utilization, exercise, sun protection, breastfeeding, substance use, HIV/sexually transmitted infection prevention behaviors and use of contraceptives, mammography, use of safety helmets, and use of seat belts (Montano & Kasprzyk, 2008). As predicted, the core constructs of TPB have been found to predict healthy eating such as fruit and vegetable intake and to explain consumption of low-fat milk (Butterfield-Booth & Reger, 2004). Attitudes and behavioral beliefs about health also have been examined within community interventions in schools and communities and found to mediate outcomes of interventions (Glanz, 2008). Theoretical constructs help explain why some people change while others do not after they complete health education programs or are exposed to communication campaigns.

Although the idea that behavioral intentions are important is central to TPB, some critics have voiced concern that intentions are too far removed to be good predictors of actual behavior. The concept of implementing intentions involves encouraging patients or people receiving an intervention to be very specific about how they would change (Montano & Kasprzyk, 2008).

Fishbein and Ajzen (Ajzen & Fishbein, 1980; Fishbein & Ajzen, 1975) have further expanded TRA and TPB to include components from other major behavioral theories and have proposed the use of an integrated behavioral model (IBM). The IBM can be used as a framework to identify specific belief targets for behavior change interventions in the previously described conceptualization of experiential and instrumental attitudes, injunctive and descriptive norms, and perceived control and self-efficacy being determined by specific underlying beliefs. Interventions built on one model construct may have effects that further affect the same or other model constructs (Montano & Kasprzyk, 2015). The IBM is a recent expansion of the TPB that is likely to be more widely used and to have a stronger empirical research base in the coming years.

Examples of Application of the Theory of Planned Behavior

The TPB provided the framework for a study of male college students in South Korea and their practice of condom use (Cha et al., 2007). A significant relationship had been reported between condom self-efficacy and intention to use condoms. Cha and colleagues examined the mediating role of condom self-efficacy and the parent–adolescent relationship, as well as the intention to use condoms and actual condom use, to determine if this was a plausible approach for a family-based intervention to improve the sexual health of this young population. A cross-sectional design was used to study the college students and their parents. The mediation analyses revealed that good mother–son communication predicted a higher intention to use condoms and a higher self-efficacy for condom use; in turn, those persons with higher condom self-efficacy had higher intentions to use condoms. After adjusting for condom self-efficacy, however, the quality of the mother–son relationship no longer predicted the intention to use condoms; rather, condom self-efficacy completely mediated the intention to use condoms by mother–son communication.

The quality of the father–son relationship did not predict the intention to use condoms, although a better relationship predicted higher condom self-efficacy for these males. The father–son relationship had an indirect effect on the intention to use condoms.

This study illustrates how different cultural practices in parenting can influence intention and behaviors. The theoretical framework also was helpful in interpreting study findings.

THE TRANSTHEORETICAL MODEL AND THE STAGES OF CHANGE

Long-term behavior change for disease prevention and management involves multiple actions and adaptations over time. For example, some people may not be ready to attempt changes in their diets, whereas others may have already begun implementing dietary modifications. The construct of *stage of change* is a key element of the transtheoretical model of behavior change, which proposes that people are at different stages of readiness to adopt healthful behaviors (Prochaska, Redding, & Evers, 2015). The notion of readiness to change, or stage of change, has been examined in health behavior research on a variety of topics assessed in many studies around the world and found useful in explaining and predicting behavior.

Stages of change is a heuristic model that describes a sequence of steps in successful behavior change: *precontemplation* (no recognition of need for or interest in change), *contemplation* (thinking about changing), *preparation* (planning for change), *action* (adopting new habits), and *maintenance* (ongoing practice of new, healthier behavior) (Prochaska, Redding, & Evers, 2008). People do not always move through the stages of change in a linear manner: They often recycle and repeat certain stages. For example, individuals may relapse and go back to an earlier stage depending on their level of motivation and self-efficacy.

The stages of change model can be used both to explain why patients might not be ready to change their behaviors and to improve the success of patient education and other behavior change interventions. Patients can be classified according to their stage of change by asking a few simple questions. In the case of dietary change, for example, the nurse might ask the following question about each patient: Is he or she interested in trying to change his or her eating patterns, thinking about changing the diet, ready to begin a new eating plan, already making dietary changes, or trying to sustain changes he or she has been following for some time? By identifying the individual's current stage, the nurse can determine how much time to spend with the patient, whether to wait until he or she is more ready to attempt active changes, whether referral for in-depth counseling or case management is warranted, and so on. Knowledge of the patient's current stage of change can lead also to appropriate follow-up questions about past efforts to change, obstacles and challenges, and available strategies for overcoming barriers or obstacles to change.

Examples of Application of the Transtheoretical Model of Behavior Change

Finnell has applied the transtheoretical model of behavior change to different behaviors in different populations (Finnell, 2003, 2005a, 2005b). Finnell's early work focused on the use of the transtheoretical model to determine whether individuals with co-occurring conditions—mental disorders and substance abuse—undergo change in a similar way to others who have been studied with the use of this model (Finnell, 2003). The presence of several conditions, including impaired decision-making abilities, disordered thought processes, and denial, which can be present with either disorder, may make it difficult for these individuals to recognize that they need assistance and to ask for it. The findings from a cross-sectional survey that was conducted in this population revealed that individuals with comorbid mental disorders and substance abuse rely on different processes as they adopt new behaviors and may need different interventions than persons who have only a substance abuse problem (Finnell, 2003).

Finnell is also applying the transtheoretical model of behavior change to the study of medication adherence among patients in a Veterans Administration inpatient facility. The stages of change concept is being used to guide the assessment of patients regarding their readiness to be adherent to antidepressant medication (Finnell, 2005b). Extensive information is provided on various websites that is dedicated to the use of this theoretical framework, including a video demonstrating the practice of applying the framework.

SOCIAL COGNITIVE THEORY

SCT—the cognitive formulation of social learning theory that has been best articulated by Bandura (1986, 1997)—explains human behavior in terms of a three-way, dynamic, reciprocal model in which personal factors, environmental influences, and behavior continually interact. Because SCT synthesizes concepts and processes from cognitive, behavioristic, and emotional models of behavior change, it can be readily applied to nutritional intervention for disease prevention and management. A basic premise of SCT is that people learn not only through their own experiences, but also by observing the actions of others and the results of those actions. Key constructs of this theory that are relevant to health behavior interventions include *observational learning*, *reinforcement*, *self-control*, and *self-efficacy* (Kelder, Hoelscher, & Perry, 2015).

Principles of behavior modification, which have often been used to promote health behavior change, are derived from SCT. Some elements of behavioral interventions based on SCT constructs of self-control, reinforcement, and self-efficacy include goal setting, self-monitoring, and behavioral contracting (Glanz & Rimer, 2005). For habitual behaviors, such as quitting smoking and improving eating patterns, goal setting and self-monitoring seem to be particularly useful components of effective interventions (Acharya, Elci, Sereika, Styn, & Burke, 2011; Burke, Styn, et al., 2009; Burke et al., 2011; Burke et al., 2012; Burke et al., 2015; Glanz, 2008; Wang et al., 2012; Zheng, Klem, et al., 2015; Zheng, Sereika, et al., 2015). Self-efficacy, or a person's confidence in his or her ability to take action and to persist in that action despite encountering obstacles or challenges, seems to be especially important for influencing health behavior change efforts (Bandura, 1997). Health providers can make deliberate efforts to increase patients' self-efficacy using three types of strategies:

1. Setting small, incremental, and achievable goals
2. Using formalized behavioral contracting to establish goals and specify rewards
3. Monitoring and reinforcing progress, including patient self-monitoring by keeping records (Ambeba et al., 2015; Burke et al., 2015; Glanz et al., 2008)

In group programs, it is possible to easily incorporate activities such as problem-solving discussions and self-monitoring that are rooted in SCT.

The key SCT construct of *reciprocal determinism* means that a person can be both an agent for change and a responder to change. Thus, changes in the environment, role models, and reinforcements can be used to promote healthier behavior. This core construct is also central to social ecological models and is more important today than ever before.

Examples of Application of Social Cognitive Theory

The implementation of interventions based on SCT is quite common among advanced practice nurses. Burke and colleagues tested different approaches to self-monitoring diet and physical activity in a behavioral weight-loss study, including use of a paper diary versus use of an electronic diary (personal digital assistant), with and without feedback messages (Burke, Elci, et al., 2009). Guided by self-regulation, also derived from SCT, the intervention built on the behavioral change strategy of self-monitoring to increase the individual's awareness of his or her behavior, which serves as a crucial step before asking a person to change current behavior. Based on specific goals set with the participant, self-monitoring provides feedback to the person on progress related to those goals. A review of progress made permits self-attribution for the progress and goal achievement. In this study, the delivery of a feedback message via the electronic diary added another element of reinforcement for reported behavior change related to eating behaviors and food selection, as well as physical activity (Ambeba et al., 2015; Burke, Styn, et al., 2009; Burke et al., 2012; Conroy et al., 2011).

Other strategies based on SCT include *role modeling*, which can be implemented by having individuals who are successful in changing behavior model the behavior for those who are learning to adopt it. Examples of successful use of this strategy include cardiac rehabilitation programs in which participants who have successfully adopted a physical activity program demonstrate their ability to exercise for individuals who are newly enrolled, as well as having a person who is credible to the patients demonstrate how to prepare a low-fat meal. It is important that the model who demonstrates the skill or behavior be credible and a person with whom the patient can identify.

Sevick and colleagues used SCT to guide the development and implementation of a diabetes self-management intervention for adults with type 2 diabetes. Their intervention included self-monitoring of the person's diet and daily blood glucose levels, use of an electronic diary in the intervention group, group sessions, and cooking demonstrations (Sevick et al., 2008). Goal setting for various components of self-management was part of the intervention; preliminary results indicate that the intervention led to improved self-management behaviors, as well as improved clinical outcomes (Sevick et al., 2012).

Example of Application of Self-Efficacy

Self-efficacy is considered part of SCT and has provided the underpinning for numerous interventions addressing behavior change. Its role in changing behavior has been reported across several behavior domains, including smoking cessation (Burke et al., 2015; Gwaltney et al., 2001; Gwaltney et al., 2002; Gwaltney, Shiffman, & Sayette, 2005; Ockene et al., 2000; Warnecke et al., 2001; Warziski, Sereika, Styn, Music, & Burke, 2008), weight loss (Butler & Mellor, 2006; Clark, Cargill, Medeiros, & Pera, 1996; Clark & King, 2000), and being more physically active (Dallow & Anderson, 2003; Desharnais, Bouillon, & Godin, 1986; Ewart et al., 1986; Moore, Dolansky, Ruland, Pashkow, & Blackburn, 2003; Pinto, Clark, Cruess, Szymanski, & Pera, 1999). Self-efficacy is described as the perception of one's capability to mobilize the motivation, cognitive resources, and courses of action required to meet given situational demands (Bandura, 1997).

One example of a self-efficacy–based intervention implemented by a cardiovascular nurse specialist is a study of individuals who were being seen for dyslipidemia and who also reported inadequate dietary adherence (Burke et al., 2005). The purpose of the randomized controlled trial was to examine whether the self-efficacy intervention improved adherence to a cholesterol-lowering diet. The intervention was delivered as an adjunct to the usual care; the comparison group received only the usual care. The behavioral intervention focused on strategies to improve self-efficacy for following the prescribed diet and included the individual setting short-term, realistic goals for behavior change to improve adherence and self-monitoring in a paper diary (e.g., eliminating high-fat snacks obtained from the vending machine at work).

At each biweekly intervention session, the nurse reviewed with the participant the goal that had been set and the participant reviewed the diary over the phone and practiced self-reinforcement for positive changes. Any progress toward goal achievement was attributed to the individual. As the person experienced success, incremental changes were made in the goals, reinforcing the strategy of *mastery*, which according to the theory is the strongest source for improving self-efficacy.

Verbal persuasion was another strategy that was used to increase self-efficacy; it was particularly well suited for the telephone delivery of the intervention. This part of the program entailed the interventionist verbally convincing the participant that she was confident in his ability to perform the new behavior.

At the end of the 14-week intervention, the researchers noted significant improvement in adherence to the recommended intake of dietary cholesterol and total and saturated fat. In addition, there was a significant improvement in serum low-density lipoprotein cholesterol, with significantly greater improvements occurring in the intervention group (Burke et al., 2005).

SOCIAL ECOLOGICAL MODELS

Social ecological models focus on the factors affecting behavior and provide guidance for developing successful programs through social environments. These models emphasize multiple levels of influence (such as individual, interpersonal, organizational, community, and public policy spheres) and the idea that behaviors both shape and are shaped by the social environment (McLeroy, Bibeau, Steckler, & Glanz, 1988; Sallis & Owen, 2015).

The principles of social ecological models are consistent with SCT concepts that suggest initially creating an environment that is conducive to change is important to making it easier to adopt healthy behaviors. Given the widespread problems associated with the unhealthy lifestyles followed by many people today, as well as these lifestyles' role in chronic diseases such as diabetes and lung disease, more attention is being devoted to increasing the health-promoting features of communities and neighborhoods. Examples of environmental change strategies to promote healthful behaviors that are based on social ecological models include reducing exposure to secondhand smoke and the consumption of high-calorie, high-fat foods in large portions. Changing the healthcare system by giving providers such as doctors and nurses reminders and incorporating health counseling into primary care are other examples of the application of social ecological models to health behavior.

REPRESENTATIONAL APPROACH

The RA, a theoretical perspective on patient education developed by Donovan and Ward, is a patient-centered intervention theory that links existing health psychology and educational theory to specific psycho-educational interventions (Donovan & Ward, 2001; Donovan et al., 2007). Leventhal's common-sense model (CSM) of illness representations (Leventhal, Meyer, & Nerenz, 1980; Leventhal, Nerenz, & Steeler, 1984) provided the centerpiece of this theoretical framework, which also drew upon educational theory of conceptual change (Hewson & Thorley, 1989; Posner, Strike, Hewson, & Gertzog, 1982).

The RA was developed to increase the probability that individuals will experience conceptual change. It consists of seven elements:

1. Representational assessment
2. Exploration of individuals' concerns and misconceptions or any gaps
3. Creation of conditions for conceptual change
4. Introduction of new information
5. Setting of goals and development of management strategies
6. Summarization
7. Evaluation of strategy and revision (Donovan & Ward, 2001; Donovan et al., 2007)

These key elements of RA use the CSM to focus on what patients or individuals know and understand about their health problems, which guides the clinician in eliciting these individuals' illness representations. The elements derived from theories of conceptual change center on how patients learn new information and behaviors, which helps ensure that the information is presented in ways that will be not only understood by the individual, but also accommodated and acted on by that person.

The RA requires the provider to elicit and understand the individual's preexisting representations of illness before he or she provides any new information to the patient. In this way, both the clinician and the patient have the opportunity to recognize voids, misunderstandings, and confusion in the patient's representation. It is also important for the clinician to understand the individual's representations of the health problem so the clinician can give new information in an individualized manner that is specific, highly relevant, and more likely to be accepted by the patient as intelligible, plausible, and fruitful. The efficacy of interventions based on the RA has been supported by evidence from controlled randomized clinical trials conducted by nurse investigators studying other patient populations (Donovan, Ward, Sherwood, & Serlin, 2008; Donovan et al., 2007; Heidrich et al., 2009; Song et al., 2005; Song et al., 2009; Ward et al., 2008; Ward et al., 2009).

Example of Application of the Representational Approach

In one study using the RA, an advanced practice nurse employed a novel delivery mode in a program referred to as the WRITE Symptoms (a *Written Representational Intervention To Ease Symptoms;* Donovan et al., 2007). This study evaluated the feasibility and acceptability of delivering the intervention to women with recurrent ovarian cancer via a secure Internet messaging service. It compared the changes in symptom representation, symptom interference with life activities, and quality of life in the group whose members received the WRITE Symptom intervention to a group of patients who received usual care. Participants in this study selected several symptoms they wished to address, and the process and content of the intervention session was closely aligned with the seven elements of the RA described earlier in this section (Donovan et al., 2014).

What was novel about this study was that instead of face-to-face sessions or interviews, the research nurse and study participants communicated through postings on private message boards. This approach permitted each study participant, the researcher, and the clinicians caring for the individual to have more time and greater flexibility to communicate with one another in assisting the participant to manage her symptoms. For example, each participant had a secure bulletin board—a special place where she could go to correspond with the clinicians and work on her symptom management. Use of this approach also permitted the clinician to follow the message thread, review the content, and respond with recommendations when time permitted. Also, because the information exchange could be voluminous and complex, it permitted each party time to process the material; the asynchronous messaging allowed the clinicians time to review the participant's specific concerns and respond with an individualized reply.

In summary, the strength of the RA to patient education is that it was derived from Leventhal's CSM and models of conceptual change in a thoughtful and purposeful evolution. Because it links existing theory and specific interventions, and because it relies on a clear theoretical framework, the RA can be applied to an array of clinical problems. Nurses play a key role in the delivery of patient education; this relatively new approach to patient education provides an organized framework with the seven elements providing sound structure. For the nurse researcher, the framework needs further empirical exploration and testing of the seven elements to determine if all seven are essential for successful outcomes (Donovan et al., 2007, 2008, 2014).

CROSS-CUTTING CONCEPTS

The various theories that can be used for health behavior change interventions are not mutually exclusive. Perhaps not surprisingly, they share several constructs, and common issues cut across multiple theories (Glanz & Oldenburg, 2001). It can be challenging to sort out the key issues in various models. This section focuses on important issues and constructs across models.

The Patient's View of the World: Perceptions, Cognitions, Emotions, and Habits

The first key point is that successful health behavior change depends on a sound understanding of the patient's (or consumer's) view of the world (Glanz, 2008). For health professionals who work with patients and provide them with advice on health and lifestyle, adherence to treatment is often disappointingly poor, even in response to relatively simple medical advice. Such poor adherence often arises because patients do not have the necessary behavioral skills to make lifestyle changes or to follow a medication regimen. Following a heart attack, for example, patients might well understand the importance of adopting changes to their lifestyle yet be unable to make those changes. In other circumstances, patients might not understand the importance of such changes and may even believe that these changes pose an additional risk to their health. In still other circumstances, a patient might be experiencing depression or anxiety, such that emotional dysfunction will be a major barrier to compliance.

Traditionally, it has been assumed that the relationship between knowledge, attitudes, and behavior is a simple and direct one. In the past, many prevention and patient education programs have been based on the premise that if people understand and believe in the health consequences of a particular behavior, they will modify it accordingly. Research conducted over the past 30 years has revealed a much different finding, however: The relationships between knowledge, awareness of the need to change, intention to change, and an actual change in behavior are very complex, indeed.

Ideally, each patient should be treated as an individual with unique circumstances and health history. Even so, epidemiological research indicates that certain demographic subgroups differ in terms of risk factors and health behaviors. Understanding these population trends can help prepare a provider to work with various types of patients. For example, younger persons may feel invulnerable to coronary events, and older adults may be managing multiple chronic conditions. An active middle-aged professional may place returning to his previous level of activity above important health protective actions. These examples serve as a reminder that the provider must be sensitive to group patterns, yet avoid stereotyping in the absence of firsthand evidence about an individual. Within this general context, various theories and models can guide the search for effective ways to reach and positively motivate patients.

Behavior Change as a Process

Sustained health behavior change involves multiple actions and adaptations over time. Some people may not be ready to attempt changes, some may be thinking about attempting change, and others may have already begun implementing behavioral modifications. One central issue that has gained wide acceptance is the simple notion that *behavior change is a process, not an event.* The idea that behavior change occurs in a number of steps is not particularly new, but it has gained wider recognition in the past few years. Indeed, various multistage theories of behavior change date back more than 50 years to the work of Lewin, McGuire, Weinstein, Marlatt, and Gordon, and others (Glanz et al., 2015). Put simply, it is important to think of the change process as one that occurs in stages. It is not a question of someone deciding one day to stop smoking and the next day becoming a nonsmoker for life. Most people will not be able to make long-term changes in their health behaviors easily. The average successful quitter has tried multiple times before quitting successfully.

The notion of readiness to change, or stage of change, has been examined in health behavior research and found useful in explaining and predicting a variety of types of behaviors. Prochaska, Velicer, DiClemente, and their colleagues (e.g., 1988) have been leaders in formally identifying the dynamics and structure of change that underlie both self-mediated and clinically facilitated health behavior change. The construct of stages of change described earlier in this chapter is a key element of the transtheoretical model of behavior change; it proposes that people are at different stages of readiness to adopt healthful behaviors (Prochaska et al., 2008).

While the stages of change construct cuts across various circumstances of individuals who need to change or want to change, other theories also address these processes. The remainder of this section looks across various models to illustrate four key concerns in understanding the process of behavior change: (1) motivation versus intention, (2) intention versus action, (3) changing behavior versus maintaining behavior change, and (4) the role of biobehavioral factors.

Motivation Versus Intention

Behavior change is challenging for most people, even if they are highly motivated to change. As noted earlier in this chapter, the relationships between knowledge, awareness of the need to change, intention to change, and an actual change in behavior are very complex. For individuals who are coping with disease and illness, and who are often having to make very significant changes to their lifestyle and other aspects of their lives, this challenge is even greater. According to the transtheoretical model, people in the precontemplation stage are neither motivated nor planning to change, those in the contemplation stage intend to change, and those in the preparation stage are acting on their intentions by taking specific steps toward the action of change (Prochaska et al., 2008). The importance of intentions is emphasized in the TPB (Montano & Kasprzyk, 2008).

Intention Versus Action

The transtheoretical model makes a clear distinction between the contemplation and preparation stages and the stage in which overt action takes place (Prochaska et al., 2008).

A further application of this distinction comes from the TPB (Ajzen, 1991; Montano & Kasprzyk, 2008). Although the TPB proposes that intentions are the best predictor of behaviors, researchers are increasingly focusing attention on implementation intentions as being more proximal and even better predictors of behavior and behavior change (Gollwitzer, 1999).

Changing Behaviors Versus Maintaining Behavior Change

Even when there is good initial compliance with a lifestyle change program, such as quitting smoking or changing diet, relapse is very common. It is widely recognized that many overweight persons are able to lose weight initially, only to regain it within a year. Thus it has become clear to researchers and clinicians that undertaking initial behavior changes and maintaining behavior change require different types of strategies. The transtheoretical model's distinction between the action and maintenance stages implicitly addresses this phenomenon (Prochaska et al., 2015). Long-term maintenance of behavior change requires developing self-management and coping strategies, as well as establishing new behavior patterns that emphasize perceived control, environmental management, and improved self-efficacy. These strategies consist of an eclectic mix drawn from SCT (Bandura, 1986), the TPB (Montano & Kasprzyk, 2015), applied behavioral analysis, and the forerunners of the stages of change model.

Biobehavioral Factors

The behavioral and social theories described thus far have some important limitations, many of which are only now beginning to be understood. Notably, for some health behaviors—especially addictive or addiction-like behaviors—there are other important determinants of behavior, which may be physiological or genetically determined. Among the best known are the addictive effects of nicotine, alcohol, and some drugs. Physiological factors increase psychological cravings and create withdrawal syndromes that may impede even highly motivated persons from changing their behaviors (e.g., quitting smoking or not consuming alcoholic beverages). Some behavior changes—for example, weight loss—also affect energy metabolism and make long-term risk factor reduction an even greater challenge than it would be if it depended on cognitive-behavioral factors alone. Research into the psychobiology of appetite, for instance, offers intriguing possibilities for better understanding biobehavioral models of food intake (Glanz, 2008).

Control Over Behavior and Health: Control Beliefs and Self-Efficacy

Sometimes, control beliefs and self-efficacy hold people back from achieving better health. These deterrents to positive health behavior change are commonplace and can be found in several models of health behavior, including SCT and the TPB. One of the most important challenges for these models—and ultimately for the nurses who apply them—is to enhance perceived behavioral control and increase self-efficacy, thereby improving patients' motivation and persistence in the face of obstacles.

APPLICATIONS IN NURSING AND NURSING RESEARCH

The examples provided throughout this chapter illustrate how nurses use theory to guide their research and also serve as exemplars of theory application. In selecting a theory to guide one's research, it is important to understand how the framework will shape the entire research process and, where applicable, how it will influence intervention design. It is not sufficient to identify a behavioral theory or model to guide one's conceptual background; the theory needs to guide the variables that will be measured and the measurement tools to assess the variables.

Once the data are collected, the theory should help interpret the findings; in other words, the findings should be placed in the context of the theoretical framework. For example, Charron-Prochownik and colleagues (2001) interpreted girls' reported perceptions of risk for reproductive complications and their limited knowledge related to this issue as part of their study. The findings led to the development of an instrument that was true to the theory, and subsequently, an intervention was developed that was consistent with the HBM framework. Thus a theory is not just a statement but rather a thread or theme that is consistently interwoven throughout a study.

As advanced practice nurses use behavioral change theories as part of their research and practice, they will contribute to the greater understanding and refinement of the constructs that compose the theory. For example, the work by Ward and Donovan and their colleagues is refining an adaptation of the illness representation model. In a similar way, other nurse researchers can make valuable contributions to the theoretical basis of their practice though multiple paths of study.

DISCUSSION QUESTIONS

1. Explain the multiple levels of influence that affect patients' health-related behaviors and the implications for using an ecological perspective in developing health education/ promotion programs in outpatient healthcare settings.
2. What are the major differences between *explanatory* theories and *change* theories?
3. The idea of health behavior change as a *process*—not an event—cuts across several behavior change theories. Explain how this idea can be put into action for either adherence with diabetic treatment and self-management regimens or smoking cessation, using constructs from either the stages of change or the TPB.

REFERENCES

Acharya, S. D., Elci, O. U., Sereika, S. M., Styn, M. A., & Burke, L. E. (2011). Using a personal digital assistant for self-monitoring influences diet quality in comparison to a standard paper record among overweight/obese adults. *Journal of the American Dietetic Association, 111*(4), 583–588.

Ajzen, I. (1991). The theory of planned behavior. *Organizational Behavior and Human Decision Processes, 50*(2), 179–211.

Ajzen, I., & Fishbein, M. (1980). *Belief, attitude, intention, and behavior.* Reading, MA: Addison-Wesley.

Ambeba, E. J., Ye, L., Sereika, S. M., Styn, M. A., Acharya, S. D., Sevick, M. A., et al. (2015). The use of mHealth to deliver tailored messages reduces reported energy and fat intake. *Journal of Cardiovascular Nursing, 30*(1), 35–43.

Bandura, A. (1986). *Social foundations of thought and action: A social cognitive theory.* Englewood Cliffs, NJ: Prentice Hall.

Bandura, A. (1997). *Self-efficacy: The exercise of control.* New York, NY: W. H. Freeman.

Bartlett, S. J., Lukk, P., Butz, A., Lampros-Klein, F., & Rand, C. S. (2002). Enhancing medication adherence among inner-city children with asthma: Results from pilot studies. *Journal of Asthma, 39*(1), 47–54.

Berg, J., Dunbar-Jacob, J., & Rohay, J. M. (1995). Assessing inhaler medication adherence using an electronic monitoring device: Revisited. *Annals of Behavioral Medicine, 17*(Suppl.)(S128 (Abstract)).

Berg, J., Dunbar-Jacob, J., & Sereika, S. M. (1997). An evaluation of a self-management program for adults with asthma. *Clinical Nursing Research, 6*(3), 225–238.

Burke, L. E., Conroy, M. B., Sereika, S. M., Elci, O. U., Styn, M. A., Acharya, S. D., et al. (2011). The effect of electronic self-monitoring on weight loss and dietary intake: A randomized behavioral weight loss trial. *Obesity (Silver Spring), 19*(2), 338–344.

Burke, L. E., Dunbar-Jacob, J., Orchard, T. J., & Sereika, S. M. (2005). Improving adherence to a cholesterol-lowering diet: A behavioral intervention study. *Patient Education and Counseling, 57*(1), 134–142.

Burke, L. E., Elci, O. U., Wang, J., Ewing, L. J., Conroy, M. B., Acharya, S. D., & Sereika, S. M. (2009). Self-monitoring in behavioral weight loss treatment: SMART trial short-term results. *Obesity (Silver Spring), 17*(Suppl. 2), 828-P.

Burke, L. E., Ewing, L. J., Ye, L., Styn, M., Zheng, Y., Music, E., et al. (2015). The SELF trial: A self-efficacy-based behavioral intervention trial for weight loss maintenance. *Obesity (Silver Spring), 23*(11), 2175–2182.

Burke, L. E., Styn, M. A., Glanz, K., Ewing, L. J., Elci, O. U., Conroy, M. B., et al. (2009). SMART trial: A randomized clinical trial of self-monitoring in behavioral weight management-design and baseline findings. *Contemporary Clinical Trials, 30*(6), 540–551.

Burke, L. E., Styn, M. A., Sereika, S. M., Conroy, M. B., Ye, L., Glanz, K., et al. (2012). Using mHealth technology to enhance self-monitoring for weight loss: A randomized trial. *American Journal of Preventive Medicine, 43*(1), 20–26.

Burkhart, P. V., Rayens, M. K., Oakley, M. G., Abshire, D. A., & Zhang, M. (2007). Testing an intervention to promote children's adherence to asthma self-management. *Journal of Nursing Scholarship, 39*(2), 133–140.

Burns, A. (1992). The expanded health belief model as a basis for enlightened preventive health care practice and research. *Journal of Health Care Marketing, 12*(3), 32–45

Butler, P., & Mellor, D. (2006). Role of personal factors in women's self-reported weight management behaviour. *Public Health, 120*(5), 383–392.

Butterfield-Booth, S., & Reger, B. (2004). The message changes belief and the rest is theory: The "1% or less" milk campaign and reasoned action. *Preventive Medicine, 39*(3), 581–588.

Cha, E. S., Kim, K. H., & Doswell, W. M. (2007). Influence of the parent–adolescent relationship on condom use among South Korean male college students. *Nursing and Health Sciences, 9*(4), 277–283.

Charron-Prochownik, D., & Downs, J. (2009). *READY-Girls*. Pittsburgh, PA: University of Pittsburgh.

Charron-Prochownik, D., & Downs, J. (2016). *Diabetes and reproductive health for girls*. Alexandria, VA: American Diabetes Association.

Charron-Prochownik, D., Ferons-Hannan, M., Sereika, S., & Becker, D. (2008). Randomized efficacy trial of early preconception counseling for diabetic teens (READY-Girls). *Diabetes Care, 31*(7), 1327–1330.

Charron-Prochownik, D., Hannan, M. F., Sereika, S. M., Becker, D., & Rodgers-Fischl, A. (2006). How to develop CD-ROMs for diabetes education: Exemplar "Reproductive-Health Education and Awareness of Diabetes in Youth for Girls" (READY-Girls). *Diabetes Spectrum, 19*(2), 110–115.

Charron-Prochownik, D., Sereika, S. M., Becker, D., Jacober, S., Mansfield, J., White, N. H., . . . Trail, L. (2001). Reproductive health beliefs and behaviors in teens with diabetes: Application of the expanded health belief model. *Pediatric Diabetes, 2*(1), 30–39.

Charron-Prochownik, D., Sereika, S. M., Becker, D., White, N. H., Schmitt, P., Powell, A. B., 3rd, et al. (2013). Long-term effects of the booster-enhanced READY-Girls preconception counseling program on intentions and behaviors for family planning in teens with diabetes. *Diabetes Care, 36*(12), 3870–3874.

Charron-Prochownik, D., Wang, S. L., Sereika, S. M., Kim, Y., & Janz, N. K. (2006). A theory-based reproductive health and diabetes instrument. *American Journal of Health Behavior, 30*(2), 208–220.

Clark, M. M., Cargill, B. R., Medeiros, M. L., & Pera, V. (1996). Changes in self-efficacy following obesity treatment. *Obesity Research, 4*(2), 179–181.

Clark, M. M., & King, T. K. (2000). Eating self-efficacy and weight cycling: A prospective clinical study. *Eating Behaviors, 1*(1), 47–52.

Conroy, M. B., Yang, K., Elci, O. U., Gabriel, K. P., Styn, M. A., Wang, J., . . . Burke, L. E. (2011). Physical activity self-monitoring and weight loss: 6-month results of the SMART trial. *Medicine and Science in Sports and Exercise, 43*(8), 1568–1574.

Cook, P. F., McCabe, M. M., Emiliozzi, S., & Pointer, L. (2009). Telephone nurse counseling improves HIV medication adherence: An effectiveness study. *Journal of the Association of Nurses in AIDS Care, 20*(4), 316–325.

Dallow, C. B., & Anderson, J. (2003). Using self-efficacy and a transtheoretical model to develop a physical activity intervention for obese women. *American Journal of Health Promotion, 17*(6), 373–381.

DeBusk, R. F., Miller, N. H., Superko, H. R., Dennis, C. A., Thomas, R. J., Lew, H. T., et al. (1994). A case-management system for coronary risk factor modification after acute myocardial infarction. *Annals of Internal Medicine, 120*(9), 721–729.

Desharnais, R., Bouillon, J., & Godin, G. (1986). Self-efficacy and outcome expectations as determinants of exercise adherence. *Psychological Reports, 59*(3), 1155–1159.

Donovan, H. S., & Ward, S. (2001). A representational approach to patient education. *Journal of Nursing Scholarship, 33*(3), 211–216.

Donovan, H. S., Ward, S., Sherwood, P., & Serlin, R. C. (2008). Evaluation of the Symptom Representation Questionnaire (SRQ) for assessing cancer-related symptoms. *Journal of Pain Symptom Management, 35*(3), 242–257.

Donovan, H. S., Ward, S. E., Sereika, S. M., Knapp, J. E., Sherwood, P. R., Bender, C. M., et al. (2014). Web-based symptom management for women with recurrent ovarian cancer: A pilot randomized controlled trial of the WRITE Symptoms intervention. *Journal of Pain Symptom Management, 47*(2), 218–230.

Donovan, H. S., Ward, S. E., Song, M. K., Heidrich, S. M., Gunnarsdottir, S., & Phillips, C. M. (2007). An update on the representational approach to patient education. *Journal of Nursing Scholarship, 39*(3), 259–265.

Ewart, C. K., Stewart, K. J., Gillilan, R. E., Kelemen, M. H., Valenti, S. A., Manley, J. D., & Kelemen, M. D. (1986). Usefulness of self-efficacy in predicting overexertion during programmed exercise in coronary artery disease. *American Journal of Cardiology, 57*(8), 557–561.

Finnell, D. S. (2003). Use of the transtheoretical model for individuals with co-occurring disorders. *Community Mental Health Journal, 39*(1), 3–15.

Finnell, D. S. (2005a). Building a program of research based on the transtheoretical model. *Journal of Addictions Nursing, 16*(1–2), 13–21.

Finnell, D. S. (2005b). Promote medication adherence, one stage at a time. *Current Psychiatry, 4*(8), 88.

Fischl, A. F., Herman, W. H., Sereika, S. M., Hannan, M., Becker, D., Mansfield, M. J., et al. (2010). Impact of a preconception counseling program for teens with type 1 diabetes (READY-Girls) on patient–provider interaction, resource utilization, and cost. *Diabetes Care, 33*(4), 701–705.

Fishbein, M., & Ajzen, I. (1975). *Belief, attitude, intention, and behavior: An introduction to theory and research.* Reading, MA: Addison-Wesley.

Glanz, K. (2008). Current theoretical bases for nutrition intervention and their uses. In A. M. Coulston & C. J. Boushey (Eds.), *Nutrition in the prevention and treatment of disease* (2nd ed., pp. 127–138). Amsterdam, Netherlands: Elsevier.

Glanz, K., & Oldenburg, B. (2001). Utilizing theories and constructs across models of behavior change. In R. Patterson (Ed.), *Changing patient behavior: Improving outcomes in health and disease management* (pp. 25–40). San Francisco, CA: Jossey-Bass.

Glanz, K., & Rimer, B. K. (2005). *Theory at a glance: Application to health promotion and health behavior* (2nd ed.). National Cancer Institute, National Institutes of Health, U.S. Department of Health and Human Services (NIH Pub. No. 05-3896). Washington, DC: National Institutes of Health.

Glanz, K., Rimer, B. K., & Viswanath, K. (2008). *Health behavior and health education: Theory, research, and practice* (4th ed.). San Francisco, CA: Wiley/Jossey-Bass.

Glanz, K., Rimer, B. K., & Viswanath, K. (2015). *Health behavior: Theory, research, and practice* (5th ed.). San Francisco, CA: Wiley/Jossey-Bass.

Golden, S., & Earp, J. A. (2012). Social ecological approaches to individuals and their contexts: Twenty years of Health Education and Behavior interventions. *Health Education and Behavior, 39*(3), 364–372.

Gollwitzer, P. M. (1999). Implementation intentions: Strong effects of simple plans. *American Psychologist, 54*(7), 493–503.

Gwaltney, C. J., Shiffman, S., Norman, G. J., Paty, J. A., Kassel, J. D., Gnys, M., et al. (2001). Does smoking abstinence self-efficacy vary across situations? Identifying context-specificity within the Relapse Situation Efficacy Questionnaire. *Journal of Consulting and Clinical Psychology, 69*(3), 516–527.

Gwaltney, C. J., Shiffman, S., Paty, J. A., Liu, K. S., Kassel, J. D., Gnys, M., & Hickcox, M. (2002). Using self-efficacy judgments to predict characteristics of lapses to smoking. *Journal of Consulting and Clinical Psychology, 70*(5), 1140–1149.

Gwaltney, C. J., Shiffman, S., & Sayette, M. A. (2005). Situational correlates of abstinence self-efficacy. *Journal of Abnormal Psychology, 114*(4), 649–660.

Haskell, W. L., Alderman, E. L., Fair, J. M., Maron, D. J., Mackey, S. F., Superko, H. R., et al. (1994). Effects of intensive multiple risk factor reduction on coronary atherosclerosis and clinical cardiac events in men and women with coronary artery disease. The Stanford Coronary Risk Intervention Project (SCRIP). *Circulation, 89*(3), 975–990.

Heidrich, S. M., Brown, R. L., Egan, J. J., Perez, O. A., Phelan, C. H., Yeom, H., & Ward, S. E. (2009). An individualized representational intervention to improve symptom management (IRIS) in older breast cancer survivors: Three pilot studies. *Oncology Nursing Forum, 36*(3), E133–E143.

Hewson, P. W., & Thorley, N. R. (1989). The conditions of conceptual change in the classroom. *International Journal of Science Education, 11*(5), 541–553.

Hochbaum, G. M. (1958). *Public participation in medical screening programs: A socio-psychological study*. Washington, DC: U.S. Department of Health, Education, and Welfare.

Jorstad, H. T., von Birgelen, C., Alings, A. M., Liem, A., van Dantzig, J. M., Jaarsma, W., et al. (2013). Effect of a nurse-coordinated prevention programme on cardiovascular risk after an acute coronary syndrome: Main results of the RESPONSE randomised trial. *Heart, 99*(19), 1421–1430.

Kelder, S. H., Hoelscher, D., & Perry, D. L. (2015). How individuals, environments and health behaviors interact: Social cognitive theory. In K. Glanz, B. K. Rimer, & V. Viswanath (Eds.), *Health behavior: Theory, research, and practice* (5th ed., pp. 159–181). San Francisco, CA: Jossey-Bass.

Kipnis, D. (1994). Accounting for the use of behavior technologies in social psychology. *American Psychologist, 49*(3), 165–172.

Leventhal, H., Meyer, D., & Nerenz, D. (1980). The common-sense representation of illness danger. In S. Rachman (Ed.), *Medical psychology* (Vol. II, pp. 7–30). New York, NY: Pergamon Press.

Leventhal, H., Nerenz, D., & Steeler, D. (1984). Illness representations and coping with health threats. In A. Baum & J. Singer (Eds.), *Handbook of psychology and health* (Vol. IV, pp. 221–252). New York, NY: Erlbaum.

Matarazzo, J. D., Weiss, C. M., Herd, J. A., Miller, N. E., Weiss, S. M., & Wiley, J. (1984). *Behavioral health: A handbook of health enhancement and disease prevention*. New York, NY: Wiley.

McKenzie, K., & Chang, Y. P. (2015). The effect of nurse-led motivational interviewing on medication adherence in patients with bipolar disorder. *Perspectives in Psychiatric Care, 51*(1), 36–44.

McLeroy, K. R., Bibeau, D., Steckler, A., & Glanz, K. (1988). An ecological perspective on health promotion programs. *Health Education Quarterly, 15*(4), 351–377.

Michie, S., West, R., Campbell, R., Brown, J., & Gainforth, H. (2014). *ABC of theories of behavioural change*. Great Britain: Silverback Publishing.

Montano, D. E., & Kasprzyk, D. (2008). Theory of reasoned action, theory of planned behavior, and the integrated behavioral model. In K. Glanz, B. K. Rimer, & K. Viswanath (Eds.), *Health behavior and health education: Theory, research, and practice* (4th ed., pp. 68–96). San Francisco, CA: Jossey-Bass.

Montano, D. E., & Kasprzyk, D. (2015). Theory of reasoned action, theory of planned behavior, and the integrated behavioral model. In K. Glanz, B. K. Rimer, & V. Viswanath (Eds.), *Health behavior: Theory, research, and practice* (5th ed., pp. 95–124). San Francisco, CA: Jossey-Bass, Inc./Wiley.

Moore, S. M., Dolansky, M. A., Ruland, C. M., Pashkow, F. J., & Blackburn, G. G. (2003). Predictors of women's exercise maintenance after cardiac rehabilitation. *Journal of Cardiopulmonary Rehabilitation, 23*(1), 40–49.

Ockene, J. K., Emmons, K. M., Mermelstein, R. J., Perkins, K. A., Bonollo, D. S., Voorhees, C. C., & Hollis, J. F. (2000). Relapse and maintenance issues for smoking cessation. *Health Psychology, 19*(1 Suppl), 17–31.

Painter, J. E., Borba, C. P., Hynes, M., Mays, D., & Glanz, K. (2008). The use of theory in health behavior research from 2000 to 2005: A systematic review. *Annals of Behavioral Medicine, 35*(3), 358–362.

Pinto, B. M., Clark, M. M., Cruess, D. G., Szymanski, L., & Pera, V. (1999). Changes in self-efficacy and decisional balance for exercise among obese women in a weight management program. *Obesity Research, 7*(3), 288–292.

Posner, G. J., Strike, K. A., Hewson, P. W., & Gertzog, W. A. (1982). Accommodation of a scientific conception: Toward a theory of conceptual change. *Science Education, 66*(2), 211–227.

Powell, B. J., McMillen, J. C., Proctor, E. K., Carpenter, C. R., Griffey, R. T., Bunger, A. C., et al. (2012). A compilation of strategies for implementing clinical innovations in health and mental health. *Medical Care Research and Review, 69*(2), 123–157.

Prochaska, J. O., Redding, C., & Evers, K. (2008). The transtheoretical model of behavior change. In K. Glanz, B. K. Rimer, & K. Viswanath (Eds.), *Health behavior and health education: Theory, research, and practice* (4th ed., pp. 97–121). San Francisco, CA: Jossey-Bass.

Prochaska, J. O., Redding, C. A., & Evers, K. E. (2015). The transtheoretical model and stages of change. In K. Glanz, B. K. Rimer, & V. Viswanath (Eds.), *Health behavior: Theory, research, and practice* (5th ed., pp. 125–148). San Francisco, CA: Jossey-Bass.

Ruppar, T. M., Cooper, P. S., Mehr, D. R., Delgado, J. M., & Dunbar-Jacob, J. M. (2016). Medication adherence interventions improve heart failure mortality and readmission rates: Systematic review and meta-analysis of controlled trials. *Journal of the American Heart Association, 5*(6). doi:10.1161/JAHA.115.002606

Saffi, M. A., Polanczyk, C. A., & Rabelo-Silva, E. R. (2014). Lifestyle interventions reduce cardiovascular risk in patients with coronary artery disease: A randomized clinical trial. *European Journal of Cardiovascular Nursing, 13*(5), 436–443.

Sallis, J. F., & Owen, N. (2015). Ecological models of health behavior. In K. Glanz, B. K. Rimer, & V. Viswanath (Eds.), *Health behavior: Theory, research, and practice* (5th ed., pp. 43–64). San Francisco, CA: Jossey-Bass.

Sevick, M. A., Korytkowski, M., Stone, R. A., Piraino, B., Ren, D., Sereika, S., et al. (2012). Biophysiologic outcomes of the Enhancing Adherence in Type 2 Diabetes (ENHANCE) trial. *Journal of the Academy of Nutrition and Dietetics, 112*(8), 1147–1157.

Sevick, M. A., Stone, R. A., Novak, M., Piraino, B., Snetselaar, L., Marsh, R. M., et al. (2008). A PDA-based dietary self-monitoring intervention to reduce sodium intake in an in-center hemodialysis patient. *Patient Preference and Adherence, 2*, 177–184.

Song, M. K., Kirchhoff, K. T., Douglas, J., Ward, S., & Hammes, B. (2005). A randomized, controlled trial to improve advance care planning among patients undergoing cardiac surgery. *Medical Care, 43*(10), 1049–1053.

Song, M. K., Ward, S. E., Happ, M. B., Piraino, B., Donovan, H. S., Shields, A. M., & Connolly, M. C. (2009). Randomized controlled trial of SPIRIT: An effective approach to preparing African-American dialysis patients and families for end of life. *Research in Nursing and Health, 32*(3), 260–273.

Tabak, R. G., Khoong, E. C., Chambers, D. A., & Brownson, R. C. (2012). Bridging research and practice: Models for dissemination and implementation research. *American Journal of Preventive Medicine, 43*(3), 337–350.

Wang, J., Sereika, S. M., Chasens, E. R., Ewing, L. J., Matthews, J. T., & Burke, L. E. (2012). Effect of adherence to self-monitoring of diet and physical activity on weight loss in a technology-supported behavioral intervention. *Patient Prefer Adherence, 6*, 221–226.

Ward, S. E., Donovan, H., Gunnarsdottir, S., Serlin, R. C., Shapiro, G. R., & Hughes, S. (2008). A randomized trial of a representational intervention to decrease cancer pain (RIDcancerPain). *Health Psychology, 27*(1), 59–67.

Ward, S. E., Serlin, R. C., Donovan, H. S., Ameringer, S. W., Hughes, S., Pe-Romashko, K., & Wang, K. K. (2009). A randomized trial of a representational intervention for cancer pain: Does targeting the dyad make a difference? *Health Psychology, 28*(5), 588–597.

Warnecke, R. B., Morera, O., Turner, L., Mermelstein, R., Johnson, T. P., Parsons, J., et al. (2001). Changes in self-efficacy and readiness for smoking cessation among women with high school or less education. *Journal of Health and Social Behavior, 42*(1), 97–110.

Warziski, M. T., Sereika, S. M., Styn, M. A., Music, E., & Burke, L. E. (2008). Changes in self-efficacy and dietary adherence: The impact on weight loss in the PREFER study. *Journal of Behavioral Medicine, 31*(1), 81–92.

Zheng, Y., Klem, M. L., Sereika, S. M., Danford, C. A., Ewing, L. J., & Burke, L. E. (2015). Self-weighing in weight management: A systematic literature review. *Obesity (Silver Spring), 23*(2), 256–265.

Zheng, Y., Sereika, S. M., Ewing, L. J., Danford, C. A., Terry, M. A., & Burke, L. E. (2015). Association between self-weighing and percent weight change: Mediation effects of adherence to energy intake and expenditure goals. *Journal of the Academy of Nutrition and Dietetics, 116*(4), 660–666.

Chapter 12

Theories Focused on Interpersonal Relationships

Sandra Nelson

INTRODUCTION

In the first two editions of this text, this chapter presented three concepts of interpersonal relations as nursing theory and the related frameworks of nurse theorists:

- *Interpersonal relationship:* Peplau's theory of interpersonal nursing (1952), Orlando Pelletier's nursing process discipline theory (1961), and Travelbee's human-to-human relationship model (1966)
- *Humanism/caring:* Paterson and Zderad's humanistic nursing theory (1976)
- *Existentialism/phenomenology:* Watson's theory of human caring (1979), later known as the theory of transpersonal caring or transpersonal caring science (1999); Newman's theory of health as expanding consciousness (1992); and Parse's man-living-health theory, originally introduced in 1981 and later renamed the theory of "humanbecoming" (1992)

Five non-nursing theories and theorists relating to interpersonal relations were also discussed:

- *Interpersonal relations* (Harry Stack Sullivan)
- *Humanism* (Carl Rogers)
- *Existentialism* (Viktor Frankl and Rollo May)
- *Positive psychology* (Martin Seligman and Mihaly Csikszentmihalyi)
- *Transpersonal psychology* (Anthony Sutich)

Finally, recovery-oriented care (also known as recovery-oriented systems of care) was introduced as a paradigm shift in the nation's approaches to behavioral and mental healthcare systems of care and treatment. This care approach was discussed as an interpersonal relationship concept that needed to find a "home" among other nursing theories or conceptual frameworks and practice specialties.

In this third edition, the preceding theories and frameworks of the identified nurse and non-nurse theorists are presented. Recovery-oriented care and trauma-informed care have emerged to represent paradigm shifts in the nation's behavioral and mental healthcare systems but still await inclusion within nonbehavioral and mental healthcare nursing research and practices. These two conceptual systems are continued in this third edition as proposed interpersonal relationship systems that *should*, again, profoundly influence, if not undergird, nursing research and advanced nursing practice with regard to healthcare systems for women veterans of the military.

Fundamentally, all interpersonal theorists believe that anxiety arises from experiences in relationships with significant others. They emphasize the importance of social forces, or what one does in relation to others, rather than internal or biological factors. Many of these theorists have asserted that adult mental disorders stem from impaired interpersonal relationships during childhood. Because of the dynamics of interpersonal relationships, understanding these concepts enables nurses to form healthy relationships with their clients at various developmental stages and to influence their patients' ability to adapt to environmental stressors (Antai-Otong, 2008, p. 41).

Interpersonal relationship theories and concepts in health care grew primarily from the research of psychiatrist Harry Stack Sullivan (1892–1949) and several other neo-Freudian psychiatrists (e.g., Karen Horney, Erik H. Erikson, Erich Fromm, and Frieda Fromm-Reichmann) who developed a theory of interpersonal relationships, or interactional relations. Sullivan viewed humans as social beings requiring the support and nurture of their environment, and childhood development as being directly influenced by the interpersonal relations found in a person's social and cultural environment. Essentially, all human processes occur in interrelationships; none occur in isolation.

A SIGN OF THE TIMES: 1800S TO 1970S

Nurses writing about nursing between the late 1800s and 1950s addressed all aspects of knowing, perhaps without recognizing it (Chinn & Kramer, 2008, p. 29). Firmly committed to her ideals, Florence Nightingale and subsequent nurse theorists maintained that knowledge developed and used by nursing must be distinct from medical knowledge (Chinn & Kramer, 2008, p. 31). However, throughout most of the first half of the 20th century, the approach to nursing was based largely on medical knowledge. Nurses, taught by physicians, were instructed in what physicians thought they needed to know to carry out the medical regime for the patient. Even the advent of university education did not change the educational approach for nurses as curricula continued to be organized around medical specialty areas (Newman, 1972).

In the 1950s, conceptual frameworks in nursing were based primarily on theories developed from other disciplines. Many of these theories were deemed of value to nursing, but some degree of caution had to be exercised to make certain that the theory used was examined from the perspective of nursing in nursing situations (Walker & Avant, 2004). The shift toward a concept of nursing knowledge as predominantly scientific began in the 1950s and took strong hold in the 1960s (Chinn & Kramer, 2008, p. 45). Throughout the second half of the 20th century, three major trends contributed to evolving directions in the development of nursing knowledge: (1) utilization of theories borrowed from other disciplines, (2) development of conceptual frameworks defining nursing, and (3) development of middle-range theory linked to practice (Chinn & Kramer, 2008, p. 47).

Conceptual frameworks for nursing education and practice proliferated in the 1960s and 1970s. The movement of psychiatric care into community settings, which followed on the heels of the development of new psychotropic medications, contributed to the theoretical focus on the importance of interpersonal communication—a focus notable in the works of Peplau, Orlando, and Travelbee. Writings in the 1960s and 1970s made significant contributions to the development of theoretical thinking in nursing that not only formed the basis for curricula but also guided research and focused practice. The nursing process also replaced the rule- and principle-oriented approaches that were grounded in a medical model in which the nurse functions as the physician's assistant (Alligood & Tomey, 2010, pp. 48–49).

INTERPERSONAL RELATIONS

Hildegard Peplau (1909–1999): The Theory of Interpersonal Nursing

Peplau, one of Sullivan's students and a pioneering psychiatric nurse, developed her theory of interpersonal relations from Sullivan's interpersonal findings. When Peplau's *Interpersonal Relations in Nursing* was published in 1952, nursing was not considered to be a profession, nor was psychiatric nursing (Peplau's chosen specialty practice area) viewed as separate from and independent of medicine and psychiatry (Vandemark, 2006). Indeed, the publication of her book and theory was delayed 4 years because of concern that it was unacceptable for a nurse to publish a book without a physician coauthor (Sills, 1999). In her theory and early writings, Peplau used the term *counseling* to describe the role of the nurse-therapist because the idea of a nurse as therapist was unacceptable (O'Toole & Welt, 1989).

The Interpersonal Relationship Process

Peplau proposed three phases (orientation, working, and resolution) and six nursing roles in the nurse–patient relationship (stranger, resource person, teacher, leader, surrogate, and counselor). Peplau (1952, 1992) carefully explained that "the nurse–patient relationship has a starting point, proceeds through definable phases, and being time-limited, has an end point" (1952, p. 14). In delineating these roles and phases, Peplau described the mechanisms the nurse uses in facilitating the interpersonal process. The original working phase has two subphases: (1) identification and (2) exploitation. Most current publications list four phases: (1) preorientation or preparation, (2) orientation, (3) working, and (4) termination (resolution). Also, *phases* are often referred to as *stages*.

The core concepts of Peplau's theory were the phases of the nurse–client relationship:

1. *Preorientation:* client data-gathering and "autodiagnosis" phase
   - Nurse gathers healthcare and other information about the client.
   - Nurse engages in autodiagnosis (confronts own thoughts and feelings, preconceptions, and attitudes about the particular client or illness/disorder).
2. *Orientation:* problem- or issue-defining phase (Peplau, 1997, pp. 163–164)
   - Introductions are made; nurse and client become acquainted.
   - The pair begin building trust and rapport.
   - Questions are asked and issues clarified.
   - Nurse and client convey needs, expectations, and limitations to each other.
   - Contracting occurs; outcome criteria are established and a plan of care is formulated.
   - Time limits for interactions/visits are clarified and agreed upon.
   - Termination stage outcomes/behaviors are considered.
3. *Working:* major therapeutic activity phase
   - *Identification subphase*
     - Nurse serves as counselor and advocate.
     - Specific problems to be addressed are outlined.
     - Nurse commits to work on specific problems that require immediate attention.
     - Client takes responsibility for behavior and actively works toward change.
   - *Exploitation subphase*
     - Nurse acts as teacher, advocate, resource person, and leader.
     - Client takes on new behaviors and tries them out in safe environment(s).
     - Available resources are identified and put to use.
4. *Resolution:* relationship closure phase (Peplau, 1997, pp. 163–164)
   - Nurse helps prepare client and situation(s) for termination.
   - Nurse and client reduce interaction times; client functions more independently.
   - Nurse and client come to a mutual agreement regarding resolution of issues.
   - Needs are met and resolution of issues summarized.
   - Follow-up instructions are given.
   - Client has health maintenance plan.

Peplau developed tasks associated with the stages of personality development as described by Freud and Sullivan. These tasks, which are outlined in **Table 12-1**, had to be learned to achieve a mature personality.

Table 12-1   Peirau's Stages of Personality Development

Age	Stage	Major Developmental Task
Infancy	Learning to count on others	Learning to communicate in various ways with the primary caregiver in order to have comfort needs fulfilled
Toddlerhood	Learning to delay satisfaction	Learning the satisfaction of pleasing others by delaying self-gratification in small ways
Early childhood	Identifying oneself	Learning appropriate roles and behaviors by acquiring the ability to perceive the expectations of others
Late childhood	Developing skills in participation	Learning the skills to compromise, compete, and cooperate with others; establishing a more realistic view of the world and a feeling of one's place in it

When psychological tasks are successfully learned at each era of development, biological capacities are used productively and relations with people lead to productive living. When not successfully learned, they carry over into adulthood and attempts at learning continue in devious ways, more or less impeded by conventional adaptations that provide a superstructure over the baseline of actual learning (Peplau, 1991, p. 166).

Peplau's theory development was influenced by Sullivan's research and findings related to anxiety, self system, and modes of experiencing (discussed in greater detail later in the chapter). She also drew upon concepts in learning theory and developmental psychology, as well as the ideas of such humanistic psychologists as Carl Rogers, Abraham Maslow, and Rollo May (Gastman, 1998; Peplau, 1952, 1992, 1997).

Peplau's contribution to nursing's history and practice is immeasurable. She was the first nurse to initiate a significant move from an intrapsychic, Freudian emphasis within psychiatric mental health nursing and a dominant focus on physical care within general nursing to an interpersonal focus on both. She was also the first nurse to synthesize nursing theory from other scientific fields, such as Sullivan's theory. Peplau's theory emerged largely from clinical observations, is inductive, and is derived from the phenomenological domain of nursing practice. She regarded the nurse as a professional with "particular expertise" (Fawcett, 2005, p. 531) and sought to have nursing identified as a profession with a unique focus. She differentiated the nursing profession from other healthcare professions—especially physicians.

Peplau was also instrumental in guiding the development of the definition of nursing that was to be permanently represented in nursing's declaration of a social contract with society, the American Nurses Association's (ANA) *Nursing: A Social Policy Statement* (ANA, 1980, 2003).

- "Nursing is the diagnosis and treatment of human responses to actual or potential health problems" (ANA, 1980, p. 4).
- "Nursing is the protection, promotion and optimization of health and abilities, prevention of illness and injury, alleviation of suffering through *the diagnosis and treatment of human response*, and advocacy in the care of individuals, families, communities and populations" (ANA, 2003, p. 5).

In addition, Peplau was the first nurse to suggest the essential relationship between therapeutic use of self and the outcome of patient well-being (Haber, 2000, p. 60). She emphasized the treatment milieu as it affects clients' mental health and nursing's role in milieu therapy. She was instrumental in designing the first *Statement on Psychiatric-Mental Health Nursing Practice* (ANA, 1967) that preceded the development of other specialty area scope of practice statements.

She was a harbinger of the nursing process, as indicated by her statement: "Nursing is a significant, therapeutic interpersonal process. It functions cooperatively with other human processes that make health possible for individuals in communities" (Peplau, 1952, p. 16). She developed a theory that is adaptable to any area of nursing (practice, education, and research) and any nursing specialty area where the end purpose is meeting patients' needs (Perese, 2012).

According to Fawcett (2005, p. 531), Peplau did not devote much attention to the environment but noted the importance of culture on the formation of personality and increasing multi-ethnicity as a contemporary world factor that nurses should include in their information gathering, especially when it is about cultures other than one's own (Peplau, 1997, p. 162).

Sills (2000) celebrated Peplau's "influence in the evolutionary processes of increasing professionalization of nursing in America," crediting her with the fact that "The social policy statement for the first time in nursing's history states the phenomenological focus of nursing" (p. 33).

Peplau on Nursing Education

The central task of the basic professional school of nursing is viewed as the fullest development of the nurse as a person who is aware of how she functions in a situation. (Peplau, 1952, p. xii)

The purpose of Peplau's book on interpersonal relations in nursing was to promote recognition of the importance of the nurse's personality in this context. She stated that "the basic task of nursing education should not be concern for the patient but rather development of each nurse as a person who wants to nurse patients in a helpful way" (p. xii). Thus, the direction for this development is maturity (Vandemark, 2006).

Peplau on Nursing Practice

The nurse–patient relationship is the primary human contact that is central in a fundamental way to providing nursing care. (Peplau, 1997, p. 163)

The one-to-one nurse–client relationship, also known as the therapeutic nurse–client relationship, is the situation in which clients can accomplish developmental tasks such as learning to trust and collaborate, and practicing healthy communication and behaviors. Peplau's teachings are still relevant to practice in understanding and guiding decisions in the one-to-one relationship and individual counseling. In the relationship, the nurse uses theoretical understandings, personal attributes, and appropriate clinical techniques to provide opportunities for a corrective emotional experience for clients (Kneisl & Trigoboff, 2009, p. 775). The goal transcends any particular nursing specialty. Analysis of Peplau's works illuminates a scholarship of nursing practice that remains relevant today (Reed, 1996, p. 29).

Peplau on Nursing Research

Peplau's interpersonal relationship in nursing theory was originally identified as a conceptual framework. Peplau also referred to it as a middle-range theory or a partial theory. She proposed that her theory is useful as an interpersonal process applicable to all nurses' practice (Peplau, 1991, p. 261). McCamant (2006) asked, "Is Peplau's model still relevant today?" (p. 336). In response she insisted, "Peplau's theory was predicated on the recognition that nurses have more actual direct patient contact than any other healthcare professional. . . . The theory occurs precisely in the expected order, despite abbreviated interactive time between nurse and patient" (p. 336). As Kneisl and Trigoboff (2009) comment, "Some say that these phases are ancestors of the nursing process" (p. 25). Peplau's work on nurse–patient relationships is so well known globally that it continues to influence how nursing practice is viewed and evaluated (Johnson & Webber, 2010). Moreover, the interpersonal process is no longer limited to nursing.

Critique of Peplau's theory, similar to critiques of Sullivan's theory, suggests that her theory has not been supported by sufficient empirical investigation and has not yet been tested in terms of its relevance for multidisciplinary, or interprofessional, practice. For the theory to gain credibility within the dynamics of the multidisciplinary team, it must be tested through a robust research design involving various diagnostic groups and practice settings. Until then, the theory's utility remains questionable (Mohr, 2008).

Ida Jean Orlando Pelletier (1926–2007): Nursing Process Discipline Theory

Orlando Pelletier's study grew out of her dissatisfaction with the possibility that nursing care was governed by organizational rules rather than attention to clients' needs and her desire to offer nursing students a theory of effective nursing practice. In her first book, *The Dynamic Nurse Patient Relationship: Function, Process and Principles* (Orlando, 1961), she identified her work as a theory of effective nursing practice; however, in the preface to her 1990 reprint, she wrote:

> If I had been more courageous in 1961, when this book was first written, I would have pro-posed it as "nursing process theory" instead of as a "theory of effective nursing practice." A "deliberative" process was presented as a guide for nurses to practice "effectively." Conversely, an "automatic" process was shown to be "ineffective." "Effectiveness" was conceptualized and illustrated as "improvement" in the patient's behavior. The "improvement" stemmed from the fact that the deliberative process made it possible for the nurse to identify and meet the patient's *need for help.* (p. vii)

In answering questions about the elements of effective care and nursing actions, she conducted a study to evaluate what is good and bad nursing practice. From an analysis of approximately 2,000 recorded nurse–patient interactions, Orlando identified three areas of concern for nursing: (1) nurse–patient relations, (2) the nurse's professional role, and (3) the identity and development of knowledge that is distinctly nursing (Orlando, 1961; Tyra, 2008). She also was able to link effective nursing care to the nurse's knowledge of patient needs that are validated by patient response (Johnson & Webber, 2010). In 1972, Orlando wrote *The Discipline and Teaching of Nursing Process (An Evaluative Study)*, in which she renamed her deliberative nursing process as a nursing process discipline, emphasizing the importance of deliberative nursing actions—a process that assists the nurse to consciously identify and respond to patient needs on the basis of the meanings that are validated between nurse and client (Kneisl & Trigoboff, 2009)—to the need for every student nurse to receive special training in the deliberative nursing process. The purpose of the training "is to change the responsiveness of the nurse from the one described as personal and automatic to one [that] is disciplined and professional" (p. 33).

Orlando then published the final version of her theory, the nursing process discipline theory. According to Johnson and Webber (2010), although Orlando's theory of nursing process discipline resembles the nursing process used in practice, it is not the same. Not only does her theory require more comprehensive interaction and involvement between nurse and patient, but her process is also "reflexive and circular, occurring during encounters with patients, not the linear process taught in nursing education" (Rittman, 2001, p. 12).

Orlando believed that nursing is an interpersonal process involving a nurse's interaction with an ill individual to meet an immediate need. The nursing situation was identified as consisting of (1) the person's behavior, (2) the nurse's reaction, and (3) nursing actions appropriate to the person's need. Essential nursing activities include an automatic nursing process and a deliberative nursing process. The automatic nursing process involves several nursing process activities that are "without discipline" (Orlando Pelletier, 1990, p. vii), meaning that "some automatic activities are ordered by the doctor; others are concerned with routines of caring for patients, and still others are based on principles pertinent to protecting and fostering the health of people in general" (Orlando Pelletier, 1990, p. 60). This nursing process, even if correct, does not meet the patient's need for help.

The deliberative nursing process comprises nursing process activities that are "with discipline" (Orlando Pelletier, 1990, p. vii), meaning nurse-initiated process activities done to ascertain how the patient is affected by what she says or does (Orlando, 1961, p. 67). These activities include instructions, suggestions, directions, explanations, information, requests, and questions directed toward the client; making decisions for the client; and shaping the client's immediate environment. For Orlando Pelletier (1990), only "deliberation is needed to determine whether the activity actually achieves its intended purpose and whether the patient is helped by it" (p. 60).

Fundamentally, Orlando Pelletier believed that nursing is unique and that licensure gives nurses the authority to work independently from medicine. Thus, the nurse is accountable directly to the individual receiving care (Chinn & Kramer, 2008; Johnson & Webber, 2010). According to Schmieding (n.d.),

> Orlando was one of the first to use field methodology to develop her theoretical perspectives long before it was accepted as appropriate. From participant-observer notes, she derived an ingenious conception of the elements and relationships involved as the nurse determines the meaning of the patient's immediate behavior. (p. viii)

Her contribution to nursing practice helped nurses focus on the whole patient rather than on diseases or institutional demands, improved nurses' decision-making skills, provided for more effective resolution of staff and staff–physician conflicts, and promoted a more positive nursing identity and unity (Tyra, 2008). Her ideas continue to be useful today, and current research supports her model (Boyd, 2008; Potter & Bockenhauer, 2000).

Joyce Travelbee (1926–1973): The Human-to-Human Relationship Model

While Peplau drew upon the works of neo-Freudian psychiatrists, Travelbee credited discussions with existential psychologists and philosophers such as Viktor Frankl and Rollo May as significantly influencing her thinking and allowing her to bring an existential perspective to nursing (Meleis, 2007).

As a result of psychiatric nursing experiences in a Catholic charity hospital, Travelbee came to believe that the care given in these types of institutions lacked compassion. She argued that nursing needed a "humanistic revolution" and a renewed focus on caring as central to nursing. It was her belief that unless nurses became more aware of the value of caring as the basic goal of the nursing profession, consumers of nursing would demand the services of a new and different kind of healthcare worker (Moses, 1994; Travelbee, 1966).

She proposed that nursing's caring goal was to assist an individual, family, or community to prevent or cope with the experiences of illness and suffering and, if necessary, find meaning in these experiences, with the ultimate goal being the presence of hope (Travelbee, 1966, 1971). The concept of hope was defined as "a mental state characterized by the desire to gain an end or accomplish a goal combined with some degree of expectation that what is desired or sought is attainable" (Travelbee, 1971, p. 77). Her original conceptualization of hope was directed toward clients with psychiatric illness, but she later expanded her concept to long-term physical illnesses.

Travelbee (1969) described understanding as acknowledging the uniqueness of the ill person. She contended that understanding was "a force which can provide the ill person with the necessary endurance and courage to face the inevitable problems which lie before him" (p. 81). Focusing her attention on individuals who must learn to live with chronic illness, she believed that the nurse's spiritual values and philosophical beliefs about suffering would determine the extent to which the nurse could help ill people find meaning in these situations (Boyd, 2008).

Similar to Peplau and Orlando, Travelbee (1966, 1971) emphasized the importance of communication in the phases of the nurse–client relationship and described the instrument for delivery of the process of one-to-one nursing as the therapeutic use of self. However, as Travelbee focused on the *meaning* in nurse–client interactions, "her unique synthesis of their ideas differentiated her work from theirs in terms of the therapeutic human-to-human relationship between nurse and patient" (Alligood & Tomey, 2010, p. 61; Kneisl & Trigoboff, 2009). She insisted that nursing is defined and accomplished through the relatedness found in the human-to-human relationship and successfully working through the phases of initial encounter, emerging identity, empathy, sympathy, and rapport (Moses, 1994, p. 200).

Travelbee's Phases of the Nurse–Client Relationship

Travelbee described the nurse–client relationship in terms of the following phases:

- *Original encounter:* Emotional knowledge colors the impressions and perceptions of both nurse and patient during initial encounters. The task is to "break the bond of categorization in order to perceive the human being in the patient and vice versa" (Travelbee, 1966, p. 133).
- *Emerging identities:* Both nurse and patient begin to transcend their respective roles and perceive uniqueness in each other. Tasks include separating oneself and one's

experiences from others and avoiding "using oneself as a yardstick" by which to evaluate others. Barriers to such tasks may be caused by role envy, lack of interest in others, inability to transcend the self, or refusal to initiate emotional investment (Travelbee, 1966, p. 139).

- *Developing feelings of empathy:* Empathy means sharing another's psychological state but standing apart and not sharing another's feelings; it is characterized by "the ability to predict the behavior of another." When empathizing, the warmth and urge to action are not present (Travelbee, 1966, p. 143).

- *Developing feelings of sympathy:* This means sharing, feeling, and experiencing what others are feeling and experiencing. This phase demonstrates emotional involvement and discredits objectivity as dehumanizing. The task of the nurse is to translate sympathy into helpful nursing actions (Travelbee, 1964, p. 70.) Sympathy "implies a desire, almost an urge to help or aid an individual in order to relieve his distress" (Rich, 2003, p. 202; Travelbee, 1964, p. 68).

- *Rapport:* All previous phases culminate in rapport, defined as all those experiences, thoughts, feelings, and attitudes that both the nurse and the client undergo and are able to perceive, share, and communicate (Travelbee, 1964, 1966, pp. 133–162).

The Empathy Versus Sympathy Disagreement

Travelbee believed that it was as important for the nurse to sympathize as it was to empathize if the nurse and patient were to develop a human-to-human relationship. In 1964, Travelbee, in an article titled "What's Wrong With Sympathy?," expressed dismay that nursing, as a profession, was losing its value of sympathy and compassion in response to comments by nurses that "they were too busy to be sympathetic" (p. 68).

According to Rich (2003), Travelbee believed that nursing students should be encouraged to experience sympathy when caring for patients; sympathy and compassion are at the heart of nursing. Sympathy, to Travelbee, involves an act of courage on the part of the nurse because he or she is risking pain (p. 203). Travelbee outlined several dangers of sympathy that nurses are cautioned about: becoming too soft-hearted, overidentifying with patients, developing a distorted sense of pity, causing harm to the patient, or having their will become paralyzed (Rich, 2003).

Of current interest is the continuing acceptance of empathy as a teachable skill and crucial helping component in therapeutic nurse–patient interactions and the "demise" of sympathy as influential (Ancel, 2006; Reynolds & Scott, 1999). While there are a number of definitions of empathy and approaches to implementation, the most commonly cited and used, even among nurses, is drawn from the works of the humanistic psychologist Carl Rogers (discussed later; Reynolds & Scott, 2000); there is little reference to Travelbee's theory, her phases of the nurse–client relationship, or sympathy as a critical component in interpersonal relationships. Rich (2003), revisited Travelbee's question and wrote,

> In an age of technology, where many people feel the impact of individual isolation and existential aloneness, it is worth revisiting Travelbee's reasons why nurses may avoid feelings of sympathy. A focus on compassion may be a similar and acceptable alternative. (p. 202)

With regard to updating Travelbee's perspective on compassion, Rich stated, "We may find the Eastern philosophy idea of compassion may be more acceptable to the nursing profession" (p. 203).

Unfortunately, Travelbee's model was never subjected to empirical testing, and, because her investigations were based on direct observations, interviews, and documented analysis, it is not possible to summarize the wealth of her empirical findings. Nonetheless, her reports presented clear descriptive statements that illustrated her human-to-human theory (Moses, 1994). Her use of the interpersonal process in nursing intervention and her focus on suffering and illness helped to define areas of concern for psychiatric mental health nurses (Kneisl & Trigoboff, 2009, p. 38). She is also credited with greatly influencing the hospice movement and being far ahead of her time when, in 1949, she called for natural childbirth, prenatal instruction, father participation in birth process, and rooming-in. While her view of humanity, uniqueness, existential encounters, and nursing is highly congruent with values in psychiatric-mental health nursing, Travelbee (1969) believed that the human-to-human relationship process is central to all nursing.

A SIGN OF THE TIMES: 1970S TO THE PRESENT

In the 1970s and 1980s, there was a noticeable shift to themes and patterns that characterize the essence of caring in nursing practice. Frameworks changed from reflecting functional nursing roles to unfolding the essence of what nursing is. The common, significant thread is the primacy of human interaction in creating human health and wholeness (Chinn & Kramer, 2008, pp. 52–55).

Nursing frameworks began to be influenced by nurse scientists who benefited from early funding of doctoral education and received training in anthropology and sociology. This education is reflected in the works of Rogers, Parse, and Newman, whose theoretical perspectives are linked to developments in modern physics that moved beyond earlier system concepts of equilibrium (Chinn & Kramer, 2008, p. 49). The progression of nursing research and theory development has been influenced by two philosophies: *modernism* and *postmodernism*. As Johnson and Webber (2010) articulate, "Put simply, whereas the focus in modernism was on proving theory, the focus of postmodernism was on the development of new theory through the discovery of meaning without empirical evidence" (p. 239). Of particular significance, the postmodern view represents an epistemological shift in nursing theory development to include the modernistic search for the truth and validity of empirical findings but also the exploration of phenomenological findings unique to human beings and their experiences (Johnson & Webber, 2010, pp. 239–240).

HUMANISM/CARING

Josephine Paterson (1924–Present) and Loretta Zderad (1925–Present): Humanistic Nursing Theory (1976)

Out of necessity nursing, as a profession, reflects the qualities of the culture in which it exists. In our culture for the past quarter of a century nursing has been assailed with rapid economic, technological, shortage-abundance, changing scenes' vicissitudes. In the individual nurse these arouse turmoil and uncertainty. These cultural stirrings inflame that part of the nurse's spirit capable of chaotic conflict and doubt. Often she questions her professional identity. "Just what is a nurse?" Her nurse colleagues, other professionals, and nonprofessionals freely, directly and indirectly on television, in the theater, through the news media and the literature, pummel her with their multitudinous varied views. As searching, wondering, reflecting, relating microcosms within this perplexing health nursing world for longer than a quarter of a century, we present this book. Descriptively we view the chapters as hard-wrung, philosophical foundations, synthesized extracts from our lived experiences. (Paterson & Zderad, 1976, p. ix)

In 1960, Paterson and Zderad were not impressed with the objective nature of empirical science that represented human beings as predictable objects. They believed that understanding how people experience their existence could facilitate their nursing work. The humanistic approach has its roots in existentialist thought, and both philosophies (humanism and existentialism) assert a broad view of human beings and their potential. Thus they selected humanistic-existential philosophy to inform their developing theory.

In 1976, Paterson and Zderad proposed that nurses consciously and deliberately approach nursing as an existential experience. They suggested that the science of nursing would be built over time by compilation and complementary synthesis of phenomenological descriptions of experiences in the nursing situation. They spoke of humanistic nursing as a framework that recognizes the uniqueness of each human being and "a quality of being that is expressed in the doing" (Paterson & Zderad, 1978, p. 13).

The term *humanistic nursing* was selected thoughtfully to designate the theoretical pursuit to reaffirm and floodlight this responsible characteristic as fundamentally inherent to all artful-scientific nursing. Humanistic nursing embraces more than a benevolent technically competent subject–object one-way relationship guided by a nurse on behalf of another. Rather, it dictates that nursing is a responsible searching, transactional relationship whose meaningfulness demands conceptualization founded in a nurse's existential awareness of self and of the other. As Paterson and Zderad (1988) stated, "Nursing is an experience lived between human beings" (p. 3). Humanistic nursing, then, is neither a break with nor a repetition of nursing's past. It is neither a rejection of nor a satisfaction with nursing's present state. Rather it is an awakening to the possibilities of shaping our nursing world here and now and for the future (Paterson & Zderad, 1976, preface).

Within the construct of humanistic theory, the act of nursing is understood in terms of both the nurse and the patient—often experienced and described as a "call and response" relationship (Decker-Brown, 2003, para. 14). The client calls for nursing care with an expectation that care will be provided or an unmet need will be satisfied. The nurse responds with the intention of providing the care or satisfying the unmet need. The nurse is concerned with the client's unique expression of the body related to its position in time and space (Paterson & Zderad, 1988, p. 29). Authentic presence is expressed when the nurse goes beyond being an object within the perceptual field of the client.

The goal of humanistic nursing is not attainment of mere health or *well-being*, but rather attainment of a state of dynamic *more-being* (Praeger & Hogarth, 1985). The object is for the nurse to assist the client to become *more*, to realize a potential not yet attained in the present moment of their interaction. Health is conceptualized as a process of becoming whatever is possible for the human being. Nursing phenomena are those things that nurses think are important and to which they must pay close attention; they are experienced as nurturing, being nurtured, or the process between these two reference points. While humanistic nursing focuses on the intersubjectivity experience, the most important activity for the nurse to engage in may be the use of self, or presence, with the client (Frisch & Frisch, 2011). Paterson and Zderad (1988) outlined 12 behaviors for providing comfort to a client. (See **Box 12-1**.)

According to Kneisl and Trigoboff (2009), Paterson and Zderad (1976, 1988) were a decade ahead of their time in rejecting a mechanistic cause and effect view of nursing science and urging instead that observations of the experiences of nurses in practice should be the basis of any useful nursing theory. Theirs is a highly abstract theory with a major focus on the process of interaction or dialogue between nurse and client (Kneisl & Trigoboff, 2009, p. 26).

EXISTENTIALISM

Jean Watson (1940–Present): Theory of Human Caring

Watson wrote *Nursing: Philosophy and Science of Caring* in 1979. In 1996, Watson stated that she had continued to refine her original theory "until this moment in history" (p. 141). It is clear that, over a decade later, she is still refining her theory. In exploring the progression of "refining" over the years, a relationship in her theory and publications can be traced to many of her revealed personal life situations. Her classic work is in the process of being updated.

Box 12-1   Twelve Humanistic Nursing Behaviors for Providing Comfort

1. The nurse introduces herself to the client by name, which supports the client's dignity, worth, and individual identity and is essential for an authentic subject–subject relationship.
2. The nurse provides information about the client's situation as the client seeks it or when the nurse perceives the client is puzzled about what is happening. The nurse's action is based on the existential belief that the client has the right to know and make choices about his own life, and such choices are shaped by honest information.
3. The nurse accepts the client's expression of feelings by verbalizing this acceptance when appropriate. This validates clients' right to feelings and can help them learn appropriate ways to express feelings.
4. The nurse accepts the client's expression of feeling by staying with him or doing something for the client when a verbal expression of acceptance by the nurse is not appropriate. The message conveyed is that the patient's feelings are valid but a better method of expressing the feeling is socially desirable. By remaining with the client, the nurse validates the feeling and may model a more appropriate behavioral expression.
5. The nurse expresses authentic positive feelings for the client when appropriate. The purpose of this action is to refute negative self-concepts that the client may hold.
6. The nurse supports the client's rights to have loving relationships with family members, staff, and other clients.
7. The nurse shows respect for clients as persons who have rights to make choices as their capabilities permit.
8. The nurse helps clients consider current expression of feelings and behaviors in the light of previous life experiences. This behavior enables clients to formulate self-understanding by recognition of patterns that may be helpful or unhelpful to their healing.
9. The nurse encourages clients to express themselves openly so that the nurse can respond in a helpful and therapeutic manner.
10. The nurse verifies the intuitive grasp of how the client experiences events by asking questions and making comments to the client, and then observing the client's response.
11. The nurse encourages realistic (not false) hope through discussing the positive outcomes that might occur if the client were to engage in a therapeutic opportunity.
12. The nurse supports the client's self-image with concrete examples.

Modified with permission of the National League for Nursing, Washington DC, from Paterson, J. G., & Zderad, L. T. (1988). *Humanistic nursing.* New York, NY: National League for Nursing.

Watson credited Jungian psychology, feminist theory, and Maslow's psychological concept of self-actualization as influencing her early theory development. Carl Rogers received credit for much of her thinking on therapeutic relationships and communication through his work in identifying congruency, empathy, and warmth as foundational to a caring relationship that conveys authenticity and genuineness and facilitates the client's expression of emotions. More recently, Watson acknowledged drawing heavily on the sciences, humanities, Buddhism, and Eastern philosophies that provide a phenomenological-existential and spiritual orientation to theory development (Watson, 1995, 1999, 2005). Influential nurse theorists were Peplau, Henderson, Leininger, Rogers, Newman, and, especially, Nightingale (Watson, 1985, 1997, 2005).

Watson (1996) claimed that her theory of human caring is metaphysical, explaining that "it goes beyond the rapidly emerging existential-phenomenological approaches in nursing, to perhaps a higher level of abstraction and sense of personhood incorporating the concept of the soul and transcendence" (p. 141). Clearly, the life events of the theorists discussed in this chapter have been influential in outlining and clarifying their various philosophical or conceptual approaches; Watson's personal journey in particular has been a significant influence on the development and directions of her theory. She indicated that the building blocks of her theory and concepts were "derived from clinically inducted, empirical experiences, combined with my philosophical, intellectual and experiential background; thus, my earlier work emerged from my own values, beliefs, and perceptions about personhood, life, health, and healing" (Watson, 1997, p. 49). Initially Watson (1979, 1988) differentiated nursing and medicine by stating that *curing* is the domain of medicine, and *caring* is the domain of nursing. From her original discussion of holistic human caring, her thoughts have evolved to a model of the transpersonal caring relationship (Watson, 1999, 2002, 2005).

Watson (1996) indicated that the transpersonal caring relationship depends on a moral commitment to human dignity, wholeness, caring, and healing. It also depends on the nurse's (1) orientation to affirming the significance of the person; (2) ability to realize, detect, and connect with the spirit of another; (3) ability to realize the other's state of being in the world and to feel a union with that other; and (4) caring, healing modalities to potentiate comfort, wholeness, and harmony, including promoting inner healing and own life history and ability to care for self.

Caring-healing within her theory is based on kindness, concern, love of self and others, and the ecology of the earth and involves what she terms *carative* factors: a humanistic-altruistic value system, faith-hope, and sensitivity to self and others (Watson, 1999). Her theory emphasizes sensitivity to self and values clarification regarding personal and cultural beliefs that might pose barriers to transpersonal caring. Establishing a helping and trusting human care relationship is pivotal to her theory. In 2003, Watson expanded self-care to include the ability to forgive self and others, to be grateful for life and its blessings, and to surrender and let go of ego, accepting experiences without seeking control.

In her recent work, Watson (2005) developed the notion of spiritual environment and the interconnectedness of all things, including the connection between natural healing approaches, self-knowledge, self-control, self-caring, self-healing potential, and caring, healing relationships with self and others. Her theory is philosophically congruent with contemporary global approaches to health and health promotion (Falk-Rafael, 2000; Pilkington, 2007).

While Watson's emphasis on caring is not unique, the strength of her emphasis on the embodied spirit is. She set a very high standard for nurses to follow and has brought a number of important concepts into her theoretical work. Her curative approach is deeply aligned with spiritual as well as existential and phenomenological philosophical concepts and subjects more abstract than many nurses wish to pursue. However, Watson's theory continues to evolve and to attract the attention of many, as nurses are drawn to the holistic and spiritual nature of the theory (Kneisl & Trigoboff, 2009, p. 26).

According to Boyd (2008),

> Watson's theory is especially applicable to the care of those who seek help for mental illness. This model emphasizes the importance of sensitivity to self and others, the development of helping and trusting relations, the promotion of interpersonal teaching and learning, and provision for a supportive, protective and corrective mental, physical, sociocultural and spiritual environment. (p. 71)

Frisch and Frisch (2011), however, cautioned,

> Despite the strong therapeutic potential of nursing intervention based on caring, the withdrawn, angry, suspicious, and depressed person may be very slow to enter into this kind of mutuality. The nurse. . . . must be willing to persevere, to consult with colleagues and mentors,. . . . to carefully examine her own feelings and responses, and. . . . consider a switch in theory and approach. (p. 309)

The basic premises of transpersonal caring are outlined here:

1. Being human is about more than a physical body. It includes an embodied spirit; a consciousness that supports sharing between and beyond persons; a unity of mind, body, and spirit, expressed as *mindbodyspirit*; and a connected oneness of the person, nature, and the universe.
2. There is a human–environment energy field that includes caring-healing consciousness.
3. Consciousness is energy; forgiveness and surrender are the highest level of consciousness.
4. Modalities that arise from caring-healing involve the mind, the hands, the heart, and the soul.
5. The process and relationships linking caring-healing are sacred, and the nurse can provide a sacred healing environment.
6. Viewing the connectedness of all (subject, object, environment, person, and all living things) is unitary consciousness; unbroken wholeness is the ultimate form of healing, and transcendence is love (Frisch & Frisch, 2011, p. 32).

Watson adapted her 10 carative factors from Yalom's 11 curative factors. She later enhanced the factors to include clinical caritas processes that offered ways in which the 10 factors could be implemented in the clinical setting. *Caritas* is a Latin word meaning to "cherish, appreciate, or, give special attention to" (Alligood & Tomey, 2010, p. 97).

Margaret Newman (1933–Present): Theory of Health as Expanding Consciousness

Every person in every situation, no matter how disorganized and hopeless it may seem, is part of the universal process of expanding consciousness. (Newman, 1992, p. 45)

Newman began developing her theory of expanding consciousness as a result of caring for her mother throughout a long period of illness. During this period and years of learning in undergraduate and graduate school, she came to realize that "long term illness can be dealt with if a person's consciousness is expanding"—essentially gaining a deeper appreciation for life and having more meaningful relationships (Newman, 1992, p. 45). In 1994, Newman wrote,

> Basic among these learnings was that illness reflected the life pattern of the person. And that what was needed was the recognition of the pattern and acceptance of it for what it meant to that person. Years later I came to the conclusion that health is the expansion of consciousness. It frightens me to think that I might have missed that revelation, it is so important to me now. But even my fear is unwarranted because the gist of all that I am saying is that one can trust the evolving pattern, that it is a pattern of evolving, expanding consciousness *regardless* of what form or direction it may take. This realization is such that illness and disease have lost their demoralizing power. (p. xxiii)

Newman's (1990) major theoretical concepts are health, patterns and pattern recognition, consciousness, expanding consciousness, and movement–space–time. As she stated, "Patterning of persons in interaction with the environment is basic to my view that consciousness is a manifestation of an evolving pattern of person-environment interaction" (p. 38). Newman's theory is derived from Martha Rogers's (1970) life process model, now known as the science of unitary human beings (1994): "Rogers's insistence that health and illness are simply manifestations of rhythmic fluctuations of the life process led me to view health and illness as a unitary process moving through variations of order-disorder" (Newman, 1990, p. 38).

Newman (1994) realized that her theory was "a radical departure from traditional concepts of health" and that "the essence of the theory required a 180-degree turn in thinking about health" (p. xv). In her theory, health is a synthesis of the fusion of disease and nondisease—being well and being ill. Disease and nondisease are each reflections of a larger wholeness that takes on a new and different form that is not diminished by illness and thus creates a new concept of health. Health and the evolving pattern of consciousness are the same and viewed as "a transformative process to more inclusive consciousness" (Newman, 2008, p. 16).

Newman (2008) specified five major assumptions (stated in part here):

1. Health encompasses conditions heretofore described as illness or, in medical terms, pathology.
2. These pathological conditions can be considered a manifestation of the total pattern of the individual.

3. The pattern of the individual that eventually manifests itself as pathology is primary and exists before structural or functional changes.
4. Removal of the pathology in itself will not change the pattern of the individual.
5. If becoming "ill" is the only way an individual's pattern can manifest itself, then that is health for that person.

In Newman's view, the focus of nursing is on the nurse–client relationship. Clients get in touch with the meaning of their lives through identification of meanings in the process of their evolving patterns of relating. Newman (2008) stated, "The emphasis of the process is on knowing/caring through pattern recognition" (p. 10). The nurse facilitates pattern recognition by forming relationships with clients at critical points in their lives and connecting with them in authentic ways. In an expansive discussion, Newman (2008) asserted the following:

> In nursing, the emphasis is on relationship: relationships within the client's life and between the nurse and client as being integral to nursing. A relationship may be symmetrical, complementary, or asymmetrical. A *symmetrical* relationship is one in which the action of one part escalates the action of the other, as in competition. *Complementary* relationships tend to move toward equilibrium: the action of one balances the action of another. . . . An *asymmetrical* relationship is one of growth, evolvement, and transcendence. Movement of a symmetrical or complementary relationship to an asymmetrical one requires additional information and new insight, an expansion of consciousness. (p. xv)

According to Newman, pattern recognition is the essence of practice and the task of intervention. She explained in 1994, "The more expanded the consciousness of the nurses, the more readily they [are] able to enter into a transformative relationship with clients" (p. 18). Expanding consciousness is described as insight and the recognition of patterns. Newman suggested that nurses will be transformed by nursing theory and, thereby, will become transforming partners with clients (Vandemark, 2006, p. 606).

For Newman, research is praxis or practice. In 2003, she wrote, "Nursing praxis integrates theory, research, and practice. It is art, science and practice" (p. 242). Theory, practice, and research are viewed as a process rather than as separate nursing domains. Newman called for a specific curriculum and focus of education for nurses using the theory. The new curriculum must reflect the shift in worldview from the traditional views of health and illness to the transformative expectation of pattern recognition. As Newman (2008) explained, "Attention to the nature of transformative learning will help to establish the priorities of the discipline" (p. 73). Newman espoused the professional doctorate degree as a requirement for professional practice, one that "requires a strong arts and sciences background as pre-professional education. . . . and brings students with added personal maturity" (p. 127).

Vandemark (2006) cautioned that for advanced practice (psychiatric) nurses providing psychotherapy to clients, the need for self-awareness is more acute and more specific to their practice. The development of insight and self-awareness vis-à-vis the practice of psychotherapy is a significant responsibility for professional schools of nursing to leave to the individual nurse. Although the role of the psychiatric advanced practice nurse includes individual and family therapy, many existing psychiatric nurse practitioner programs have no courses or practicum experiences in patient-centered psychotherapy (Wheeler & Haber, 2004). While psychiatric clinical nurse specialist programs often do include course work in individual and group or family therapy and accompanying clinical supervision, this mentorship is, as Peplau counseled, focused on the content of the nurse's interaction with the patient, not the interpersonal dynamics of the nurse.

Rosemarie Rizzo Parse (Year of Birth Unknown–Present): Humanbecoming Theory

Parse's theory of "humanbecoming" (1992) was originally introduced as the man-living-health theory (1981). Parse developed her theory of humanbecoming with tenets from existential-phenomenological philosophers, primarily Heidegger, Sartre, and Merleau-Ponty (Parse, 1981, 1998) and the work of Martha Rogers (1970). Although Parse initially labeled her work a theory, in 1998, to extend Rogers's work and add greater density to the philosophical underpinning, she changed her label from a theory to a *school of thought*. Although it is "consistent with Rogers' principles and postulates about unitary human beings and it is consistent with major tenets and concepts from existential-phenomenological thought, it is a new product, a different conceptual system" (Parse, 1998, p. 135).

The theory was originally guided by three principles incorporating the central ideas of meaning, rhythmicity, and transcendence (Parse, 1981, 1995, 1998). Recently, and within the context of rapidly changing technological developments and cost efficiencies in health care, she has further emphasized the idea of indivisible co-creation by joining the word "human" and "becoming" to form the term *humanbecoming* (Parse, 2007). The wording of the three principles has changed slightly for clarification, but the meanings remain unchanged. The three principles are (1) structuring meaning, (2) configuring rhythmical patterns of relating, and (3) co-transcending with possibles (Parse, 2007). Underlying the three principles are the postulates of illimitability—"indivisible unbounded knowing extended to infinity" (Parse, 2007, p. 308); paradox—"lived rhythms" (p. 308); freedom—"contextually construed liberation"; and mystery—"the unexplainable" (p. 308).

Parse's (1998) first set of nine assumptions about humans and becoming were later synthesized into three assumptions related to humanbecoming (2007):

1. *Humanbecoming* is freely choosing personal meaning with situation, intersubjectively living value priorities.
2. *Humanbecoming* is configuring rhythmical patterns of relating with *humanuniverse*.
3. *Humanbecoming* is co-transcending illimitably with emerging possibilities.

Although Parse did not include nursing in her metaparadigm, she challenged the traditional medical view of nursing and has distinguished the discipline of nursing as a unique, basic science focused on human lived experience. Nursing's goal consists of being with or in the presence of mutual nurse–client processes to understand and value the meaning of the client's lived experience and assimilate preferences and beliefs that influence healthcare choices and preference (Parse, 1998). The nurse also uses a nonjudgmental approach and reveres the client's expertise in knowing what is best for him or her within the nurse–client relationship. The nurse uses her true presence with the client to establish mutual processes and ensure shared decision making with the client to assess behavior, identify treatment choices, develop a client-centered treatment plan, and observe changing health patterns. Exhibiting true presence by the nurse involves mindfulness to the client.

Parse views health as inseparable and irreducible from both human and universe. Health is humanbecoming. It is structuring meaning, configuring rhythmical patterns of relating, and co-transcending with possibles (Parse, 2007). Humans are intentional beings and by nature live a seamless symphony throughout the life span. People are involved with the universe in directing their personal becoming through relationships with others. Individuals live in the moment within the presence of mutual processes with the universe structures that are multidimensional. Mutual processes enable persons to manage their lives and health through the freedom and right to make choices and live their lives as they choose (Parse, 1998, 2002). Environment includes the universe and mutual processes. Humans are in mutual process with the universe structure or with others who are with the individual.

Quality of Life Versus Health

Quality of life is explicit in Parse's theory (1994). Quality of life is "the indivisible human's view on living moment to moment as the changing patterns of shifting perspectives weave the fabric of life through the human-universe interconnectedness" (p. 17). It is a subjective, global perception of the meaning of one's lived experiences in the moment. It fluctuates moment to moment in co-creation with the universe (Parse, 1994). Parse has used words such as *shifting*, *changing*, and *in-the-moment* in reference to quality of life. The personal nuances of the nurse–person process enhance quality of life (Parse, 1994).

The concept has been well-developed through extensive research. Parse and colleagues have explicitly described quality of life to inform understanding as it is constituted in different contexts. Understanding promotes nurses' ability to be with people in ways that honor their lived experiences. Parse's contribution to quality of life has pragmatic utility for the discipline of nursing because it articulates the goal of nursing practice.

Fawcett (2005) explained that the term *metaparadigm* is the result of Masterman pointing out that Kuhn's use of the term *paradigm* had multiple meanings and that "one reflected a metaphysical rather than scientific notion or entity" (p. 4). According to Fawcett (2005),

"The metaparadigm is the most abstract set of central concepts for the discipline of nursing (i.e., human beings, environment, health and nursing)" (p. 4). In relating contemporary practice needs to nursing's current metaparadigm, Phillips (1995) stated the following:

> A clear definition of quality of life is important to nursing knowledge development because it guides the art of practice. Defining quality of life from a holistic perspective is also important to nursing because it reflects contemporary practice and it helps nurses to understand the inherent indivisibility of life and its qualities. (pp. 100–101)

Plummer and Molzahn (2009) conducted a critical review and comparison of the concept, quality of life, as it is conceptualized in the contemporary nursing theories of Peplau, Rogers, Leininger, King, and Parse. The goal of the study was twofold: (1) to enhance clarity of the concept from a nursing perspective and (2) to assess the usefulness of the concept to nursing science. Each theoretical "perspective was compared to the others in order to identify commonalities, similar themes, and differences" (p. 135). According to Plummer and Molzahn (2009), the findings "contributed to the understanding of the interconnectedness of the person, relationships, and environment with quality of life" (p. 140). Thus, Plummer and Molzahn (2009) summarized, "Given the breadth of nursing practice and the value of the concept for nursing . . . it is appropriate to consider replacing health as a metaparadigm concept with quality of life" (p. 140).

NON-NURSING THEORIES FOCUSED ON INTERPERSONAL RELATIONSHIPS

Interpersonal Relations Theory

Interpersonal philosophy defines personality as behavior that can be observed within interpersonal relationships. Interpersonal theorists emphasize the socialization of humans throughout their developmental stages. Failure to proceed through these stages satisfactorily lays the foundation for later maladaptive behavior. Supporters believe that unsatisfactory interpersonal relations are the primary cause of maladaptive behaviors. The interpersonal perspective also is concerned with the anxiety-arousing aspects of interpersonal relationships. At present, no systemic view of human nature and behavior is based entirely on interpersonal theory or the social context in which people live and work. The closest approximation may be the viewpoint developed by the neo-Freudian psychologist Harry Stack Sullivan. Several nursing theories also can be classified as interpersonal relations theory (see **Table 12-2**).

Harry Stack Sullivan (1892–1949): Theory of Interpersonal Relations

Sullivan believed that all human processes occur in interrelationships; none occur in isolation. His research and practice broke with Freudian theories and research in that he based his primary work on direct and verifiable observations. In his words, one must pay attention to the "interactional," not the "intrapsychic" (Sullivan, 1953, p. 3). Sullivan's

Table 12-2   Interpersonal Theories and Theorists

Theory/Discipline	Theorist	Therapeutic Process
Interpersonal (Psychiatry)	Harry Stack Sullivan	The purpose of all behavior is to get needs met through interpersonal interactions, not personality reconstruction as in psychodynamic theories. He coined the terms *participant observer* and *security operations*.
Nurse–Patient Relationship (Nursing)	Hildegard Peplau	Influenced by Sullivan's theory. First nurse theorist to describe the nurse–client relationship as the foundation for the professional practice of psychiatric nursing. Used the technique of process recording to facilitate communication and interpersonal skill building. Synonymous with the concept of the helping relationship as used in counseling.
Nursing Process Theory (Nursing)	Ida Jean Orlando	Study grew out of her dissatisfaction with the possibility that nursing care was governed by organizational rules rather than attention to client needs and her desire to offer nursing students a theory of effective nursing practice. She was also able to link effective nursing care to the nurse's knowledge of patient needs that are validated by patient response(s).
Human-to-Human Relationship Model (Nursing)	Joyce Travelbee	Focuses on meaning in the nurse–client relationship and the relief of client suffering through the use of communication skills within the phases of the nurse–client relationship.

approach laid the groundwork for understanding the specific social context, environment, and relationship(s) in which an individual interacts/interacted with other human beings.

In addition, Sullivan (1953) outlined a stage theory of interpersonal development that comprises life processes. Each stage prepares an individual for the next stage; failure to successfully navigate a stage could severely limit personality development and a person's potential for a successful life (**Table 12-3**). Sullivan believed that cultural environment greatly shapes personality and that personality development does not end at 5 years of age, as espoused by Freud, but continues until young adulthood. In essence, Sullivan emphasized the pervasive interaction between the organism and the environment as well as the tasks of personality development.

Sullivan introduced several new terms and concepts that became influential to the care of individuals and nursing. One concept critical to the organization of behavior is the *self system*, a construct that includes three components: the *good me*, the *bad me*, and the *not me*. The self system is built from the child's experience and provides tools that enable people to deal with the tasks of avoiding anxiety and establishing security. Sullivan emphasized the

Table 12-3 Sullivan's Stages of Interpersonal Development

Age	Stage	Task/Key Concept
Birth to 18 months (to appearance of speech)	Infancy	Experiences anxiety in interaction with mother figure; learns to use maternal tenderness to gain security and avoid anxiety. Major task is gratification of needs.
18 months to 6 years (first speech to need for playmates)	Childhood	Learns to delay gratification in response to interpersonal demands; uses language and action to avoid anxiety.
6–9 years	Juvenile	Develops peer relationships; uses environment outside the family to shape self. Learns competition, cooperation, and compromise.
9–12 years	Preadolescence	Develops caring relationship with same-sex peer, chum relationships, and the ability to collaborate with another person.
12–14 years	Early adolescence	Develops interest in and satisfactory relationships with persons of opposite sex; develops a sense of identity that is separate and independent from parents.
14–21 years	Late adolescence	Establishes a self-identity. Has satisfying relationships; direct sexual impulses.
>21 years	Adulthood	Achieves independence within society. Establishes a love relationship.

development of the self-system *personification* that includes all related attitudes, feelings, and concepts about oneself or another acquired from extensive experience. Other major concepts introduced into psychiatric literature include interpersonal security and the term *significant other* (Antai-Otong, 2008, p. 41).

Sullivan (1953, p. 25) believed that poor relationships cause anxiety and serve as the basis for all emotional problems:

> One of the greatest mysteries of human life, [is] how some unfortunate people carry on in the face of apparently overwhelming difficulties, whereas other people are crushed by comparatively insignificant events, contemplate suicide, perhaps actually attempt it. This is to be understood on the basis not of the particular "objective" events which bring about the circumstance of success under great hardship or self-destruction; it is to be understood on the basis of the self system, the organization of experience reflected to one from the significant people around one—which determines the personal characteristics of those events. In no other fashion can we explain the enormous discrepancy between people's reaction to comparable life situations. (Sullivan, 1947, p. 11)

Haber, Krainovich-Miller, McMahon, and Hoskins (1997, p. 94) caution nurses that Sullivan's interpersonal theory remains empirically unverified and nurses should take care when generalizing from his theory to the client.

Humanistic Theory

Humanistic philosophy/psychology focuses on the personal worth of the individual and the essential role of human values. The person is a "work in progress." Humanistic psychology took root in the United States in the Cold War era. Humanistic psychology has been described as a broad spectrum of approaches to treatment that arose as a spirited challenge to the rival orthodoxies of Freudian theory.

Carl Rogers (1902–1987): Humanistic Psychology and Client-Centered Therapy

Rogers' greatest contribution has not been in giving us a technique to fix people, but in creating a new form, a new definition of relationship in which people can function more fully and be more self-determining. (Farson, 2001, p. 201)

Carl Rogers, along with Abraham Maslow and Rollo May, was a forerunner in the identification of humanistic psychology as a person-centered approach involving specific values that emphasize the individual, choice, responsibility, and creativity (Rogers, 1980). However, Maslow and May eventually went on to carry the banner of humanistic psychology and focus on ideas of self-actualization rather than Rogers's emphasis on the treatment of sick persons.

The five fundamental building blocks of humanistic psychology can be identified as follows:

1. Actualizing human potentialities for creativity and growth
2. Regarding the person in the here and now
3. Emphasizing the centrality of self
4. Placing significance of experience as well as behavior
5. No assumptions of disease process, unconscious motivation, or developmental history.

Carl Rogers is now best known for his contributions to experience-oriented therapy, which focuses on the client's experiences as an agent for producing change. This therapy engages the client in new interactions and ways of being within the therapeutic situation. His therapy was originally called nondirective, was later renamed client-centered, and is now known as Rogerian therapy; even so, the terms *nondirective* and *client-centered* are still commonly used.

In Rogerian therapy, the client is viewed as the expert about himself or herself. As Rogers (1962) explained, "It is *client* who knows what hurts, what directions to go, what problems are crucial, what experiences have been deeply buried" (p. 422). As such, the therapist serves as a supportive facilitator. Rogers (1962) stated,

> Constructive personality growth and change comes about only when the client perceives and experiences a certain psychological climate in the relationship. The conditions which constitute this climate. . . . are feelings or attitudes which must be experienced by the counselor and perceived by the client if they are to be effective. Those I have singled out as being essential are: a sensitive empathic understanding of the client's feelings and personal meanings; a warm, acceptant prizing of the client; and unconditionality in this positive regard. (p. 422)

Rogers's healthy person is "fully-functioning" and possesses the following qualities: (1) openness to experience, (2) existential living, (3) organismic trusting, (4) experiential freedom, and (5) creativity.

According to Farson (2001), Rogers has given us a way to be with one another, an ethical basis for human interaction, guidelines for important considerations in assessing not just the outcome but the process of a relationship, a different way in which we think about human relationships, the expectations we have about intimate personal contact, the nature of interpersonal and organizational behavior, and the right to self-determination. Professionals from education, religion, counseling, nursing, medicine, psychiatry, law enforcement, race relations, and social work, to mention only a few disciplines, have taken his humanistic theory and client-centered techniques more seriously than those in psychology. Unfortunately, in spite of its demonstrated impact, Rogers's work has been corrupted over the years by practitioners who have discovered the technique but not the philosophy. According to Farson (2001),

> His is essentially a linear theory, as opposed to a curvilinear one; maximizing rather than optimizing. His concepts, like most in humanistic psychology, are based on the idea of 'the more the better' as opposed to 'there can be too much of a good thing.' Rogers would have you believe that the more congruence, the more honesty, the more intimacy, the more closeness, the more empathy, the better. Sounds good, but with most linear thinking, it fails in the extreme. . . . For a revolutionary, Rogers has paid precious little attention to role, power, status, culture, politics, history, systems, technology, and perhaps most significantly, the paradoxical quality of human experience. (pp. 200–201)

There are several commonalities in humanistic psychology and existential psychotherapy, as noted by Burston (2003):

- "Suffering might have a 'redemptive' function, pointing the person toward a more authentic, integrated existence, rather than being a mere nuisance to be eliminated so he (or she) can get on with the *real* business of living" (p. 313).
- "Existential psychotherapy and humanistic psychology share a core conviction [of] the role of self-authorship or self-determination in the formation of our character and conduct.

According to this view, we are never entirely determined by our past experiences. Personal choice plays a significant role in who we are and what we become" (pp. 313–314).

- "To varying degrees, and in different ways, [both humanistic psychology and existential psychotherapy] draw on an older, European tradition of literary and philosophical humanism" (p. 314). (See **Table 12-4.**)

Existentialism/Phenomenology

Existential philosophy seeks meaning of life or of human experience. It is based on the doctrine that existence takes precedence over essence; humans are totally free to act and responsible for their acts. What counts are acts performed. Decision making is not based on knowledge; instead, knowledge is the result of decision making. These theories claim that physical laws are not enough to explain the complexities of human behavior. Existentialists

Table 12-4 Humanistic and Existential Philosophies and Theories

Therapy	Therapist	Therapeutic Process
Rational emotive	Albert Ellis	This type of cognitive therapy confronts "irrational beliefs" that prevent the individual from accepting responsibility for self and behavior.
Logotheraphy	Viktor Frankl	This therapy is designed to help individuals assume personal responsibility. The search for meaning (*logos*) in life is a central theme, as is the magnitude of love: "The salvation of man is through love and in love" (1963, pp. 58–59).
Reality	William Glasser	The need for identity through responsible behavior is the therapeutic focus. Individuals are challenged to examine ways in which their behavior thwarts their attempts to achieve life goals.
Positive psychology	Martin E. P. Seligman and Mihaly Csikszentmihalyi	This theory focuses on prevention. It is a new approach to improving health that focuses on "health strengths," instead of the traditional emphasis on diagnosis, treatment, and prevention of disease. The premise is that positive health is a buffer against physical and mental illness.
Transpersonal psychology	Abraham Maslow, Stanislav Grof, and Anthony Sutich	The concern is with the "study of humanity's highest potential, and the recognition, understanding, and realization of unitive, spiritual, and transcendent states of consciousness" (Lajoie & Shapiro, 1992, p. 231). Issues considered in transpersonal psychology include spiritual *self-development*, *peak experiences*, *mystical experiences*, *systemic trance*, and other *occult* experiences of living.

are more subjective than other theorists. Creativity, individual initiative, and self-fulfillment are important personality factors. *Phenomenology*, the study of one's subjective experiences/perceptions, is one aspect of existential thought.

Viktor Frankl (1905–1997): Logotherapy

Frankl was a Viennese psychiatrist and neurologist who developed his own existential philosophy and therapeutic technique known as logotherapy, which involves an application of the principles of existential philosophy to clinical practice. It is the term *meaning* that framed Frankl's therapeutic work. Logotherapy postulates a *will to meaning*; it proceeds *from* the spiritual, whereas existential analysis proceeds *toward* the spiritual. When comparing his therapy to Freud and Adler's therapies, Frankl suggested that Freud essentially postulated a *will to pleasure* as the root of all human motivation and Adler a *will to power*.

Frankl's theory and therapy grew out of his experiences in Nazi death camps. Watching who did and did not survive (given an opportunity to survive!), he concluded that the philosopher Friedrich Nietzsche (1961) was right: "He who has a *why* to live for can bear with almost any *how*" (p. 121). Frankl saw that people who had hopes of being reunited with loved ones, or who had projects they needed to complete, or who had great faith, tended to have better chances of survival than those who had lost all hope. Frankl's first book was published in 1946 in German and translated into English in 1959 under the title *From Death Camp to Existentialism*. In 1963 this book was revised to include the basic concepts of logotherapy and redistributed under the title *Man's Search for Meaning*.

For Frankl, the essence of human motivation is the *will to meaning* (*Der zum Sinn*). When meaning is not found, the individual becomes "existentially frustrated." This frustration may or may not lead to clinical pathology. *Logotherapy* (from the Greek word *logos*, meaning "study," "word," "spirit," "God," or "meaning") is the method of psychotherapy for treating what Frankl termed an *existential vacuum*, which manifests itself mainly in a state of boredom. Frankl identified two types of symptoms for treatment: one he called *noogenic neurosis* (*noos* being Greek for "of the spirit or mind"), which emerges from conflicts involving existential problems. The other chief dynamic of the existential vacuum is *existential frustration*, which arises from failures and disappointments related to the will to meaning.

Rollo May (1909–1994): Existentialism

I have described the human dilemma as the capacity of man to view himself as object and as subject. My point is that both are necessary—necessary for psychological science, for effective therapy, and for meaningful living. I am also proposing that in the dialectical process between these two poles lie the development, and the deepening and widening, of human consciousness. (May, 1967, p. 20)

Existentialism. . . . is the endeavor to understand man by cutting below the cleavage between subject and object which has bedeviled Western thought and science since shortly after the Renaissance. (May, 1967, p. 11)

Rollo May was an American psychologist who, although a Congregationalist minister, preferred psychology. He introduced existential perspectives into the United States and is credited with being one of the editors of *Existence*, the first U.S. book on existential psychology, published in 1958, which highly influenced the emergence of American humanistic psychology.

While he accepted many Freudian psychodynamic principles (such as neurosis, repression, and defense), May believed that individuals could be understood only in terms of their subjective sense of self. He was influenced by American humanism theory and was interested in reconciling existential psychology with other approaches, especially Freud's. May believed that abnormal behavior is often just a stratagem for protecting the *center*, the subjective sense of self, against perceived threats. Persons may give up on self-growth if they perceive that their center is threatened and retreat to the secure, known center. As May put it in 1967, this is "a way of accepting nonbeing. . . . in order that some little being may be preserved" (p. 75). May also was concerned with people's loss of faith in values. If we lose our commitment to a set of values, he contended, we will feel lonely and empty. Life will be meaningless. In his view, we must ultimately take responsibility for ourselves and find meaning in our lives.

May identified four stages of development: (1) innocence, (2) rebellion, (3) ordinary, and (4) creative. *Innocence* is the pre-self-conscious stage of the infant. An innocent does have a degree of will in the sense of a drive to fulfill his or her needs. *Rebellion* is the childhood and adolescent stage of developing one's ego or self-consciousness. The rebellious person wants freedom but does not yet have full understanding of the responsibility that goes with it. Teenagers may want to spend their allowance in any way they choose, yet they still expect the parent to provide the money and will complain about unfairness if they do not get it. *Ordinary* is the normal adult ego. Adults have learned responsibility but find it too demanding and so seek refuge in conformity and traditional values. The *creative* stage is the authentic adult, the existential stage, beyond ego and self-actualizing.

May believed that knowing we will die gives life meaning. It reminds us that we must do something now, or never do anything. He also believed that anxiety is a force that could be channeled within the individual, thereby enabling the person to achieve and live a meaningful life. This knowledge was tested when, after surviving tuberculosis, he decided that struggling against the disease had been the key to remaining alive. His perpetual anxiety and fear of dying had been helpful, he determined, because it kept him from becoming resigned to death.

May wrote about this experience in his first major book, *The Meaning of Anxiety* (1950), and continued to express his philosophical and therapeutic approaches in a number of subsequent books between 1953 and 1981.

Positive Psychology

Positive psychology was founded on the belief that people want more than an end to suffering. People want to lead meaningful and fulfilling lives, to cultivate what is best within themselves, and to enhance their experiences of love, work, and play. The aim of positive psychology is to begin to catalyze a change in the focus of psychology—that is, to move away from a preoccupation with only repairing the worst things in life and toward building positive qualities. At the subjective level, the field of positive psychology is about valued subjective experiences: well-being, contentment, and satisfaction (in the past); hope and optimism (for the future); and flow and happiness (for the present). At the individual level, it is about positive individual traits: the capacity for love and vocation, courage and interpersonal skill, aesthetic sensibility, perseverance, forgiveness, originality, future-mindedness, spirituality, high talent, and wisdom. At the group level, it is about the civic virtues and the institutions that move individuals toward better citizenship: nurturance, altruism, civility, moderation, tolerance, and work ethic. At the forefront of this approach is the issue of prevention (Seligman, 2002).

Three pillars undergird the three central concerns of positive psychology: (1) positive experiences, (2) positive individual traits, and (3) positive institutions. Understanding positive emotions entails the study of contentment with the past, happiness in the present, and hope for the future. Understanding positive individual traits consists of the study of the strengths and virtues: the capacity for love and work, courage, compassion, resilience, creativity, curiosity, integrity, self-knowledge, moderation, self-control, and wisdom. Understanding positive institutions entails the study of the strengths that foster better communities, such as justice, responsibility, civility, parenting, nurturance, work ethic, leadership, teamwork, purpose, and tolerance.

According to Seligman and Csikszentmihalyi (2000, p. 5), the major psychological theories have changed to undergird a new science of strength and resilience. No longer do the dominant theories view the individual as a passive vessel responding to stimuli; rather, individuals are now seen as decision makers, with choices, preferences, and the possibility of becoming masterful, officious, or, in malignant circumstances, helpless and hopeless (p. 8).

Seligman prodded psychologists to study life's joys, and in 2002, he wrote a book outlining his theory of authentic happiness, which posited that happiness could be analyzed into three different elements that one chooses for their own sake: *positive emotion*, *engagement*, and *meaning*.

Since its inception, the science of positive psychology has moved into areas of practice and research that ensure "human beings are seen as possessing essential freedom, or psychological determinism," in any sort of situation (Seligman, 2002, p. 10). Positive psychology theory and initiatives have been applied across a number of healthcare domains. However, as research proceeded, Seligman (2008) began seeing certain limitations to the concept of happiness as a positive emotion. People did not find joy or happiness in succeeding or in accomplishment. Thus, in 2011, Seligman announced that authentic happiness as a theory was overrated; happiness actually had certain limitations and he regretted creating the "authentic happiness" title. Essentially people did not find aesthetic satisfaction, or meaning, in an accomplishment. Seligman (2011) concluded, "They wanted to win for its own sake, even if it brought no positive emotion" (p. 8).

In 2011, Seligman announced the creation of a new theory of positive psychology, "well-being" or "flourishing," which measures not only one's mood at the moment but also relationships with others and the sense that something worthwhile is being accomplished. Seligman also created PERMA, an acronym for what he defines as the five crucial elements of well-being: *p*ositive emotion, *e*ngagement (the feeling of being lost in a task), *r*elationships, *m*eaning, and *a*ccomplishment—each pursued for its own sake (pp. 16–18). As he explained, "Well-being cannot exist just in your own head: Well-being is a combination of feeling good as well as actually having meaning, good relationships and accomplishment" (2011, p. 16). He offered the following interpretation of his well-being theory:

> If we just wanted positive emotions, our species would have died out a long time ago. . . . We have children to pursue other elements of well-being. We want meaning in life. We want relationships. . . . My view of positive psychology is that it describes rather than prescribes what human beings do. . . . I don't want to mess with people's values. I'm not saying it's a good or a bad thing to want to win for its own sake. I'm just describing what lots of people do. One's job as a therapist is not to change what people value, but given what they value, to make them better at it. (Seligman, 2011, p. 26)

Transpersonal Psychology

Transpersonal psychology is an academic discipline, not a religious or spiritual movement, developed from earlier schools of psychology, including psychoanalysis, behaviorism, and humanistic psychology. There is a strong connection between the transpersonal and the humanistic approaches to psychology. This is not surprising, according to Aanstoos, Serlin, and Greening (2000), given that transpersonal psychology started off within humanistic psychology (pp. 23–24).

Lajoie and Shapiro (1992) suggested that transpersonal psychology "is concerned with the study of humanity's highest potential, and with the recognition, understanding, and realization of unitive, spiritual, and transcendent states of consciousness" (p. 231). Issues considered in transpersonal psychology include spiritual self-development, peak experiences, mystical experiences, systemic trance, and other occult experiences of living. Transpersonal psychology was developed in an attempt to describe and integrate the experience of mysticism within modern psychological theory. Types of mystical experience examined vary greatly but include religious conversion, altered states of consciousness, trance, and other spiritual practices. Although Carl Jung and others explored aspects of the spiritual and transpersonal in their work, Miller (1998, pp. 541–542) notes that Western psychology has had a tendency to ignore the spiritual dimension of the human psyche.

Transpersonal psychology is associated with New Age beliefs (Friedman, 2000). Although the transpersonal perspective has many overlapping interests with theories and thinkers associated with the term *New Age*, it is still problematic to place transpersonal psychology within such a framework. Indeed, associations between transpersonal psychology and the New Age movement have probably contributed to the failure of the nation's professional psychological authority, the American Psychological Association (APA), to establish formal recognition of transpersonal psychology in the United States. A significant breakthrough in this area was the successful establishment of a Transpersonal Psychology Section within the British Psychological Society (the United Kingdom's professional equivalent to the APA) in 1996, cofounded by David Fontana, Ingrid Slack, and Martin Treacy, the first section of its kind.

Today transpersonal psychology also includes approaches to health, social sciences, and practical arts such as process art. Transpersonal perspectives are being applied to such diverse fields as psychology, psychiatry, anthropology, sociology, pharmacology (Scotton, Chinen, & Battista, 1996), and social work theory (Cowley & Derezotes, 1994). Transpersonal therapies are included in many therapeutic practices.

Criticisms of transpersonal psychology have come from several commentators. For example, Rollo May, discussed earlier in the chapter, disputed the conceptual foundations of transpersonal psychology (Aanstoos et al., 2000, p. 25). Albert Ellis (1989), the cognitive psychologist and humanist, questioned transpersonal psychology's scientific status and its relationship to religion and mysticism. Friedman (2000) criticized the field of transpersonal psychology for being underdeveloped as a field of science, placing it at the intersection between the broader domain of inquiry known as transpersonal studies (which may include a number of unscientific approaches) and the scientific discipline of psychology.

RECOVERY-ORIENTED SYSTEMS OF CARE

Change is enviable; growth is optional. (Tavis Smiley, personal communication, May 2013)

The goal of recovery is not to become normal. The goal is to embrace the human vocation of becoming more deeply, more fully human. (Deegan, 1996)

Background

Within the literature, *recovery*, as a term, has been described by a number of professional disciplines and used to mean an approach, a model, a philosophy, a paradigm, a movement, a vision, and a myth (Roberts & Wolfson, 2004; Whitwell, 1999). As a healthcare concept, recovery is also not new. In health care, substance use and mental disorders treatment as well as "lived recovery" have been identified and discussed for decades. Yet now, the push toward recovery-oriented care lies at the core of the Substance Abuse and Mental Health Services Administration's (SAMHSA's) mission, and fostering development of recovery-oriented systems of care and services is a Center for Substance Abuse Treatment priority. Allott, Loganathan, and Fulford (2003) insist that the present claims of the recovery movement being a new paradigm are "probably exaggerated, as it represents a rediscovery of practices initiated more than 200 years ago" (p. 41).

In the U.S. healthcare system, recovery indicates a normal adaptation process of healing, improvement, or mending, to mention a few meanings. Globally, interest in recovery has been a focus for mental health services in the United Kingdom and New Zealand for several decades. Anthologies of personal stories of recovery have been used by governments and professionals as a means of combating stigma and reasserting a focus on *personal* perspectives (Lapsley, Waimarie, & Black, 2002; Leibrich, 1999). New Zealand's mental health services have been based on a recovery-centered blueprint, "which has led them to become a wellspring of ideas and guidance on recovery-based practice" (O'Hagen, 2001; Roberts & Wolfson, 2004).

In 1999, the U.S. Surgeon General set recovery as the focus of mental health policy (U.S. Department of Health and Human Services, 1999). Recovery-oriented care was originally envisioned as "the most important aim of behavioral health [meaning substance use and alcohol] services" (President's New Freedom Commission, 2003). In 2005, O'Connell, Tondora, Croog, Evans, and Davidson identified the elements of a recovery-oriented environment among alcohol and substance users. At that time, SAMHSA maintained separate definitions for mental disorders and substance use disorders. Noticeable disparity in care services and opportunities available caused considerable disagreement between the two areas. Mental health clients, practitioners, and other stakeholders confronted SAMHSA administrators about the limitation in scope of transformation services designation. After several conferences held between SAMHSA administrators and mental health participants, O'Connell and colleagues (2005) identified the elements of a recovery-oriented environment (see **Box 12-2**).

According to Roberts and Wolfson (2004), "Recovery is usually taken as broadly equivalent to 'getting back to normal' or 'cure,' and by these standards few people with severe mental illness recover" (p. 37). The goal of the discussions with SAMHSA was to achieve inclusion for the mentally ill and a redefinition of what recovery means to those with severe mental health problems. Roberts and Wolfson (2004) explained the importance of this redefinition:

> Redefinition of recovery as a process of personal discovery, of how to live (and to live well) with enduring symptoms and vulnerabilities, opens the possibility of recovery to all. The "recovery movement" argues that this reconceptualization is personally empowering, and raises realistic hope for a better life alongside whatever remains of illness and vulnerability. (p. 37)

Box 12-2   The Elements of Recovery-Oriented Environments
Encourages individuality; Promotes accurate and positive portrayals of psychiatric disability while fighting discrimination; Focuses on strengths; Uses a language of hope and possibility; Offers a variety of options for treatment, rehabilitation, and support; Supports risk-taking, even when failure is a possibility; Actively involves service users, family members, and other natural supports in the development and implementation of programs and services; Encourages user participation in advocacy activities; Helps develop connections with communities; and Helps people develop valued social roles, interests and hobbies, and other meaningful activities.

Reproduced from O'Connell, M., Tondora, J., Croog, G., Evans, A., & Davidson, L. (2005). From rhetoric to routine: Assessing perceptions of recovery-oriented practices in a state mental health and addiction system. *Psychiatric Rehabilitation Journal, 28*(4), 378–386. Reprinted with permission.

Box 12-3   The Vision and Values of Recovery-Oriented Care
Recovery is a personal and individualized process of growth that unfolds along a continuum, and there are multiple pathways to recovery. People in recovery are active agents of change in their lives and not passive recipients of services. People in recovery from mental illness and/or addiction disorders often note the important role of family and peer support in making the difference in their recovery. The values of recovery-oriented mental health and addictions systems are based on the recognition that each person is the agent of his or her own recovery and all services can be organized to support recovery. Person-centered services offer choice, honor each person's potential for growth, focus on a person's strengths, and attend to the overall health and wellness of a person with mental illness and/or addiction.

Reproduced from Gagne, C. A., White, W., & Anthony, W. A. (2007). Recovery: A common vision for the fields of mental health and addictions. *Psychiatric Rehabilitation Journal, 31*(1), 32–37. Published by the American Psychological Association. Reprinted with permission.

In a 2007 article, Gagne, White, and Anthony described the vision and values of recovery-oriented care that intersect the addiction and mental health fields, as shown in **Box 12-3,** and concluded that recovery should serve as the organizing construct for service provision and for systems improvement.

Finally, SAMHSA published the *Working Definition of Recovery From Mental Disorders and/or Substance Use Disorders,* which provided a unified working definition of recovery and set of recovery principles (see **Box 12-4**) designed to "help advance recovery opportunities for all Americans and help to clarify these concepts for peers, families, funders, providers, and others."

Box 12-4 Working Definition of Recovery

A process of change through which individuals improve their health and wellness, live a self-directed life, and strive to reach their full potential.

Four Major Dimensions Supporting a Life in Recovery

Health: overcoming or managing one's disease(s) as well as living in a physically and emotionally healthy way

Home: a stable and safe place to live

Purpose: meaningful daily activities, such as a job, school, volunteerism, family caretaking, or creative endeavors, and the independence, income, and resources to participate in society

Community: relationships and social networks that provide support, friendship, love, and hope

10 Guiding Principles of Recovery

Recovery emerges from hope: The belief that recovery is real provides the essential and motivating message of a better future—that people can and do overcome the internal and external challenges, barriers, and obstacles that confront them.

Recovery is person-driven: Self-determination and self-direction are the foundations for recovery as individuals define their own life goals and design their unique path(s).

Recovery occurs via many pathways: Individuals are unique, with distinct needs, strengths, preferences, goals, culture, and backgrounds, including trauma experiences that affect and determine their pathway(s) to recovery. Recovery is built on the multiple capacities, strengths, talents, coping abilities, resources, and inherent value of each individual. Recovery pathways are highly personalized. They may include professional clinical treatment, use of medications, support from families and in schools, faith-based approaches, peer support, and other approaches. Recovery is nonlinear, characterized by continual growth and improved functioning that may involve setbacks. Because setbacks are a natural, though not inevitable, part of the recovery process, it is essential to foster resilience for all individuals and families. Abstinence from the use of alcohol, illicit drugs, and nonprescribed medications is the goal for those with addictions. Use of tobacco and nonprescribed or illicit drugs is not safe for anyone. In some cases, recovery pathways can be enabled by creating a supportive environment. This is especially true for children, who may not have the legal or developmental capacity to set their own course.

Recovery is holistic: Recovery encompasses an individual's whole life, including mind, body, spirit, and community. The array of services and supports available should be integrated and coordinated.

Recovery is supported by peers and allies: Mutual support and mutual aid groups, including the sharing of experiential knowledge and skills, as well as social learning, play an invaluable role in recovery.

Recovery is supported through relationship and social networks: An important factor in the recovery process is the presence and involvement of people who believe in the person's ability to recover; who offer hope, support, and encouragement; and who also suggest strategies and resources for change.

Recovery is culturally based and influenced: Culture and cultural background in all of its diverse representations including values, traditions, and beliefs are keys in determining a person's journey and unique pathway to recovery. Services should be culturally grounded, attuned, sensitive, congruent, and competent, as well as personalized to meet each individual's unique needs.

Recovery is supported by addressing trauma: Services and supports should be trauma-informed to foster safety (physical and emotional) and trust, as well as promote choice, empowerment, and collaboration.

(Continues)

Recovery involves individual, family, and community strengths and responsibility: Individuals, families, and communities have strengths and resources that serve as a foundation for recovery.

Recovery is based on respect: Community, systems, and societal acceptance and appreciation for people affected by mental health and substance use problems—including protecting their rights and eliminating discrimination—are crucial in achieving recovery.

For further detailed information about the new working recovery definition or the *guiding* principles of recovery please visit http://www.samhsa.gov/recovery/.

Reproduced from SAMHSA's Blog. (2012a). *SAMHSA's working definition of recovery.* Retrieved from http://store .samhsa.gov/shin/content/PEP12-RECDEF/PEP12-RECDEF.pdf.

Recovery and Trauma-Informed Care

Another reality emerged among the care and service considerations for persons with behavioral and mental health needs—trauma as a near universal experience of individuals with behavioral and mental health problems. Greater than 90% of people served in public and mental health settings have histories of repeated exposure to trauma and violence; many patients reported a history of trauma and abuse most commonly having occurred in childhood (National Council for Behavioral Health, 2012). Individuals with histories of physical and sexual abuse and other types of trauma-inducing events often experience mental health and co-occurring disorders such as chronic health conditions, substance abuse, eating disorders, and HIV/AIDS, as well as contact with the criminal justice system. According to SAMHSA (2012b), "Although exact prevalence estimates vary, there is a consensus in the field that most consumers of mental health services are trauma survivors and that their trauma experiences help shape their responses to outreach and services." When expanding the recovery construct to other inclusive concepts, the generalizability of the recovery framework to include trauma emerges. Yet Ragins (2010) states,

> Ultimately to recover one must achieve some meaningful role apart from the destruction [trauma]. . . . Becoming a [trauma] victim is not a recovered role, and frankly, neither is [trauma] survivor. After achieving increased hopefulness, inner strength and self-responsibility, these traits are applied to meaningful roles apart from the [trauma]. (p. 3)

Despite Ragins's (2010) statement, trauma-informed care, by definition, is a strength-based framework that is grounded in an understanding of the responsiveness to the *impact of trauma*; emphasizes physical, psychological, and emotional safety for both providers and survivors; and creates opportunities for survivors to rebuild a sense of control and empowerment. It is an approach *made by providers* to engaging people with histories of trauma that recognizes the presence of trauma symptoms and acknowledges the role that trauma has played in their lives (see **Box 12-5**).

Box 12-5   Trauma-Informed Care
Trauma-specific interventions are designed to address the consequences of trauma in the individual and to facilitate healing. Treatment programs generally recognize the following: • The survivors' need to be respected, informed, connected, and hopeful regarding their own recovery • The interrelation between trauma and symptoms of trauma (e.g., substance abuse, eating disorders, depression, and anxiety) • The need to work in a collaborative way with survivors, family and friends of the survivor, and other human services agencies in a manner that will empower survivors and consumers

Reproduced from Substance Abuse and Mental Health Services Administration. (2012b). *Welcome to the National Center for Trauma-Informed Care.* Washington, DC: SAMHSA.

In all of these environments, the goal of care is to change the paradigm from one that asks, "What's wrong with you?" to one that asks, "What has happened to you?" According to SAMHSA (2012b),

> When a human service program takes the step to become trauma-informed, every part of its organization, management, and service delivery system is assessed and potentially modified to include a basic understanding of how trauma affects the life of an individual seeking services. Trauma-informed organizations, programs, and services are based on an understanding of the vulnerabilities or triggers of trauma survivors that traditional service delivery approaches may exacerbate, so that these services and programs can be more supportive and avoid re-traumatization.

Thus, a *recovery-oriented system* now describes and coordinates the delivery of care for individuals with substance use *and* mental disorders *and* trauma-related issues.

Conclusions About the Recovery-Oriented System of Care

As health care continues to change rapidly, the need for change in our traditional nursing roles has never been more apparent. Traditional models of health care have focused on curing illness. Right now, recovery is primarily viewed as a cross-cutting framework unifying mental health and substance use disorder treatments. However, recovery should be envisioned as an overarching framework for practice development and focus for all healthcare treatment. It has been suggested that practitioners need to change their practice in a number of ways, including (to mention only a few):

- We need to get out of the "treatment box" and accept that treatment is only one part of recovery; we must implement value-based approaches to care.
- Language use has to change to facilitate the value-based focus of recovery. To this end, Jensen et al. (2013) champion the use of person-first language.
- We must view and approach the expected change as a process, with starts and stops, not a destination; and we must remember, the purpose of recovery is *hope*—a movement from hopelessness to hopefulness.

Again, change is inevitable; growth is optional.

Building a Framework for Recovery-Oriented Care and Trauma-Informed Care

Quality of life is "the indivisible human's view on living moment to moment as the changing patterns of shifting perspectives weave the fabric of life through the human-universe interconnectedness." It is a subjective, global perception of the meaning of one's lived experiences in the moment. It fluctuates moment to moment in co-creation with the universe. (Parse, 1994, p. 17)

Today, health care must be client-driven (meaning *person*-driven). Nurses must always be at the forefront of changes to provide quality, cost-effective care for the betterment of the client, family, and community. Evidence of effective recovery-oriented, trauma-informed interventions or best practices in nursing is limited. Effectiveness of existing recovery-oriented interventions, programs, or models of care needs to be evaluated (Sheedy & Whitter, 2009). Munhall (2011) states,

The sands of science itself are shifting as more and more scientists, including nurse scientists, realize that science cannot be a field of absolute and final truth but is an endeavor focused on *illuminating an ever-changing body of ideas* . . . . Some consider this shift a "grievous loss" while others consider it "exhilarating and liberating." (pp. 12–13)

Preparation for the inevitable paradigm change in nursing science and practice, as outlined by Whall (2005), is more a matter of what Munhall (2011, p. 46) called a "*perspective development* than an anticipation of a specific occurrence."

Recovery is about the lived experience and understanding the lived experience. It is not what is wrong with a person, but rather what has happened to the person; in essence, as a lived experience, the only way out is to go through it (Anthony, 2008; Beck, 2011). Clinicians must remember "recovery is not a step-by-step process but rather is viewed as nonlinear, a growth experience with setbacks. Instead of focusing on the illness, the recovery process is strength based" (Boyd, 2012, pp. 17–18). As Boyd (2012) explains, "The patient and clinician in partnership facilitate recovery by managing the illness, strengthening coping abilities, and building resilience for life's challenges" (p. 17).

As the opening statement to this section offers—change is inevitable; *growth* is optional. While the immediate national push to integrate recovery-oriented systems of care is focused on, or seemingly limited to, being a framework for transforming mental and behavioral health, exciting implications for nursing and advanced practice nurses emerge to identify and expand recovery-oriented, trauma-informed nursing care in all areas of practice, not just psychiatric mental health and substance use practice. This push is well within nursing's capacity to exert considerable influence to broaden the scope of needed services.

According to Moller and McLoughlin (2013), "One could argue that the American Nurses Association's (ANA) definition of general nursing epitomizes the recovery philosophy but has not been recognized as so" (p. 114). Dual-diagnosis patients can also have comorbid diseases. Advanced practice nurses representing any specialty practice area or population group can use recovery-oriented, trauma-informed focused care approaches with any patients, not just those with behavioral and/or mental health problems.

Oftentimes in finding new ways of thinking about transforming care practices to meet emerging social trends and discipline needs, a reassessment of one's philosophy of nursing, theory of nursing, and tenets of nursing practice is required. As Munhall (2011) stated, "The future of nursing knowledge development requires nurses to blend philosophical aspects with the emerging social trends and needs in the discipline" (p. 46). As explained by Polifroni (2011), in outlining the continental philosophy of science,

> Human science deals with persons and their connectedness to the world in which they live and the lived experiences of their life. . . . The continental philosophy of science. . . . is concerned with the connection of an idea to the world around the idea and its historical context. [This philosophy] is not about theories or truths, but rather about relationships among people, ideas, meanings, and their historical connectedness. [Like patient assessment, it] requires an examination of historical context as much as it does what is happening in the present time. [One's belief] is not cause and effect, but rather in connectedness and the often used adage, "Past is prologue." (p. 14)

Zuzelo (2011) asserted that "nursing practice is. . . . built upon the premise that experiences are individual and unique. . . . As a result, nursing requires a pluralistic, multimethod approach to its knowledge-building endeavors" (p. 538). Newman (2008) insisted, "The link between nursing science [postmodernism, neomodernism], theory [interpersonal theory], and what is seen [patient-driven data focused on one's lived experience] makes important differences in practice" (p. 45). Aligning nursing science, interpersonal theory, and recovery care seems to be an attainable goal at all levels of nursing, particularly advanced practice specialties. Any successful alignment ought to be highly generalizable across all practice areas.

It is common to find nursing theories or conceptual frameworks classified in a number of ways. Today, although research and practice still are not always connected, there is absolute awareness that nursing practice is also a process of knowledge development. The goal of recovery-oriented nursing care transcends any particular disagreement.

Attempting to provide a cursory outline for building a framework for recovery-oriented research and practice using SAMHSA's principles and guidelines and Polifroni's (2011) idea of the past being prologue leads to a review of the works of such previously mentioned influential interpersonal nurse theorists as Joyce Travelbee (human-to-human relationship model), Margaret Newman (theory of health as expanding consciousness), and especially Rosemarie Rizzo Parse (humanbecoming theory). As Parse (1998) stated, "Nursing's goal consists of being with or in the presence within mutual nurse–client processes to understand

and value the meaning of the client's lived experience and assimilate preferences and beliefs that influence health care choices and preference" (p.14).

In Parse's view, health is inseparable and irreducible from both human and universe. Humans are intentional beings and, by their very nature, live a seamless symphony throughout the life span. People are involved with the universe in directing their personal becoming through their relationships with others. Individuals live in the moment within the presence of mutual processes with the universe structures that are multidimensional. In turn, these mutual processes enable persons to manage their lives and health through the freedom and right to make choices and live their lives as they choose (Parse, 1998, 2002). The environment includes the universe and mutual processes. Humans are engaged in mutual processes with the universe structure or with others who are with the individual. Thus, Plummer and Molzahn summarized, "Given the breadth of nursing practice and the value of the concept for nursing. . . . it is appropriate to consider replacing health as a metaparadigm concept with quality of life" (p. 140).

These interpersonal theories continue to provide integrative theoretical perspectives that are important for advanced nursing practice and *should* drive or actually undergird nursing research as new knowledge continues to evolve.

THE NEW NORMAL: WHAT IS OLD IS NEW AGAIN

Expanding Recovery-Oriented Care and Trauma-Informed Care to Military and Veteran Care

Background

Recovery is a process of change through which individuals improve their health and wellness, live self-directed lives, and strive to reach their full potential. Because setbacks are a natural part of life, one's ability to remain optimistic and maintain *hope* (the belief that challenges and conditions can be overcome) and *resilience* (an individual's ability to cope with adversity and adapt to challenges or change) is foundational to the recovery process. Thus, optimism and the ability to maintain hope are essential to resilience and the process of recovery. Recovery-oriented care addresses the whole person, supported by his or her family members and community, and is built on access to evidence-based clinical treatment and support services for all populations (SAMHSA, 2015).

The nation's behavioral and mental health organizations include recovery-oriented and trauma-informed processes as integral to their systems of care. When expanding recovery-oriented, trauma-informed frameworks/processes and systems of care to the nation's military and Veterans Health Administration (VHA) systems, a natural fit emerges. Within the military and VHA systems, *resilience* becomes the overarching concept linking these two frameworks to the military and VHA systems. According to Saltzman, Bartoletti, and Beardslee (2014),

Resilience describes one of the military's fundamental tasks: to maintain or restore individual functional capacity and well-being in the face of extreme adversity. [It] has become the organizing principle for program and service development across the U.S. Department of Defense and the various service branches. (p. 277)

Interpersonal relations theories and interpersonal relationship approaches emphasizing recovery-oriented and trauma-informed care as well as their end products—hope and resilience—are timely and relevant in the exploration of military health care. As stated by Mattocks et al. (2012), "Veterans' health must be positioned at the forefront of the biomedical research and health policy agenda" (p. 543). Areas appropriate to nursing research, theory development, and advanced practice are prominent among the care needs of women veterans, with clear imperatives among those reintegrating or transitioning back into civilian life.

Application of Interpersonal Relations Theories to Evolving Nursing Research

Trends and paradigm shifts are always occurring, and the critical questions asked by nurses cannot be limited to whether to follow along as viewpoints shift. With regard to nursing knowledge and research, the most important question to ask is: ". . . does it encourage progress in nursing?" (Rodgers, 2014, p. 33)

Peplau extended and reframed Sullivan's theory of interpersonal relations to a nursing theory and process that outlines one multidimensional central concept—the nurse–patient relationship, the core of nursing and framework for psychodynamic nursing. As Peplau (1952) stated, "Nursing is a significant, therapeutic interpersonal *process*" (p. 16), focused very specifically on person-to-person interaction(s). Further, the focus of Peplau's theory did not include pathophysiology or biological phenomena or other aspects of one's human experience. Basically, nursing practice always involves a therapeutic relationship between at least two persons—a nurse and a patient (1965, p. 274). Other nurse theorists expanded their research and theories to include physical as well as emotional or psychiatric illnesses in individuals, families, groups, and communities and reflected nurse–patient relations that transitioned from neo-Freudian to existential perspectives applied to nursing education and practice.

Today, it is probably safe to say that the concept of interpersonal relationships, nurse—patient interactions, is fundamental to *all* nursing theories. Also the "patient" can be identified as individual, family, group, or community. Travelbee's human-to-human relationship (1971) is a prime example; her original conceptualization was directed toward clients with psychiatric illness, but it was later expanded to long-term physical illnesses. As previously discussed, she proposed that the caring goal of nursing was to assist an individual, family, or community with the ultimate goal being the presence of hope (Travelbee, 1966, 1971).

Watson's theory (1985) espoused an existential orientation that features caring as "a moral ideal rather than an interpersonal technique" (p. 58). Her theory evolved into a mutually therapeutic restorative transpersonal relationship between a nurse and patient (as individuals, families, groups, or community). Then, too, Newman's theory featured evolving "patterns," expanding consciousness regardless of the form or direction it may take.

A Brief Overview of Veteran Health Care and Women's Issues

Historically, soldiers and veterans were primarily men, and Veterans Affairs (VA) healthcare services and facilities were designed to provide care for male veterans. Since the Vietnam War, increasing numbers of women have been inducted into military service and returned home (reintegrated into the community) as veterans. Most of these women veterans did not seek VA healthcare services on reintegration, likely due to the lack of gender-specific services. Instead they returned to their more familiar premilitary civilian facilities and providers. In subsequent years, the VA rushed to offer improved gender-sensitive services, yet the services continued to be marginalized (of unique concern have been reproductive care needs), and women veterans were hesitant to use VA healthcare services. Later, even with a few added women-specific services, many Gulf War I and Global War on Terrorism women veterans continued to seek treatment in their more familiar civilian community and primary care health facilities (Conard, Allen, & Armstrong, 2015).

In 2010 the VA Women's Health Research Agenda identified priorities and supporting activities designed to transform care for women veterans in six broad areas of study: (1) access to care and rural health; (2) primary care and prevention; (3) mental health; (4) postdeployment health; (5) complex chronic conditions, aging, and long-term care; and (6) reproductive health. Thus, the problem remains and many women veterans of the Iran, Iraq, and Afghanistan wars continue to seek treatment in community and primary care health facilities (Conard et al., 2015). It is also worth noting that VHA health care or insurance is not an automatic benefit to all veterans (Boyd, Bradshaw, & Robinson, 2013).

Linking Interpersonal Relationship Theories, Recovery-Oriented Care, and Trauma-Informed Care to Women Veteran Care and Nursing Practice

Enhancing Women Veteran Care and Nursing Practice

In 2016, there were 201,400 women in active military duty. Of them, about 60 were flag officers and about 92,000 were currently deployed (Department of Defense, 2016). As of July 2016, all military specialties, including active combat, had been opened to women; thus the advent of women warriors. Unfortunately, it is a well-established *reality* that deployment produces a new generation of persons; that is, the person who was deployed is not the same person who returns home. Conversely, the family left on deployment is not the same family encountered postdeployment. While women and men warriors have similar experiences in combat, women warriors are often transitioned directly back into their roles as primary caregivers for their children—more and more often as a single parent—or other family members. For those female members of armed/combat groups, some may be suffering from unrecognized, thus untreated, mental and/or physical health complications. Of unique concern are their reproductive care needs. Thus, adjustment or reintegration to civilian life after deployment requires a holistic perspective that encompasses modifying life outside the hierarchical military structure to a *different* postdeployment world (History.com, 2011).

Mattocks et al. (2012) identified three categories of stressful military experiences for women veterans—combat-related experiences, military sexual trauma, and separation from family. Similar to the chilly reception themes given the male Vietnam veterans, many women warriors interviewed expressed a sense that upon reintegration their roles and combat experiences were often minimized or widely misunderstood, or even unrecognized by family and friends. Similarly, according to Street, Vogt, and Dutra (2009), "While women Veterans faced obstacles related to seeking gender-specific VA services, they also experienced difficulty at non-VA facilities as a function of their combat Veteran status" (p. 692). Important themes echoed across many studies were feelings that the *contextual realities* of their war experiences were often misunderstood or not widely recognized by healthcare providers or in community/civilian healthcare settings (Boyd et al., 2013; Maiocco & Smith, 2016; Mattocks et al., 2012; Street et al., 2009). The concerns centered around the readiness of community healthcare providers to serve veteran populations (Murdoch et al., 2006). Street et al. (2009) explained this scenario:

> Since non-VA female healthcare providers may not have training or experience in serving Veteran populations, Veterans may be concerned that such providers will not have the knowledge or skills required to address their unique healthcare needs. While little research is available with respect to quality of non-provider care, which is likely to differ from provider to provider, it is possible that women Veterans' perceptions of their needs as unique keeps them from seeking and receiving needed post-deployment healthcare services at non-VA facilities. (p. 692)

There are certain timeless and *expected* combat exposure features of a conventional war that are not present in the current unconventional war(s). Unconventional wars feature extremely different culture practices, often untenable moral challenges where "the enemy wears no uniform, can strike without warning and can be a woman or child" (Boyd et al., 2013, p. 13). Simply stated, the military atrocities, killing, and aftermath of war, which pose even greater risks for morally questionable or ethically ambiguous situations that "may produce considerable lasting distress and inner turmoil" in many warriors—men or women—are the essential features or warzone-related contextual factors (Litz et al., 2009,

p. 696). Boyd et al. (2013), citing Luxton, Skopp, and Maguen (2010), have offered a very graphic review of the contextual features:

> There are multiple traumatic events that contribute to mental health morbidity including multi-casualty incidents (suicide bombers), IEDs, ambushes, seeing the aftermath of battle, handling human remains, friendly fire, witnessing or being involved in excessive violence, witnessing death or injury of close friend, death and injury of women and children, feeling helpless to defend or counterattack, being unable to protect/save another service member, killing at close range, and killing civilians and avoidable casualties or deaths. Combat exposure is a strong predictor of post-deployment depression and PTSD symptoms in women. (p. 13)

Too often the significance of veteran status/experiences is overlooked in primary care settings or treated as "business as usual" (Luxton et al., 2010; Mattocks et al., 2012).

Most models of the impact of war zone deployment on mental and physical health care are predicated on the experiences of male service members. Women's expanding role in combat operations presents both an opportunity and a challenge for nursing to adapt these models to effectively capture the experiences of women service members. Appropriate, timely, evidence-based interventions should increase the likelihood of healthy recovery from war-related stress, and secondary and tertiary prevention strategies are important components (Mattocks et al., 2012, p. 544).

Traumatic brain injury, PTSD, limb loss, functional gastrointestinal disorders—the two most common being irritable bowel syndrome and functional dyspepsia—and sexual trauma are signature wounds of the Iraq and Afghanistan wars. Combat-injured women suffered more facial and external injuries as well as more severe extremity injuries in contrast to nonbattle trauma (Conard et al., 2015; Department of Labor, 2010; Tsai et al., 2013). Clearly, more research is needed to characterize the nature of injuries in women and the subsequent outcomes associated with rehabilitation and reintegration across transitions of care.

With regard to nurses in the military as opposed to civilian nurses, Polomano and Stringer (2012) stated, "Civilian nurses may have difficulty envisioning the combat war zone and related health care environments" (p. 157). Unlike civilian nurses, active-duty military nurses must fulfill military requirements to maintain fitness and combat readiness and have little control over where they practice. Combat support hospitals place these nurses in "harm's way" (p. 157). According to Polomano and Stringer (2012),

> Nurses are not guaranteed safety, have limited access to needed health care resources, and are confined in unimaginable conditions of extreme temperatures without the basic necessities of daily living. Scannell-Desch and Doherty (2010) applied descriptive and phenomenological methodologies to elucidate feedback from 37 military nurses, 32 of whom were women deployed to Afghanistan and Iraq. The purpose of the study was to glean insight into these women's experiences. Seven themes emerged from the qualitative analyses of data that demonstrated

the physical and emotional toll that deployment places on military nurses and their struggles with post-deployment adjustment. (p. 157)

An article by Kelly (2010) offers more contrasts of the differences between battlefield and civilian nursing practices and environments.

Although men and women veterans will experience numerous difficulties when reintegrating into civilian life, there is a dearth of evidence-based nursing research to focus recommendations for practice related to the myriad military mental and physical healthcare needs of women veterans. A number of topic areas must be explored to understand the experiences of a new generation of women veterans (see **Box 12-6**). Understanding gender-specific issues in the postdeployment mental and physical health readjustment of Iraq and Afghanistan service members has broad potential relevance for nursing practice at all levels.

Box 12-6   Five Critical Points About Caring for Women Veterans

A review of current literature exposed the following top five points nurses and other healthcare professionals need to know about caring for women veterans.

1. Demonstrate cultural competence of the overall military subculture.
Upon joining the military and going to war, she becomes a member of a unique club that holds values and expectations generally diverse and separate from the civilian community (Dinnen, Kane, & Cook, 2014). As articulated by Captain Jill Glasenapp (2013), 101st Airborne Division, "There is no 'female' or 'male.' There is 'soldier.' We are all soldiers. We all bleed green" (Heinz Endowments, 2013).

2. Use person-first, person-centered, focused therapeutic communication skills.
No blanket assumptions should be made about the veteran's experience. Avoid using the word *what* as much as possible when questioning clients. It is very important to anticipate issues of grief and loss in service members as they return from combat. Tailor language used in conversations on the basis of cues from the client. Often, women do not identify with the term *military* or see themselves as veterans after separation. Suggest asking the women whether she was ever in the military or had a "military job."

It is now an accepted practice to say "Thank you for your service" to military persons and veterans; however, many current nurses were not alive or were very young at the time of the Vietnam War and are not aware of the reception given those soldiers on return from service. To many Vietnam soldiers, those words are tantamount to an apology (Coll, Weiss, & Yarvis, 2011; Mattocks et al., 2012; Street et al., 2009).

3. Provide recovery-oriented, trauma-informed nursing practice.
It is clear that women who have been deployed to Iraq or Afghanistan have unique health and mental healthcare needs related to their wartime experiences (Coll et al., 2011). Again, no blanket assumptions should be made about the veteran's experience(s); however, service members, even though assessed before reintegration, are returning home with undetected posttraumatic stress disorder (PTSD), military sexual trauma, depression, substance use, and other mental health disorders that emerge several months later. It is often unclear whether the symptoms occurred/existed before enlistment and deployment or developed during the deployment and reintegration processes and were never disclosed because of the stigma of having mental health problems.

(Continues)

Fears of career retribution or being prevented from returning home may preclude early reporting of physical and/or mental health issue. Reporting may also be delayed if symptoms do not emerge until several months following deployment. Development of a caring, trusting, trauma-informed, recovery-oriented relationship is particularly important for these women to be able to recount their experiences and come to terms with the impact of the experience(s). Recovery-oriented, trauma-informed care principles should undergird all specialty areas of nursing practice (Boyd et al., 2013; Maiocco & Smith, 2016).

4. Have knowledge of the Veterans Health Administration (VHA) and Community Reintegration Systems

Although VA services, for whatever reason, are underutilized by women, most VHA health care or insurance is not an automatic benefit to all veterans. Women (and men) Reservists and National Guard personnel have accessibility to military health insurance for only a limited time, after which they must purchase a civilian health insurance plan (Boyd et al., 2013; Hinojosa, Hinojosa, Nelson, & Nelson, 2010).

Build a community of practice (Wenger-Trayner & Wenger-Trayner, 2015). A growing number of people and organizations in various sectors are now focusing on communities of practice as a key to improving their performance. These learning communities are groups of people who share the desire to improve and who wish to learn and collaborate with their peers with similar missions. Participants engage in a process of collective learning in a shared domain of human endeavor. In this case, that domain concerns the needs of women who served in the U.S. military who subsequently became homeless and jobless, as well as the needs of veterans (whether male or female) who are homeless with families.

Offer general considerations in care, including connecting veterans with each other; offering practical help with specific problems related to workplace, family, friends, and finances; and attending to the broader needs as a result of the impact of both premilitary and postmilitary stressors. Understand that *family*, both military and civilian, is key to helping the war veteran reintegrate into the community. Offer women-only service spaces. Because women were reluctant to go to VA Medical Centers or settings where their male counterparts gathered, some grantees created welcoming women-only spaces that were bright, clean, and organized and that offered ample seating (Fargo et al., 2012; Murphy, 2014; Maiocco & Smith, 2016).

5. Have an understanding of homelessness among female veterans

We know that women veterans are overrepresented in the homeless population and four times more likely to be homeless than nonveteran women Fargo et al., 2012). Factors associated with women veteran homelessness are childhood adversity, trauma and/or substance abuse during military service, postmilitary abuse, adversity, relationship termination, postmilitary mental health substance abuse and/or medical problems, and unemployment. Being sexually assaulted during military service, being disabled, and screening positive for an anxiety disorder or PTSD have also been associated with homelessness. Protective factors include being a college graduate and being married (Fargo et al., 2012; Murphy, 2014; National Veterans Technical Assistance Center, 2013).

Peplau (1965) stressed the need for nurses to be able to feel within themselves the feelings that others are communicating verbally or nonverbally. They should integrate an understanding of their own behaviors and self-awareness to assist patients in identifying problems and in working toward achieving health and well-being; however, complicating reliable transfer, or comingling of interpreted feeling, is the community nurse provider's familiarity with the *realities* of war. As a new generation of women warriors return from combat, it is critical that both mental and physical healthcare providers understand this cohort's unique war zone experiences and readjustment concerns/needs to facilitate access to or development of evidence-based treatment.

Postdeployment interventions specific to women veterans must occur at multiple levels (individual, family, community) and from multiple institutions, including VA and community-based providers.

Enhancing Women Veteran Care and Nursing Education

A search of nursing textbooks revealed no discussion of prevalent war-related injuries, healthcare needs, or care facilities for veterans, especially in nonveteran community settings. The ANA House of Delegates, in 2008, voted to work with the VA to increase awareness of veteran care needs among nurses and nursing students to advance care and research in the area of veteran health. Today, veteran-related content is being included in a number of psychiatric nursing textbooks. The American Psychiatric Nurses Association has developed continuing education programs related to military mental health.

Understanding gender-specific issues in the postdeployment mental and physical health readjustment of Iraq and Afghanistan service members has broad potential relevance for nursing research, practice at all levels, and education. Within the area of mental health, women are approximately twice as likely as their male counterparts to be diagnosed with PTSD, with indications that the gender-specific risk of PTSD differs substantially by type of traumatic event.

Women's role in combat environments may not always be directly engaging with the enemy using deadly force, but their exposure to violence, the aftermath of violence, and traumatic exposures are significant factors in their subsequent health. Coupled with the rigorous environment within war zones where privacy is nonexistent, personal hygiene access is laborious, and physical hazards are overly abundant, women veterans with combat deployments are at risk for numerous and more intense health consequences. The ability of an active-duty service member to recover from the stresses and injuries of a combat deployment is linked to resiliency. The presence of self-esteem directly impacts the individual's ability to recognize and be willing to engage a healthcare system to create positive change and recovery (Crum-Cianflone & Jacobson, 2014, p. 6).

Table 12-5   Resource Websites for Veterans' Health Care and Nursing Education

American Psychiatric Nurses Association—a guide to military and PTSD resources, tips, and other resources for civilian mental health; resources for working with patients in the military; instructions for navigating the VA's mental health system; and links to webinar and podcast resources	http://www.apna.org/i4a/pages/index.cfm?pageid=4403 http://www.apna.org/i4a/pages/index.cfm?pageid=1
Veterans Access to Quality Healthcare Alliance—a resource comprised of dedicated advanced practice nursing organizations seeking to promote veterans' access to the high-quality care they deserve	https://www.veteransaccesstocare.com/
National League for Nursing—interactive, unfolding case studies and simulation scenarios that focus on veteran-centered care	http://www.nln.org/professional-development-programs/teaching-resources/veterans-ace-v/joining-forces/web-based-resources
VA Public Health Programs—information to help care for veterans	http://www.publichealth.va.gov/index.asp
Center for Women Veterans—information for women veterans	http://www1.va.gov/womenvet
American Association of Colleges of Nurses—information about the Enhancing Veterans' Care (EVC) Toolkit, a resource produced through a joint effort with the VA	http://www.aacn.nche.edu/downloads/joining-forces-tool-kit
VA Office of Academic Affiliations—information about the Military Health History Pocket Card for Clinicians, which provides applicable (and validated) questions to yield more information about a patient's service history and possible associated medical problems	http://www.va.gov/oaa/pocketcard

Table 12-5 offers online resources for nurses to learn more about the unique requirements and skills involved in caring for veterans.

BACK TO THE FUTURE

Recovery is about hope, resilience, and one's quality of life, not illness. (Sandra Nelson)

As discussed previously, in all recovery-oriented, trauma-informed environments and practices, the goal of care is to change the paradigm from one that asks, "What's wrong with you?" to one that asks, "What has happened to you?" and to then integrate the lessons learned from research into evidence-based practice and policy.

According to Whall (2002), nurses in the United States "did not focus on (or perhaps understand) the nature and importance of a paradigm shift that occurred just a few decades ago" (p. 72). Whall (2005) further offered,

> When nursing in the past was not clear concerning its meta-theoretical stance, practicing nurses at times assumed the practice values of other disciplines. The result might be described as analogous to a "rudderless ship," greatly influenced by the winds of the day and not by specific values of nursing. (p. 1)

It is well past time to move away from research using non-nursing principles and models of care. Nursing remains focused on interpersonal relationships—the interaction between client and nurse. Philosophical and paradigmatic issues foundational to nursing have gone through a shift from positivism to postmodernism and increasingly to neomodernism and existentialism. Given the movement of nursing research away from developing mechanistic models for explaining human activity, the opportunities for healthcare system growth found in recovery-oriented and trauma-informed care practices are poised to foster new directions for enhanced evidence-based military and veteran health nursing care models with immediate emphasis on women veteran health needs. This effort is important not only for enriched nursing knowledge, research, education, and practice, but also for the nation's health and well-being.

DISCUSSION QUESTIONS

1. Many recovery principles are innately embedded in the interpersonal relations philosophy and theories. Read the article "The Experience of Women Veterans Coming Back From War" by Maiocco and Smith (2016). Identify and discuss the role/importance of the civilian family and the "women warrior" military family to veteran recovery, resilience, and reintegration.
2. In the article "The Conceptual Model of Military Women's Life Events and Well-Being," Segal and Lane (2016) offer a number of recommendations for changes in policies, practices, and other mechanisms designed to optimize the well-being of military women and their families. Select and discuss one issue or policy offered or inferred.
   a. Pose a research question/hypothesis applicable to interpersonal relations theory and interpersonal relationships.
   b. How would you incorporate your findings into your practice?
3. Increasing numbers of women are enlisting in military service and direct combat duties as "women warriors." Discuss three gender-specific physical or mental health issues emerging among women veterans.
   a. Which resources, both formal services and informal social support, are most effective in creating positive effects on well-being in the aftermath of military service, especially in combat?
   b. How will these issues inform your practice? Your research?

4. According to the article "Access to Care for Women Veterans: Delayed Healthcare and Unmet Need" by Washington, Bean-Mayberry, Riopelle, and Yano (2011), data suggest that VA services are historically underutilized by women. Does the primarily male environment at VA Medical Centers play a role in the underutilization of services? If so, what changes in the delivery system are likely to improve access and participation?

5. In the article "'Homelessness and Trauma Go Hand-in-Hand': Pathways to Homelessness Among Women Veterans," Hamilton, Poza, and Washington (2011) identified a "web of homelessness vulnerability," identifying several life experiences that form interconnected factors that are predominant pathways for homelessness among women. Select one life experience identified in the "web" and build a community of practice on the basis of an interpersonal relations nursing theory or concept for our "women warriors" related to the experience.

6. Read the article "Battlefield Conditions: Different Environment but the Same Duty of Care" by Kelly (2010) and the article "Experiences of U.S. Military Nurses in the Iraq and Afghanistan Wars, 2003–2009" by Scannell-Desch and Doherty (2010). Compare and contrast the contextual realities (the differences) between battlefield and civilian nursing practices and environments.

REFERENCES

Aanstoos, C., Serlin, I., & Greening, T. (2000). History of division 32 (humanistic psychology) of the American Psychological Association. In D. Dewsbury (Ed.), *Unification through division: Histories of the divisions of the American Psychological Association, Vol. V.* Washington, DC: American Psychological Association.

Alligood, M. R., & Tomey, A. M. (2010). *Nursing theorists and their work* (7th ed.). Maryland Heights, MO: Mosby.

Allott, P., Loganathan, L., & Fulford, K. W. M. (2003). Discovering hope for recovery from a British perspective. In S. Lurie, M. McCubbin, & B. Dallaire (Eds.), International innovations in community mental health (special issue). *Canadian Journal of Community Mental Health, 21*(3).

American Nurses Association. (1967). *Statement on psychiatric-mental health nursing practice* (Publication No. S-85). New York, NY: Author.

American Nurses Association. (1980). *Nursing: A social policy statement.* Kansas City, MO: Author.

American Nurses Association. (2003). *Nursing: A social policy statement* (2nd ed.). Washington, DC: American Nurses Publishing.

Ancel, G. (2006). Developing empathy in nurses: An inservice training program. *Archives of Psychiatric Nursing, 20*(6), 249–257.

Antai-Otong, D. (2008). *Psychiatric nursing: Biological and behavioral concepts* (2nd ed.). Philadelphia, PA: F. A. Davis.

Anthony, K. H. (2008). Helping partnerships that facilitate recovery from severe mental illness. *Journal of Psychosocial Nursing, 46*(7), 25–53.

Beck, C. T. (2011). Exemplar: Teetering on the edge: A second grounded theory modification. In P. L. Munhall (Ed.), *Nursing research: A qualitative perspective* (5th ed., pp. 257–281). Sudbury, MA: Jones & Bartlett Learning.

Boyd, M. A. (2008). *Psychiatric nursing: Contemporary practice* (4th ed.). Philadelphia, PA: Lippincott Williams & Wilkins.

Boyd, M. A. (2012). *Psychiatric nursing: Contemporary practice* (5th ed.). Philadelphia, PA: Lippincott Williams & Wilkins.

Boyd, M. A., Bradshaw, W., & Robinson, M. (2013). Mental health issues of women deployed to Iraq and Afghanistan. *Archives of Psychiatric Nursing, 27*(1), 10–22.

Burston, D. (2003). Existentialism, humanism, and psychology. *Existential Analysis, 14*(2), 309–319.

Chinn, P. L., & Kramer, M. K. (2008). *Integrated theory and knowledge development in nursing* (7th ed.). St. Louis, MO: Mosby.

Coll, J. E., Weiss, E. L., & Yarvis, J. S. (2011). No one leaves unchanged: Insights for civilian mental health care professionals into the military experience and culture. *Social Work in Health Care, 50*(7), 487–500.

Conard, P. L, Allen, P. E. & Armstrong, M. L. (2015). Preparing staff to care for veterans in a way they need and deserve. *The Journal of Continuing Education in Nursing; 46*(3), 109–118.

Cowley, A. S., & Derezotes, D. (1994). Transpersonal psychology and social work education. *Journal of Social Work Education, 30*(1), 100.

Crum-Cianflone, N. F., & Jacobson, I. (2014). Gender differences of postdeployment post-traumatic stress disorder among service members and veterans of the Iraq and Afghanistan conflicts. *Epidemiologic Reviews, 36*(1), 5–18.

Decker-Brown, K. (2003). Humanistic theory information website. Retrieved from www .humanisticnursingtheory.com

Deegan, P. (1996). Recovery as a journey of the heart. *Psychiatric Rehabilitation Journal, 19*, 19–97.

Department of Labor Women's Bureau. (2010). *Trauma-informed care for women veterans experiencing homelessness: A guide for service providers.* Washington, DC: Author.

Dinnen, S., Kane, V., & Cook, J. M. (2014). Trauma-informed care: A paradigm shift needed for services with homeless veterans. *Professional Case Management, 19*(4), 161–170.

Ellis, A. (1989, February). Dangers of transpersonal psychology: A reply to Ken Wilber. *Journal of Counseling & Development, 67*(6), 336.

Falk-Rafael, R. A. (2000). Watson's philosophy, science and theory of human caring as a conceptual framework for guiding community health nursing. *Advances in Nursing Science, 23*(2), 34–49.

Fargo, J., Metraux, S., Byrne, T., Munley, E., Montgomery, A., Jones, H., & Culhane, D. (2012). Prevalence and risk of homelessness among U.S. veterans. National Center on Homelessness Among Veterans. Penn Libraries. Retrieved from http://repository.upenn.edu/cgi/viewcontent .cgi?article=1161&context=spp_papers

Farson, R. (2001). Carl Rogers, quiet revolutionary. *Education, 95*(2), 197–203.

Fawcett, J. (2005). *Contemporary nursing knowledge: Analysis and evaluation of nursing models and theories* (2nd ed.). Philadelphia, PA: F. A. Davis.

Frankl, V. E. (1963). *Man's search for meaning: An introduction to logotherapy* (I. Lasch, Trans.). New York, NY: Washington Square Press. (Earlier title, 1959, *From death-camp to existentialism.* Originally published in 1946 as *Ein Psycholog erlebt das Konzentrationslager*).

Friedman, H. (2000). *Toward developing transpersonal psychology as a scientific field*. Paper presented at Old Saybrook 2 Conference, May 11–14, 2000, State University of West Georgia.

Frisch, N. C., & Frisch, L. E. (2011). *Psychiatric mental health nursing* (4th ed.). Clifton Park, NY: Delmar.

Gagne, C. A., White, W., & Anthony, W. A. (2007). Recovery: A common vision for the fields of mental health and addictions. *Psychiatric Rehabilitation Journal, 31*, 32–37.

Gastman, C. (1998). Interpersonal relations in nursing: A philosophical-ethical analysis of the work of Hildegard Peplau. *Journal of Advanced Nursing, 28*, 1312–1319.

Haber, J. (2000). Hildegard Peplau: The psychiatric nursing legacy of a legend. *Journal of the American Psychiatric Nurses Association, 6*(2), 56–62.

Haber, J., Krainovich-Miller, B., McMahon, A. L., & Hoskins, P. P. (1997). *Comprehensive psychiatric nursing* (5th ed.). St. Louis, MO: Mosby.

Heinz Endowments. (2013). Journey to normal. Retrieved from http://www.heinz.org/Interior.aspx ?id=417&view=entry&eid=1146

Hinojosa, R., Hinojosa, M. S., Nelson, K., & Nelson, D. (2010). Veteran family reintegration, primary care needs, and the benefit of the patient-centered medical home model. *Journal of the American Family Board of Medicine, 23*(6), 770–774.

History.com staff. (2011). Women in the Vietnam War. A&E Networks. Retrieved from http://www .history.com/topics/vietnam-war/women-in-the-vietnam-war

Jensen, M. E., Pease, E. A., Lambert, K., Hickman, D. R., Robinson, O., McCoy, K. T., . . . King, J. K. (2013). Championing person-first language: A call to psychiatric mental health nurses. *Journal of the American Psychiatric Nurses Association, 19*(3), 146–151.

Johnson, B. M., & Webber, P. B. (2010). *An introduction to theory and reasoning in nursing* (3rd ed.). Philadelphia, PA: Lippincott Williams & Wilkins.

Kelly, J. (2010). Battlefield conditions: Different environment but the same duty of care. *Nursing Ethics, 17*(5), 636–645

Kneisl, C. R., & Trigoboff, E. (2009). *Contemporary psychiatric-mental health nursing* (2nd ed.). Upper Saddle River, NJ: Pearson.

Lajoie, D. H., & Shapiro, S. I. (1992). Definitions of transpersonal psychology: The first twenty-three years. *Journal of Transpersonal Psychology, 24*, 230–241.

Lapsley, H., Waimarie, L. N., & Black, R. (2002). *Kia Mauri Tau! Narratives of recovery from disabling mental health problems*. Wellington, New Zealand: Mental Health Commission.

Leibrich, J. (1999). *A gift of stories: How to deal with mental health illness*. Dunedin, New Zealand: University of Otago Press.

Litz, B. T., Stein, N., Delaney, E., Lebowitz, L., Nash, W. P., Silva, C., & Maguen, S. (2009). Moral injury and moral repair in war veterans: A preliminary model and intervention strategy. *Clinical Psychology Review, 29*, 695–706.

Luxton, D. D., Skopp, N. A., & Maguen, S. (2010). Gender differences in depression and PTSD symptoms following combat exposure. *Depression and Anxiety, 27*, 1027–1033.

Maiocco, G., & Smith, M. J. (2016). The experience of women veterans coming back from war. *Archives of Psychiatric Nursing, 30*(3), 393–399.

Mattocks, K. M., Haskell, S. G., Krebs, E. E., Justice, A. C., Yano, E. M., & Brandt, C. (2012). Women at war: Understanding how women veterans cope with combat and military sexual trauma. *Social Science and Medicine, 74*(4), 537–545.

May, R. (1950). *The meaning of anxiety* (rev. ed.). New York, NY: W. W. Norton.

May, R. (1967). *Psychology and the human dilemma.* New York, NY: W. W. Norton.

McCamant, K. L. (2006, October). Humanistic nursing, interpersonal relations theory, and the empathy-altruism hypothesis. *Nursing Science Quarterly, 19*(4), 334–338.

Meleis, A. I. (2007). *Theoretical nursing: Development and progress* (4th ed.). Philadelphia, PA: Lippincott Williams & Wilkins.

Miller, J. J. (1998). Book review: Textbook of transpersonal psychiatry and psychology. *Psychiatric Services, 49,* 541–542.

Mohr, W. K. (2008). *Psychiatric mental health nursing: Evidence-based concepts, skills, and practices* (7th ed.). Philadelphia, PA: Lippincott Williams & Wilkins.

Moller, M. D., & McLoughlin, K. A. (2013). Integrating recovery practices into psychiatric nursing: Where are we in 2013? *Journal of the American Psychiatric Nurses Association, 9*(3), 113–116.

Moses, M. M. (1994). Caring incidents: A gift to the present. *Journal of Holistic Nursing, 12,* 193–203.

Munhall, P. L. (2011). *Nursing research: A qualitative perspective* (5th ed.). Sudbury, MA: Jones & Bartlett Learning.

Murdoch, M., Bradley, A., Mather, S. H., Klein, R. E., Turner, C. L., & Yano, E. M. (2006). Women and war: What physicians should know. *Journal of General Internal Medicine, 21,* S5–S10.

Murphy, E. C., & Hans, S. (2014). Women veterans: The long journey home. Retrieved from https://www.dav.org/wp-content/uploads/women-veterans-study.pdf

National Council for Behavioral Health. (2012). Trauma-informed care. Retrieved from http://www.thenationalcouncil.org/topics/trauma-informed-care/

National Veterans Technical Assistance Center. (2013, October). Lessons learned from the U.S. Department of Labor Grantees: Homeless female veterans and homeless veterans with families. Houston, TX: Author.

Newman, M. A. (1972). Time estimation in relation to gait tempo. *Perceptual and Motor Skills, 34,* 359–366.

Newman, M. A. (1990). Newman's theory of health as praxis. *Nursing Science Quarterly, 3,* 37–41.

Newman, M. A. (1992). Nightingale's vision of nursing theory and health. In F. Nightingale, *Notes on nursing: What it is and what it is not* (commemorative ed., pp. 44–47). Philadelphia, PA: Lippincott.

Newman, M. A. (1994). *Health as expanding consciousness* (2nd ed.). New York, NY: National League for Nursing.

Newman, M. A. (2003). The world on no boundaries. *ANS Advances in Nursing Science, 26*(4), 240–245.

Newman, M. A. (2008). *Transforming presence: The difference that nursing makes.* Philadelphia, PA: F. A. Davis.

Nietzsche, F. W. (1961). *Thus spoke Zarathustra: A book for everyone and no one.* London, UK: Penguin Group.

O'Connell, M., Tondora, J., Croog, G., Evans, A., & Davidson, L. (2005). From rhetoric to routine: Assessing perceptions of recovery-oriented practices in a state mental health and addiction system. *Psychiatric Rehabilitation Journal, 28*(4), 378–386.

O'Hagan, M. (2001). *Recovery competencies for New Zealand mental health workers.* Wellington, New Zealand: Mental Health Commission.

Orlando, J. J. (1961). *The dynamic nurse patient relationship: Function, process and principles.* New York, NY: G. P. Putnam's Sons.

Orlando, J. J. (1972). *The discipline and teaching of nursing process (an evaluative study).* New York, NY: G. P. Putnam's Sons.

Orlando Pelletier, J. J. (1990). Preface to the NLN edition. In J. J. Orlando, *The dynamic nurse patient relationship: Function, process and principles* (pp. vii–viii). New York, NY: National League for Nursing.

O'Toole, A. W., & Welt, S. R. (Eds.). (1989). *Interpersonal theory in nursing practice: Selected works of Hildegard E. Peplau.* New York, NY: Springer.

Parse, R. R. (1981). *Man-living-health: A theory of nursing.* New York, NY: Wiley.

Parse, R. R. (1992). Human becoming: Parse's theory of nursing. *Nursing Science Quarterly, 5,* 35–42.

Parse, R. R. (1994). Quality of life: Sciencing and living the art of human becoming. *Nursing Science Quarterly, 7*(1), 16–21.

Parse, R. R. (1995). Nursing theories and frameworks: The essence of advanced practice nursing. *Nursing Science Quarterly, 8*(1), 1.

Parse, R. R. (1998). Moving on. *Nursing Science Quarterly, 11*(4), 135.

Parse, R. R. (2002). Transforming health care with a unitary view of human. *Nursing Science Quarterly, 15,* 46–50.

Parse, R. R. (2007). The humanbecoming school of thought in 2050. *Nursing Science Quarterly, 20,* 308.

Paterson, J. G., & Zderad, L. T. (1976). *Humanistic nursing.* New York, NY: Wiley.

Paterson, J. G., & Zderad, L. T. (1978). *The tortuous way toward nursing theory* (National League for Nursing Publication No. 15-1708). New York, NY: National League for Nursing.

Paterson, J. G., & Zderad, L. T. (1988). *Humanistic nursing.* New York, NY: National League for Nursing.

Peplau, H. (1952). *Interpersonal relations in nursing.* New York, NY: G. P. Putnam's Sons.

Peplau, H. (1991, re-issued). *Interpersonal relations in nursing: A conceptual frame of reference for psychodynamic nursing.* New York, NY: Springer.

Peplau, H. (1992). Interpersonal relations: A theoretical framework for application in nursing practice. *Nursing Science Quarterly, 5,* 13–18.

Peplau, H. (1997). Peplau's theory of interpersonal relations. *Nursing Science Quarterly, 10*(4), 162–167.

Perese, E. F. (2012). Framework for practice of advanced practice psychiatric nurses. *Psychiatric Advanced Practice Nursing: A Biopsychosocial Foundation for Practice.* Philadelphia, PA: Davis.

Phillips, J. R. (1995). Quality of life research: Its increasing importance. *Nursing Science Quarterly, 8,* 100–101.

Pilkington, F. B. (2007). Envisioning nursing in 2050 through the eyes of nurse theorists: Leininger and Watson. *Nursing Science Quarterly, 20*(1), 8.

Plummer, M., & Molzahn, A. E. (2009, December). Quality of life in contemporary nursing theory: A concept analysis. *Nursing Science Quarterly, 22,* 134–140.

Polifroni, E. C. (2011). Philosophy of science: An introduction. In J. B. Butts & K. L. Rich. *Philosophies and theories for advanced nursing practice* (pp. 3–18). Sudbury, MA: Jones & Bartlett Learning.

Polomano, R. C., & Stringer, M. (2012). Narrowing the gaps in research for women in the military and veterans. *Journal of Obstetric, Gynecologic, and Neonatal Nursing, 41,* 157–159.

Potter, M. L., & Bockenhauer, B. J. (2000). Implementing Orlando's nursing theory. *Journal of Psychosocial Nursing and Mental Health Services, 38*(13), 14–21.

Praeger, S. G., & Hogarth, C. R. (1985). Josephine E. Paterson and Loretta T. Zderad. In J. B. George (Ed.), *Nursing theories* (2nd ed., pp. 287–299). Englewood Cliffs, NJ: Prentice Hall.

President's New Freedom Commission, Mental Health. (2003). Achieving the promise: Transforming mental health care in America—final report (DHHS Publication No. SMA- 03-3832).

Ragins, M. (2010). *Four levels of recovery practice.* Bethesda, MD: Development Services Group.

Reed, P. G. (1996). Transforming practice knowledge into nursing knowledge—A revisionist analysis of Peplau. *Journal of Nursing Scholarship, 28*(1), 29–33.

Reynolds, W. J., & Scott, B. (1999). Empathy: A crucial component of the helping relationship. *Journal of Psychiatric and Mental Health Nursing, 6,* 363–379.

Reynolds, W. J., & Scott, B. (2000). Do nurses and other professional helpers normally display much empathy? *Journal of Advanced Nursing, 31,* 226–234.

Rich, K. (2003). Revisiting Joyce Travelbee's question: What's wrong with sympathy? *Journal of the American Psychiatric Association, 9*(6), 202–204.

Rittman, M. R. (2001). Ida Jean Orlando: The dynamic nurse-patient relationship. In M. E. Parker (Ed.), *Nursing theories and nursing practice.* Philadelphia, PA: F. A. Davis.

Roberts, G., & Wolfson, P. (2004). The rediscovery of recovery: Open to all. *Advances in Psychiatric Treatment, 10,* 37–48.

Rogers, C. (1962). The interpersonal relationship: The core of guidance. *Harvard Educational Review, 32*(4), 422.

Rogers, C. (1980). *A way of being.* Boston, MA: Houghton Mifflin.

Rogers, M. E. (1970). *An introduction to the theoretical basis of nursing.* Philadelphia, PA: F. A. Davis.

Rogers, M. E. (1994). Science of unitary human beings. Current perspectives. *Nursing Science Quarterly, 7,* 33–35.

Saltzman, W. R., Bartoletti, M., Lester, P., & Beardslee, W. R. (2014). Building resilience in military families. In S. J. Cozza, M. N. Goldenberg, & R. J. Ursano (Eds). *Care of military service members, veterans, and their families* (pp. 277–297). Washington, DC: American Psychiatric Publishing.

Scannell-Desch, E., & Doherty, M. E. (2010). Experiences of U.S. military nurses in the Iraq and Afghanistan wars, 2003–2009. *Journal of Nursing Scholarship,* 42(1), 3–12.

Schmieding, N. J. (n.d.). *Ida Jean Orlando's nursing process theory.* Retrieved from www.uri.edu /nursing/schmieing/orlando

Scotton, B. W., Chinen, A. B., & Battista, J. R. (Eds.). (1996). *Textbook of transpersonal psychiatry and psychology.* New York, NY: Basic Books.

Seligman, M. E. P. (2002). *Authentic happiness: Using the new positive psychology to realize your potential for lasting fulfillment.* New York, NY: Free Press (Simon & Schuster).

Seligman, M. E. P. (2008). Positive health. *Applied Psychology: An International Review, 57,* 3–18.

Seligman, M. E. P. (2011). *Flourish: A visionary new understanding of happiness and well-being.* New York, NY: Free Press (Simon & Schuster).

Seligman, M. E. P., & Csikszentmihalyi, M. (2000, January). Positive psychology: An introduction. *American Psychologist, 55*(1), 5–15.

Sheedy, C. K., & Whitter, M. (2009). Guiding principles and elements of recovery-oriented systems of care: What do we know from the research? HHS Publication No. (SMA) 09-4439. Rockville, MD: Center for Substance Abuse Treatment, Substance Abuse and Mental Health Services Administration. Retrieved from http://www.viahope.org/assets/uploads/SAMHSA_guiding_principles_Whitepaper.pdf

Sills, G. M. (1999). Hildegard E. Peplau, RN: Ed.D; FAAN: Nurse scholar, educator, leader. *Nursing Science Quarterly, 12*(3), 188–189.

Sills, G. M. (2000). Peplau and professionalism: The emergence of the paradigm of professionalism. *Journal of the American Psychiatric Nurses Association, 6*(1), 29–34.

Street, A. E., Vogt, D., & Dutra, L. (2009). A new generation of women veterans: Stressors faced by women deployed to Iraq and Afghanistan. *Clinical Psychology Review, 29*, 685–694.

Substance Abuse and Mental Health Services Administration. (2012a). *SAMHSA's working definition of recovery.* Washington, DC: SAMHSA. Retrieved from http://store.samhsa.gov/shin/content/PEP12-RECDEF/PEP12-RECDEF.pdf

Substance Abuse and Mental Health Services Administration. (2012b). *Welcome to the National Center for Trauma-Informed Care.* Washington, DC: SAMHSA. Retrieved from http://www.samhsa.gov/nctic/

Substance Abuse and Mental Health Services Administration. (2015). Recovery and recovery support. Retrieved from http://www.samhsa.gov/recovery

Sullivan, H. S. (1947). *Conceptions of modern psychiatry* (2nd ed.). Washington, DC: William Alanson White Psychiatric Foundation.

Sullivan, H. S. (1953). *The interpersonal theory of psychiatry.* New York, NY: W. W. Norton.

Travelbee, J. (1964). What's wrong with sympathy? *The American Journal of Nursing, 6*(1), 68–71.

Travelbee, J. (1966). *Interpersonal aspects of nursing.* Philadelphia, PA: F. A. Davis.

Travelbee, J. (1969). *Intervention in psychiatric nursing: Process in the one-to-one relationship.* Philadelphia, PA: F. A. Davis.

Travelbee, J. (1971). *Interpersonal aspects of nursing* (2nd ed.). Philadelphia, PA: F. A. Davis.

Tyra, P. A. (2008). In memoriam: Ida Jean Orlando Pelletier. *American Psychiatric Nurses Association, 14*(3), 231–232.

Tsai, J., Pietrzak, R. H., & Rosenheck, R. A. (2013). Homeless veterans who served in Iraq and Afghanistan: Gender differences, combat exposure and comparisons with previous cohorts of homeless veterans. *Administration and Policy in Mental Health and Mental Health Services Research, 40*, 400–405.

U.S. Department of Defense. (2016). News releases. Retrieved from http://www.defense.gov/News/News-Releases

U.S. Department of Health and Human Services. (1999). Mental health: A report of the Surgeon General. Rockville, MD: Author.

Vandemark, L. M. (2006). Awareness of self and expanding consciousness: Using nursing theories to prepare theories to prepare nurse-therapist. *Issues in Mental Health Nursing, 27*, 605–615.

Walker, L. O., & Avant, K. C. (2004). *Strategies for theory construction nursing* (4th ed.). Upper Saddle River, NJ: Prentice Hall.

Watson, J. (1979). *Nursing: Philosophy and science of caring.* Boston, MA: Little, Brown.

Watson, J. (1985). *Nursing: Human science and human care—A theory of nursing.* Norwalk, CT: Appleton & Lange.

Watson, J. (1988). *Nursing: Human science and human care—A theory of nursing.* New York, NY: National League for Nursing.

Watson, J. (1995). Post modernism and knowledge development in nursing. *Nursing Science Quarterly, 8*(2), 60–64.

Watson, J. (1996). Watson's theory of transpersonal caring. In P. J. Walker & B. Neuman (Eds.), *Blueprint for the use of nursing models: Education research, practice, and administration* (pp. 141–184). New York, NY: National League for Nursing Press.

Watson, J. (1997). The theory of human caring: Retrospective and beyond. *Nursing Science Quarterly, 10*(1), 49–52.

Watson, J. (1999). *Postmodern nursing and beyond.* Edinburgh: Churchill Livingstone.

Watson, J. (2002). *Instruments for assessing and measuring caring in nursing and health sciences.* New York, NY: Springer.

Watson, J. (2003). Love and caring: Ethics of face and hand. *Nursing Administration Quarterly, 27*(3), 197–202.

Watson, J. (2005). *Caring science as sacred science.* Philadelphia, PA: F. A. Davis.

Wenger-Trayner, E., & Wenger-Trayner, B. (2015). Introduction to communities of practice. Retrieved from http://wenger-trayner.com/introduction-to-communities-of-practice

Whall, A. L. (2002). The unrecognized paradigm shift in nursing: Implications, problems, and possibilities. *Nursing Outlook, 50*(2), 72–76.

Whall, A. L. (2005, January/February). "Lest we forget": An issue concerning the doctorate in nursing practice (DNP). *Nursing Outlook, 53*(1), 1.

Wheeler, K., & Haber, J. (2004). Development of psychiatric mental health nurse practitioner competencies: Opportunities for the 21st century. *Journal of the American Psychiatric Nurses Association, 10*(3), 129–138.

Whitwell, D. (1999). The myth of recovery from mental illness. *Psychiatric Bulletin, 23,* 621–622.

Zuzelo, P. R. (2011). Evidence-based nursing and qualitative research: A partnership imperative for real-world practice. In P. L. Munhall (Ed.), *Nursing research: A qualitative perspective* (5th ed., pp. 533–552). Sudbury, MA: Jones & Bartlett Learning.

Chapter 13

Environmental Philosophy and Theories

Steven J. Vanderheiden

INTRODUCTION

Environmental theories fall into one of two distinct but related categories: explanatory and normative. *Explanatory* environmental theories offer an account of the nature of various environmental phenomena, their relationship to human life, and the causal connections between the two. Anthropogenic climate change, for example, is a phenomenon that depends on an explanatory theory that posits climatic changes are a result of human activities and affect human welfare. This theory seeks to explain the role that various human activities play in causing and being affected by climate change, although in its strictly explanatory sense, it prescribes no particular response to the phenomenon. *Normative* environmental theories are, by contrast, prescriptive, in that they posit some set of values and recommend action on the basis of those values. Arguments in favor of endangered species protection laws made on grounds of the important value of biodiversity offer an example of the application of normative environmental theory, at least insofar as theory-based reasons are offered on behalf of biodiversity.

While explanatory environmental theories are primarily based on facts and normative environmental theories primarily on values, these two kinds of theories are often dependent on each other; that is, most explanatory theories contain at least some implicit or explicit normative elements, and all normative theories depend on at least some explanatory theories. People who defend anticruelty laws to protect nonhuman animals, for example, typically invoke explanatory claims concerning animal cognition and sentience, asserting that animals actually do suffer when treated in certain ways. Those working on primarily explanatory questions concerning animal cognition and sentience often do so with the recognition that normative judgments about how animals should be treated follow directly from their empirical theoretical research. Without the explanatory theories, there would be no grounds for believing that people could do anything to cause nonhuman animals to experience something qualitatively similar to human suffering, which is both a physical and psychological response to some loss or injury. Without the normative theories, there would be no grounds for calling this avoidable suffering wrong or unjust.

When fact-based claims aimed primarily at explanation are bundled together with normative value judgments in a coherent theoretical system, they produce environmental discourses (Dryzek, 1997). These discourses characterize problems in certain ways, focusing attention on particular attributes of some phenomena at the expense of others, and generating support for one or another prescription as the appropriate way to address the problem at hand. Some problems are described quite differently by competing environmental discourses, with divergent remedial prescriptions issuing from the distinct conceptual lens through which different discourses shed light on the problem.

For example, the problems of natural resources depletion and pollution engender a range of environmental discourses that offer various diagnoses of the root causes of these problems or, conversely, dispute their status as problems in the first place. These diagnoses of the causes or nature of environmental problems prompt recommendations for various courses of action that presumably follow from the combination of facts and values they posit.

Notably, some people find the problems of pollution and depletion to be the inevitable result of a human population that has grown too large for the carrying capacity of the planet; according to this perspective, pollution and resource depletion may be viewed as the symptoms of an overtaxed habitat, akin to the way that other animals overshoot their optimal populations and in so doing create environmental problems that threaten some of their members. Based on this discourse, which depends crucially on the idea of ecological limits to growth for its explanatory theory, the appropriate response to such problems is to limit or reduce the human population.

Other people see these problems as being caused primarily by overconsumption of resources by the affluent; to relieve these pressures, they counsel that big consumers scale back their consumption activities. Still other discourses lead to a diagnosis of problems such as those resulting from market failures, where resources are depleted because they are underpriced or heavily subsidized and pollution results from environmental externality. Yet others deny that resources are, in fact, being depleted or that pollution represents any serious threat to human health or welfare. Driving these various judgments are different explanatory theories and value systems, which together work to capture the essence of a problem and identify its proper solution.

While environmental theories are typically applied to ethics (i.e., the distinction between right and wrong actions undertaken by individual persons in the way that each of us interacts with the environment) and to politics (i.e., the just or legitimate rules or courses of action for public institutions and collective action as these decisions relate to the environment), the interaction between facts and values within environmental theories is also instructive for many healthcare decisions. An ethical question that depends on environmental theories might concern the moral permissibility of eating tuna caught with drift nets that also snare and drown dolphins; in such a case, consumer demand for the tuna that is not "dolphin safe" endangers an intelligent aquatic mammal that many think deserves some of the same protections that are afforded to humans by virtue of its similarity to us. A question for political theory might concern the limits on the allowable release into the air or water of known toxins such as sulfur dioxide or mercury, to be enforced by regulatory agencies like the Environmental Protection Agency, or the justice problems associated with locating toxic waste facilities near minority communities. Traditionally, ethical questions have been considered the provenance of environmental ethicists working in philosophy departments, while political questions have been addressed by political theorists working in political science departments. More recently, however, these disciplinary boundaries have been challenged by theorists on both sides, who often contend that ethics and politics are so intimately intertwined that such jurisdictional distinctions between them are increasingly irrelevant. If some action is morally wrong, they assert, this is relevant to politics, and vice versa.

This chapter introduces and briefly discusses several families of environmental theories, along with the implications of each family for ethical and political theories. Where relevant, implications of these environmental theories for policy making are considered. After surveying theories based on ecological limits, environmental value, holistic analysis, and distributive justice, current developments in environmental theories and their application to contemporary problems are briefly considered.

ECOLOGICAL LIMITS THEORIES

The first generation of normative environmental theories called attention to the finite stock of natural resources and capacity of the environment to assimilate pollution, drawing inferences for humans from laws of nature that were seen as applying to all species in similar ways. In one of the first works of this kind, Rachel Carson's (1962) largely explanatory work on pesticides and bird mortality called attention to the widespread dissemination of toxins within the environment and the often deadly consequences of human attempts to control aspects of the natural world.

Even more notably, Paul Ehrlich's (1968) population analysis and the "limits of growth" thesis proposed by the Club of Rome, a nonprofit international organization (Meadows, Meadows, Randers, & Behrens, 1972), established the idea of *carrying capacity* as a scientific concept with profound normative implications. According to this notion, ecological systems have the capacity to support a finite population of any given species, but beyond this threshold further growth in population is accompanied by ecological stress, decline in support capacity, ecological collapse, and the dying off of populations that "overshoot" the carrying capacity of their natural habitats. According to Ehrlich (1968), just as deer populations tend to expand beyond carrying capacity when their natural predators are eradicated, only to die back as available food becomes insufficient to support a growing population, so humans may also face ecological crises if population growth rates remain unchecked. The Club of Rome expanded this analysis through a sophisticated computer model that demonstrated increasing scarcity in a wide range of natural resources and ecological services, predicting future calamity if current trends were not corrected.

Garrett Hardin's (1968) analysis of "the tragedy of the commons" emerged from this limits literature, defending draconian intrusions into reproductive freedoms as the only solution to the population problem, which he characterized as a collective action problem that results from the absence of ownership in the environmental commons. More recent contributions to ecological limits theory include analyses of individual and group environmental impacts through the ecological footprint, which measures the resource use and waste production of a person or group based on the amount of land that would be needed to support that person's or group's consumption habits (Wackernagel & Rees, 1998). As with the first generation of ecological limits scholarship, the empirical analysis of ecological footprints—which scholars have calculated for most nations based on aggregate consumption and pollution patterns, and which several online calculators estimate for individual persons—implies specific moral judgments about permissible shares of resource production and waste assimilation capacity for each and posits that insidious harm ensues when those shares are exceeded. Recognizing an ecological limit may involve empirical measurement and projection from current trends, but it also contains a moral judgment about how persons or groups ought to control their behavior.

Ehrlich's work contains a strong prescription for sustainable population sizes, and the Club of Rome's analysis does so for sustainable consumption patterns. Ecological footprint analysis updates the role of ecological limits in setting the moral constraints on human action by noting the footprint size that is sustainable for a given population and then implicitly condemning environmental impacts that exceed this threshold. As environmental theory, then, ecological limits approaches derive implicit norms from observable facts combined with a concern for the future consequences of continuing trends, drawing their normative force from this tight connection between facts and values. If people want to avoid outcomes that all agree would be calamitous (e.g., famine, intensified conflicts over increasingly scarce resources), they suggest that patterns of behavior that the environment cannot support indefinitely must be altered. Scientific study of ecology yields the insights necessary for sustainable human living on the planet, but it also reveals the extent to which many current human activities are unsustainable and predicts dire future consequences of imprudent current action. Such theories, therefore, contribute to a discourse of environmental concern that Dryzek (1997) termed "survivalist" because of its focus on the necessary conditions for continued human survival on earth.

ENVIRONMENTAL VALUE THEORIES

The second generation of environmental theories developed accounts of value that encompass nonhumans or the environment itself as morally considerable or worthy of respect (Attfield, 1987; Taylor, 1986), giving rise to the academic field of *environmental ethics*. Value theory lies at the root of any normative claim about what ought to be done in personal or political life: It offers an account of what is genuinely important and why, of interests that must be taken into account in decision making, and of how various things or states of affairs figure into a larger hierarchy of value. Theories of environmental value aim to extend the moral value that is commonly attributed only to human beings and their experiences beyond humanity to other entities, typically supposing that the root cause of environmentally destructive behavior is a failure to adequately recognize the harm to valuable nature that such action causes. Thus, these theories bring previously excluded entities into the domain of ethics, decrying as wrong environmentally harmful actions that might previously have been condemned as imprudent but not immoral, and conferring moral status on nonhumans of various sorts, depending on the approach.

While utilitarian ethics has long held all sentient creatures to be morally valuable by virtue of their ability to experience pain, most moral and political philosophy before the advent of such approaches simply denied that nonhumans have any morally relevant interests. This conventional approach, now termed *anthropocentrism* for its assumption that only humans and their experiences have intrinsic value, was challenged by the hedonistic utilitarianism of Jeremy Bentham (1879/2007) more than two centuries ago, but the project of expanding ethics beyond human interests remained obscure until the latter half of the 20th century. Bentham's expanded moral community included the higher mammals with sufficiently advanced nervous systems that could feel pain; other approaches to environmental value theory expanded that community even further to include all or nearly all animals (Regan, 1983), all living things (Taylor, 1986), or whole ecosystems (Callicott, 1989; Leopold, 1949). In so doing, these new environmental theories challenged anthropocentrism in ethics, either on the basis of ontological claims about what constitutes a relevant difference between humans and other animals (Singer, 1975) or on the basis of empirical evidence concerning the experiences of other beings.

At the center of this challenge was a contested concept—*intrinsic* value, which non-anthropocentric environmental theories posited is at the core component of all normative judgment. Intrinsic value can, therefore, be contrasted with *instrumental* value. Things can be valuable in the latter sense when a person subjectively values them for some purpose that presumably reduces to human welfare; in contrast, things that are valuable in the former sense need no further referent to a human who values them for their service to human welfare because they are valuable in themselves. Proponents of anthropocentric value theories admit that land or nonhuman animals can have value, but they insist that this value is only instrumental to human welfare or that the capacity to confer value (a cognitive and subjective process through which estimates of worth are made) is attributable only to humans. For example, it might be seen as wrong under anthropocentric ethical theories to kill someone's dog or despoil a person's property, in that these nonhuman things are seen as having some value that would be lost through such actions, but their owners—rather than the dog or land itself—are the ones wronged by such actions. According to this view, a person can have moral duties *with respect to* nonhumans (e.g., to refrain from destroying) but cannot have duties *to* those nonhumans because they lack intrinsic value and, therefore, do not have moral status.

According to anthropocentric value theories, nonhuman nature (including individual plants or animals or whole ecosystems) has no morally relevant interests or good of its own, although persons may have interests in nature. It might be wrong to clear-cut a forest if this practice destroys someone's aesthetic appreciation of a striking landscape because human aesthetic experience can have moral value; even so, the forest has no value of its own, independent of this experience. Also, the wrongness of clearing a forest would depend on other sources of instrumental human value, such as that provided by the lumber and wood products yielded by timber harvests. Needless to say, the negative impacts of deforestation on other species would not be considered morally relevant by these accounts, except insofar as some lost species might in some way affect some human welfare interests.

Some environmental ethicists and political theorists have identified these kinds of anthropocentric value theories as the root cause of environmental degradation, suggesting that the failure to recognize intrinsic value in nature leads humans to exploit rather than conserve it. Things other than humans can be of intrinsic value, they argue, and, therefore, can be the object of moral obligations or political responsibilities, apart from any effect they might have on humans or their welfare (Goodin, 1992). Sometimes the opposing value theory to anthropocentrism is termed *ecocentrism* (for being ecosystem centered), and sometimes it is called *biocentrism* (life centered); both notions expand the notion of intrinsic value beyond humanity. Baird Callicott (1984) goes so far as to identify nonanthropocentrism with the scholarly field of environmental ethics, rejecting humanistic ethics as incompatible with ecological analysis and environmental protection. Robyn Eckersley (1992) subtitled her seminal book on environmental political theory "Toward an Ecocentric Approach" in recognition of her critique that anthropocentric political theories could not be reconciled with strong environmental protection.

Merely asserting that things other than humans contain intrinsic value does not by itself provide much guidance for environmental decision making, unless different kinds or sources of value can be meaningfully compared. For example, the construction of a hydroelectric dam that brings a new source of inexpensive electricity to a city but causes the extinction of an endangered species may not necessarily be wrong simply because that species is recognized as intrinsically valuable. The judgment made ultimately depends, instead, on how the value of cheap power for humans compares with the value of the threatened species.

Although few theorists had made serious attempts to develop a taxonomy of value that could make these kinds of comparisons feasible, Peter Singer (1975) argued that the life of a dog does have moral value, but less than that of a typical human life. Employing an updated version of Bentham's utilitarian ethics that treats pleasure as valuable and pain as bad, such that all sentient creatures have a moral interest in maximizing pleasure and minimizing pain, Singer claims that it would be morally permissible to kill a dog rather than a human if one or the other must die (if, for example, starving people and dogs on a lifeboat could be saved if they were to eat one from among their number), given the additional disutility that a human person would suffer in anticipation of his or her killing and the additional sorrow that this fate would cause for the person's family and friends. In this kind of analysis, the respective moral worth of persons and dogs depends on facts about their cognitive capacities and neural transmitters. Such facts assist in determining which of two valuable beings is more valuable than the other, which in turn dictates how ethical dilemmas are resolved.

Environmental value theories have been successful in critiquing anthropocentric biases in conventional ethical and political theories and calling attention to the pressing need to inform decision making with values that recognize the importance of human reliance on the natural world. In doing so, such approaches have spawned the scholarly fields of environmental ethics and political theory, and debates over value theory continue unabated in the scholarly journals from both fields. More recent work in both fields has turned from primarily ontological and meta-theoretical questions about value theory to the applied ethics and political theory topics through which such theories make their critical analyses. This shift in focus has been partly pragmatic and largely a result of the success of earlier scholarly work on value theory. Many philosophers now accept that nonhumans have noninstrumental value or interests that cannot be reduced to human welfare but wonder how such an account of value might inform potential solutions to current environmental problems.

HOLISTIC THEORIES

Individualistic environmental value theories constitute one approach to environmental theory, in that they aim to challenge the common presumption that things other than humans can be of intrinsic value and have moral worth. Their influence can be seen in the social movement for animal rights, for example, which asserts this sort of intrinsic value on behalf of nonhuman animals that are used in scientific research or raised on factory farms.

A subset of such theories goes even further in challenging the conventional individualistic basis of ethics by claiming that groups or whole ecosystems can have value of their own, beyond the sum of their constituent individual parts. For example, advocates of this position claim that an entire species is more valuable than all of its individual members, particularly when that species is threatened with extinction. To invoke a widely discussed case, the loss of a single snail darter may not be significant enough to halt a major construction project near its habitat, presuming that the project confers benefits to humans that outweigh any such loss, and as long as the entire species of snail darters is not threatened with extinction. When that individual snail darter is the last of its kind, however, the loss is often thought to be greater, perhaps trumping the project's economic value. Hence, legislation such as the U.S. Endangered Species Act confers no particular value on individual members of unthreatened species but places very high value on threatened or endangered species taken as a whole. Because an entire species represents an evolutionary line that cannot be replaced if it disappears, in the same way that an individual member of that species can be replaced by another member if one dies, its loss is viewed as more serious and weighty according to holistic environmental theories.

Perhaps the most famous of holistic environmental theories is Aldo Leopold's (1949) land ethic, which places ultimate moral value on whole ecosystems rather than on particular species or individual plants or animals. According to Leopold's core moral principle, "A thing is right if it tends to preserve the stability, integrity, and beauty of the biotic community. It is wrong if it tends otherwise" (p. 272). In contrast with individualistic ethics, where right and wrong are defined in terms of effects on individuals, Leopold's holism assumes that the whole "biotic community" is the relevant unit of analysis. Thus something might be right in that it is good for the whole system yet bad for one or more individual members of that community. For example, Gary Varner (1998) defends the "therapeutic hunting" of "management species" such as deer populations as bad for the individual deer that are culled in management efforts but good for the larger population of deer of which these individuals are part and also for the ecosystem on which that population depends. To the extent that Leopold's holistic value theory assumes the welfare of entire ecosystems to be more important than the welfare of their constituent members, as Callicott argues that it should, it is "holistic with a vengeance" (Callicott, 1989, p. 87).

Holistic theories need not necessarily posit that the interests of whole systems trump those of their individual members, and so they may avoid this call for sacrifice of individuals on behalf of whole systems that Callicott endorses. One might instead interpret Leopold's land ethic as asserting the moral considerability of ecosystems without in any way diminishing the moral importance of each system's individual members (Warren, 2000), much as Christopher Stone's (1974) assertion of the moral considerability of trees did not undermine the moral importance of the persons who might use those trees as resources.

Ultimately, however, such attempts to resolve the tension between holistic and individualistic value theories undermine the ability of ethical systems built with such value theories as their foundation to resolve hard cases where individual and systemic interests conflict. While still popular in some circles, such as among those philosophers embracing "deep ecology" (Devall & Sessions, 2001), holistic environmental theories have been significantly tempered by their former supporters in response to charges of advocating "environmental fascism." Today, they are more ecumenically structured, but less action guiding, in their effort to balance the sometimes competing interests of individuals and whole systems.

JUSTICE THEORIES

Whereas the previously mentioned approaches to environmental theory aim primarily to revise conventional ethics in order to take account of nonhumans in moral decision making, several other approaches to environmental theory apply to the domain of political theory and employ anthropocentric value theories when approaching environmental problems. Rather than invoking ethics on behalf of environmental protection, they work within concepts in political theory such as justice, understood in its distributive sense. *Distributive justice* theories take the distribution of "goods" and "bads" among persons to be the primary subject matter for justice, articulating principles for how those "goods" and "bads" should be distributed. For example, John Rawls's (1971) well-known account states that social goods such as income and wealth should be distributed so that inequalities in shares held by various individuals are justified only insofar as this inequality benefits society's least advantaged. Others (Anderson, 1999; Miller, 2001; Walzer, 1984) working in the distributive justice tradition claim that justice requires that a basic minimum of important social goods be available to all, or that inequalities of one kind of goods (e.g., wealth) not lead to inequalities in other kinds of goods (e.g., health). Regardless, these approaches assume that justice is an attribute of relationships between and among human persons and communities, rather than attempting to extend the concept to nonhumans.

Early efforts to theorize environmental problems through concepts of justice arose from Murray Bookchin's (1982) school of social ecology, which concentrated on the way that class divisions were often reflected in environmental problems and which saw sustainability as a component of social justice. Like social ecologists, ecofeminists (Plumwood, 1993; Warren, 2000) theorize that the root causes of environmental degradation are based in domination, whether toward women by men, toward developing countries by industrialized ones, or toward nature by industrial societies. Such theories avoid an explicitly distributive conception of justice, however.

Working within distributive justice theory, some environmental theorists have more recently seized upon the apparent injustice of the way that important environmental goods and hazards have been distributed among persons and groups of people. Robert Bullard (1990) coined the term *environmental racism* to describe the way in which hazardous waste facilities in the United States have been disproportionately located in poor neighborhoods largely populated by people of color, implicitly accusing the site selection decisions for such facilities of being unjust and giving rise to the *environmental justice* social movement. This movement later expanded the justice frame to include analysis of inequities in group recognition and participation, as well as injustice in distribution (Schlosberg, 2007), but remained primarily concerned with equity issues among human communities.

Justice-based environmental theories have been particularly prominent in areas related to the allocation of natural resources or the production of pollution, where those theories are able to specify what is unjust about certain patterns of resource use or pollution. Besides environmental justice concerns about connections between race and toxic waste, for example, justice-based environmental theories have been applied to the distribution of costs in global climate policy (Vanderheiden, 2008) and variability in the ecological footprints of nations and individual persons (Dobson, 1990). Social movements invoking the goals of "climate justice" or "environmental justice" demonstrate power- or justice-based environmental discourses and the theories on which they have been constructed. Although most such theories do not explicitly posit environmental values that are distinct from human concerns for justice, often they do endorse a program whereby environmental harm is avoided and nonhuman interests accommodated, even if the latter are not recognized as intrinsically valuable. Because they rely upon normative theories that were originally developed to articulate justified relationships among human persons and communities rather than between humans and nature, they can be more accurately called theories *for* the environment rather than *of* the environment. Nonetheless, they are action guiding and are regarded as a useful basis on which to theorize obligations with respect to the environment, and from which to design the institutions of a sustainable society.

SUMMARY

By the nature of professionalization within the scholarly fields of environmental ethics and political theory, a wide variety of apparently competing normative theories have been developed over the past four decades. Most such theories can be grouped into one of the categories described in this chapter, although proponents of competing theories within each of those categories continue to subject the validity of this taxonomy to debate. From the outside, it appears that scholars are deeply divided on questions of environmental theory and that no consensus on what constitutes the most plausible contemporary view exists. Within the field, however, there is considerable consensus on judgments concerning what are considered environmental problems and even rough agreement on how to solve those problems (Norton, 1991), even if scholars continue to disagree about why such issues are problems and what the best philosophical approach to theorizing those problems might be.

Nearly all scholars currently working within environmental ethics and political theory agree that the manner in which people understand value affects their behavior. Given this understanding, they seek to enlighten people about the nonhuman things that are, in fact, valuable to them, if not also intrinsically valuable. Most people agree on the critical need for reforming unsustainable practices, viewing sustainability as constitutive of right action and a just society, even as they disagree about the best way to incorporate such concerns into contemporary ethical and political theories. All environmental philosophers agree that environmental decision making should be more reflexive when it affects the environment, whether such decisions are personal or social and institutional, because narrowly instrumental action is widely viewed as responsible for most, if not all, current environmental problems.

Environmental theories of various kinds, like all normative theories, are designed to guide action and to bring our facts in line with our values and our values in line with facts. In this sense, they are consonant with other efforts to bring abstract knowledge to bear on practical problems in the world, and to resolve those problems in light of rationality and concern for others.

DISCUSSION QUESTIONS

1. How are facts and values related in environmental theories, and how might this relationship parallel decision making in healthcare ethics or allocation issues?
2. To what extent are environmental issues also issues of human health, and vice versa? Is environmental protection an aspect of public health?
3. Caring for the natural world is like caring for ill patients in some respects but different in others. Physicians and nurses often can know the wishes of the patients whom they treat, but can humans know how the natural world prefers to be treated? Insofar as we must hypothesize about the latter, does the way that we think about the best interests of patients who are unable to communicate their wishes resemble the way that nature's interests are considered?

REFERENCES

Anderson, E. (1999). What's the point of equality? *Ethics, 109*, 287–337.

Attfield, R. (1987). *A theory of value and obligation.* London, UK: Croom Helm.

Bentham, J. (2007). *An introduction to the principles of morals and legislation.* Mineola, NY: Dover. (Original work published 1879.)

Bookchin, M. (1982). *The ecology of freedom: The emergence and dissolution of hierarchy.* Palo Alto, CA: Cheshire Books.

Bullard, R. (1990). *Dumping in Dixie: Race, class, and environmental quality.* Boulder, CO: Westview Press.

Callicott, J. B. (1984). Non-anthropocentric value theory and environmental ethics. *American Philosophical Quarterly, 21*(4), 299–309.

Callicott, J. B. (1989). *In defense of the land ethic: Essays in environmental philosophy.* Albany, NY: SUNY Press.

Carson, R. (1962). *Silent spring.* London, UK: Hamish Hamilton; New York, NY: Fawcett Crest.

Devall, B., & Sessions, G. (2001). *Deep ecology: Living as if nature mattered.* Layton, UT: Gibbs Smith.

Dobson, A. (1990). *Green political thought.* London, UK: HarperCollins.

Dryzek, J. S. (1997). *The politics of the earth: Environmental discourses.* New York, NY: Oxford University Press.

Eckersley, R. (1992). *Environmentalism and political theory: Toward an ecocentric approach.* London, UK: UCL Press.

Ehrlich, P. R. (1968). *The population bomb.* New York, NY: Ballantine Books.

Goodin, R. (1992). *Green political theory.* Oxford, UK: Blackwell.

Hardin, G. (1968). The tragedy of the commons. *Science, 162,* 1243–1248.

Leopold, A. (1949). *A Sand County almanac.* New York, NY: Oxford University Press.

Meadows, D. H., Meadows, D. L., Randers, J., & Behrens, W. W. (1972). *The limits to growth.* New York, NY: New American Library.

Miller, D. (2001). *Principles of social justice.* Cambridge, MA: Harvard University Press.

Norton, B. (1991). *Toward unity among environmentalists.* New York, NY: Oxford University Press.

Plumwood, V. (1993). *Feminism and the mastery of nature.* London, UK: Routledge.

Rawls, J. (1971). *A theory of justice.* Cambridge, MA: Belknap Press.

Regan, T. (1983). *The case for animal rights.* London, UK: Routledge & Kegan Paul.

Schlosberg, D. (2007). *Defining environmental justice: Theories, movements, nature.* New York, NY: Oxford University Press.

Singer, P. (1975). *Animal liberation.* New York, NY: Random House.

Stone, C. D. (1974). *Should trees have standing?* Los Angeles, CA: Kaufmann.

Taylor, P. (1986). *Respect for nature.* Princeton, NJ: Princeton University Press.

Vanderheiden, S. (2008). *Atmospheric justice: A political theory of climate change.* New York, NY: Oxford University Press.

Varner, G. E. (1998). *In nature's interests? Interests, animal rights, and environmental ethics.* New York, NY: Oxford University Press.

Wackernagel, M., & Rees, W. (1998). *Our ecological footprint: Reducing human impact on the earth.* Vancouver, BC: New Society.

Walzer, M. (1984). *Spheres of justice: A defense of pluralism and equality.* New York, NY: Basic Books.

Warren, K. (2000). *Ecofeminist philosophy: A Western perspective of what it is and why it matters.* Lanham, MD: Rowman & Littlefield.

Chapter 14

Economic Theories

Sherry Hartman

INTRODUCTION

Given a budget deficit and a slowing but still growing percentage of the gross domestic product (GDP) devoted to health care, healthcare delivery and reform continue to be at the forefront of policy debate. In 2010, Congress passed historical legislation with the enactment of the Patient Protection and Affordable Care Act, commonly called the Affordable Care Act (ACA) or Obamacare. Throughout political and public discourse in the United States, differing economic philosophies and theories held by policy makers are evident. Controversy and resistance to the ACA have been pervasive and led to a Supreme Court ruling on the legislation. The act was deemed constitutional and implementation continues amid both support and opposition. In the 2016 presidential race, plans to amend or repeal the ACA factored largely into candidates' policy platforms. Ultimately, Donald Trump, whose position has been to repeal the ACA, was elected president, putting the legislation in a vulnerable position.

With the passage of the ACA, the public has become more aware of and concerned with healthcare delivery in the United States. However, commentaries continue to indicate (1) that the general public misunderstands the U.S. healthcare system and (2) that little is known about health economics and health care as a unique market situation. Having faced many classrooms of "citizens" aspiring to be nurses, I have struggled often to create some enthusiasm among undergraduate nursing students for economic ways of thinking about health care and nursing. Nurses focused on human care can easily be disconnected from the concerns of economic decisions.

The climate of the last few years has made it easier to persuade nurses that they have a stake in the public decisions being made and that they need to understand the economic arguments put forth either to justify or oppose the enacted reform, its continuing implementation, and new proposals. Advanced practice nurses, especially, beyond worrying about basic clinical skills and becoming licensed, have the professional experience to recognize both the economics of running a business and economic mandates that shape their practice every day and affect the lives of their patients (Buppert, 2015). They have to join the conversation. A favorite quip to my students was that they cannot join an ongoing conversation and say anything meaningful unless they have knowledge of what was said before they arrived. In this chapter, I attempt to lay the groundwork for taking part in the conversations based on economic theory.

Economic theory of market competition increasingly has been a major topic in the healthcare conversation, following on the heels of a general trend in the United States to view the market as efficient and government as inefficient. Opposition to the 2016 Democratic presidential candidate Bernie Sanders's proposal for a single-payer system exemplifies the latter view of government inefficiencies, including a "messy, fractious democracy" subject to powerful interest groups and a government "extremely bad at controlling costs" (McArdle & Bershidsky, 2016). The ACA somewhat increased government involvement in health care, and Sanders's single-payer proposal was considered a proposal for the federal government as sole manager of universal health care.

Commentary and debate on these programs often invoke the term "socialism," often in a pejorative sense. Understanding economics requires differentiating market economics from socialist methods and recognizing variations. Socialism is at times improperly used to describe any form of government control or intervention in production and allocation of resources. Properly used, it more narrowly refers to centralized state planning of the economy through nationalization of industry, with ownership of production and means of financing. The present U.S. healthcare system is primarily based on free market mechanisms. The only program that fits the policies of socialism—that is, the only program wholly planned and run by the government—is the Veteran's Health Administration (VHA). Providers and other workers in the VHA are employees of the government, and facilities are owned by the government. Closely related, Medicare is totally financed and services are paid for by the government. However, the government pays free market providers of those services. As a single payer, the federal government is the sole checkpoint for Medicare management. Medicare is one of many programs (e.g., workers' compensation, unemployment insurance, Social Security, health subsidies) run by the government. They are social programs, but not policies of socialism. Given that for many reasons, most experts believe the U.S. healthcare system will continue to be market driven (McArdle & Bershidsky, 2016; Reinhardt, 2013; Rice, Biles, Brown, Diderichsen, & Kuehn, 2000), the issues and inefficiencies of a socialist system are not covered in this chapter. Indeed, such a system is rare in any country. However, a balance of market forces and government intervention is relevant. Rice et al. (2000) note that in general the dichotomy between markets and government is a "false one" and each needs the other (p. 869).

Any discussion of the situation of health care begins with the process of collecting data on soaring costs, calling into question whether higher costs are related to higher quality, and making dire predictions of the consequences of failing to control costs. Some analysts and policy makers claim the competitive market as the superior option to bring efficiency to the system, as well as greater social welfare. The Reagan presidency was noted for early reforms relying on managed competition. Evidence in the 1990s indicated that increased competition did slow the growth of costs but had an ambiguous effect on efficiency, with concerns being voiced that consumers and the public were not receiving quality for their money spent and about the corporatization of health care. The numbers of uninsured and underinsured continued to increase, accompanied by claims that this increase was partially related to increased competition among insurance providers. The deep recession of the latter years of the first decade of the 2000s worsened the statistics and created a more urgent need to make decisions about healthcare resources in the United States. Implementation of the ACA addresses increased coverage, but there are conflicting claims about its effect on costs. A disappointment for many during the reform struggles was the failure to achieve universal coverage or a single-payer system. The involvement of employers and reliance on the competitive market of insurers and providers remain the mainstays of our delivery system.

Economics is considered both a social science and a foundational form of knowledge. All financial management is ultimately built on economics. In fact, accounting and finance are applied areas of microeconomics. Economic theory and research also guide policy makers, yet policy is but one familiar application of economic theory. Because it is a science of human behavior, it serves as a framework for exploring diverse phenomena. For example, Wagoner (2012) interestingly used previous economic theory to explore the generation of economic theory. Exploring the relationships between economic theory and nursing administration, researchers have found that economic theory is useful in the study of allocation of scarce nursing resources (Bartel, Beaulieu, Phibbs, & Stone, 2014; Jones & Yoder, 2010; Turkel & Ray, 2000; Uchida-Nakakoji, Stone, Schmitt, Phibbs, & Wang, 2016). This chapter aims to provide advanced practice nurses with broad and general understandings of the lens through which such varied application occurs. Using Fawcett's (1998) definitions, the chapter will look at how economists approach and examine phenomena of interest, conceptual models, and grand theories. It will also introduce the area of economic analysis, which is an application of economic concepts considered increasingly necessary in healthcare cost analysis and control, included in parts of the ACA, and thus, of interest to nursing.

The steps in theory analysis provided by nurse theorists (e.g., Fawcett, 2005; Parse, 2005) were inspiration for the discussion sequence in this chapter. Theories are best understood when attention is paid to their history and assumptions before turning to the concepts and relationships that make up the theory content. I cannot hope to present a comprehensive evaluation and critique of economic theory in this brief chapter, but I believe this is a helpful starting point.

Some healthcare economists raise serious objections to the prospect of relying on competition in health care, as economic theory would prescribe. It is especially important for advanced practice nurses to be aware of the potential problems with market competition.

Rice is one economist widely referenced for his arguments showing the misunderstanding of economic theory as it applies to health (Rice, 1998; Rice et al., 2000). He stated, "It is vitally important that we get our theory right when applying economics to health—and the key to this understanding is the validity of the assumptions" (1998, p. 6). After identifying assumptions and presenting the major concepts, several core assumptions that support concepts, relationships, and principles of marketplace competition are critiqued and then rationale is given for why they are invalid, often making specific reference to the case of health services.

THE HISTORY AND BEGINNINGS OF MAINSTREAM ECONOMICS

Although humankind has long engaged in reflection related to commerce and market exchange, modern economic thought developed only as society became increasingly industrialized. The move away from agrarian relationships to an industrial economy resulted in more socially interdependent relationships. Economics sought to understand the exchange of resources, which were assumed to be limited. Scarcity of resources is a basic assumption of economics. *Scarcity* is the concept of finite resources and infinite wants. Broadly, it means not having enough resources to satisfy all the needs or wants of humankind. Scarcity also means that resources have alternative uses. What is not spent on health care can be spent on food, education, recreation, and the like. Scarcity leads to rationing or competition for the limited resources.

Without scarcity, the science of economics would not exist. When people freely have all they want and need, there are no choices or exchanges to make, and no trade-offs among possible alternatives, and, therefore, no economic problem. The healthcare debate occurring today would not be necessary if there were no scarcity of health resources and no unmet needs for health care.

The phenomenon of interest for economics is human behavior in the choices and interactions taken to overcome the problem of scarce resources with alternative uses. Interestingly, one nurse scholar has grasped the assumption of scarcity itself as a problem and urges the use of quantum physics theory to assume abundance instead; with this perspective, we would see the human situation differently (Dunham-Taylor & Pinczuk, 2015). For the most part, economists do not question that the assumption of scarcity is valid, although abundance economics is not unheard of in the field and has even been considered discussion worthy at Harvard University (Heskett, 2006). Mainstream scarcity economics is addressed in this chapter.

Contemporary economics consists of many schools and branches, with variants existing within even orthodox economics. A significant amount of work in mainstream economics is applied economics using simple theoretical concepts. However, both applied and theoretical economics can be identified as microeconomics or macroeconomics. As implied, the difference between the two fields lies in the scale of focus.

- *Microeconomics* explains the behavior of individual markets and small economic units, such as individual household consumers, firms that produce goods or services, or governmental agencies, to see how they behave within a market. Individual behaviors often are considered in the aggregate. Areas examined could include human capital, competition policy, problems of industry, and the role of government in resource allocation. For example, microeconomic study of firms in the market underlies financial concepts such as normal profit, fixed costs, and variable costs.

- *Macroeconomics* allows economists to look at the "big picture" market, considering the aggregate functions of all the markets within the larger focus. Such issues as growth, unemployment, monetary policy, deficits, and inflation are of concern in macroeconomics.

Economic theory as it is known today is derived from schools of thought from the last few centuries that have become the building blocks for today's economic thinking. Ideas have been revised and some discarded, only to be revived later. **Table 14-1** offers

Table 14-1 Major Schools of Thought in Economic Theory

16th to 17th century: Mercantilism	Accumulation of gold and silver made a nation wealthy, and those who did not have these items naturally could obtain them only by selling more than they bought from abroad. Leaders intervened in the market with tariffs and subsidies to regulate trade and commercial activities. Promoted a materialist perspective.
18th century: Physiocratic	Reaction against the many trade regulations. French theorists opposed promoting trade, saw agriculture as the source of economic wealth, and advocated a laissez-faire policy (minimal government interference).
1776: Classical	Adam Smith publishes *The Wealth of Nations* in 1776. Land, labor, and capital are identified as factors of production contributing to a nation's wealth. The ideal economy is a self-regulating market guided by an "invisible hand," which leads self-interested individuals to produce the greatest good for society. The classical view adopted a laissez-faire policy but disagreed that only agriculture was productive. David Ricardo focused on income distribution among landowners, workers, and capitalists. Landowners conflict with labor and capital. Population and capital growth pushing against a fixed land supply raises rents and lowers wages and profits. Thomas Robert Malthus explained low living standards with the idea of diminishing returns. Rapid population growth against limited land meant diminishing returns to labor. Chronic low wages kept the standard of living from rising above the subsistence level for most of the population. Malthus questioned whether a market economy would tend to produce full employment. Unemployment is caused by too much saving, rather than too little spending in the economy. John Stuart Mill opposed earlier classical thinking that income from the market is necessarily distributed by the market and noted the differences between the two roles of the market. The market is efficient at allocating resources but not at distributing income. Society must intervene in the distribution of income.

(Continues)

Table 14-1   Major Schools of Thought in Economic Theory (*Continued*)

1960s to late 1900s: Marginalists	Added demand as a factor in determining price to the classicists' theory that production costs determine price. Demand depends on satisfaction gained from goods and services. Marginalists offered the basic analytical tools of demand, supply, and utility and developed a framework to use these tools. In a free market, the factors of production receive returns equal to their contribution—an idea used to justify distribution of income: People earn what their labor or property contribute to production.
Mid-19th century: Marxists	Capitalism is a phase of development, which will eventually destroy itself. At that point, private property will not exist. All production belongs to labor; workers are exploited by capitalist owners, who deny them a fair share of production. Competition for profit leads to adoption of more machinery. The resulting unemployed will rise up and seize the means of production.
Mid-19th century: Institutionalists	Individual behavior reflects a larger social context influenced by cultures. Economic self-interest is rejected as a primary motivation. Institutionalists argued against laissez-faire policy and advocated more equitable income distribution via government intervention and social reform.
Mid-19th century: Keynesians	John Maynard Keynes broke with convention with his General Theory of Employment, Interest and Money (1936). The Keynesian view argues against the classical view that falling wages and prices in a recession will eventually restore full employment. Instead, low prices and wages are seen as depressing income and preventing spending. Government should intervene in a recession to increase total spending. The Keynesian view remains the core of macroeconomic analysis.

Modified from SNBCHF. (2013). Major schools of economic theory. Retrieved from http:// snbchf.com/economic -theory/major-schools-of-economics/

an abbreviated look at these benchmarks in history. Current thought is commonly called *neoclassical economics*, which builds on the ideas of Keynesian theory and the work of classic thinkers. It is also often called *mainstream economics*. The concepts and principles presented in this chapter come from mainstream economics.

In the history of economics, the specialty of *healthcare economics* is a recently developed field. The origins of this field are credited to Nobel Prize–winning economist Kenneth Arrow (1963) based on his article published in *The American Economic Review* (Peterson, 2001; Savedoff, 2004). Arrow clarified the conceptual distinctions between health and other goals. Those factors that differentiate health economics from other areas include amount of government intervention, intractable uncertainty in many areas, asymmetrical information, and externalities. Among his many contributions, Arrow is especially well known for his theoretical insights on the economics of uncertainty. He argued that uncertainties in the incidence of disease and the efficacy of treatments lead to inefficient allocation of resources, which force nonmarket institutions to compensate for these inequalities. Hammer, Haas-Wilson, and Sage (2001) claimed that even decades after the publication of Arrow's seminal article and the introduction of more competitive forces as means to control costs, the same questions remain:

> What is the proper role of markets in delivering health care services? Can we base our health care system exclusively on private competition? What place should be reserved for government or for social mechanisms such as professionalism, nonprofit status or trust? Do these "non-market institutions" help markets overcome uncertainty, or do they replace markets that have failed because of information asymmetry? How does one define the proper boundary between market and non-market institutions? (p. 836)

Such questions fall within the realm of *normative economics*, which advocates for what ought to be and then judges how well the performance of a market or outcome of economic policies conforms to those values. The field of *welfare economics* deals with issues that are considered normative economics. *Positive economics*, in contrast, describes "facts" or "what is." Rice (1998) pointed out that unlike other social sciences, which predominately study and describe how people behave, prescription is more prevalent in positive economics such that "in economics one commonly sees the word 'ought' (e.g., people ought to maximize their utility otherwise they are being 'irrational'; to maximize social welfare a society 'ought' to depend on a competitive marketplace)" (p. 38).

In summary, early classical economists developed a full explanation of abstract, general laws or principles of the operation, functioning, and process of the liberal economy. That economy was a system consisting of free "private" producers, consuming households, and competitive markets. The neoclassical economists developed superior analysis of the economy with fuller solutions to many of the problems. Branches of specialized areas of economics exist, and healthcare economics is a relatively new specialized application of economic thought. However, a consensus that market forces, as theorized by traditional economics, are appropriate for healthcare services delivery is yet to be attained.

ASSUMPTIONS OF ECONOMIC THEORY

Advanced practice nurses in select fields are likely to have used clinical applications of some of the assumptions of classical economic theory in the form of social exchange theory. An example is study of provider interactions with patients and their attitudes to risk (Roth, Trautman, & Voskort, 2016). In *social exchange theory*, assumptions that were held about individuals in economic exchange relationships have been adapted to explain human interactions in all social contexts (Bielkiewicz, 2002). In addition to scarcity, as discussed in the

Table 14-2   Twelve Assumptions of Economic Theories

1. There are no externalities of consumption.

2. Individuals know what is best for themselves.

3. Individuals use reason to determine a balance in their choices.
   - They have the cognitive ability.
   - They have the time.

4. Individuals seek to maximize benefits and minimize costs of alternative choices (the most useful product or greatest reward for the lowest price).

5. Individual preferences are revealed by choices.

6. Individual preferences can be ranked.

7. Preferences are determined and stable over time.

8. Consumers have full and perfect information with which to make good choices.

9. Consumers know, with certainty, the results that will follow their choices.

10. Supply and demand are independently determined.

11. No one firm dominates the marketplace.

12. Firms seek to maximize profits.

Modified from Rice, T. (1998). *The economics of health reconsidered*. Chicago, IL: Health Administration Press.

previous section, several assumptions are held in economics. Rational behavior is a major assumption. Aspects of assumed rational behavior and other assumptions relevant to health care are summarized in **Table 14-2**. These assumptions will be revisited in the discussion of the concept of market failure, introduced in the following section.

CONCEPTS, RELATIONSHIPS, AND PRINCIPLES IN ECONOMIC THEORIES

Markets

Markets are the means by which buyers and sellers engage in trade. A market economy is based on private ownership of scarce resources. The market facilitates the efficient allocation of scarce resources through interactions of individual buyers and businesses that produce and sell goods or services.

Within the market, consumers seek to maximize their *utility*, which is determined by the bundle of goods they possess. They purchase their ideal bundle of goods based on preferences, the price, and their available resources. Consumers must make *trade-offs*, giving up some of one thing they like to get another thing. When they have reached their maximum utility given their resources, they quit trading.

Producers in the market seek to *maximize profits*, just as consumers seek to maximize utility. The profit motive drives producers' decisions. They purchase inputs and turn them into outputs through a production process. Firms seek to produce as much as they can by using the least costly mix of inputs. The two most important classes of inputs are *labor* and *capital*. Thus, production theory indicates that firms will try to use their inputs in the most efficient way and make output choices to maximize profits. Their actions are also socially desirable in conserving inputs and producing only what consumers will use.

Competition in the marketplace is the mechanism for setting price and quality. Producers compete for buyers of their products. Marketplaces that operate most efficiently will flourish; those that do not have satisfied consumers will close down. Price is the most common basis for competition, but competition can also be based on technical quality, amenities, access, and other factors if prices are stable.

Efficiency is an important concept related to production in the market. Efficiency refers to the practice of maximizing the production of goods or services while minimizing the resources required for their production (Penner, 2011). *Technical efficiency* is attained when a firm produces a maximum output with a given amount of inputs. *Economic efficiency* (production efficiency) occurs when the mix of inputs used to produce maximum output is the least costly possibility. Alternatively, given a certain cost for inputs, the outputs are maximized. *Allocative efficiency* entails minimizing the amount and thus the costs of inputs or using a set amount of inputs to produce outputs of greater value. At the level of the economy as a whole, allocative efficiency is a state of the market rather than a firm.

Eventually, an economy could reach the point where it is impossible to make someone better off (i.e., improve welfare) without making someone else worse off; this situation is referred to as *Pareto optimality*. According to economic theory of the market, under ideal conditions, a free or competitive market will reach a *competitive equilibrium* that is Pareto optimal. However, a Pareto optimal competitive equilibrium ensures only allocative efficiency, not equity. Equilibrium could occur in which one person has nearly all the output, while another has almost no output. Society may be better off with an inefficient use of resources and a better distribution of income (output).

The Production Possibility Curve

Economic analysis often is carried out under the assumption of economic efficiency. The *production possibility curve* measures the quantities of two goods that can potentially be produced with currently available resources and technology. It is a graphic representation of the trade-offs between the two goods. Points on the curve represent alternative combinations of inputs that will produce the maximum output. Points that lie above the curve are impossible production; points that lie inside the curve represent inefficient production. The production possibility curve depicts possibilities with fixed amounts of resources and technology. If either increases as the result of economic growth, the curve would shift outward to the right, indicating the potential for producing greater amounts of both products.

Opportunity cost is a concept related to the trade-offs that are made in the marketplace and made evident on the production possibility curve. A consequence of scarcity is that when resources are used to buy or produce one product, they are not available for other goods. Opportunity cost is the value of the forgone alternative service or product.

Demand

Demand is the force that drives market competition. Demand is the quantity a buyer is willing to purchase at various prices. The amount of a commodity that is produced is determined by the demand for it. In addition, in economic theory, demand forms the basis for evaluating economic welfare. The things people demand are, by definition, those goods and services that allow for their highest level of welfare given their available resources. If all individuals act and choose to maximize their utilities within their incomes, then society as a whole will also be at a welfare maximum.

Demand is represented by a demand schedule of the quantities a buyer is willing to purchase at different prices. When plotted on a graph, these data form a *demand curve*. According to the *law of demand*, as the price goes up, the quantity demanded goes down— an inverse relationship. Two kinds of changes can be depicted with the graph of a demand curve. A *change in the quantity* demanded is a movement *along the demand curve*. If a price changes from $2.00 to $4.00, for example, the quantity demanded moves to the left (down) along the curve, a decrease. A *change in demand* is represented by a *shift in the demand curve*: The quantity demanded will have changed at all prices. A shift of the curve to the *left* will mean that at all possible prices, the quantity demanded is *less*. A *right*ward shift means that at all possible prices, the quantity demanded is *greater*. It is important to keep these differences clear. Only one thing will change the quantity demanded (change along the curve): a change in price. There are several reasons why demand could change and shift.

Reasons for Demand to Shift

Shifters are factors other than price that influence the quantity demanded. Income has a powerful influence: Greater income equals greater demand at all prices. Goods for which changes in demand vary directly with income are called *normal goods*. If an increase in income is related to a decrease in quantity demanded, then the product is labeled as an *inferior good*. Similar to the effect seen with increases in income, insurance increases the quantity of covered services demanded because they are largely paid for by the insurer.

The price of related goods is another demand shifter. A *substitute* is any good that satisfies the same needs as the original product. If the price of a good rises and a substitute is available, demand will decrease for the original good as it is replaced with the substitute.

A good can also be related as a *complement*, a good closely related to a specific good or service. If the price goes up for one product, the demand curve for its complement will shift to the left (less demand), and vice versa.

Changes in preferences can shift demand, such as decreased demand for cigarettes as more consumers quit smoking. A shift may also occur from circumstances that change expectations; for example, a recession and fear of unemployment will shift the demand curve for goods with long-term payments to the left. Illness would make a person's demand curve shift to the right, as his or her demand for health care rises at all price levels.

Utility

Utility is a term used by economists to describe the pleasure or satisfaction that a consumer obtains from consumption of goods or services. This subjective measure is dependent on the consumer's tastes, preferences, beliefs, culture, and values. Although the concept of utility is derived from classical utilitarianism, modern economists reject the utilitarian assumption that utility can be measured or that one person's utility can be compared to another's.

The utility received from consuming a particular amount of a good is a consumer's total utility. *Marginal utility* is the addition to total utility that consuming just one more unit of the good or service brings to the individual. The *law of diminishing marginal utility* states that as consumption increases, marginal utility will decrease. Once an individual is saturated, additional consumption adds no additional utility. Eyeglasses are an example. One set provides a certain utility and a second set used as a spare will have a good deal of utility, but a fourth or fifth pair will be of much less use, and a tenth would hold no utility at all. The notion of marginal utility can also be illustrated with this example. If you have three apples, you have a total utility (enjoyment) from eating all of them. But the third will not be quite as "good" because you are already full—so your enjoyment of it is less than your enjoyment of the others. The third apple, then, contributes less to total enjoyment (utility). Marginal utility is what the last apple (unit) added to the total—always the smallest amount of all units. (Note: Usually, never say "always," because there is *always* some exception case!)

Supply

Supply is the quantity of a good or service that producers are able and willing to sell at a particular price. Like demand, supply determines market price and quantities. The *law of supply* states that there is a direct relationship between the price of goods and the amount supplied: As price increases, the quantity supplied will increase.

Similar to consumer demand, a seller's quantity supplied can be depicted with a supply schedule and a graph. A change in the quantity supplied is a *movement along the supply curve* because of a change in the price. A change in demand is represented by a *shift of the supply curve*. A shift of an original supply curve to a new curve located to the left results in a reduced supply at all prices. A shift to the right indicates an increased supply at all prices.

Reasons for Supply to Shift

Several factors can cause a shift in the supply curve. Two notable ones are changes in the prices of inputs and technology. Prices for inputs of labor, materials, and services from facilities can increase the costs of production. If inputs become cheaper, the supply curve will shift to the right and a greater quantity will be supplied at all prices. Conversely, higher prices for supplies will increase costs of production, so the supply curve will shift to the left, indicating less quantity supplied. Cost is highly important to producers. Producers are interested in total costs (the costs of all inputs needed to produce a given level of output), and they are interested in average costs (the total costs of production in a time period divided by the quantity produced in the same period). *Marginal cost* is the increase in total costs given one more unit of output. The *law of increasing costs* maintains that marginal costs increase with increased output, so total costs increase at an increasing rate as production increases. The corollary is the law of diminishing returns.

Technology-related changes can also cause a shift in the supply curve. For example, a technological breakthrough could lower the cost of production, shifting the curve outward to the right. Technology in health care can also be used to increase well-being and comfort, but not to reduce costs of production.

If there is a change in the number of suppliers of a product or if existing suppliers increase their capacity, total supply will increase and shift the supply curve to the right. For any single supplier of several products, if prices for one product fall and it becomes less profitable, the supplier will produce more of the profitable goods, thereby increasing the available supply of those goods and moving the supply curve to the right.

Equilibrium

Although demand and supply can be analyzed separately, in the market, decisions of producers interact with decisions of consumers. Supply and demand set the prices paid by consumers and the quantities of the goods and services delivered to them. When the demand for a product equals the supply for a product, the market is considered to be in *equilibrium*.

A simple narrative of what economists depict with graphs and equations is presented here. To demonstrate equilibrium, the supply and demand curves are plotted on one graph. Equilibrium is the point at which the two curves intersect. The intersection marks a point of equilibrium price and equilibrium quantity supplied. If a demand or supply shift occurs (for any of the reasons discussed previously), the appropriate curve will shift; along with the increase or decrease in either demand or supply, the equilibrium point will change to indicate a higher or lower price and higher or lower quantity demanded, as necessary. The relationships described and often shown on graphs allow economists to gather data and describe and make predictions about market activity. They can answer questions such as these: How has the price of a product changed? What caused it to change? What are the resource allocation implications of the changes?

Disequilibrium occurs when the quantities supplied and demanded do not balance. A *surplus* occurs when there is an excess of quantity supplied or a drop in the quantity demanded. A *shortage* is a market situation in which quantity demanded is greater than quantity supplied. In either of these instances of disequilibrium, market forces are put in play. The automatic actions of buyers and sellers, acting independently of one another, move the market price toward equilibrium. In a shortage, consumers are willing to pay more and then prices rise; in response to these higher prices, suppliers increase the quantity produced. In a surplus, producers lower the price, consumers buy more, and the market moves back to equilibrium.

Elasticity

In addition to theorizing about how equilibrium prices change as supply and demand change, economists have developed explanations of how demand and supply change in response to changes in prices and incomes. Such responsiveness is measured by *elasticity* of demand or supply. Both can be calculated by formulas:

$$\text{Price elasticity of demand} = \frac{\text{Percent change in quantity demanded}}{\text{Percent change in price}}$$

$$\text{Price elasticity of supply} = \frac{\text{Percent change in quality supplied}}{\text{Percent change in price}}$$

When the price elasticity of the demand ratio is greater than 1 (the percent change in quantity demanded is greater than the percent change in price), demand is said to be price elastic, meaning that it is very responsive to price changes. If the change in quantity demanded is smaller than the price change, the ratio is less than 1 and demand is price inelastic, or not very responsive to price. The same relationships hold for supply elasticity.

The same formulas can be used to determine income elasticity. To calculate the ratio, one would replace "change in price" with "change in income." Elasticity of demand for income is positive for a normal good: As income rises, demand rises. It is negative for an inferior good: With greater income, there is less demand for the good.

MARKET FAILURE

Economists who advocate the superiority of competitive marketplaces base their preferences on what would happen in an ideal, pure market. Based on the concepts and principles that have been described so far, in an ideal market the following occurs: On the demand side, consumers have a variety of choices for goods and services to purchase. For individual consumers in the health marketplace, these include choices among insurers, doctors, hospitals, home health agencies, pharmacies, medical equipment suppliers, and so on. Consumers maximize their satisfaction through self-motivated behavior and pick the quality they want for the price they are willing to pay. Income, tastes, preferences, and information about the product are all factors that influence their choices.

Consumers' choices reveal to suppliers whether their products are priced correctly and are of appropriate quality. Suppliers then adjust the price and quality of their goods to satisfy consumers. For suppliers in a competitive industry, there are strong incentives to minimize the costs of making their products and services. They can then be priced competitively to sell in the marketplace. Suppliers must be innovative and respond to customers' perceptions of quality.

These two behaviors—*benefit-maximizing behaviors of consumers* and *profit-maximizing behaviors of suppliers*—through the mechanism of the market produce the best patterns of production and consumption for society. Because each individual has attained the best outcome that can be personally reached, the welfare of all is socially optimal (Hartman & Bauman, 2016).

For the market to work in the manner described here, the assumptions listed in Table 14-2 must hold. Economic theorists recognize that the realities of the market often are not in accordance with the assumptions, creating *market failure*. In a failed market, the necessary competition does not occur as it should. Consumers and producers fail to take necessary actions and to make optimal choices. Market mechanisms fail to produce the best outcomes for achieving the best use of resources. Fair allocation, quality and cost control, and setting of social priorities that enhance social welfare—all of which are posited to be the gains associated with an effective market—are not realized. In practice, economic theory does not operate in the pure form; such markets do not exist.

ASSESSING ASSUMPTIONS FOR VALIDITY

Externalities, addressed in the first assumption in Table 14-2, represent uncompensated consequences to the utility of others when an individual produces or consumes some goods and services (Penner, 2011). The example of vaccinations is cited often to illustrate a positive externality. A consumer who gets a flu shot benefits other members of society who are less likely to get the flu when more people are vaccinated. Public consumption of tobacco creates a negative externality by creating a harmful environment for others.

Rice (1998) presented two more examples of externalities found in the market: one positive, one negative. Through an argument too long to summarize here, he showed that status concerns relative to others create demand in the market, thereby causing an overproduction of goods and services that convey status. Such increased production, however, does not encourage redistribution of wealth such that society is better off. The case of a positive externality is concern about others: An individual wants to help others. The problem with giving, which increases the individual's utility, is that if many individuals want to help others, soon too many people are tempted to become *free riders*. In a competitive market where caring for the poor and giving are voluntary, it will seem to people that their relatively small portion of caring/giving does not have an impact, so they will cease to care/give. As more people follow this path, too little money is redistributed. Rice discussed how taxes and subsidies could be a remedy in this case, but the point made here is the market operates inefficiently because of an externality: One person's desire to give has consequences for others' willingness to do so.

There are several challenges to the assumptions about individual actors in the market system. Assumptions 2 to 4 in Table 14-2 can be considered problems with rational decision making and perfect information. There are reasons to doubt that individuals do know what is best for themselves (Rice, 1998). It takes considerable time to work through Rice's carefully constructed evidence; just a sampling is summarized here with reasons why Assumptions 2, 3, 4, 8, and 9 are not met.

For Assumption 2, being the best to judge one's own welfare, Rice maintained that the many rules of society intended to hinder individual choice demonstrate that we make many public choices for other people for two reasons: (1) We believe that some individuals will not choose wisely on their own, and (2) in some cases, there are experts who know more. Some people do not choose wisely because they make decisions to enhance their status; others need protection from their obviously foolish waste of money.

Regarding Assumption 8, having full and perfect information, Rice included these points: (1) Authors in journal articles frequently call for more consumer education; (2) studies indicate that patients do not act as consumers by becoming aware of costs, seeking information, and shopping around for services; and (3) little evidence shows that consumers understand concepts of managed care and reimbursement. Brill (2013) presented an in-depth look at the maze of pricing mechanisms followed by hospitals starting with greatly inflated *chargemaster* rates, which are charged to self-pay patients and used as a starting point for discount negotiations with insurers. It is impossible for patients to negotiate the maze knowing these costs before delivery of care and therefore shop around for options and review their insurance limits. The complexity has created a need for specialists who are hired by consumers as *billing advocates* to negotiate discounts and drop unreasonable charges.

On knowing the consequences of consumption decisions, Assumption 9, Rice pointed out that for individuals to determine they made the right choices, they must answer many counterfactual questions, such as "Would the result have been different if I had seen a different physician than the one I sought?" (p. 73). Knowing what is best for themselves and having adequate information about options does not mean that individuals act rationally on that knowledge, as Assumption 3 would indicate. Rice cited several examples, such as informed smokers who continue to smoke, concluding, "When cognitive dissonance is important there is little reason to suppose that people will act in a rational manner" (p. 77). Regarding the expectation that patients are capable of using cognitive skills, Penner (2011) noted some physical and psychological barriers that can exist. In addition, emergency needs do not allow time for reasoned action. Consumers who are not knowledgeable or informed cannot make rational decisions and thus cannot act on their own behalf to maximize their utility, as Assumption 4 indicates. A further confounding of Assumption 4 is inherent in our system of third-party payers. Insurance lowers the price of care for individuals such that they are relatively price insensitive. The resulting increase in demand for care over what it would be without insurance is labeled *moral hazard* (Fuchs, 2015).

Another consideration here is the notion of *preferences*. To analyze this issue, Rice (1998) turned to both game theory and the concept of commitment. *Game theory* illustrates the importance of interdependencies between people, making the point that behavior that will make two individuals better off in their real preferences is not the behavior that will reveal those preferences (p. 79). *Commitment* can compel individuals to choose something they are committed to over an alternative that yields a higher welfare such that true preference is not evident. Assumptions 5, 6, and 7 in Table 14-2 are not met.

Assumption 10 brings up the problem of supplier-induced demand. In economic theory, it is assumed that supply and demand are independent of one another. Power lies with the consumer, but, in reality, physician suppliers are often viewed as agents acting on behalf of their clients. Thus consumer demand is subject to artificial demand, commonly called *supplier-induced demand* (Shi & Singh, 2015). In some cases, physicians own laboratories and invest in healthcare organizations, which can affect their impartiality in recommending the use of those resources. This problem, according to Rice (1998), is one of the most studied in all of health economics. He drew the conclusion that in spite of the difficulty of testing for demand inducement, sufficient evidence exists to doubt the independence of demand and supply curves in the physician's market. It is questionable whether Assumption 10 is valid.

For the market to work, Assumption 11 must be true or else market power will lead to market failure (Penner, 2011). A monopoly occurs when there are only a few competitors in the market, which cooperate to control production and service. Some monopolies are natural, such as when a rural hospital is the only community provider of acute care. In contrast, consolidation among healthcare networks of hospitals and multispecialty group practices gives large market shares to these groups. Mergers such as these create massive local market leverage. The ACA created policy to encourage savings through sharing in integrated provider groups called accountable care organizations (ACOs). ACOs promote coordination but also increase the likelihood of anticompetitive conditions (Baicker & Levy, 2013). Ramirez (2014) outlined the necessary efforts of the Federal Trade Commission (FTC) to balance consolidation trends in health care with prevention of mergers that will reduce needed competition. Assumption 11 is too often in question.

Do firms seek to maximize profits, as Assumption 12 declares? Notably, many providers in the healthcare arena operate on a nonprofit basis. (Again, there is a vast literature collection on this subject.) Managers in health, like their counterparts in other sectors, often seek to fulfill their firm's goals and objectives (i.e., quality care), rather than maximizing the firm's overall profit. Even if owners of a healthcare firm do want to maximize profits, they typically hire others as their agents to accomplish this task but, for differing reasons, some agents are not motivated, efficient, or trustworthy enough to meet those expectations. Assumption 12 is another often-refuted assumption.

The point behind enumerating the several ways in which the assumptions of market theory do not hold in the markets for healthcare products is to indicate the need for intervention in the market to overcome these failures. Policy and regulation, such as FTC antitrust enforcement to prevent monopoly and quality reporting and price transparency efforts to increase consumer choice information, are designed with economic concepts in mind to improve market functioning. The healthcare market needs assistance to work completely as theory would predict.

ECONOMIC ANALYSIS OF CLINICAL AND MANAGERIAL INTERVENTIONS

So far the chapter has reviewed the following topics: (1) the history of economic theory development, (2) the identification of assumptions that form the foundations for economic theory, (3) the major concepts and principles from mainstream economics, and (4) an assessment of the validity of some of the key assumptions. The chapter next addresses an important area of application of economic theory—economic analysis of interventions.

The startling increases in healthcare costs in recent decades and the many efforts to control them have dramatically increased the relevance of economic analysis of clinical interventions. In the ACA health reform bill passed by Congress in early 2010, considerable resources were designated for increased funding of comparative-effectiveness research in health care. However, the ACA has restrictions on use of cost-effectiveness studies to guide reimbursement decisions. Garber and Sox (2010) outline the methods and benefits of including cost-effectiveness with the closely related comparative-effectiveness analysis. Achievement of the same or better outcomes accompanied by smaller cost increases saves money for payers and increases profits for providers. In capitated systems, where keeping enrollees healthy is key to profitability, discovering strategies to increase disease prevention, self-care, or adherence to clinically beneficial treatments can also have payoffs. Economics, the field that was born out of the problem of scarcity, has developed methods to assist society in using scarce resources more wisely.

Healthcare administrators are finding that those methods for production and labor cost identification and measurement used successfully by business firms in the private sector now need to be adopted by or adapted in the healthcare arena. An analysis of interventions is designed to support decision makers, but not to make decisions. *Analysis* provides the framework for understanding data and information.

Four types of cost analysis are common, each with its own strengths and weaknesses. The individuals conducting the analysis need to know what each type of analysis accomplishes and what the relative advantages and disadvantages of each are so that they can choose the most appropriate approach. It is also important as a clinician to be able to interpret, and make decisions based on, study findings.

Cost Analysis

A major contribution of economics to analysis is *cost analysis*. There are three tasks in measuring: (1) clarifying the perspective taken, (2) identifying the resources used, and (3) identifying the opportunity costs of those resources. Which costs are relevant depends on the stakeholder involved. Customers, managers, boards, clinicians, and a healthcare system will all identify costs from their perspective. The authority for conducting such studies in the United States is the Panel on Cost Effectiveness in Health and Medicine, which was convened in 1993 by the U.S. Public Health Service (Chang, Price, & Pfoutz, 2001). This panel first recommended assuming the broadest perspective—society as a whole. This approach recognizes all costs, no matter where or to whom they accrue.

Costs equal the volume of resources used for an intervention multiplied by the opportunity costs of those resources (Lee, 2009). To capture all costs, constructing a clinical pathway and developing a good clinical understanding of an intervention itself are helpful. Opportunity cost usually is equivalent to what was paid for a resource, but if it is old or no longer available, valuation of its best alternative use has to be filled in as a substitute. Costs include both *direct costs* and *indirect costs*. For health services, three categories of costs are included: (1) the cost of an intervention, (2) costs borne by patients and their families, and (3) external costs borne by the rest of society. Some costs must be *discounted*. In economics, in recognition of the "time value of money," a dollar today is more valuable than a dollar in the future. Thus, any expenditures or costs incurred in the future must be discounted back to a *present value* using a *discount rate*.

Cost of illness studies estimate the total monetary effects of a specific disease or condition. This information is used for public planning and to estimate the costs of health care and the financial burden of disease and illness.

Cost minimization analysis is the simplest comparison analysis. Only two steps are needed: (1) identifying the expected costs for each option and (2) showing that the lowest-cost option has outcomes at least equal to the outcomes for the alternative. It can be difficult sometimes to show evidence that the outcomes are comparable or that the lowest-cost option is superior or at least equal.

Cost–benefit analysis is a method used to compare benefits in terms of disease prevention with the costs of a program. In this analysis, benefits are measured in monetary terms.

Cost–benefit analysis is the principal method used to evaluate decisions involving public expenditures. Decisions are biased toward alternatives providing the greatest net benefit, which is the greatest level of economic efficiency. One of the drawbacks of using this method in health care is the difficulty of placing a dollar value on outcomes, such as pain or loss of life. Methods developed by economists in this regard are quite controversial (Lee, 2009).

In conducting a *cost-effectiveness analysis*, which is sometimes considered a more acceptable alternative for health care, a ratio is calculated in which health outcome is measured in health-related units, such as number of infections avoided or years of life saved. The cost for the treatment or intervention is measured in dollars, so results are presented on the basis of cost per case prevented or cost per life saved. The point is to compare the relative value of different interventions in creating better health or longer life. Costs of alternative interventions are compared based on a single nonmonetary outcome.

SUMMARY

Healthcare professionals who become familiar with the content of this chapter will experience a sense of comfort when they enter into a conversation with others about economics and health care. Although this attempt at an orderly presentation could seem to confine economics to a static set of beliefs, it is a mistake to think that the real-world conversation will be confined to a narrow or orthodox set of ideas. Any explanation of core ideas tends to be a backward look, but, as is the case with nursing theory, at any point in time, a successful discipline will have hundreds of new ideas being tried and tested.

Collander, Holt, and Rosser (2004) stated over 10 years ago that they expected new ideas to change the way economics is done. Their interviews with "cutting-edge" economists provided evidence that the orthodoxy of economic thought—rationality, greed, and equilibrium—was being challenged by another set of assumptions—purposeful behavior, enlightened self-interest, and sustainability. According to these authors, theories and ideas from a "new economics" are already recognizable to other professionals and the lay public. The popular press is discussing behavioral economics, agent-based models, evolutionary game theory, and experimental economics. It is exciting to consider how the specialized field of healthcare economics will be influenced by insights brought by new and revised theories. Equally encouraging is the availability of large data sets and dramatic growth in computing power in recent years that allow researchers in economic analysis to make greater sense of economic information (Jones, Rice, d'Uva, & Balia, 2012). We remain hopeful that we will apply new knowledge wisely to achieve society's goals, or at least to achieve improved efficiency and equity in health care.

DISCUSSION QUESTIONS

1. One of the assumptions of economic theory is that producers of products and consumers of products act independently of one another, without influencing one another. Is this

assumption valid in health care? How do providers and consumers act? Are they independent? Is there any incursion of the provider into the consumer role? Of the consumer into the production role? Think about economic theory and how well the "production of health" conforms to the theory.

2. In theory derivation, one can shift terminology or structure from one theoretical field or context to another. Which concepts or principles from economic theory could be useful to conceptualize phenomena of interest to nursing?

3. From the individual's point of view, what conditions determine the allocation between health and other goods?

4. Can the often volatile pattern of human behavior ("sinning against health as long as health is good; sacrificing everything for health when health is bad") be brought into line with rationality? Or are individual preferences inconsistent, implying that medical experts should perhaps determine the appropriate amount of preventive behaviors?

5. Can the economic concept of substitution be applied to health production even though situations can easily be envisioned in which only medical services (rather than one's own health-enhancing efforts) offer the prospect of improvement?

6. Is there a research question from your practice that could be situated in an economic framework for study? Which sorts of nursing questions can you imaginatively explore using economic concepts and analysis?

REFERENCES

Arrow, K. (1963). Uncertainty and the welfare economics of medical care. *The American Economic Review, 53*, 941–973.

Baicker, K., & Levy, H. (2013). Coordination versus competition in health care reform. *The New England Journal of Medicine, 369*(9), 789–791.

Bartel, A. P., Beaulieu, N. D., Phibbs, C. S., & Stone, P. W. (2014). Human capital and productivity in a team environment: Evidence from the healthcare sector. *American Economic Journal: Applied Economics, 6*(2), 231–259.

Bielkiewicz, G. M. (2002). Theories from the sociological sciences. In M. McEwen & E. M. Wills (Eds.), *Theoretical basis for nursing* (pp. 229–249). Philadelphia, PA: Lippincott Williams and Wilkins.

Brill, S. (2013, February 20). Bitter pill: Why medical bills are killing us. *Time*. Retrieved from http://www.uta.edu/faculty/story/2311/Misc/2013,2,26,MedicalCostsDemandAndGreed.pdf

Buppert, C. (2015). *Nurse practitioner's business practice and legal guide* (5th ed.). Burlington, MA: Jones & Bartlett Learning.

Chang, C. F., Price, S. A., & Pfoutz, S. K. (2001). *Economics and nursing: Critical professional issues*. Philadelphia, PA: F. A. Davis.

Collander, D. E., Holt, R. P. F., & Rosser, J. B. (2004). *The changing face of economics: Conversations with cutting edge economists*. Ann Arbor, MI: University of Michigan Press.

Dunham-Taylor, J., & Pinczuk, J. Z. (2015). *Financial management for nurse managers* (3rd ed.). Burlington, MA: Jones & Bartlett Learning.

Fawcett, J. (1998). *The relationship of theory and research* (3rd ed.). Philadelphia, PA: F. A. Davis.

Fawcett, J. (2005). *Contemporary nursing knowledge: Analysis and evaluation of nursing models* (2nd ed.). Philadelphia, PA: F. A. Davis.

Fuchs, V. R. (2015). Major concepts of health care economics. *Annals of Internal Medicine, 162,* 380–383.

Garber, A. M., & Sox, H. C. (2010). The role of costs in comparative effectiveness research. *Health Affairs, 35(6),* 1805–1811.

Hammer, P. J., Haas-Wilson, D., & Sage, W. M. (2001). Kenneth Arrow and the changing economics of health care. Why Arrow? Why now? *Journal of Health Policy, Politics, and Law, 26,* 835–849.

Hartman, S., & Bauman, D. (2016). Economics of health care. In K. S. Lundy & S. Janes (Eds.), *Nursing in the community: Caring for the public's health* (3rd ed., pp. 157–185). Burlington, MA: Jones & Bartlett Learning.

Heskett, J. (2006). What happens when the economics of scarcity meets the economics of abundance? *Working knowledge: A first look at faculty research.* Harvard Business School. Retrieved from http://hbswk.hbs.edu/item/5469.html#original

Jones, A. M., Rice, N., d'Uva, T. B., & Balia, S. (2012). *Applied health economics* (2nd ed.). London, UK: Routledge Taylor and Francis Group.

Jones, T. L., & Yoder, L. (2010). Economic theory and nursing research: Is this a good combination? *Nursing Forum, 45,* 40–53.

Lee, R. H. (2009). *Economics for healthcare managers* (2nd ed.). Chicago, IL: Health Administration Press.

McArdle, M., & Bershidsky, L. (2016, January 22). Health care's continental divide. *Bloomberg View.* Retrieved from https://origin-www.bloombergview.com/articles/2016-01-22/health-care-s-continental-divide

Parse, R. R. (2005). Parse's criteria for evaluation of theory with a comparison of Fawcett's and Parse's approaches. *Nursing Science Quarterly, 18,* 135–137.

Penner, S. (2011). *Introduction to health care economics and financial management.* Philadelphia, PA: Lippincott Williams & Wilkins.

Peterson, M. A. (2001). Editor's note: Kenneth Arrow and the changing economics of health care. *Journal of Health Policy, Politics, and Law, 26,* 823–828.

Ramirez, E. (2014). Antitrust enforcement in health care—controlling costs, improving quality. *The New England Journal of Medicine, 371,* 2245–2247.

Reinhardt, U. (2013, November). A conversation with Uwe E. Reinhardt, PhD: Health care deserves more respect. *Managed Care.* Retrieved from http://www.managedcaremag.com/archives/2013/11/conversation-uwe-e-reinhardt-phd-health-care-deserves-more-respect

Rice, T. (1998). *The economics of health reconsidered.* Chicago, IL: Health Administration Press.

Rice, T., Biles, B., Brown, E. R., Diderichsen, F., & Kuehn, H. (2000). Reconsidering the role of competition in health care markets: Introduction. *Journal of Health Policy, Politics, and Law, 25(5),* 863–873.

Roth, B., Trautman, S. T., & Voskort, A. (2016). The role of personal interaction in assessment of risk attitudes. *Journal of Behavioral and Experimental Economics, 63,* 106–113.

Savedoff, W. D. (2004). Kenneth Arrow and the birth of health economics. *Bulletin of the World Health Organization, 82.* Retrieved from http://www.scielosp.org/scielo.php?pid=S0042-96862004000200012&script=sci_arttext

Shi, L., & Singh, D. A. (2015). *Delivering health care in America: A systems approach* (6th ed.). Burlington, MA: Jones & Bartlett Learning.

Turkel, M. C., & Ray, M. A. (2000). Relational complexity: A theory of the nurse-patient relationship within an economic context. *Nursing Science Quarterly, 13*, 307–313.

Uchida-Nakakoji, M., Stone, P. W., Schmitt, S., Phibbs, C., & Wang, Y. C. (2016). Economic evaluation of registered nurse tenure on nursing home resident outcomes. *Applied Nursing Research, 29*, 89–85.

Wagoner, R. E. (2012). The social construction of theoretical landscapes: Some economics of economic theories. *American Journal of Economics and Sociology, 71*, 1186–1204.

Chapter 15

Theories of Organizational Behavior and Leadership

Sandra Bishop

INTRODUCTION

> Theories are used in management not to mirror reality but to help explain it. They may do so deductively by helping us to slot the behavior of organizations into categories, but they must also do so inductively by providing the concepts through which we can see new things, and so make better diagnoses. (Mintzberg, 1989)

Theories of organizational behavior "are important because they continue to influence the assumptions people in organizations make" (Daft & Noe, 2001, p. 6). Theories of organizational behavior and leadership have an interesting history, and the unique principles and processes of each theory have remained substantially consistent in application over time. Although the earlier organizational behavior theories are not as popular as they were in times past, they remain the foundation for more contemporary theories. This chapter provides an overview of the classical, neoclassical, and modern organizational theories.

CLASSICAL ORGANIZATIONAL THEORY

History reveals that thinking about organizations began in the ancient civilizations, such as with the Sumerians (Sullivan & Decker, 2005). Organizational thinking continued sporadically but remained mostly unfamiliar until the Industrial Revolution, when the school of thought evolved to one of organizational structure and efficiency where individuals functioned with extremely defined tasks to accomplish the main purpose of the organization (see **Box 15-1**).

Box 15-1 Classical Theory
Classical theorists pioneered ideas related to organizational behavior and leadership. As their theories were conceived, a merger of the concepts of scientific management, administrative theory, and bureaucratic theory began to occur. Considering these concepts, answer the following questions: 1. Are the principles of scientific management useful today in the healthcare industry? If so, where and how? If not, explain why. 2. Is a bureaucracy necessary to minimize chaos in today's healthcare organizations? Defend your answer.

Frederick Winslow Taylor: Principles of Scientific Management

The determination of the best method of performing all of our daily acts will, in the future, be the work of experts who first analyze and then accurately time while they watch the various ways of doing each piece of work and who finally know from exact knowledge—and not from anyone's opinion—which method will accomplish the results with the least effort and in the quickest time. (Taylor, cited in Crainer, 2003, p. 49)

Frederick Winslow Taylor first addressed his views of management in the classic book *The Principles of Scientific Management*, written in 1911. Taylor conducted extensive studies of steel workers and analyzed each worker's task in relation to the tools used, the design of the tools, how the worker held and used the tools, and so on. Taylor theorized that there was one best way to accomplish each step in the production of work, and he applied the scientific method to discover that best way. Taylor believed that managers should be as detailed with the assignment of tasks and supervising workers as workers should be with the structure of task performance. In his view, increased productivity, rewards, and salaries should be tied to production. The manager's responsibility, then, is to scientifically determine the best way to do a job, to select the best employee for the job, to train the employee, and to share the responsibility for results with the workers. This stepwise management practice became known as *Taylorism*.

At the time when Taylor was developing his ideas, workers and managers generally were considered to have opposing ideals and values. Moreover, managers did not take responsibility for the work of their subordinates. Taylor contended, however, that workers and managers shared the responsibility for production. Taylor's systemized methods for dividing work for workers and managers into the smallest elements and standardizing assignments were intended to maximize efficiency.

When scientific management first became popular in the early 20th century, its methods replaced rule-of-thumb standards and traditional methods. Unfortunately, Taylor's methods had an unintended effect: Many jobs were changed into a succession of dull tasks, and many people believed that such methods diminished the role of the manager. Some workers disliked Taylor's approach because it standardized procedures and thus prohibited creativity in much of their daily work. Taylor's critics argued that scientific management dehumanized workers and placed people second to production. Other people supported his work and believed that his methods greatly improved the working conditions of the era (Johnson, 2009). Whether Taylor's methods were appreciated or not, he certainly changed the way organizational leaders viewed workers and managers.

Taylor also is credited with being the first theorist to contribute to the organization and technology of the factory system, such as through the introduction of assembly lines (Nelson, 1980). Taylor's management principles continue to be translated into today's workplace in the form of employee education, goal setting, and performance incentives (McShane & Von Glinow, 2005).

Henri Fayol: General Principles of Administration

Management . . . is neither an exclusive privilege nor particular responsibility of the head or senior members of the business; it is an activity spread, like all other activities, between head and members of the body corporate. (Fayol, as cited in Parker & Ritson, 2005, p. 182)

Henri Fayol is considered to be the first author to develop a complete administrative theory. In the early 1900s, Fayol suggested that management consists of 14 basic but flexible universal principles: (1) specialization and division; (2) formal authority based on the job, not the person; (3) discipline; (4) unity of command, one boss per person; (5) unity of direction, orders coming from one boss; (6) group interests over individual interests; (7) fair and equitable pay; (8) centralizing communication and authority; (9) scalar chain; (10) an orderly work environment; (11) equity; (12) stability of personnel; (13) individual initiative; and (14) esprit de corps—harmony and unity in the organization (Johnson, 2009).

Fayol recognized that management is universal, no matter what the industry. In particular, Fayol considered administration to be the "art of managing people" (Breeze, 1981, p. 102), and in his theory he stressed the concepts of coordination and specialization. He also included the concepts of organizing, planning, controlling, and coordinating in his theory of management. The 14 principles, along with these concepts, were the foundation for his approach to organizational design, chain of command, and span of control (Brunsson, 2008).

Although Fayol's principles were based on his own experiences rather than on empirical research, he offered a language to communicate management theory. As a consequence, he is credited with initiating a move toward management thought that focuses on management of the total organization. Unlike Taylor and his followers, who prescribed sets of all-encompassing principles, Fayol hoped to arouse debate from which a substantial theory of management might emerge (Parker & Ritson, 2005).

Max Weber: Bureaucratic Theory

Bureaucratic and patriarchal structures are antagonistic in many ways, yet they have in common the most important peculiarity: permanence. (Weber, as cited in Eisenstadt, 1968, p. 3)

During roughly the same era that Taylor and Fayol were developing scientific management and principles for management, Max Weber was developing a theory of bureaucracy. Weber's bureaucratic theory extended Taylor's theory and emphasized the need to reduce ambiguity and diversity in organizations. Weber believed in the value of a hierarchical structure and recognized the significance of specialization and the necessity of division of labor. In addition, he endorsed the idea of promotion based on merit and impersonal rules. Three forms of legitimate authority were identified in his theory: (1) rational or legal authority, (2) traditional authority, and (3) charismatic authority. Weber believed that having rational or traditional authority is most stable for administrators (Johnson, 2009). He considered bureaucracies to be suitable settings in which administrators could use rational authority because bureaucratic organizations are bound to analyzable rules (Eisenstadt, 1968).

As one of the founders of social science, Weber defined bureaucracy as "the means of carrying 'community action' over into rationally ordered 'societal action'" (Weber, cited in Eisenstadt, 1968, p. 75). Bureaucracy, in his view, was considered a tool or power instrument. In a bureaucracy, he suggested, the importance of individuals is not emphasized, but rather the rules and offices of the organization are valued. The established offices and policies remain part of the organization, even if individuals holding offices are not. According to Weber, a good bureaucrat worries about the means, not the ends (Hargreaves, 2006). Thus, in contrast to a process of aristocratic ascendancy, bureaucrats should be selected for office based on their skills, not on their ancestry (Sager & Rosser, 2009). Weber believed that the masses cannot rule without chaos; once it is well established, a bureaucracy is seen as a tool to combat chaos that is difficult to destroy. Over the years, Weber's work has been criticized for not distinguishing between position or line authority and staff or expert authority.

NEOCLASSICAL ORGANIZATIONAL THEORIES

Human Resource Theory: The Hawthorne Experiments

The point of view which gradually emerged from these studies is one from which an industrial organization is regarded as a social system. (Roethlisberger & Dickson, 1967, p. 551)

One of the more powerful movements in the development of human relations theory stemmed from a study conducted at the Western Electric plant in Hawthorne, Illinois, a city bordering Chicago. Serendipitously, though the study was begun under the auspices of interest in worker efficiency and output, the data from the Hawthorne study bridged scientific management and human relations theories. The large Western Electric organization covered a wide range of occupations and amassed a huge array of equipment. In 1924, researchers working in conjunction with the National Research Council of the National Academy of Sciences undertook a study at the Hawthorne plant with the purpose of determining the "relation of quality and quantity of illumination to efficiency in industry" (Roethlisberger & Dickson, 1967, p. 14). Essentially, the initial research question guiding the study was "Does increased lighting intensity increase productivity?" Careful attention was given to the selection of workrooms and types of illumination used. The study was done experimentally with test and control groups and produced surprising results—high intensity, low intensity, or no change in intensity of lighting seemed to have no relationship to the workers' output. However, the researchers believed that something "screwy" was happening with the experiments. They wondered if the unexpected results were related to the researchers, the workers, or the data. Rather than being discontinued, the research was continued for more than 10 years. Study methods such as observation and interviews were added to the experimental methods to learn about the thoughts and feelings of the workers.

From the results of the study emerged a new view of organizations as large social systems. Two major functions of the organization were identified: the production of a product and satisfaction among the individual workers in the organization. From these functions, researchers identified two facets of the overall organization: a technical organization (e.g., products, tools, materials) and a human organization (satisfied workers; Roethlisberger & Dickson, 1967).

Critics of the Hawthorne study concluded that the Industrial Revolution had caused workers to lose a sense of work-related security and camaraderie. Although researchers originally planned to manipulate the esthetics of the work environment and determine how such changes affected quality and productivity, they soon discovered that *any* change that involved increased attention to employees was sufficient to improve productivity. In other words, it was the attention to employees and the study itself that made the difference—a phenomenon now known as the *Hawthorne effect* (Johnson, 2009). As stated by Filley and House (1969), "Perhaps the most lasting contribution of the Hawthorne studies themselves was their emphasis on the proposition that a human problem to be brought to a human solution requires human data and human tools" (p. 23).

The Economy of Incentives

Careful inspection of the observable actions of human beings in our society—their movements, their speech, and the thought and emotions evident from their action and speech—shows that many and sometimes most of them are determined or directed by their connection with formal organizations. (Barnard, 1938, p. 3)

Chester Barnard (1938) also studied and theorized about individuals and their relationships in organizations. Like the Hawthorne researchers, Barnard came to view workers as having social, behavioral, and psychological dimensions. Barnard introduced one of the first neoclassical theories by defining an organization as "a system of consciously coordinated personal activities or forces" (p. 72). Coordinated activities, he suggested, include the physical environment, the social environment, individuals, and other variables. Barnard argued that organizations cannot operate if individuals do not communicate and are not willing to contribute to common goals (Hellriegel & Slocum, 1976). He viewed organizations as systems that should be treated as a whole because all of their parts are related in a significant way. In addition, Barnard viewed organizations as hierarchies with defined authority and clear communication linkages. The success of each organization was linked to the leader's ability to generate a cohesive environment.

Other aspects of Barnard's work focused on fair treatment of workers and humane leadership. His work informed much later research on job design, participative decision making, worker satisfaction, culture, behavior, supervision, and groups, to name a few areas. Barnard is considered a transitional theorist because his theory contains elements drawn from both classical and neoclassical methods (Barnard, 1938).

The Proverbs of Administration

The anatomy of the organization is to be found in the distribution and allocation of decision-making functions. The physiology of the organization is to be found in the processes whereby the organization influences the decisions of each of its members—supplying these decisions with their premises. (Simon, 1976, p. 220)

When Herbert Simon dissected the administrative principles proposed by Taylor and Fayol, he decided that they were contradictory. In developing his own theory, Simon considered a description of administrative situations and the weight of administrative criteria. He viewed the primary administrative situations to be allocation of functions and formal structures of authority. After investigating the science of administration, Simon proposed that administrative science can be theoretical and practical. He viewed the behaviors of human beings in organized groups as the sociology of administration. Thus, Simon proposed that the practical science of administration "consists of propositions as to how men would behave if they wished their activity to result in the greatest attainment of administrative objectives with scarce means" (Simon, 1976, p. 253).

Simon (1976) believed that "the hierarchy of means and ends is as characteristic of the behavior of organizations as it is of individuals" (p. 63). In other words, the work at one level in the organization serves as the means to accomplish the end purpose of the level above it in the organizational hierarchy. These hierarchal relationships are seen as guiding

Box 15-2   Neoclassical Theory

Neoclassical theorists focused on the behavior of workers, speaking to the issues intrinsic to classical theory, such as rigidity and structured work environments. Classical theory squelched workers' growth and creativity, whereas neoclassical theory exhibited a concern for workers. Based on these points, answer the following questions:

1. Are the results of the Hawthorne study relevant to advanced nursing practice today? Explain your answer.
2. How are authority and leadership differentiated? What subconcepts can be used to characterize each of these broad concepts?
3. Do nurses today respond more positively to authority or leadership?
4. Identify and discuss examples of healthcare organizations and departments that use the principles of neoclassical theory.

decision making from the bottom up. In his work, Simon (1976) defined the means–end chain sequence of related elements, from behavior to resulting values.

Whereas Taylor and Simon were attentive to workers, Weber and Fayol focused on the organization. All of these theorists believed that the role of administration is to maintain balance within the organization. Consequently, they emphasized managers' ability to manipulate workers and their environments.

The neoclassical theorists viewed hierarchies, principles, authority, rules, and goals as important concepts. These theorists focused on the behavior of workers (see **Box 15-2**).

MODERN ORGANIZATIONAL THEORIES

Contingency Theory

The most successful organizations tended to maintain states of differentiation and integration consistent with the diversity of the parts of the environment and the required interdependence of these parts. (Lawrence & Lorsch, cited in Filley & House, 1969, p. 97)

The classical and neoclassical theorists' position was that conflict should be avoided because it causes an imbalance in the organization. In contrast, contingency theorists consider conflict to be an inescapable occurrence and believe that it should be actively managed. They suggested that the environment in which conflict exists complements organizational performance. Environment, according to this view, includes the influences of objects, people, and ideas outside of the organization.

Paul Lawrence and Jay Lorsch

In 1967, Lawrence and Lorsch considered organizations as social systems. As such, they viewed contingency theory to be a fit between individual predispositions, internal characteristics, and external conditions, including environmental uncertainty. Lawrence and Lorsch asserted that there is no best way to organize; instead, each organization's environment determines the structure that results in best performance. The environmental variables or contingencies affecting this determination include such determinants as size, geography, technology, and uncertainty. The organizational structures that are considered to be contingent on these variables are differentiation, decentralization, the degree of formalization, and integration (Johnson, 2009; Sullivan & Decker, 2009). Integration includes the internal relationships of organizational members and is influenced by "the nature of the task being performed, the form of relationships, rewards, and controls, and the existing ideas within the organization about how a well-accepted member should behave" (Filley & House, 1969, p. 95). Integration also incorporates the quality of collaboration. The formality of departments and between organizations may be differentiated, based on how members of each department utilize different interests and viewpoints; because of their differences, they often find it difficult to reach consensus (Filley & House, 1969).

To Lawrence and Lorsch, "the environment of the organization determines both the character and degree of differentiation and the mode of integration" (Filley & House, 1967, p. 96). They foresaw that competitive demand and environmental uncertainty have an effect on each organization's differentiation and integration in terms of its interpersonal orientation, goals, and perception of time. In their research conducted at a group of plastics factories, Lawrence and Lorsch found that "the state of differentiation in the effective organization was consistent with the diversity of the parts of the environment, while the state of integration achieved was consistent with the environmental demands for interdependence" (p. 98).

Fred Fiedler

Leadership performance depends then as much on the organization as it depends upon the leader's own attributes. (Fiedler, 1967, p. 281)

Fred Fiedler's contingency model proposed that group performance was based on a balance between the leader's style and his or her level of control. To measure leadership style, Fiedler developed an instrument called the least preferred coworker (LPC) questionnaire. After assessing their leadership style, Fiedler matched leaders with situations. Three contingency dimensions were identified that determined leadership effectiveness: (1) leader–member relations, (2) task structure, and (3) position power. The results of Fiedler's research showed that the better the relationship between the leader and the member, the more structured the job and the stronger the position power or leader control. In other words, the best leadership style depends on situational control. From this evidence, Fiedler developed a model to match leaders with situations. Advocates of Fiedler's findings contended that there was sufficient evidence to support Fiedler's model, although the LPC scores were not stable and the questionnaire was not well understood (Robbins & Judge, 2007).

Organizational Configuration Framework

Large politicized organizations are increasingly allowed to sustain themselves by political means, threatening the destruction, not of the single spent organization, but of the whole society of organizations instead. (Mintzberg, 1989, p. 367)

Henry Mintzberg began his research in 1966 in an attempt to describe what managers do, with the goal of using different words and concepts than those presented by Fayol. During his research, Mintzberg observed chief executives, from both medium and large organizations, for 1-week periods. Based on his findings, he presented two sets of conclusions: characteristics of managerial work and the basic content of the manager's work. Six characteristics were deemed to be significant skills needed by managers to enable them to administer in a complex organization:

1. The manager performs a great quantity of work at an unrelenting pace.
2. Managerial activity is characterized by variety, fragmentation, and brevity.
3. Managers prefer issues that are current, specific, and ad hoc.
4. The manager sits between his or her organization and a network of contacts.
5. The manager demonstrates a strong preference for verbal media.
6. Despite the preponderance of obligations, the manager appears to be able to control his or her own affairs (Mintzberg, 1971, pp. B102–B103).

Managers were considered to function in three distinct roles: (1) interpersonal roles (figurehead, leader, liaison), (2) informational roles (nerve center, spokesperson, disseminator), and (3) decision-making roles (entrepreneur, resource allocator, disturbance handler, negotiator).

Mintzberg (1971) questioned whether management should be considered a profession or a science. To be defined as a profession, there should be an associated body of knowledge or science. Mintzberg did not believe that his research proved that a science of management exists, as managers "do not work according to procedures that have been prescribed by scientific analysis" (p. B107). Consequently, he recommended greater and more refined definition and study of managerial roles as the first step toward the development of a scientific base for management.

Mintzberg (1989) also sought to classify types of organizational structure and power: "We can no more talk of *the* organization than we can talk of *the* mammal, no more prescribe one best way to run all organizations than prescribe one pair of glasses for all people" (p. 93). He noted that organizational theory was not dependent on recognition of strict boundaries, but rather often shifted to reflect organizational power struggles. Mintzberg contended that the organization is the total of all the ways labor is coordinated, while divided into distinct tasks. The six coordinating mechanisms were identified as (1) mutual adjustment, (2) standardization of work processes, (3) direct supervision, (4) standardized work outputs, (5) standardized labor skills, and (6) standardized labor norms. As part of his work, Mintzberg developed a model of organizational structures that considers combinations of environmental complexity and stability. The four broad categories on his matrix are (1) decentralized bureaucratic, (2) centralized bureaucratic, (3) decentralized organic, and (4) centralized organic. The horizontal axis of the model contrasted organic and bureaucratic structures: Bureaucratic structures represent more stable environments, and organic structures represent more dynamic environments (Matheson, 2009).

One of the more innovative organizations described by Mintzberg is the *adhocracy*: a high-technology organization characterized by a basic orientation of entrepreneurship (indicating dependence on a variety of workers to achieve strategic initiatives). Adhocracy was described as a structure appropriate for the current (information) age, albeit one that is difficult for the machine bureaucracy to comprehend.

For an organization to be innovative, one of two basic forms of adhocracy must be engaged: *operating adhocracy* or *administrative adhocracy*. As Mintzberg (1989) explains, "The operating adhocracy innovates and solves problems directly on behalf of its clients. . . . For every operating adhocracy, there is a corresponding professional bureaucracy, one that does similar work but with a narrower orientation" (p. 201). In contrast, administrative adhocracy takes on projects to serve itself, "to bring new facilities or activities on line, as in the administrative structure of a highly automated company" (Mintzberg, 1989, p. 203). The administrative adhocracy, unlike the operating adhocracy, creates an apparent distinction between its operating core and administrative component.

General Systems Theory

The only meaningful way to study an organization is to study it as a system. (von Bertalanffy, 1969a, p. 9)

Ludwig von Bertalanffy introduced general systems theory in the late 1950s. According to von Bertalanffy, when the theoretical frameworks for various scientific disciplines become isolated from one another, communication between them becomes difficult. He suggested that, in fact, a common element in all frameworks can be found crossing the periphery of physics, biology, sociology, psychology, and so on—namely, systems. The central theme in his work is that nonlinear relationships may exist between variables. As a consequence, a small change in one variable may cause a significant change in another. The nonlinear concept introduced by von Bertalanffy added to the complexity of understanding organizations (Johnson, 2009).

Von Bertalanffy believed the task of biology is to determine the laws of biological science, which in turn requires an understanding of all levels of an organism. This systems theory of the organism, called organismic biology, later was understood as general systems theory. In outlining systems theory, von Bertalanffy "gave mathematical descriptions of system properties (such as wholeness, sum, growth, competition, allometry, mechanization, centralization, finality, and equifinality), derived from the system description by simultaneous differential equations" (von Bertalanffy, 1969b, p. 412). As a practicing biologist, von Bertalanffy sought to develop a theory of open systems. According to Drack (2009), his definition of the open system is one that maintains itself "through a continuous flux of matter and energy, by assimilation and dissimilation, and is distant from true equilibrium, and able to supply work" (p. 566). Von Bertalanffy also described the principle of ontogenesis, which was later recognized as a key concept underlying hierarchy or progressive organization.

Von Bertalanffy (1969a) defined an organization as an "alien to the mechanistic world" and noted that characteristics of organizations "are notions like those of wholeness, growth, differentiation, hierarchical order, dominance, control, competition, etc." (p. 47). Unlike biological theories, which can be quantitatively measured, organizations lend themselves to more qualitative review, according to von Bertalanffy. He discussed general systems theory as it relates to individuals, education, and science. His general systems theory propelled organizational theory into the era of open systems thinking, where the environment plays a major role.

Change Theory

Kurt Lewin

> To be stable, a cultural change has to penetrate all aspects of a nation's life. The change must, in short, be a change in the cultural atmosphere, not merely a change of a single item. (Lewin, cited in Burnes, 2004, p. 980)

Kurt Lewin, a behavioral scientist, outlined a model for change used by industry in the 1940s. His force field model included the steps of unfreezing, moving, and refreezing. In this model, change is described as a dynamic force within the organization that moves in opposing directions. A driving force pushes participants toward change, while participants use a restraining force to push back the change being directed their way. Lewin viewed change as a dynamic balance of these forces, not an event. *Unfreezing* is the act of destabilizing old behaviors and is a necessity for old behaviors to be unlearned or discarded.

Once this step is accomplished, the manager may consider the method that will result in the least resistance in moving a change forward. *Moving* enables individuals and groups to switch to more acceptable behaviors. *Refreezing* involves a return of the dynamic force field and a new quasi-stationary state of equilibrium (Hellriegel & Slocum, 1976; Sullivan & Decker, 2009).

Lewin had a strong, ethical belief in democratic values in society and democratic institutions. His pioneering work set the standard for behavioral science and group issues in organizations.

Peter Drucker

One cannot manage change. One can only be ahead of it. (Drucker, 1999, p. 73)

Peter Drucker (1999) addressed change process and theory in his book *Management Challenges for the 21st Century*. Because he considered change to be unavoidable, Drucker was convinced that organizations that do not embrace change will not survive. A *change leader* knows how to look for change, can find the right change, and understands the effects of change, both internal and external to the organization.

The first step in the process identified by Drucker is to establish change policies that will enable the organization to abandon yesterday and know how to act on abandonment. The second step is to create change through a policy of systematic innovation. This step facilitates looking for windows of opportunity. The third step focuses on piloting—that is, the use of pilot studies to test the reality of the change. The final step is change and continuity: "Change and continuity are thus poles rather than opposites" (Drucker, 1999, p. 90). To successfully adopt the role of change leader, an organization needs to establish internal and external continuity and find the right balance between rapid change and continuity.

Theories X, Y, and Z

The normal science of management is long since in need of a new paradigm. (Ouchi, 1981, p. 220)

Douglas McGregor: Theory X and Theory Y

The social psychologist Douglas McGregor criticized both classical and human relations theories as being insufficient to address workplace realities. He developed a general characterization of their principles in a theory that he dubbed theory X. Theory X is based on beliefs that the average person dislikes work and tries to avoid it; most people have to be coerced or threatened to do a job; and the average person wishes to avoid responsibility, yet wants security. McGregor distinguished theory X from propositions that he named theory Y, which is based on the following assumptions regarding human nature:

- The expenditure of effort at work is as natural as rest and play.
- Humans do have a measure of self-control and self-direction, and coercion is not the only means to bring about effort.
- A direct product of effort is the satisfaction of ego and meeting of self-actualization needs.
- The average person can seek and accept responsibility under proper conditions.
- There are significant variations in individuals' degree of ingenuity, creativity, and imagination.
- The average person's potential is not utilized in modern industrial life.

People who accept McGregor's analysis also essentially accept Maslow's hierarchy of needs. Theory X includes the assumption that lower-order needs in Maslow's hierarchy govern behavior, and theory Y includes the assumption that human behavior is governed by higher-order needs. Unfortunately, there was no evidence to confirm either theory (Filley & House, 1969; Robbins & Judge, 2007).

William Ouchi: Theory Z

While theory X and theory Y were developed as a criticism of the work of classical organizational theorists, theory Z was derived by William Ouchi in the 1970s from his work comparing the work ethic and industry in the United States to the work ethic and industry in Japan. Trust, loyalty, and commitment are key employee elements in theory Z. Companies that adhere to theory Z principles, like their Japanese counterparts, have long-term employees; establish evaluation and promotion policies based on complex, subtle, and intimate peer evaluation; and allow for unique career path development. In these companies, decision making is consensual and participative. Such companies also have a holistic orientation and an egalitarian atmosphere, where relationships tend to be informal and emphasize that "whole people deal with one another at work, rather than just managers with workers and clerks with machinists" (Ouchi, 1981, p. 79). Theory Z organizations are considered to be clans rather than bureaucracies, given the ongoing interchange between employees' social and work life.

Ouchi proposed 13 steps as necessary to become a theory Z organization:

1. Understand roles in the type Z organization. Read, discuss, and have open discussions about the substance of theory Z.
2. Audit the company's philosophy. The company philosophy expresses the values to live and work by.

3. Involve company leadership in the design of desired management philosophy. Organizational change cannot occur without support of the hierarchy.
4. Implement the chosen philosophy by constructing incentives and structures. The structure should be a guide to cooperation and subtlety.
5. Support interpersonal skills development. Recognize problem-solving and decision-making patterns of interaction.
6. Test the system. Internal and external testing of the organization is not easy but is necessary to measure success.
7. Allow for union involvement. If there is a union involved, the union must have an understanding of the emerging work relationships and organizational structure.
8. Stabilize employment. This step is a direct result of policy. Slow evaluation and promotion are pivotal factors in stabilization of employees.
9. Develop a system for slow evaluation and promotion. Employees will learn that promotions and salary increases are based on performance over time.
10. Expand career path development. A mingling of expertise benefits everyone and allows for a program of career circulation.
11. Plan for implementation at the first level—management first, and then lower-level employees. Change cannot take place unless those who rate higher in the hierarchy offer an invitation to lower-level employees to do so.
12. Seek areas for implementation. Utilize areas that have shown commitment and productivity.
13. Allow for the development of holistic relationships. These relationships are a consequence of organizational integration (Ouchi, 1981).

The logic of these steps is seen as the equivalent of going from A to Z and reaching every worker in the organization. This process encourages greater productivity and efficiency, which will thrive unless the process is thwarted intentionally by top managers or a union that is threatened. Critics of theory Z, however, suggest that this philosophy may make organizations more sexist or racist (based on Japanese philosophy), the proposed changes may be difficult given certain aspects of U.S. culture, and a decline in professionalism by employees may occur. Although they are not composed of a homogeneous group of people, organizations should find innovations that balance integration and freedom (Shafritz, Ott, & Jang, 2005).

Modern theorists of organizational behavior recognized that conflict, change, and structure are inherent in all organizations. They considered organizations as systems and cultures working in an environment of certain mingled with uncertainty (see **Box 15-3**).

Box 15-3   Modern Theories of Organizational Behavior

With the ideas of the modern theories of organizational behavior in mind, answer the following questions:

1. Describe a healthcare organization from a systems perspective.
2. Research change theory in scholarly literature and on the Internet. Evaluate how change occurs within the organization where you work. Does change occur according to a theory of change?
3. Can change be static or is it always dynamic? In other words, are the terms *static* and *change* contradictory?
4. Give examples of organizational change that you have personally experienced, and explain how the involved organizations managed change.
5. Compare and contrast concepts and propositional statements that can be drawn from theories X, Y, and Z. Which of these theories is most closely aligned with your worldview? Defend your position. Which of these theories do you believe is most useful to advanced nursing practice? Explain.

SUMMARY

The discussion in this chapter only touches the tip of the iceberg of organizational behavior and leadership. Each organization has its own culture, structure, and environment (internal and external) in which it operates. Is there a theory that fits all situations? Certainly not. What has been learned over the years of theory development is that both products and people are of equal importance and that organizations must plan and operate with both in mind.

REFERENCES

Barnard, C. I. (1938). *The functions of the executive*. Cambridge, MA: Harvard University Press.

Breeze, J. D. (1981). Henri Fayol's basic tools of administration. *Proceedings of the 41st Annual Meeting of the Academy of Management, 101,* 101–105.

Brunsson, K. H. (2008). Some effects of Fayolism. *International Studies of Management and Organization, 38*(1), 30–47.

Burnes, B. (2004). Kurt Lewin and the planned approach to change: A re-appraisal. *Journal of Management Studies, 41*(6), 977–1002.

Crainer, S. (2003). One hundred years of management. *Business Strategy Review, 14*(2), 41–49.

Daft, R. L., & Noe, R. A. (2001). The scope of organizational behavior. In *Organizational behavior* (pp. 1–36). Fort Worth, TX: Harcourt College Publishers.

Drack, M. (2009). Ludwig von Bertalanffy's early system approach. *Systems Research and Behavioral Science, 26,* 563–572.

Drucker, P. F. (1999). *Management challenges for the 21st century*. New York, NY: HarperCollins.

Eisenstadt, S. N. (Ed.). (1968). *Max Weber: On charisma and institution building*. Chicago, IL: University of Chicago Press.

Fiedler, F. E. (1967). *The theory of leadership effectiveness.* New York, NY: McGraw-Hill.

Filley, A. C., & House, R. J. (1969). *Managerial process and organizational behavior.* Englewood Cliffs, NJ: Prentice Hall.

Hargreaves, S. (2006). Latham, Weber and compassion. *IPA Review, 58*(1), 20–21.

Hellriegel, D., & Slocum, J. W. (1976). *Organizational behavior* (2nd ed.). St. Paul, MN: West.

Johnson, J. A. (2009). *Health organizations: Theory, behavior, and development.* Sudbury, MA: Jones & Bartlett.

Matheson, C. (2009). Understanding the policy process: The work of Henry Mintzberg. *Public Administration Review, 69*(6), 1148–1161.

McShane, S. L., & Von Glinow, M. A. (2005). *Organizational behavior: Emerging realities for the workplace revolution* (3rd ed.). New York, NY: McGraw-Hill/Irwin.

Mintzberg, H. (1971). Managerial work: Analysis from observation. *Management Science, 18*(3), B97–B110.

Mintzberg, H. (1989). *Mintzberg on management: Inside our strange world of organizations.* New York, NY: Free Press.

Nelson, D. (1980). *Frederick W. Taylor and the rise of scientific management.* Madison, WI: University of Wisconsin Press.

Ouchi, W. (1981). *Theory Z: How American business can meet the Japanese challenge.* Reading, MA: Addison-Wesley.

Parker, L. D., & Ritson, P. A. (2005). Revisiting Fayol: Anticipating contemporary management. *British Journal of Management, 16,* 175–194.

Robbins, S. P., & Judge, T. A. (2007). *Organizational behavior* (12th ed.). Upper Saddle River, NJ: Pearson/Prentice Hall.

Roethlisberger, F. J., & Dickson, W. J. (1967). *Management and the worker: An account of a research program conducted by Western Electric Company, Hawthorne Works, Chicago.* Cambridge, MA: Harvard University Press.

Sager, F., & Rosser, C. (2009). Weber, Wilson, and Hegel: Theories of modern bureaucracy. *Public Administration Review, 69*(6), 1136–1147.

Shafritz, J. M., Ott, J. S., & Jang, Y. S. (2005). *Classics of organization theory.* Independence, KY: Cengage Learning.

Simon, H. A. (1976). *Administrative behavior* (3rd ed.). New York, NY: Macmillan.

Sullivan, E. J., & Decker, P. J. (2005). How organizations are designed. In *Effective leadership and management in nursing* (6th ed.). Upper Saddle River, NJ: Pearson/Prentice Hall.

Sullivan, E. J., & Decker, P. J. (2009). *Effective leadership and management in nursing* (7th ed.). Upper Saddle River, NJ: Pearson/Prentice Hall.

Taylor, F. W. (1911). *The principles of scientific management.* New York, NY: Harper & Brothers.

von Bertalanffy, L. (1969a). *General system theory: Foundations, development, applications.* New York, NY: George Braziller.

von Bertalanffy, L. (1969b). The history and status of general systems theory. *Academy of Management Journal, 15*(4), 407–426. Reprinted from Klir, G. J. (1972). *Trends in general systems theory.* New York, NY: Wiley-Interscience.

Chapter 16

Theoretical Approaches to Quality Improvement

Patsy Anderson

INTRODUCTION

Numerous theories about how to improve the quality and performance of organizations have emerged over the last 50 years. Today there is so much information available about quality theory and measurement that users of this information are becoming confused. One of the *Essentials* in the American Association of Colleges of Nursing's (2006) *The Essentials of Doctoral Education for Advanced Nursing Practice* is "Organizational and Systems Leadership for Quality Improvement and Systems Thinking" (p. 10). As part of their responsibilities, advanced practice nurses now need to understand total quality management, methods for process improvement, quality process tools and techniques, and performance measurement systems. These elements can be divided into quality theories and methods for measuring quality. This chapter provides an overview and the historical context for quality theories that are useful for leadership, management, and practice.

Nurses know that concepts used in theories need to be defined. If 20 people were asked to define quality, they probably would give 20 different answers. This is not surprising given that, for many years, even experts in quality improvement have differed in their conceptualization of quality and the ways in which it can be improved. According to Crosby (1984), quality is "conformance to requirements" (p. 60). Deming (2000) never specifically defined quality but noted that "quality should be aimed at the needs of the consumer, present and future" and that quality "begins with the intent, which is fixed by management" (p. 5). Florence Nightingale viewed quality from an absence of perspective. An interesting aside is that Pirsig (1974/1999), in his cult classic *Zen and the Art of Motorcycle Maintenance: An Inquiry Into Values*, described how the indefinable nature of quality quite literally contributed to driving him mad.

Nightingale was one of the first persons who should be credited with developing a theoretical approach to quality improvement. She was followed in this endeavor by Ernest Codman and Avedis Donabedian, both of whom developed methods to study quality in health care. Healthcare industry leaders, particularly The Joint Commission, have based much of their quality improvement initiatives on the work of Codman and Donabedian, as well as on the work of leaders who focused on developing quality initiatives in the manufacturing industry, such as W. Edwards Deming, Joseph M. Juran, and Philip B. Crosby. This chapter focuses on the work of these pioneers in the field of quality improvement and management.

FLORENCE NIGHTINGALE

Florence Nightingale (1820–1910) was born into a rich, upper-class British family and became known worldwide as a nurse and as a statistician. One of her well-known contributions to health care occurred during the Crimean War (1853–1856). Nightingale left for Scutari, Turkey, on October 21, 1854, along with her Uncle Sam Smith and her nurses. Once she arrived in Turkey, she found deplorable conditions in the hospitals (General Hospital and Barracks Hospital). The Barracks Hospital was situated over a network of blocked cesspools, and privies overflowed into the hallways. Nightingale began to suspect that more soldiers were dying of disease than were being killed during battle. In January 1855, conditions were so poor that 1,000 out of 1,174 men died (Dossey, 1999).

As part of her assessment of hospital conditions, Nightingale began keeping detailed records of wounds, diseases, and deaths. In her records, deaths were divided by causes, such as contaminated food and water, lack of supplies, and organizational problems. In March 1855, the British Sanitation Commission and Nightingale began to work on improving the quality of sanitation and environmental conditions at the hospital.

During the 4 months before initiating her joint work with the Sanitation Commission, Nightingale had begun organizing the nurses and improving hospital supplies, general cleanliness, and the soldiers' welfare. Within 3 months, she and her associates were able to reduce wounded soldiers' death rates from 43 deaths per 1,000 to 2 per 1,000 (Dossey, 1999).

After she left Turkey in 1856, Nightingale began to work tirelessly toward implementing hospital reform in England. During the Crimean War, she had used new statistical analysis techniques to identify problems and to plan improvements. These tools and techniques essentially represented one of the first attempts to measure the quality of patient care. Later, Nightingale used her experiences in the Crimea as a basis for her reform work in England. Six months after he met with Nightingale in 1856, Lord Panmure, the British Secretary of State for War, formally requested that she submit a report about her observations related to the sanitary requirements of the army and the medical care and treatment of the sick and wounded in the Crimea. This report became an 830-page document titled "Notes on Matters Affecting the Health, Efficiency, and Hospital Administration of the British Army" (Small, 1999). It was during this same period that Nightingale developed her polar diagram, which was used to document the number of soldiers' deaths caused by battle compared to the number of soldiers who died from iatrogenic hospital causes. Pie charts similar to Nightingale's polar diagram remain important tools used in quality management today.

Nightingale revolutionized quality management by demonstrating the value of objectively measuring and mathematically analyzing mortality data so that the results could be used to improve patient outcomes. Quality care for Nightingale was the absence of factors that hinder the reparative process of disease. These hindrances were identified as mostly environmental things such as lack of fresh air, lack of light, and inappropriate room temperature (Nightingale, 1969/1860). In addition, for Nightingale, the environment included nurses' behaviors, such as chattering and wearing petticoats that rustled. She focused on eliminating those irritating environmental factors that often went unnoticed by nurses, but bothered patients. These environmental irritants needed to be eliminated, she suggested, so that patients would be in the best condition for healing to occur.

ERNEST CODMAN

Ernest Codman (1869–1940), a physician and surgeon, is known for his work in hospital reform and outcomes management in patient care. Codman was trained at Harvard Medical School and Massachusetts General Hospital; while at the hospital, he began what is believed to be the first morbidity and mortality conferences. He left the hospital after he and members of the Boston medical community were unable to reach agreement about his idea for evaluating surgeon competency.

In 1890, Codman proposed the end-result system of hospital standardization. Under this system, hospital staff tracked every patient treated at a hospital to determine whether the treatment was effective. The system required a determination of the appropriate time frame for tracking. If the treatment was not effective, the staff would then attempt to determine why, so that similar patient cases could be treated successfully in the future. Using this method from 1900 to 1910, Codman reviewed 600 abdominal surgery cases treated at Massachusetts General Hospital—not by diagnosis, but by physician. The benefits of having these results were so convincing that the medical staff agreed to conduct research and to improve their surgical skills and share the results with others.

In 1914, in protest of the surgical seniority system, Codman resigned from Massachusetts General Hospital. He believed that patient outcomes—not seniority—should be the basis for a surgeon's promotion. He continued to anger his fellow surgeons by advocating that the quality of surgical operations should be evaluated based on patient outcomes. In his system, indicators were identified and classified based on whether problems were related to organizational factors, clinician factors, or patient factors. Codman tracked the occurrence frequency for each factor and used the data to target an evaluation and correction of variables so that preventable problems did not reoccur. His system was not exactly "high tech." All of the data were recorded on 3-by-5-inch index cards.

Because of this controversial work and criticism he received from the Boston Medical Society during a conference on hospital efficiency, members of the medical community eventually ostracized Codman. In 1911, Codman opened his own hospital called The End Result. During a visit to England in 1912, he was appointed chair of the Committee for the Standardization of Hospitals of the American College of Surgeons. This committee monitored and developed hospital quality standards. The committee continued to function until 1950, at which time the American Medical Association and the American Hospital Association renamed the committee The Joint Commission (originally The Joint Commission on Accreditation of Healthcare Organizations). In 1996, The Joint Commission established the Codman Award, which is given to a healthcare organization or professional person for achievement in the use of process and outcome measures to improve organizational performance and, ultimately, the quality and safety of care provided to the public (Joint Commission, 1996).

W. EDWARDS DEMING

W. Edwards Deming (1900–1993) was a formidable figure in the field of quality improvement. Notably, he was the primary quality consultant credited with revolutionizing Japanese industry after World War II and helping Japanese companies achieve an unprecedented level of quality in their products and productivity.

Deming was educated as a physicist, obtaining a doctorate at Yale University in 1928. As a result of his work at the U.S. Department of Agriculture and his statistical expertise, he was sent to Japan in 1946 immediately after the war ended to study agricultural production and related problems. Deming was able not only to help Japanese businesses with statistical methods for quality improvement but also to improve the Japanese people's level of confidence in their products. He convinced the Japanese industrial leaders and workers that if they used his methods, in 5 years they would be able to capture the world market (Walton, 1986). Before his work with the Japanese, their products were considered cheap and of low quality.

When he returned from Japan, Deming tried to convince U.S. industrial leaders to implement the same theories and tools that he had implemented in Japan. However, it took much longer for Americans to appreciate his methods than it did to convince the Japanese. In contrast to the priorities established by Japanese industries after World War II, U.S. industries at that time focused on goals related to quantity rather than quality. In the late 1970s, competition from the Japanese automobile industry, especially Toyota, began to capture the attention of U.S. industry leaders. Deming became nationally known when he was featured in an NBC White Paper and television broadcast called "If Japan Can, Why Can't We?"

Deming stressed that focusing on the process is more important than focusing on the product. He found that inspection, reprocessing, and customer complaints were more costly than ensuring that a process is done correctly the first time (Walton, 1986). The Deming system is based on continuous improvement and statistical methods that must be embraced by top executives and implemented throughout an organization. Deming's theory of quality is encapsulated in his famous 14 points for management that he thought would be the basis for transforming U.S. industry. These 14 points were developed to be widely applicable to organizations of all sizes and missions, both service and manufacturing. A discussion of each of the 14 points based on Deming's (2000) work follows.

Point 1: Create constancy of purpose for improvement of product or service. To fulfill this aim, organizations, while not ignoring the problems of today such as budget, employment, and public relations, must deal with the more challenging problems of tomorrow. Coping with future problems requires constancy of purpose. This constancy of purpose entails not allowing the desire for immediate profit to hurt the organization's long-term improvement and competitiveness. For long-term improvement to occur, management must innovate by allocating resources for long-term planning, by using resources for research and education, and by continually improving the design of its products and services. Regarding constant improvement, Deming reminded managers that their obligation never stops. These actions are as essential in the healthcare field as they are in any other industry.

Point 2: Adopt the new philosophy. The "new philosophy" to which Deming referred is quality improvement as it was being practiced in Japan after World War II. Adopting this philosophy meant stopping the bad practices that American industry had adopted. Deming believed that leaders in U.S. organizations and companies should no longer accept the level of mistakes, defects, and ineffective supervision and management that were being tolerated. Deming did not limit this challenge to management but rather stated that government must remove obstacles to U.S. industry's competitive position as well.

Point 3: Cease dependence on mass inspection. Using a system based on mass inspection leads to a need for rework. It implies that defects are expected to occur and will need to be fixed or in some way repaired. Although inspection may be necessary for safety and accuracy, especially in certain very complex processes and products, reliance on inspection means that attention is not focused on improvements that would make the outcome right the first time.

Point 4: End the practice of awarding business on the basis of price tag alone. Price does not indicate quality. When an item purchased is not of high quality, high costs may result from its use. Deming suggested that long-term relationships with single vendors will elicit loyalty, trust, and, in the long run, lower costs. Even if an organization uses a single vendor, however, unwanted variations may still be introduced into the products and services.

Point 5: Improve constantly and forever the system of production and service. One way to explain this point is to discuss what it does not mean. It does not mean solving immediate problems as they arise. Rather, it means making an ongoing commitment to ensure that quality is built in at the development stage and that all existing processes are continually studied and revised to improve their outputs. Deming argued that improvement does not occur simply by allocating money for quality; rather, knowledge is the key. The better the understanding that managers and others have about the processes employed, the more effective change will be. Using reliable statistical methods to study processes is also necessary.

Point 6: Institute training and retraining. Deming stressed two kinds of training. First, managers must be trained in the complete functioning of the organization and in the concepts of quality improvement, especially focusing on reducing variations rather than on meeting specifications. Second, appropriate training and placement of staff members will ensure that their rich talents are not squandered. Appropriate training for staff members and managers includes (1) ensuring that there is training, (2) making sure that the means of training is effective, and (3) ending the practice of having staff trained by other staff who may themselves have acquired bad habits because of poor training. Training should be ongoing while evidence indicates that it is still helpful, and training should occur when circumstances require it. Continuing education is a part of the culture in health care. This education should include the tenets of quality improvement and statistical control.

Point 7: Institute leadership. Managers must, Deming said, not supervise but lead. To do this, managers must remove barriers that make it difficult for workers to take pride in their work. Managers also must know how to do the work that they supervise. To lead, managers must not treat every problem as a fire to be put out, but rather must look toward making systems improvements. Finally, leaders should not accept numerical fallacies, especially the notion that all workers should meet the average. In fact, not everyone can be average; some people will always be below average. This truth is demonstrated in statistical normal distribution.

Point 8: Drive out fear. Fear is inherent in the bad apple approach to quality and in the perception that quality is something imposed by outside forces peering over the shoulder of each member of the organization. In health care, there tends to be underreporting of medication and medical errors because of the fear of retaliation from organization leaders and managers. This underreporting, in turn, can lead to unintended consequences for both patients and organizations.

Point 9: Break down barriers between staff areas. The structure of an organization can work against quality improvement; lack of communication between people in various departments and services can impede improvement and cause problems. In health care, this is especially true. The coordination of, for example, nursing, anesthesia, surgery, and postanesthesia care is crucial for any surgical procedure. As another example, communication between professional and administrative staff is essential when contemplating equipment purchases or changes in procedures. In addition, the process by which systems are studied and improved requires close cooperation of all involved parties, regardless of their work department or service area. Removing such barriers can mean a change in the culture of an organization.

Point 10: Eliminate slogans, exhortations, and targets for the workforce. Deming emphasized that such tactics are meaningless without a plan to back them up. Also, they generate frustration by asking workers to improve without providing the necessary means to make such improvements.

Point 11: Eliminate numerical quotas. Organizational managers typically set rates of production for the average worker. If one considers the normal distribution curve, it is evident why this pattern occurs. Setting production levels, however, can result in undesired outcomes, such as various types of loss, disorganization, dissatisfaction, and turnover. In some organizations, the production rates are set based on the work of the overachiever, which puts even greater stress on workers and creates organizational problems. Quotas for managers are equally problematic, such as those engendered by the practice of management by objectives. Often these goals are not accompanied by plans, and if the system itself is not stable, a goal is meaningless.

Point 12: Remove barriers to pride of workmanship. Deming listed several specific barriers. For example, a system in which an annual performance evaluation is linked to a pay increase for salaried workers focuses on the end product, and the end of the stream—not on leadership to help people. The resultant effect is fear and self-preservation, rather than action to improve the organization. Barriers to staff having a sense of pride arise when staff members are treated as if they are commodities, they are powerless to communicate their ideas and knowledge to management, and when they do not know what is expected of them. "Quick fix" solutions to mitigate these barriers do not work. Instead, managers must demonstrate over a period of time that action will be taken to improve systems, that there is no continuing hunt for bad apples, and that there is a commitment to the long-term survival and improvement of the organization.

Point 13: Institute a rigorous program of education and retraining. As stated under Point 6, ongoing education of the sort practiced in the healthcare field is essential for people to fully develop and effectively use their talents. In addition, as the organization changes because of quality improvement activities, reeducation becomes necessary to help people adapt to the changing environment.

Point 14: Take action to accomplish the transformation. Deming believed that managers would struggle in trying to comply with all of the previous 13 points. To deal with this problem, he suggested that managers organize as a team to meet the challenges. Every employee and manager of an organization should be taught how to improve quality continually, and this initiative must come from the top down.

In addition to proposing these 14 points, Deming also identified seven deadly diseases that afflict many organizations and prevent their transformation toward quality improvement. He thought that the cure of these diseases would require a complete change in the Western style of management. These seven deadly diseases include issues such as an emphasis on short-term profits, frequent mobility of managers, and excessive medical costs (Walton, 1986).

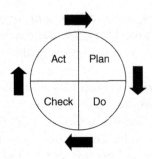

Figure 16-1 The PDCA cycle.

Deming identified several statistical processes that could be used to implement his theory. Among those statistical methods are flow diagrams to identify work processes; cause and effect diagrams that display all factors that contribute to a problem and their relationships to outcomes; statistical process control, which is used to evaluate special and common causes of process outcomes; and the Shewhart cycle.

The Shewhart cycle—named for Walter A. Shewhart, who developed it in the 1920s—is the most widely used planning and improvement process in the field of quality management. It was introduced in Japan by Deming, which explains why it is sometimes called the Deming cycle. This quality improvement framework is used to carry out ongoing processes focused on assessing, planning, acting, monitoring and evaluating, reassessing, and acting again. Given its purpose of effecting change quickly, it is often called the rapid improvement cycle; however, its most familiar designation is the *PDCA cycle*, where the initials stand for the four components of the cycle: plan, do, check, and act (see Figure 16-1).

The *plan* step involves studying a process, deciding what could improve it, and identifying data to help in the evaluation. The *do* step tests the proposed change by data simulation or small-scale trial. In the *check* step, the change is evaluated and modification of the changed process occurs. In the *act* step, the tested change is implemented to improve the process. These steps may be repeated to increase knowledge and process improvement. Using this model, the change process can be rapidly implemented (Deming, 2000). By using the PDCA task table (**Box 16-1**), any organization or individual will be successful in making changes to a process.

JOSEPH M. JURAN

Joseph M. Juran (1904–2008) was another consultant credited with leading the quality revolution in Japan. Through the Juran Institute, he conducted public and in-house seminars for managers throughout the world. Juran's legacy continues to be carried out by the Juran Institute.

Box 16-1 PDCA Task Table			
Plan	**Do**	**Check**	**Act**
Select improvement opportunity.	Map out and implement a trial run.	Analyze the results.	Adopt, adapt, or abandon the change.
Analyze current situation or process.	Collect the data.	Compare data with predictions.	Monitor.
Identify root causes.	Document problems and unexpected observations.	Summarize what was learned.	Hold the gains.
Generate and choose solutions (who, what, where, when, how).	Begin data analysis.		

Juran promoted ideas relating to the integration of quality improvement into corporate plans, with quality being defined as fitness for purpose rather than conformance to specification, teamwork, delighting customers, and problem solving. Juran suggested that quality has a dual meaning. In one sense, quality refers to freedom from deficiencies or, put in more realistic terms, reduction in error rates. In another sense, quality refers to product features. Juran identified freedom from deficiencies as reduced rework, reduced need for inspection, and reduced customer dissatisfaction. Reduced deficiencies, he noted, tend to lower costs. Product features, by comparison, are intended to meet customers' needs and produce customer satisfaction. Higher quality, in terms of product features, makes products more appealing to consumers, increases sales, increases competitiveness, and often increases costs. This distinction is especially applicable to health care (Juran, 1989). According to Juran, these two aspects of quality are not polar opposites. Rather, to satisfy customers, a product must both have the features they desire and be as free from deficiencies as possible. One or the other aspects, by itself, does not constitute high quality.

The primary foundation of Juran's quality process is the Juran trilogy (Juran, 1989). The Juran trilogy consists of three components: (1) quality planning, (2) quality control, and (3) quality improvement. The starting point is *quality planning*, which entails developing a process that will meet established goals and current operating conditions. Quality planning involves building quality—in terms of both freedom from deficiencies and increased desirability of product features—into processes and products. *Quality control* is focused on maintaining the status quo—that is, reducing variation in processes and products. To help evaluate quality control, quality control limits should be established; Juran advocated using a feedback loop in the control process. *Quality improvement* is the purposeful action taken by upper management to introduce new processes into the system (Juran, 1992). **Box 16-2** provides a synopsis of Juran's primary concepts.

Box 16-2 Juran's Primary Quality Improvement Concepts		
Quality Planning	**Quality Control**	**Quality Improvement**
Identify the customers (internal and external).	Choose control subjects.	Prove the need for improvement.
Determine customer needs.	Choose units of measurement.	Identify specific projects for improvement.
Develop product features that respond to customer needs, both products and services.	Establish measurement.	Organize to guide the projects.
Establish quality goals that meet customers' and suppliers' needs at minimum costs.	Establish standards of performance.	Organize for diagnoses—for discovery causes.
Develop processes that can produce needed product features.	Interpret the difference (actual versus standard).	Diagnose to find the causes.
Improve process capability— the ability of the process to meet the quality goals under operating conditions.	Take action on the difference.	Prove remedies. Prove that remedies are effective under operating conditions. Provide for control to hold the gains.

Data from Stephens, K. S., & Juran, J. M. (2004). *Quality and a century of improvement. Milwaukee*, WI: ASQ Quality Press.

PHILIP B. CROSBY

Philip B. Crosby (1926–2001) rose from line inspector at International Telephone and Telegraph to corporate vice president, giving him a unique understanding of quality from various points of view. In 1979, Crosby's book *Quality Is Free* was published and became a best seller in the field of quality management. Like Deming, Crosby emphasized the importance of systems knowledge and improvement, the pitfalls of inspection, and the need for statistical quality control.

Crosby defined quality in simple and absolute terms. The principal strength of Crosby's theory is the attention it gives to transforming the quality culture of an organization. As Crosby (1992) wrote in his book, *Completeness: Quality for the 21st Century*, "The problem with quality has always been management's lack of understanding of their responsibility for causing a culture of prevention in their company" (p. xi). He believed that quality is a matter of philosophy, rather than just being based on techniques and statistics. Quality, he suggested, should not be delegated from leaders to another group. It is the job of leadership to have quality actually become part of the fabric of the organization.

Crosby thought that quality means conformance to carefully determined requirements and not to goodness. By stressing individual conformance to requirements, he involved everyone in the organization in his process. While working on his theory, Crosby observed that organizations that are determined to improve their processes but fail to accomplish this have five common characteristics:

1. They called their effort a program instead of a process.
2. They aimed most of their quality efforts toward the lower operational levels.
3. They employed quality control staff who were cynical.
4. They used training materials that sometimes perpetuated an error or had a detrimental effect on quality.
5. They were impatient for results (Crosby, 1984).

Crosby began his theory with four basic concepts or absolutes of a quality improvement process. These absolutes answer four questions: (1) What is quality? (2) What kind of system is needed to cause quality? (3) Which performance standard should be used? and (4) What kind of measurement system is required? (Crosby, 1984, p. 58).

The first absolute is that "the definition of quality is conformance to requirements" (p. 59). In regard to their work, Crosby argued that everyone should "do it right the first time" (DIRFT) (p. 59). For this first absolute, he believed that management has the basic tasks of establishing the requirements that employees are asked to meet, supplying the resources for the employees to meet the requirements, and spending time encouraging and helping the employees meet the requirements. His contention was that when it is evident that the management supports DIRFT, then everyone will DIRFT.

The second absolute is that "the system of quality is prevention" (p. 66). Crosby asserted that checking for goodness after the fact is a waste of resources and that prevention is successful if everyone understands key processes. The ideal system for producing quality, he suggested, focuses on prevention, not appraisal. The service industry, which includes healthcare organizations, was found to have greater difficulty with prevention than the manufacturing industry because it is more challenging to identify organization-wide problems. For service industries, Crosby advocated the use of a statistical quality control process. This process requires that each variable of the process be identified and measured. When a variable begins to move out of control, it can then be adjusted back. Such a process consists of a measurement technique relying on charts that identify the upper and lower control limits, with the section between the limits being defined as the tolerance level for the process (Crosby, 1984).

The third absolute is that "the performance standard is zero defects" (p. 74). According to Crosby, "A company is an organism with millions of little seemingly insignificant actions that make it all happen. Each and every little action has to be done just as planned in order to make everything come out right" (p. 74). He argued that when a company does not encourage everyone to DIRFT, deviation from performance standards will occur, and these deviations ultimately become acceptable practices. Organizations of all kinds, he suggested, help their employees fail to meet performance standards by allowing or overlooking percentages of errors in certain tasks. For example, in hospitals today, certain levels of medication errors are expected to occur. Leaders or quality managers are satisfied when errors do not reach a pre-identified error limit. Crosby noted that it is interesting that people seem willing to accept a certain percentage of errors in some areas of an organization, but not in the areas of finance and payroll. In regard to finance and payroll, the expectation is that error rates will be zero (Crosby, 1984).

The fourth absolute is "the measurement of quality is the price of nonconformance" (p. 83). Crosby divided the cost of quality into two parts: the price of nonconformance (PONC) and the price of conformance (POC). The PONC includes the expenses involved in doing things wrong. He found that this PONC usually represents 20% or more in manufacturing companies and 35% or more in service organizations. The POC is what is spent for quality outcomes; it includes professional quality functions, all preventive measures, and quality education. According to Crosby, the POC represents 3% to 4% in a well-managed organization. Crosby encouraged individuals to keep track of the cost of quality because this is a persuasive way to measure quality and to demonstrate the value of quality improvement.

Beyond these four absolutes, Crosby proposed a vaccine to provide "antibodies that will prevent hassle" (p. 6). This quality vaccine is a clear picture of the characteristics of an organization that fulfills the principles of quality improvement. To administer this vaccine, managers must be determined to implement quality improvement, must educate all employees in quality improvement, and must be dedicated to a long-term process of implementing quality improvement rather than looking for a quick or easy fix. The vaccination consists of a combination of certain key ingredients divided into the five categories of integrity, systems, communications, operations, and policies (Crosby, 1984).

AVEDIS DONABEDIAN

Another 20th-century healthcare professional who had an important impact on the development of quality improvement theory and practice was Avedis Donabedian (1919–2000). Donabedian was born in Beirut, Lebanon. He came to the United States and received a master's degree in public health from Harvard University in 1955. He subsequently taught epidemiology and social medicine at New York Medical College. Later, Donabedian went to the University of Michigan School of Public Health, where he taught the principles of quality measurement.

Donabedian was one of the first people to concentrate on quality issues as they pertain to the healthcare industry. He focused on total quality management using an approach similar to the one used by Joseph Juran in his work outside the healthcare industry. Donabedian believed that quality in health care is defined by structure, process, and outcomes. In his work, structure was conceived as the environment in which services are provided and includes material and human resources. Process was described as the steps involved in the provision of medical services, and outcomes were measured by various criteria according to the particular study in progress. According to Donabedian (1988), these factors were all affected by the ambiguities of cost, public expectations, and resource limitations.

Donabedian's quality improvement process accounts for the difficulty of standardizing care-caused variances in populations of patients and among healthcare providers. He also recognized that different clinical practices could achieve the same outcome. The role of the quality manager in health care, he suggested, is to find the most efficient and legitimate processes to arrive at the greatest benefit at the least cost for the patient (Donabedian, 1990). Donabedian was the first recipient of the Codman Award from The Joint Commission. The National Database of Nursing Quality Indicators (American Nurses Association, 2013) is based on Donabedian's model.

SUMMARY

The quest for quality in health care will continue. As the United States seeks to provide quality health care to all of its citizens, the U.S. healthcare industry and the federal government are developing outcomes measurement systems, practice standards, and reimbursement based on performance. While quality improvement experts differ somewhat in their approaches, their theories share several common characteristics.

Quality Is Driven by Organization Leaders

Experts agree that leaders must be committed to quality improvement if an organization-wide program is to be successful. Leaders must embody the principles of quality improvement if they expect staff to commit themselves to the desired cultural shift. The manager's job is to remove barriers that prevent staff from providing quality services all of the time.

Customer-Mindedness Permeates the Organization

A new definition of the customer must be articulated throughout the organization. According to Deming (2000), each organization has both internal and external customers. External customers for healthcare organizations, for example, include patients, physicians, and insurance companies. Internal customers include people such as the staff who work in the organization, as well as the departments receiving services from other departments within the organization.

An Emphasis on Process Improvement

At the heart of quality improvement is a body of knowledge and tools referred to as *systems thinking* that emerged over the last half-century. Systems thinking is a framework for seeing interrelationships rather than discrete things, for seeing patterns of change rather than static snapshots (Senge, 1990). By taking a systematic view, the many processes and factors that affect outcomes become clear—for example, protocols, guidelines, and management systems. Adopting a quality improvement philosophy involves rejecting the idea that people are the problem and, instead, shifts the focus toward looking at the organization's systems.

Deming believed that most employees want to do the best job they can, but the systems they work in often prevent them from doing so. He concluded that 85% of the problems detected are systems based and only 15% can be traced to the worker (Deming, 2000). Organizations that implement quality improvement, when necessary, form teams composed of members across functional or departmental lines to examine and reexamine clinical and administrative processes and to analyze how these processes might be improved. However, all process improvements do not necessarily require the formation of a team. Juran, for instance, believed that teams sometimes are vulnerable to *groupthink*, a phenomenon that can hinder effective work on issues of quality improvement. A sign that quality improvement is beginning to infiltrate an organization is when management and staff begin to use the concepts in their everyday activities.

Formal Process Improvement Methods and Tools

To guide process improvement efforts, organizations use time-tested scientific methods and statistical tools. When improvement is needed, staff measure and analyze the current process to determine the root cause or primary reason that the process is inadequate; they then take action toward improvement based on that analysis. Organizations use a variety of tools for quality improvement purposes, such as flowcharts, cause and effect diagrams, and control charts.

Involvement of All Employees

Quality improvement is a cultural transformation that begins with a slow change in attitudes, which is then gradually realized in improved outcomes, staff morale, and patient care. It requires a commitment from everyone in the organization, from the housekeeper to the chief executive officer. A quality improvement department or a subcommittee cannot shoulder all of the responsibility for the institution's ultimate survival. One way in which this wide-scale, shared involvement is most visible is in the makeup and dynamics of teams. Quality improvement empowers staff by providing them with the methods and structure to approach their jobs, and empowered employees are better prepared to participate in quality improvement activities.

RESOURCES

In today's ever-changing healthcare industry, quality improvement remains highly relevant. All healthcare organizations need to evaluate the quality of their services for their own improvement or for external reviewers and payers. Listed here are accreditation organizations that evaluate the quality of care provided by healthcare organizations:

Accreditation Association for Ambulatory Health Care (AAAHC)
http://www.aaahc.org

AAAHC is a U.S. organization that accredits ambulatory healthcare organizations, including ambulatory surgery centers, office-based surgery centers, endoscopy centers, and college student health centers, as well as health plans, such as health maintenance organizations and preferred provider organizations.

Accreditation Commission for Health Care (ACHC)
http://www.achc.org

ACHC is a U.S. nonprofit accrediting organization. Home care health providers established it to create an accreditation option that was more focused on the needs of small providers.

Centers for Medicare and Medicaid Services (CMS)
http://www.cms.gov

CMS is a federal agency within the U.S. Department of Health and Human Services that administers the Medicare program and works in partnership with state governments to administer Medicaid, the State Children's Health Insurance Program, and health insurance portability standards.

Community Health Accreditation Partner (CHAP)
http://www.chapinc.org

CHAP is a U.S. nonprofit accrediting body for community-based healthcare organizations.

DNV Healthcare
http://dnvaccreditation.com

DNV Healthcare is a leading provider of international hospital accreditation, infection risk management, and standards development. The company was approved in 2008 by the CMS to accredit acute care hospitals in the United States and since then has also been granted CMS deeming authority for critical access hospitals. It is part of the larger multinational group Stiftelsen Det Norske Veritas (DNV).

Healthcare Facilities Accreditation Program (HFAP)
http://www.hfap.org

HFAP is a U.S. nonprofit organization that provides accreditation programs for hospitals, clinical laboratories, ambulatory surgical centers/office-based surgery, and critical access hospitals. In addition, HFAP accredits mental health and physical rehabilitation facilities and provides certification for primary stroke centers.

Healthcare Quality Association on Accreditation (HQAA)

http://www.hqaa.org

HQAA is a U.S. nonprofit healthcare accrediting body that provides an accreditation option specifically designed for durable medical equipment (DME) companies. These company types include DME, infusion and compounding pharmacies, medical practice, facility-based ventilator units, and third-party billing.

National Committee for Quality Assurance (NCQA)

http://www.ncqa.org

NCQA is a U.S. nonprofit organization designed to improve healthcare quality. NCQA manages voluntary accreditation programs for individual physicians, health plans, and medical groups.

The Compliance Team

http://www.thecomplianceteam.org

The Compliance Team is a U.S. for-profit organization that runs the "Exemplary Provider" accreditation programs. The Compliance Team accredits all types of DME, including respiratory, mobility, wound care, orthopedic, prosthetics, orthotics, diabetic, ostomy, and incontinence supplies, as well as DME point-of-service providers including pharmacy, home care, podiatrists, and orthopedic surgeons. The Compliance Team has accredited approximately 5,000 DME providers in the United States and Puerto Rico.

The Joint Commission

http://www.jointcommission.org

The Joint Commission is a U.S.-based nonprofit organization that accredits more than 19,000 healthcare organizations and programs. It accredits ambulatory care, behavioral care, critical access hospitals, home care, hospitals, laboratory services, nursing and rehabilitation centers, and international organizations.

DISCUSSION QUESTIONS

1. What does the concept of quality mean?
2. How is quality defined in nursing literature?
3. Does mass inspection improve the quality of care delivered by people working in the healthcare industry? Support your answer.
4. Is the goal of zero defects realistic in health care? Support your answer.
5. How are evidence-based practice and quality management related?

REFERENCES

American Association of Colleges of Nursing. (2006). *The essentials of doctoral education for advanced nursing practice*. Washington, DC: Author.

American Nurses Association. (2013). Nursing quality (NDNQI). Retrieved from http://www.nursingquality.org/data

Crosby, P. (1979). *Quality is free*. New York, NY: McGraw-Hill.

Crosby, P. (1984). *Quality without tears: The art of hassle-free management*. New York, NY: McGraw-Hill.

Crosby, P. (1992). *Completeness: Quality for the 21st century*. New York, NY: Penguin Books.

Deming, W. E. (2000). *Out of the crisis*. Cambridge, MA: MIT Press.

Donabedian, A. (1988). The quality of care: How can it be assessed? *Journal of the American Medical Association, 260,* 1743–1748.

Donabedian, A. (1990). The seven pillars of quality. *Archives of Pathology and Laboratory Medicine, 114,* 1115–1118.

Dossey, B. M. (1999). *Florence Nightingale*. Springhouse, PA: Springhouse.

The Joint Commission. (1996). *A study in hospital efficiency as demonstrated by the case report of the first five years of a private hospital*. Oakbrook Terrace, IL: Author.

Juran, J. M. (1989). *Juran on leadership for quality*. New York, NY: Free Press.

Juran, J. M. (1992). *Juran on quality by design*. New York, NY: Free Press.

Nightingale, F. (1969/1860). *Notes on nursing: What it is, and what it is not*. New York, NY: Dover Publications.

Pirsig, R. M. (1999). *Zen and the art of motorcycle maintenance: An inquiry into values* (25th anniversary ed.). New York, NY: Vintage. (Originally published in 1974)

Senge, P. M. (1990). *The fifth discipline: The art and practice of the learning organization*. New York, NY: Doubleday.

Small, H. (1999). *Florence Nightingale: Avenging angel*. New York, NY: Palgrave Macmillan.

Stephens, K. S., & Juran, J. M. (2004). *Quality and a century of improvement*. Milwaukee, WI: ASQ Quality Press.

Walton, M. (1986). *The Deming management method*. New York, NY: Putnam.

Chapter 17

Theories Focused on Health Equity and Health Disparities

Tori Baker

INTRODUCTION

Advanced practice registered nurses should lead the way in addressing social justice issues, especially in achieving health equity. Theories and models that explain how health disparities arise and offer avenues for achieving health equity support efforts in that regard. This chapter provides an introduction to the history of health disparities in the United States. It follows with models and theories developed to explain how health disparities arise. It finishes with theories, models, and approaches used to achieve health equity.

HEALTH EQUITY AND HEALTH DISPARITIES

Disparities in Health Status

Health equity might justifiably be called the salient health issue in the United States of last 30 years, certainly of the early 21st century, taking a key role in the discussion of research, policy, and teaching in every area of health and clinical care. In 1985, the U.S. Department of Health and Human Services presented the data on what clinicians must have felt to be an obvious problem, publishing a landmark report establishing that Blacks and other American minorities suffered worse mortality and morbidity than Whites experience. This issue was not a new one, just newly reemerged (Quinn, 2001; Quinn & Thomas, 2001). The evidence spoke, though, and the following decades have brought unprecedented national attention to the issue in terms of studying the problem and developing possible solutions. Studies began to proliferate, resulting in hundreds of reports highlighting data on the problem and solutions. Reports citing the need for interventions to reduce or eliminate racial and ethnic disparities—and, increasingly, disparities among other populations—have been issued by virtually every major health-related federal agency (e.g., Agency for Healthcare Quality and Research, 2016; Centers for Disease Control and Prevention, 2013; Centers for Medicare and Medicaid, 2016; National Institute on Minority Health and Health Disparities, n.d.), foundation (e.g., Robert Wood Johnson Foundation, 2015; W. K. Kellogg Foundation, 2016), professional association (e.g., American Association of Nurse Anesthetists, 2016; American College of Nurse-Midwives, 2007; American Dental Association, 2004; American Hospital Association, n.d.; American Medical Association, 2016; American Nurses Association, 1998; American Public Health Association, 2000; Goldstein et al., 2011), and health educational program accrediting agency (e.g., American Association of Critical-Care Nurses, 2015; American Dental Education Association, 2015; Association of American Medical Colleges, 2009; Association of Schools and Programs of Public Health, 2016; National League for Nursing, 2016).

Hundreds of reports have highlighted data on the problem and solutions, most saliently *Unequal Treatment*, the 2003 Institute of Medicine (IOM) report summarizing data on racial and ethnic healthcare disparities and recommended solutions (Anderson, Roundtable on the Promotion of Health Equity and the Elimination of Health Disparities, Board on Population Health and Public Health Practice, & IOM, 2003 with an update in 2012). Important agencies have been established during this time as well, including the Office of Minority Health of the Centers for Disease Control and Prevention (in 1988) and the National Institute on Minority Health and Health Disparities (in 2010). Furthermore, health disparities have featured as key content of Healthy People goals since 2000 (Thomas, Quinn, Butler, Fryer, & Garza, 2011).

Racial and ethnic disparities in U.S. infant mortality rate provide an early, continuing, and compelling example of health disparities. The World Health Organization (Kramer, 1987) and the IOM both issued classic documents in the 1980s seeking the causes of and considering solutions for low birth weight (Krans & Davis, 2012), a major contributor to infant mortality and a key indicator of racial and ethnic health disparities. The work on this issue continues today, as infant mortality rates overall drop over time (an indicator of improving health), but gaps in the rates between groups persist (an indicator of continuing disparities) (**Figure 17-1**). African American babies die twice as often as European American babies, and American Indian babies 50% more often. As Wise pointed out, each baby's death is a "shame," but the rates overall are "shameful" (2003). The issue of racial and ethnic disparities in U.S. infant mortality rates, and particularly research into Black infant mortality rates, provides us with some of the earliest and best developed epidemiologic and theoretical work in this area of scholarship, including many of the models and theories included in this chapter.

Definitions of what constitutes a health disparity vary somewhat, although all capture the population-based nature of the problem. The National Institutes of Health defines health disparities as differences in "the overall rate of disease incidence, prevalence, morbidity, mortality, or survival rates in the population as compared to the health status of the general

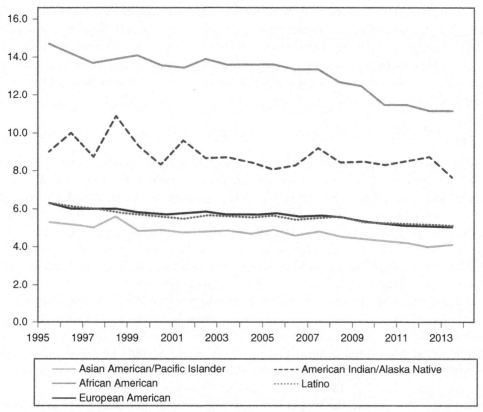

Figure 17-1 U.S. infant mortality rates by race and ethnicity. Disparities persist.

Data from CDC/NHCS National Vital Statistics System.

population" (n.d.). This definition captures the important characteristic, that of differences between populations, rather than between individuals. This definition also well captures the health aspect of the issue in its many manifestations. Unfortunately, the definition misses the ethical component, the injustice that underlies the differences. Healthy People 2020 captures the justice element in its definition of health equity, noting that health equity involves attaining "the highest level of health for all people," "valuing everyone equally," and addressing "avoidable inequalities, historical and contemporary injustices, and the elimination of health and health care disparities" (n.d.). Scholars of health equity have stressed that health disparities constitute more than differences; they constitute *preventable* differences, *inequitable* differences (e.g., Braveman, 2014; Dahlgren & Whitehead, 2006a; Marmot & Allen, 2014). Health disparities present us with not just a health issue, but an issue of social justice.

These definitions focus on preventable difference between populations, without specifying any particular population. Healthy People 2020 points out health disparities in populations defined by a variety of characteristics, including "sex, sexual identity, age, disability, socioeconomic status, and geographic location" (n.d.). Nonetheless, understanding of how disparities operate and how we might achieve equity has come most frequently from racial and ethnic health disparities.

Race

The human genome project changed our view of the biological world (Tripp & Grueber, 2011). In the case of race as a biological concept, it clarified for many a controversy of generations, finally putting to rest for most scientists (at least) the idea of race as biology. Anthropologists proposed the concept of biological (and measurable) races in the 19th century—Caucasian, Asian, African, and American Indian. Efforts to standardize the measurement of such races consistently failed, and the concept should have withered. Consider, for example, what would be the genetic common link for every Asian—that is, everyone from Mongolia, Japan, India, Thailand, Iran, Syria, etc.; the variation is far too grand to permit a genetic marker, or even a series of markers. Yet, the idea of biologically based races meshed well with our social norms, and it has hung on as science despite all evidence against it (Goodman, 2000; Montagu, 1942). The Human Genome Project showed that no racial genes could be identified and more variation could be found within races than between them, along with other excellent evidence against race as a biologic or genetic concept (Goodman, 2000, **Table 17-1**). Even today, though, while scientists mostly agree that race is social, not genetic, the lay public frequently continues to think of race as biologic.

Not only is viewing race as a matter of biology incorrect, but it can also be harmful, including in clinical applications. The approval of the drug BiDil offers an example of how the concept of race as biologic can cloud clinical thinking. Trials of this combination of cardiac medications did not show clear benefits in populations used in the earliest studies. When a subpopulation of Blacks was analyzed, statistically significant results were obtained. The statistical differences were almost certainly due to a different prevalence of some genetic characteristic in the two populations studied, not their races. Instead of further investigating the genetic difference that caused BiDil to work in some populations, the company sought (and obtained) FDA approval for Black men. Some White men also benefit from BiDil, and some Black men do not, as admitted by the trial investigators themselves. Later, impairments in nitric oxide–mediated cardiovascular function were proposed as the true mediator of which patients benefited from BiDil, an impairment with a higher prevalence among Blacks (Cole et al., 2011). By not investigating the true difference between the groups based on their cardiac physiology, by using race as a proxy for a prevalence of cardiac differences, the drug was approved for the wrong population (reviewed in Kahn, 2009). BiDil was approved for Blacks, rather than for patients who had the genetic capacity to benefit from

Table 17-1   Arguments for Race as a Social Concept (Goodman, 2000)

- The concept requires unchanging types. Humans evolve and the races change. Species do not change with this speed.
- The variation between races is continuous, not categorical. Skin color, for example, changes on a continuum. There are not only Black and White people, but also an entire palette of skin colors, and which color belongs to a "race" often cannot be defined. Can a Black person have freckles? Is an Asian Indian with dark skin really an African?
- Variations do not stay in one group. Africans may be tall or short, have flat or narrow noses, have straight or kinky hair, and still be dark skinned. Each race has the whole range of intelligence, and all other human characteristics. Physical characteristics occur in all the races, at different prevalences.
- Within-group variation is almost the same as between-group variation. This is where the Human Genome Project really put some numbers into the discussion. While prevalences of certain characteristics do vary between populations, the presence of all characteristics can be found in all races, indeed in almost all smaller populations, as well.
- No system of measurement or classification for races works. All systems vary with time and place. Some people are classified at birth as one race and at death as another. (Did they convert?)
- Race is classified differently in different places. A person in South Africa might be classified as "Colored" and in the United States as "Black," and as something else somewhere else. There is no agreement on what constitutes each race; the social context, not biology, defines these categorizations.

Not long after the Human Genome Project finished its work, Goodman (2000) summarized the arguments for race as a social concept. He points out why considering race as biology is a myth, and a harmful one.

Data from Goodman, A. H. (2000). Why genes don't count (for racial differences in health). *American Journal of Public Health, 90*(11): 1699–1702.

it, which can be tested. This erroneous marketing of the medication discourages clinicians from trying it with patients other than Black ones and may blind clinicians to Black patients who are not responding to treatment with BiDil.

Disparities in Clinical Care

Given the nature of the problem, differences between populations, health disparities do not immediately show themselves in the examination room. They can be hard for clinicians to see when caring for individuals. And most clinicians believe they give appropriate care across the board, no matter the characteristics of the person in their care.

Data dispute the idea that clinicians provide equal care to all patients, however, showing that both clinical systems and individual clinicians give different standards of care to people based on their race, gender, and (likely) other characteristics. Schulman's group (1999) demonstrated bias when physicians applied standards of care differently in managing chest pain for the same symptoms and objective findings for "patients" (actually recorded actors) of different genders and races: Black women were significantly less likely to get appropriate referrals for cardiac catheterization when compared with White men. These findings shocked people, making national headlines at the time (Goldstein, 1999).

Likewise, the report *Unequal Treatment* (2003) made national headlines when the IOM issued it (Stolberg, 2002), showing that even in the presence of access to care, racial and ethnic healthcare disparities could be shown in every clinical area of care. "Some of us on the committee were surprised and shocked at the extent of the evidence," said the report chair (Stolberg, 2002). In fact, data support that one's health status is more closely related to the race one seems to be to others (*socially assigned* race) than the race one identifies with personally (Jones et al., 2008). This supports the findings that clinicians and clinical systems do not treat every population with equal standards of care.

BIASED CARE MODEL

This bias in care probably works in more than one way (well summarized by Matthew, 2015). First, not all differences in care are disparities, as *Unequal Treatment* maps out for us. Some differences arise more naturally from differences in needs and preferences of individuals or populations. But, clearly, some differences are disparities that arise out of unjust causes, both from structural and individual forms of bias against the population of interest (as in **Figure 17-2**).

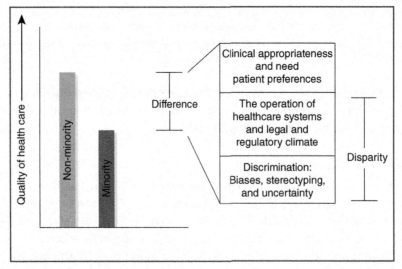

Figure 17-2   Model for components of differences in health care.

Gomes and McGuire's model clarifies how disparities comprise a subset of differences from unjust causes, and disparities may be further subdivided into structural and individual forms of bias (2001, as cited in Smedley, Stith, & Nelson, 2003, p. 4).

Reproduced from Gomes, C., & McGuire, T.G. (2001). Identifying the sources of racial and ethnic disparities in health care use. Unpublished manuscript.

Many researchers have investigated the structural and individual forms of bias. Many of these investigations take into account patient trust and preferences and patient–clinician interaction, keeping in mind that clinicians and patients make their decisions in relationship to one another. These investigations have given rise to models of how aspects of bias may function to affect decisions about care. Matthew (2015) summarizes those findings, pointing out six mechanisms that operate for individual clinicians to bias their care, contributing to racial and ethnic health outcomes disparities. She used the mechanisms to develop the biased care model (see **Figure 17-3**), noting key times in which implicit bias may affect patient care and the mechanisms through which the bias manifests:

- **Implicit bias before the clinical encounter**
  - *Mechanism 1: Clinicians' biased perceptions negatively impact minority patient outcomes* (Matthew, 2015, pp. 79–98). (Note that Matthew uses the term *physician*, and many of the studies do focus on physician practices. Here we have opted to use the more inclusive term for providers of care, *clinician*.) Clinical providers bring "stored social knowledge" (p. 79) to the encounter, containing implicit bias and stereotypes that affect communication and decisions. An example Matthew provides is the story of the doctor who admits that she must have this implicit bias that "comes out in peculiar ways . . . [such as] when it turns out that the patient who's African American turns out to be the son of a prominent official in the government" and she is surprised (p. 80). These unchallenged and unacknowledged assumptions affect the care clinicians give. Such assumptions will typically harm care, obscuring an individual's specific needs and expressed preferences, where stereotypes obscure the findings of a clinical encounter as well as clinical training.
  - *Mechanism 2: Clinicians' implicit biases can lead to discriminatory statistical interpretation* (Matthew, 2015, pp. 98–105). Clinical providers may let a known prevalence of a disease or condition in a particular group drive their diagnosis, rather than using it as a starting point to find out the individual situation of the patient at hand. A provider may not pursue a diagnosis because it has lower prevalence in a population, despite the clinical picture of the individual patient. Or, conversely, clinicians may be overly inclined to diagnose problems known to have increased prevalence in the group to which the patient belongs. For example, depression has a lower prevalence among Blacks than among Whites. When this mechanism of bias in interpretation of statistics operates, the difference in prevalence can bias clinicians against making the diagnosis in Black patients; that is, the clinician may not recognize symptoms of depression in a Black patient, thereby missing an important opportunity for timely treatment.

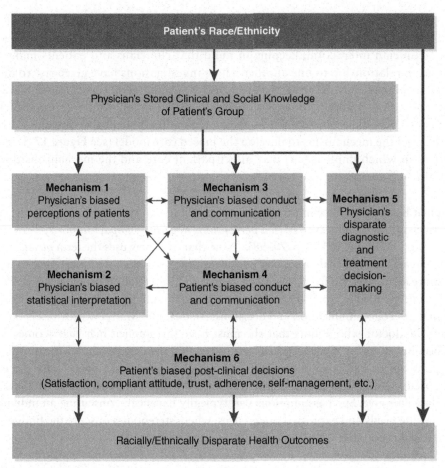

Figure 17-3 The Biased care model.

Matthew (2015) drew on current findings about clinical bias to create a model of clinical bias. It shows the interactions of six different mechanisms of bias in clinical encounters, contributing to racial and ethnic health disparities.

Reproduced from Matthew, D. B. (2015). *Just medicine: A cure for the racial inequality in American health care.* New York, NY: New York University Press.

- Implicit bias during the clinical encounter
  - *Mechanism 3: Clinicians' implicit biases influence their conduct and communication* (Matthew, 2015, pp. 107–118). Matthew well summarizes the extensive data demonstrating that both verbal and nonverbal communication can be quite different for patients of different backgrounds and that it can result in lower quality of care and poorer health outcomes. Differences have been demonstrated in interviewing,

interruptions, information giving, courtesy, and empathy. These differences can affect patient satisfaction, adherence to advice, and health outcomes.

- *Mechanism 4: Patients' implicit biases influence their conduct and communication with clinicians* (Matthew, 2015, pp. 119–127). Unfortunately, data also demonstrate that clinician bias in conduct and communication engenders negative response in patients. Distrust of clinical care can lead to less active participation on the part of patients and other negative changes in communication, in a downward spiral of poor exchange of information.
- **Implicit bias beyond the clinical encounter**
  - *Mechanism 5: Clinicians' implicit biases influence their diagnostic and treatment decisions* (Matthew, 2015, pp. 130–140). Matthew reports the multiple studies that support bias against racial and ethnic minorities in terms of recommendations made to them by their clinical providers. These biases do seem to be largely unconscious. Many providers argue that they do not happen at all. But, the data contradict that belief.
  - *Mechanism 6: Implicit biases influence patients' satisfaction, adherence, compliance, and follow-up* (Matthew, 2015, pp. 140–149). Another response to distrust of care can be lack of adherence to recommendations and/or less utilization of appropriate services, even in the presence of access to care.

Of course, these mechanisms do not exist in a vacuum, but are interrelated in the ongoing process of clinical care. Matthew has brought together her review of these data in the model shown in Figure 17-3, which describes the many ways these mechanisms interact.

Matthew also presented good news, pointing out that research also suggests that implicit biases can be changed with the right interventions. She summarized recent data addressing interventions to eliminate bias in clinical care, integrating the interventions into her framework of explanatory mechanisms of individual implicit bias and using them to work toward healthcare equity (see **Figure 17-4**):

- *Type A intervention: stereotype negation training* (Matthew, 2015, pp. 159–162). This type of training goes beyond basic cultural competence trainings, seeking to train in negative responses to negative stereotypes, negating them consciously.
- *Type B intervention: promoting counter-stereotypes* (Matthew, 2015, pp. 162–164). This type of training goes beyond negating stereotypes, replacing them with positive associations, such as with famous and admired persons from the target group.
- *Type C intervention: social and self-motivation* (Matthew, 2015, pp. 165–169). Interestingly, personal motivation and peer pressure can both provide support for reducing personal implicit biases. Matthew cites studies that demonstrate where subjects believe that bias is socially unacceptable they behave in less biased ways, showing more control over implicit bias than one might have suspected.

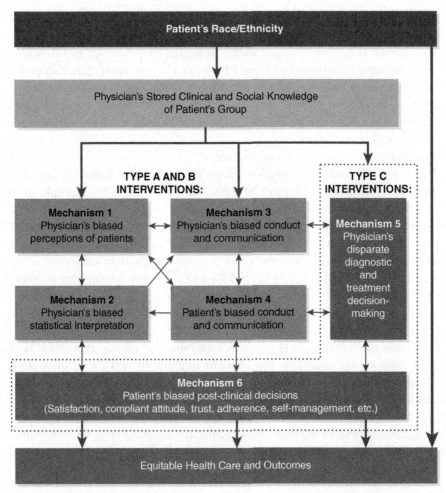

Figure 17-4 The biased care model with integration of interventions to eliminate bias in clinical care and achieve health equity.

Matthew (2015), again drawing from current findings about clinical bias, modified her model of clinical bias to incorporate existing interventions to mitigate or eliminate clinical bias and contribute to equitable healthcare and health outcomes.

Reproduced from Matthew, D. B. (2015). *Just medicine: A cure for the racial inequality in American health care.* New York, NY: New York University Press.

SOCIAL DETERMINANTS OF HEALTH MODELS

Trajectory of Health Inequities

Matthew's biased care model focuses on mechanisms that create health disparities at the level of an individual clinical encounter and interventions to remedy the problem. Remember, though, that health disparities operate on a population level. Likewise, the causes of health disparities work at many levels beyond the individual encounter. Accordingly, achieving health equity requires interventions at many levels, many systematic, rather than individual, in nature. The trajectory of health inequities (**Figure 17-5**) illustrates the increasing importance of the social determinants of health, taking two steps back from the clinical encounter, into the community, where people spend most of their lives and where the biggest influence on health outcomes and health disparities lies.

Ecological Models

Public health typically uses a more contextual perspective of health than does clinically focused health, more clearly taking into account social determinants of health, factors that tend to be invisible to those of us working in the examining room. Such models are sometimes called ecological. Whitehead, Dahlgren, and Gilson (2001) helped bring these factors into clearer focus with an ecological model they called multilevel (**Figure 17-6**), now frequently adopted to clarify the many influences of health on both individuals and populations. This model and similar characterizations of the social determinants of health can be used to broaden the areas used to understand how disparities arise as well as what to target when interventions to achieve health equity are designed. If attention stays focused exclusively on more individual levels of the model, such as individual risk factors, many of the areas that increase disparities will not be addressed. Success requires also addressing levels of broader influence, such as those of living conditions or socioeconomic conditions, which encompass factors like institutional racism, access to care, or social networks.

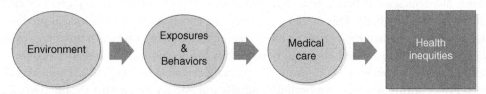

Figure 17-5   Trajectory of health inequities: taking two steps back.

Reproduced from Cohen, L., & Iton, D. (2009). A time of opportunity: Local solutions to reduce inequities in health and safety. Retrieved from http://www.preventioninstitute.org/component/jlibrary/article/id-81/127.html.

The Main Determinants of Health

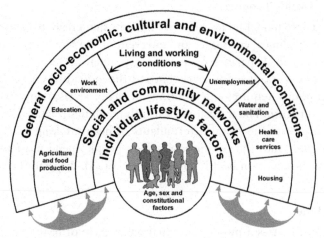

Figure 17-6   Multilevel model of social determinants of health.

Dahlgren and Whitehead (2006b) proposed this conceptualization of the social determinants of health in 1993, an ecological view of health used by public health, shown here in an updated version. This model and others that bring the social determinants of health into focus have been used to explain both how health disparities arise and how to achieve health equity (e.g., Kaplan, Everson, & Lynch, 2000).

From Dahlgren, G., & Whitehead, M. (1993). Tackling inequalities in health: what can we learn from what has been tried? Working paper prepared for the King's Fund International Seminar on Tackling Inequalities in Health, September 1993, Ditchley Park, Oxfordshire. London, King's Fund, accessible in: Dahlgren, G., & Whitehead, M. (2007). European strategies for tackling social inequities in health: Levelling up Part 2. Copenhagen: WHO Regional office for Europe: http://www.euro.who.int/__data/assets/pdf_file/0018/103824/E89384.pdf.

These social determinants of health also have important influences on health disparities and must also be addressed.

Ecological models such as Dahlgren and Whitehead's frequently serve to clarify how health disparities arise, broadening our perspective from the immediately obvious characteristics of individuals. This model pulls back the lens from the physiological processes and individual characteristics to take into account the influence on health outcomes of the characteristics of social and community networks, living conditions, and socioeconomic, cultural, and environmental conditions (i.e., social determinants of health). These broader levels affect health outcomes for both individuals and populations across the life span. The authors stress, "This model for describing health determinants emphasizes interactions: individual lifestyles are embedded in social norms and networks, and in living and working conditions, which in turn are related to the wider socioeconomic and cultural environment" (Dahlgren & Whitehead, 2006b, p. 20).

Infant mortality rates provide an example of how this model may be used to explain racial health disparities. Using this example, each level in the model can be explained as follows:

- **Age, sex, and constitutional factors**
  - Infants born to mothers older than 40 years or to teen mothers are more likely to die in infancy (Mathews, MacDorman, Thoma, & Division of Vital Statistics, 2015).
  - Infant mortality varies enormously by race and ethnicity, with Black babies dying at double the rate of White babies nationally and American Indian babies at rates 50% higher than Whites (Mathews et al., 2015). These disparities have widened over the last decade, as rates overall have dropped (Mathews et al., 2015). (See Figure 17-1.)
- **Individual lifestyle factors**
  - Maternal smoking, alcohol, and illegal drugs all contribute to higher rates of infant mortality (Collins & David, 2009).
- **Social and community networks**
  - Babies born to single mothers are 73% more likely to die in their first year than those born to married mothers (Mathews et al., 2015), possibly a reflection of the social networks linked to families with two parents.
- **Living and working conditions**
  - Lower maternal education levels are linked to higher rates of infant mortality (Collins & David, 2009; U.S. Department of Health and Human Services, Centers of Disease Control and Prevention, National Center for Health Statistics, Division of Vital Statistics, 2016).
  - Later start to prenatal care and lack of insurance are linked to higher rates of preterm birth (Anum, Retchin, Garland, & Strauss, 2010), which is tightly linked to infant mortality (Anum et al., 2010; Collins & David, 2009; Mathews et al., 2015).
  - Lifelong residence in a poor, urban community contributes to low birth weight, also linked tightly to infant mortality (reviewed in Collins & David, 2009).
- **General socioeconomic, cultural, and environmental conditions**
  - Racism has been implicated in maternal stress leading to preterm delivery and low birth weight (Kramer & Hogue, 2009; Love, David, Rankin, & Collins 2010; Spong, Iams, Goldenburg, Hauck, & Willinger 2011; Witt et al., 2014), leading risk factors for infant mortality. Low-birth-weight babies suffer infant mortality rates 25 times higher than other babies (Mathews et al., 2015). Low birth weight is implicated in two-thirds of all infant deaths (Krans & Davis, 2012), and preterm delivery in one-third (Callaghan, MacDorman, Rasmussen, Qin, & Lackritz, 2006).
  - Low socioeconomic status contributes to a higher rate of infant mortality (reviewed in Collins & David, 2009).

Dahlgren and Whitehead's multilevel model also helps us to develop interventions to achieve health equity. Families Forward Resource Center in Denver, Colorado, provides a community-based example of a program that addresses reducing Black infant mortality and disparities in infant mortality using a many-pronged approach (Families Forward Resource Center, n.d.). Black infants in Colorado died at 2.7 times the rate of White infants in 2014 (Colorado Department of Public Health and Environment, 2016), higher than the national disparity of 2.2 as of 2013 (Mathews et al., 2015). Families Forward addresses the Black infant mortality rate in terms of social determinants of health at all levels of the multilevel model:

- **Age, sex, and constitutional factors**
  - The Resource Center offers services to African American families, those at highest risk for infant mortality.
- **Individual lifestyle factors**
  - Courses are offered on parenting, couples communication, fathering, financial literacy, nutrition, and exercise.
- **Social and community networks**
  - The youth development work includes the Youth Leadership Squad, a program in which small groups of youth learn to work together on community projects.
- **Living and working conditions**
  - The Resource Center helps identify resources for families, including food, housing, utilities, crisis intervention, access to care, and other public and private benefits.
- **General socioeconomic, cultural, and environmental conditions**
  - The Resource Center participates in the Community Action Network of organizations and individuals working to address institutional-level interventions to reduce infant mortality, including addressing racism and increasing community support networks and systems of advocacy.

INTERGENERATIONAL EFFECTS MODELS

Popular culture tells us to live in the present. The "Just say 'No'" to drugs campaign of the 1980s emphasized taking charge in the present (Ronald Reagan Presidential Foundation and Library, 2010), without much emphasis on history or contextual factors. Nike tells us to "Just Do It!" and we buy into the message (Martin, 2013). We should "Get over it!" (whatever happened in the past) and move on (to our future) (Phrase Finder, n.d.).

Contrary to this view, data tell us that our history lives on in us, with health at birth partly predicting education, income, and disability long term (Aizer & Currie, 2014). In fact, even our mother's history lives on in us, with maternal disadvantage predicting health at birth (Aizer & Currie, 2014). As such, several models have emerged to explain how history operates to perpetuate health disparities—our own history, as well as our family's and our community's.

Not surprisingly, this view of enduring effects has the most influence in models used to understand perinatal health disparities. In the early programming model, Barker (Barker, Osmond, & Law, 1989) theorized that insults in an individual's earliest experiences affect health long into adulthood (e.g., Fall, Vijayakumar, Baker, Osmond, & Duggleby, 1995). Much of his research focused on cardiovascular disease as a result of early experiences, with adult children born to European women pregnant during famine in World War II serving as cases in point (Barker, 2004). This model does not focus particularly on health disparities, but works well as a framework for understanding their etiology.

The weathering hypothesis (Geronimus, 1992) suggests that "the health status of women may begin to deteriorate in detectable ways in young adulthood as a response to perpetual social and environmental insult or prolonged active coping with stressful circumstances" (Geronimus, 2002), particularly racism. Multiple studies have since supported this model, well reviewed by Williams and Mohammed (2009) and Collins and David (2009).

Particularly striking early support for this theory came from a study of birth weight data in the state of Illinois (David & Collins, 1997). This study supported the hypothesis that U.S.-born Blacks experience particular lifetime stress, not only compared with U.S.-born Whites but also compared with African-born Blacks. The data from 15 years of births in Illinois showed that the weights of babies born to African immigrants much more closely resembled the weights of U.S.-born White babies than U.S.-born Black babies. Since the African immigrant births came from the western African regions from which most slaves were kidnapped, these data undermined the hypothesis that U.S.-born Black babies were genetically inclined to smaller weights. In addition, it gave support to the hypothesis that U.S.-born Blacks have particularly stressful life experiences, leading to low-birth-weight babies, more often than do either African-born Blacks or U.S.-born Whites. These authors and others since have summarized subsequent data supporting the hypothesis that racism and lifetime stress seem the most likely explanation for racial perinatal health disparities (e.g., Hobel, Goldstein, & Barrett, 2008; Kramer & Hogue, 2009; Love et al., 2010; Spong et al., 2011; Witt et al., 2014).

Bringing together these two models about the enduring effects of early experiences (fetal programming and weathering), Lu and Halfon (2003) proposed the life course model to explain perinatal health disparities. According to this model, birth outcomes and racial disparities in birth outcomes require looking well beyond the period of pregnancy, throughout the maternal life course. In this respect, the model draws on early programming. But, by bringing in the data on the ill effects of social stress highlighted in the weathering model, the life course model brings in all the social determinants of health. The life course model has taken hold very strongly in the maternal child health literature (e.g., Braveman, 2014; Love et al., 2010; Lu et al., 2010). In a call to use this model for sweeping reforms to improve maternal child outcomes (Lu et al., 2010), clinical researchers called for strengthening health care, but also for reforms to social institutions, such as "creating social capital in African American communities," "undo[ing] racism," and "clos[ing] the education gap."

INTERVENTION MODELS

The social determinants of health models and the intergenerational effects models highlight the need to go well beyond clinical care to find interventions to achieve health equity. As in so many clinical issues, the examination room provides only a start to solutions; achieving health lies well beyond the clinical arena. Two models provide more guidance for interventions to achieve health equity, both in the clinical setting and in wider arenas.

Critical Race Theory

Critical race theory came out of legal scholarship and has since spread to other disciplines (Delgado & Stefancic, 2012, p. 6). In legal scholarship, the theory provides a framework for understanding how legal scholarship and opinions have developed, particularly in terms of civil rights. Work using this theory has focused on the "law's role in the construction and maintenance of social domination and subordination." Starting in the 1980s, critical race theorists have been developing analyses that take into account the sometimes invisible "role of deep-seated racism in American life" (Crenshaw, 1995, p. xi). Early work analyzed topics such as affirmative action (Kennedy, 1990), tribal rights (Torres & Milun, 1990), and equal protection under the law (Lawrence, 1987).

In public health, critical race theory provides both a framework to understand mechanisms by which health disparities arise and interventions to eliminate them. Ford and Airhihenbuwa (2010) reconceptualized the theory as "an iterative methodology for helping investigators remain attentive to equity while carrying out research, scholarship, and practice." They argue convincingly that to date work analyzing the etiology of health disparities and appropriate interventions for health equity rarely has taken into account the complexities of race and racism. They apply concepts from earlier critical race theory scholarship to public health for purposes of better analysis and intervention for health equity (see **Table 17-2**). They point out that their theory differs from theories in other disciplines in that it provides both explanation of phenomena and methodology for intervention. In Table 17-2, applications have been added to Ford and Airhihenbuwa's concepts and definitions, using the public health issue of disparities in the rates of Black infant mortality.

Table 17-2 Concepts of Critical Race Theory as Applied to Racial Disparities in Infant Mortality (adapted from Ford & Airhihenbuwa, 2010)

Concept	Definition	Application to Infant Mortality Disparities
Public health	The art (i.e., practice) and science (i.e., research) of protecting and improving the health of communities	Certainly, this constitutes a public health problem. We have already defined health disparities and health equity as issues of populations, rather than individuals. So reducing racial disparities in infant mortality would constitute an issue of "protecting and improving the health of communities."
Centering in the margins	Making the perspectives of socially marginalized groups, rather than those of people belonging to dominant race or culture, the central axis around which discourse on a topic revolves	Since Black (and American Indian) communities suffer the disparities in infant mortality rates, these communities should be leading the discourse on explanations and solutions. Leaders from other communities, including health professionals, should be following their lead.
Critical consciousness	Digging beneath the surface of information to develop deeper understandings of concepts, relationships, and personal biases	Many discussions of infant mortality focus on proximal causes, such as sudden infant death syndrome or preterm delivery. To get at solutions, explanations and solutions must "take two steps back" (as in the trajectory of health inequities [Cohen & Iton, 2009] or the maternal life course models [Lu & Halfon, 2003]) and consider social determinants of health and racism as the causes of infant mortality.
Experiential knowledge	Ways of knowing that result from critical analysis of one's personal experiences	Qualitative data from families and communities should carry substantial weight as explanations are formed and solutions sought.
Ordinariness	The nature of racism in post–civil rights society: that is, integral and normal rather than aberrational	Black infant mortality has maintained between double and triple the rates for Whites for decades, becoming an accepted norm. At times, researchers proposed that Black babies are genetically smaller, that this was normal for them. Until this theory was debunked by evidence (as explained in the chapter), it supported the notion that infant mortality rate disparities were "normal."

(Continues)

Table 17-2   Concepts of Critical Race Theory as Applied to Racial Disparities in Infant Mortality (adapted from Ford & Airhihenbuwa, 2010) (Continued)

Concept	Definition	Application to Infant Mortality Disparities
Praxis	Iterative process by which the knowledge gained from theory, research, personal experiences, and practice inform one another	Public health critical race theory recommends praxis as the road forward. The coalition of organizations in which Families Forward participates might provide an example of this approach, where different groups and individuals make sense together of personal experiences, data, theory, and practice, seeking solutions for their communities.
Primacy	Prioritizing the study of racial influences on outcomes	Given the growing evidence of the effects of racism on health, and on pregnancy outcomes in particular, and given the enormous contribution of low birth weight and preterm birth to infant mortality rates, study of infant mortality must take into account racism. To date, few (if any) studies of infant mortality or racial disparities in infant mortality study the effects of racism.
Race consciousness	Explicit acknowledgment of the workings of race and racism in social contexts or in one's personal life	
Social construction of race	The endowment of a group or concept with a delineation, name, or reality based on historical, contextual, political, or other social considerations	This concept reminds us that race is a social, not biological, construction. Looking for biological reasons for racial disparities in infant mortality proved a low-yield approach. Addressing issues of culture, social class, or other social determinants of health should yield more results.

Ford and Airhihenbuwa adapted and expanded concepts from earlier critical race theory scholarship (presented in Delgado & Stefancic, 2001) to the needs of research, practice, and scholarship in public health.

Data from Ford, C. L., & Airhihenbuwa, C. O. (2010). Critical Race Theory, race equity, and public health: Toward antiracism praxis. *American Journal of Public Health, 100*(S1): S30–5.

Health Equity Action Research Trajectory (HEART)

The trajectory of work around health disparities over the last few decades has been characterized in a conceptual model as having three distinct phases (Kilbourne, Switzer, Hyman, Crowley-Matoka, & Fine, 2006). In the first phase, epidemiologists define the problem, using data to demonstrate health disparities of populations in terms of health status, care, and outcomes. In this phase, researchers ask if health disparities exist and, if they do, to what extent. In this phase health disparities are investigated epidemiologically, in terms of disparities in prevalence of conditions, disparities in health care, and disparities in health outcomes. All of these issues contribute to the overall disparities in the health status of any given population. Then, in the second phase, theorists understand the problem, by

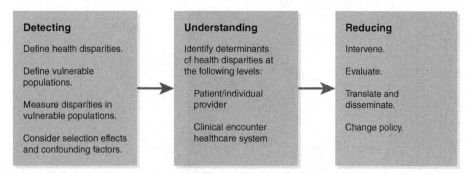

Figure 17-7 Kilbourne's group's three phases of the disparities research agenda.

Kilbourne et al. (2006) proposed a model of research into health disparities with three sequential phases.

Reproduced from Kilbourne, A. M., Switzer, G., Hyman, K., Crowley-Matoka, M., & Fine, M. J. (2006). Advancing health disparities research within the health care system: A conceptual framework. *American Journal of Public Health, 96*, 2113–21. Published by The American Public Health Association.

hypothesizing and testing theories that explain how these various disparities arise. Finally, scholars and practitioners investigate effective solutions that translate evidence to that date into policy answers (**Figure 17-7**).

Thomas's group (Thomas et al., 2011) expanded this model. They divide the third phase into two, first providing solutions and then taking action. They point out that "research is urgently needed that builds the evidence base of effective and culturally appropriate interventions for racial and ethnic minority populations." They report that scholarship has entered well into the third generation, research focusing on interventions. But, they report, that work has failed to make many inroads into achieving health equity because it generally focuses on clinical conditions. Race, they point out, is treated mainly only in terms of cultural implications and rarely in terms of the impact of racism (Thomas et al., 2011). An ever-growing body of research points to racism as lying at the root of racial and ethnic health disparities (e.g., Jones et al., 2008; Krieger et al., 2010; Williams & Mohammed, 2009). Translational, third-generation research often does focus on community engagement and multidisciplinary contributions, which is necessary. But typically this does not suffice. Without addressing encompassing issues of race, third-generation research falls short, both in vision and in results (Thomas et al., 2011).

Thomas's group posits that more explicit work in this aspect of solutions will be required to achieve health equity—that attention must be paid to both health and racism to eliminate disparities. They propose an expanded model of a research trajectory, the health equity action research trajectory (HEART) (**Figure 17-8**). This model provides the needed emphasis provided by a fourth phase, where findings from previous phases can be used to take action. In this fourth phase, they incorporate several elements: critical race theory,

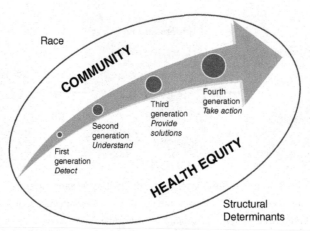

Figure 17-8   Health equity action research trajectory (HEART).

Thomas et al. (2011) proposed a model of research that recognizes that finding solutions and implementing them require different actions and skills. Racism and race require particular attention in the fourth phase, taking action. In this phase, the authors integrate critical race theory into their model of health equity research.

Reproduced from Thomas, S. B., Quinn, S. C., Butler, J., Fryer, C. S. & Garza, M. A. (2011). Toward a fourth generation of disparities research to achieve health equity. *Annual Review of Public Health, 32,* 399–416. *Annual Review of Public Health* by Annual Reviews. Reproduced with permission of Annual Reviews.

focus on multiple levels of intervention, and reflective practice. **Table 17-3** provides an example of how their approach incorporates critical race theory.

Multilevel intervention models should be enhanced by incorporating fourth-generation research. As we have seen in the multilevel model, health disparities operate at many levels. Thus, to reduce health disparities, the social determinants of health must be addressed at many levels. Interventions often do not operate at more than one level. Thomas's group argues for using ecological models (such as Dahlgren and Whitehead's) in the design of interventions to achieve health equity.

Finally, the authors of this model point out the need for reflective practice, not just of clinicians, but also of researchers. Nursing educators often agree, recommending personal reflection in nursing preparation (e.g., Benner, Sutphen, Leonard, & Day, 2010), as do many other educators (reviewed in Horton-Deutsch, McNelis, & Day, 2012). Cultural theorists in particular stress the importance of reflection for work across cultures (e.g., Campinha-Bacote, 2002, 2007). Applying the concept of reflection to public health practitioners and researchers, Thomas's group says the following:

> We have to move beyond the mere synthesis and application of awareness, knowledge, and sensitivity gained from a discrete end point like a cultural competence workshop to the belief that one can be committed to self-reflection and critique over one's life span. We describe this process as *cultural confidence.* Cultural confidence is a lifelong process based on the individual's self-reflection about their personal biases and prejudices.

Table 17-3 Applying Public Health Critical Race Praxis (Thomas et al., 2012)

PHCR Principles	Definition	Selected Third-Generation Healthy Black Family Project Intervention Components	Proposed Fourth-Generation Healthy Black Family Project Intervention Components
Race consciousness	Deep awareness of one's racial position; awareness of racial stratification processes operating in color-blind contexts	Engaged health professionals and researchers to conduct health education and clinical outreach to HBFP participants by working in local barber shops and beauty salons, followed by debriefing discussions, as part of the urban immersion program	Engage all health professionals, researchers, and staff working with HBFP in the Undoing Racism Workshop series
Primacy of racialization	The fundamental contribution of facial stratification to societal problems, the central focus of CRT scholarship on explaining racial phenomena	Completed a qualitative CBPR study with HBFP members that integrated community voices with quantitative data on grocery store practices and policies shaped by structural racism and resulting in poor access to full-service grocery stores in segregated black neighborhoods	Mobilize consumer demand for access to full-service grocery stores in black neighborhoods using data from mixed-methods research to posit a social justice alternative to the prevailing market justifications for the food desert status quo
Race as social construct	Significance that derives from social, political, and historical forces	Created HBFP and its associated media campaign in a deliberate way to overcome the negative image of black families as a means to seize race and the family as positive constructs	Although the HEZ was established on the basis of historical geographic patterns of racial segregation, poverty, and unearned disadvantages, use the mass media platform to redefine the HEZ as the geographic space for targeted investments designed to promote social cohesion and direct political power needed to achieve health equity

(Continues)

Table 17-3 Applying Public Health Critical Race Praxis (Thomas et al., 2012) (*Continued*)

PHCR Principles	Definition	Selected Third-Generation Healthy Black Family Project Intervention Components	Proposed Fourth-Generation Healthy Black Family Project Intervention Components
Ordinariness of racism	Racism is embedded in the social fabric of society		After the Undoing Racism Workshops, health professionals, researchers, and HBFP members meet to work jointly on the development of a study of how exposure to racism impacts their mental health
Structural determinism	The fundamental role of macrolevel forces in driving and sustaining inequities across time and contexts; the tendency of dominant group members and institutions to make decisions or take action that preserves existing power hierarchies	Created the HEZ using census and national health data to identify residential racial segregation, poverty, and chronic disease to target HBFP	Create a Black Leadership Commission on Health Equity charged with developing an advocacy agenda with leadership from community members focused on addressing racialized structural determinants that could eliminate disparities
Social construction of knowledge	The claim that established knowledge within a discipline can be reevaluated using antiracism modes of analysis		Develop a community-driven request for proposals for academic researchers to engage in relevant research on problems identified by the community
Critical approaches	To dig beneath the surface; to develop a comprehensive understanding of one's biases		Engage health professionals and researchers to participate in community-based dialogue with HBFP participants about race and the impact of racism on research recruitment
Intersectionality	The interlocking nature of co-occurring social categories (e.g., race and gender) and the forms of social stratification that maintain them		Engage HBFP male participants in the examination of how race, gender, and current structure of activities impact male involvement in HBFP

CBPR = community-based participatory research, CRT = critical race theory, HBFP = Healthy Black Family Project, HEZ = Health Empowerment Zone.

This group proposed using public health critical praxis, a version of critical race theory, to guide interventions meant to achieve health equity. In this table they give examples of how this approach might work.

Reproduced from Thomas, S. B., Quinn, S. C., Butler, J., Fryer, C. S. & Garza, M. A. (2011). Toward a fourth generation of disparities research to achieve health equity. *Annual Review of Public Health, 32*, 399–416. *Annual Review of Public Health* by Annual Reviews. Reproduced with permission of Annual Reviews.

IMPLICATIONS FOR ADVANCED PRACTICE

Models used to explain health disparities and design interventions for health equity have arisen relatively recently. Unlike the models in some fields, which may span generations, models in this field have been developing only over the last 20 or 30 years, some far more recently. These new models have much to offer advanced practice nursing, at the clinical and professional levels.

As clinicians, we should be aware of implicit bias and of the interventions available to us to mitigate it. We all grow up with cultural beliefs and biases. The good news is that we can learn and grow, and we can do better.

As a profession, we have a duty to advocate for our patients, speaking out about the abundant data and models that show that racism does hurt our patients. Both implicit bias and structural racism contribute to racial and ethnic health disparities, and it will take all of us to work to correct the problems. As we learn more about racial and ethnic disparities, we also learn about other populations, and we can do better across the board.

SUMMARY

Achieving health equity and eliminating health disparities have been the project of generations of healthcare providers, researchers, and theorists. This chapter defines some of the terms needed for study of this issue and reviews some of the data demonstrating its importance. The biased care model, models using the social determinants of health, and those addressing intergenerational effects help explain how disparities arise. Models for intervention help lead us to achieve health equity. All the models can inform advanced nursing practice, leading to excellence in care, research, and leadership.

DISCUSSION QUESTIONS

1. Consider how the issues of health equity and health disparities are by nature a matter of differences in "the overall rate of disease incidence, prevalence, morbidity, mortality, or survival rates in the population as compared to the health status of the general population" (National Institutes of Health, n.d.). What do such differences mean in clinical practice? How do you know if you see a health disparity? What can you do to eliminate them in a clinical encounter?

2. What are the most important health disparities in your community? Where does your community do well? (Often state or local health departments will highlight these strengths in community assessments, or you might find them in Healthy People reports.) Do you have racial disparities in infant mortality? Disparities in access to care in rural areas? What about maternal mortality rates? Cancer death rates? Cancer detection rates? Sexually transmitted infection rates? Once you have an idea where

your community has the most work to do, how does your own practice fit in? Where can you provide leadership?

3. The concept of race permeates our cultures. When in your practice has it clouded your clinical judgment, leading you to miss important information?

4. The biased care model offers many avenues for improvement of clinical care. Would any of them be useful to implement in your clinical agency? What would it take to begin that process?

5. Social determinants of health models (such as the trajectory of health inequities model and the multilevel model) ask us to "take two steps back" and consider the context from which our patients come. Clinicians often find this easy to overlook, thinking about what can be seen in the examination room. What questions or other data do you gather in your practice that would increase your data on social determinants of health? What can you do with those data?

6. Critical race theory and HEART offer a roadmap for community-based interventions to achieve health equity. What might be first steps to take in your community? What persons or organizations might want to take them?

REFERENCES

Agency for Healthcare Research and Quality. (2016). 2015 national healthcare quality and disparities report and 5th anniversary update on the National Quality Strategy. Retrieved from http://www.ahrq.gov/sites/default/files/wysiwyg/research/findings/nhqrdr/nhqdr15/2015nhqdr.pdf

Aizer, A., & Currie, J. (2014). The intergenerational transmission of inequality: Maternal disadvantage and health at birth. *Science*, *344*, 856–861.

American Association of Critical-Care Nurses. (2015). Mission and values. Retrieved from https://www.aacn.org/about-aacn/about-aacn-cert-corp

American Association of Nurse Anesthetists. (2016). Diversity, inclusion, and equity. Retrieved from http://www.aana.com/resources2/professionalpractice/Documents/Diversity%20Inclusion%20and%20Equity.pdf

American College of Nurse-Midwives. (2007). Reducing health disparities. Retrieved from http://www.midwife.org/ACNM/files/ACNMLibraryData/UPLOADFILENAME/000000000112/Health_Care_Disparities_Issue_Brief_10_07.pdf

American Dental Association. (2004). State and community models for improving access to dental care for the underserved: A white paper. Retrieved from http://www.ada.org/~/media/ADA/Advocacy/Files/topics_access_whitepaper.ashx

American Dental Education Association. (2015). Need for diversity. Retrieved from http://www.adea.org/GoDental/Dentistry_101/Need_for_Diversity.aspx

American Hospital Association. (n.d.). Eliminating racial and ethnic disparities. Retrieved from http://www.aha.org/advocacy-issues/disparities/index.shtml

American Medical Association. (2016). Reducing disparities in health care. Retrieved from http://www.ama-assn.org/ama/pub/physician-resources/public-health/eliminating-health-disparities.page

American Nurses Association. (1998). Discrimination and racism in health care. Retrieved from http://www.nursingworld.org/MainMenuCategories/Policy-Advocacy/Positions-and-Resolutions/ANAPositionStatements/Position-Statements-Alphabetically/Copy-of-prtetdisrac14448.html

American Public Health Association. (2000). Effective interventions for reducing racial and ethnic disparities in health. Retrieved from http://www.apha.org/policies-and-advocacy/public-health-policy-statements/policy-database/2014/07/29/07/40/effective-interventions-for-reducing-racial-and-ethnic-disparities-in-health

Anderson, K. M., Roundtable on the Promotion of Health Equity and the Elimination of Health Disparities, Board on Population Health and Public Health Practice, & Institute of Medicine. (2012). *How far have we come in reducing health disparities: Progress since 2000: Workshop summary.* Washington, DC: National Academies Press.

Anum, E. A., Retchin, S. M., Garland, S. L., & Strauss, J. F. (2010). Medicaid and preterm births in Virginia: An analysis of recent outcomes. *Journal of Women's Health, 19*(11), 1969–1975.

Association of American Medical Colleges. (2009). Addressing racial disparities in health care: A targeted action plan for academic medical centers. Retrieved from https://members.aamc.org/eweb/upload/addressing%20racial%20disparaties.pdf

Association of Schools and Programs of Public Health. (2016). Addressing health disparities. Retrieved from http://www.aspph.org/discover/#addressing-health-disparities

Barker, D. J. (2004). The developmental origins of well-being. *Philosophical Transactions of the Royal Society of London, 359,* 1359–1366.

Barker, D. J., Osmond, D., & Law, C. M. (1989). The intrauterine and early postnatal origins of cardiovascular disease and chronic bronchitis. *Journal of Epidemiology and Community Health, 43*(3), 237–240.

Benner, P., Sutphen, M., Leonard, V., & Day, L. (2010). *Educating nurses: A call for a radical transformation.* San Francisco, CA: Jossey Bass.

Braveman, P. (2014). What are health disparities and health equity? We need to be clear. *Public Health Reports, S2*(129), 5–8.

Callaghan, W. M., MacDorman, M. F., Rasmussen, S. A., Qin, C., & Lackritz, E. M. (2006). The contribution of preterm births to infant mortality rates in the United States. *Pediatrics, 118*(4), 1566–1573.

Campinha-Bacote, J. (2002). The process of cultural competence in the delivery of health care services: A model of care. *Journal of Transcultural Nursing, 13*(3), 181–184.

Campinha-Bacote, J. (2007). *The process of cultural competence in the delivery of healthcare services: The journey continues.* Cincinnati, OH: Transcultural Care Associates.

Centers for Disease Control and Prevention. (2013). CDC health disparities and inequalities report—United States, 2013. *Morbidity and Mortality Weekly Report, 62*(Suppl 3), 1–186.

Centers for Medicare and Medicaid. (2016). CMS Office of Minority Health. Retrieved from https://www.cms.gov/About-CMS/Agency-Information/OMH

Cohen, L., & Iton, D. (2009). A time of opportunity: Local solutions to reduce inequities in health and safety. Retrieved from http://www.preventioninstitute.org/component/jlibrary/article/id-81/127.html

Cole, R. T., Kalogeropoulos, A. P., Georgiopoulou, V. V., Gheorghiade, M., Quyyumi, A., Yancy, C., & Butler, J. (2011). Hydralazine and isosorbide dinitrate in heart failure: Historical perspective, mechanisms, and future directions. *Circulation, 123,* 2414–2422.

Collins, J. W., & David, R. J. (2009). Racial disparity in low birth weight and infant mortality. *Clinics in Perinatology, 36,* 63–73.

Colorado Department of Public Health and Environment. (2016). Colorado Health Information Dataset (CoHID). Retrieved from http://www.chd.dphe.state.co.us/cohid/Default.aspx

Crenshaw, K. W. (1995). Mapping the margins: Intersectionality, identity politics, and violence against women of color. In K. Crenshaw, N. Gotanda, N. Peller, & K. Thomas (Eds.), *Critical race theory: The key writings that formed the movement.* New York, NY: The New Press.

Dahlgren, G., & Whitehead, M. (2006a). Concepts and principles for tackling social inequities in health: Levelling up (part 1). Copenhagen, Denmark: World Health Organization. Retrieved from http://www.who.int/social_determinants/resources/leveling_up_part1.pdf

Dahlgren, G., & Whitehead, M. (2006b). European strategies for tacking social inequities in health: Levelling up (part 2). Copenhagen, Denmark: World Health Organization. Retrieved from http://www.euro.who.int/__data/assets/pdf_file/0018/103824/E89384.pdf

David, R. J., & Collins, J. W. (1997). Differing birth weight among infants of U.S.-born Blacks, African-born Blacks, and U.S.-born Whites. *New England Journal Medicine, 337,* 1209–1214.

Delgado, R., & Stefancic, J. (2012). *Critical race theory: An introduction.* New York, NY: New York University Press.

Fall, C. H. D., Vijayakumar, M., Baker, D. J. P., Osmond, C., & Duggleby, S. (1995). Weight in infancy and prevalence of coronary heart disease in adult life. *British Medical Journal, 310,* 17–20.

Families Forward Resource Center. (n.d.). Families Forward Resources Center [website]. Retrieved from http://www.familiesforwardrc.org

Ford, C. L., & Airhihenbuwa, C. O. (2010). Critical race theory, race equity, and public health: Toward antiracism praxis. *American Journal of Public Health, 100*(S1), S30–S35.

Geronimus, A. T. (1992). The weathering hypothesis and the health of African American women and infants: Evidence and speculations. *Ethnicity and Disease, 1,* 207–221.

Geronimus, A. T. (2002). Black-White difference in the relationship of maternal age to birth weight: A population-based test of the weathering hypothesis. In LaVeist, T. A. (Ed.), *Race, ethnicity, and health: A public health reader.* San Francisco, CA: Wiley.

Goldstein, A. (1999, February 25). Race, sex disparity found in heart care. *The Washington Post.* Retrieved from http://www.washingtonpost.com/wp-srv/national/daily/feb99/heart25.htm

Goldstein, M. S., Scalzitti, D. A., Craik, R. L., Dunn, S. L., Irion, J. M., Irrgang, J., . . . Shields, R. K. (2011). The revised research agenda for physical therapy. *Physical Therapy, 91*(2), 165–174.

Goodman, A. H. (2000). Why genes don't count (for racial differences in health). *American Journal of Public Health, 90*(11), 1699–1702.

Healthy People 2020. (n.d.). Disparities. Retrieved from https://www.healthypeople.gov/2020/about/foundation-health-measures/Disparities

Hobel, C. J., Goldstein, A. M., & Barrett, E. S. (2008). Psychosocial stress and pregnancy outcome. *Clinical Obstetrics and Gynecology, 51*(20), 333–348.

Horton-Deutsch, S., McNelis, A. M., & Day, P. O. (2012). Developing a reflection-centered curriculum for graduate psychiatric nursing education. *Archives of Psychiatric Nursing, 26*(5), 341–349.

Jones, C. P., Truman, B. I., Elam-Evans, L. D., Jones, C. A., Jones, C. Y., Jiles, R., . . . & Perry, G. S. (2008). Using "socially assigned race" to probe White advantages in health status. *Ethnicity & Disease, 18*, 496–504.

Kahn, J. (2009). Beyond BiDil: The expanding embrace of race in biomedical research and product development. *St. Louis University Journal of Health, Law and Policy, 3*(61), 61–92.

Kaplan, G. A., Everson, S. A., & Lynch, J. W. (2000). The contribution of social and behavioral research to an understanding of the distribution of disease: A multilevel approach. In B. D. Smedley & S. L. Syme (Eds.), *Promoting health: Intervention strategies from social and behavioral research.* Committee on Capitalizing on Social Science and Behavioral Research to Improve the Public's Health, & Institute of Medicine Division of Health Promotion and Disease Prevention. Washington, DC: National Academy Press.

Kennedy, D. (1990). A cultural pluralist case for affirmative action in academia. In K. Crenshaw, N. Gotanda, N. Peller, & K. Thomas (Eds.), *Critical race theory: The key writings that formed the movement.* New York, NY: The New Press.

Kilbourne, A. M., Switzer, G., Hyman, K., Crowley-Matoka, M., & Fine, M. J. (2006). Advancing health disparities research within the health care system: A conceptual framework. *American Journal of Public Health, 96*, 2113–2121.

Kramer, M. R., & Hogue, C. R. (2009). What causes racial disparities in very preterm birth? A biosocial perspective. *Epidemiology Review, 31*, 84–98.

Kramer, M. S. (1987). Determinants of low birth weight: Methodological assessment and meta-analysis. *Bulletin of the World Health Organization, 65*(5), 663–737.

Krans, E. E., & Davis, M. M. (2012). Preventing low birthweight: 25 years, prenatal risk, and the failure to reinvent prenatal care. *American Journal of Obstetrics and Gynecology, 206*(5), 398–403.

Krieger, N., Carney, D., Lancaster, K., Waterman, P. D., Kosheleva, A., & Banaji, M. (2010). Combining explicit and implicit measures of racial discrimination in health research. *American Journal of Public Health, 100*, 1485–1492.

Lawrence, C. R. (1987). The word and the river: Pedagogy as scholarship as struggle. In K. Crenshaw, N. Gotanda, N. Peller, & K. Thomas (Eds.), *Critical race theory: The key writings that formed the movement.* New York, NY: The New Press.

Love, C., David, R. J., Rankin, K. M., & Collins, J. J. (2010). Exploring weathering: Effects of lifelong economic environment and maternal age on low birth weight, small for gestational age, and preterm birth in African-American and White women. *American Journal of Epidemiology, 172*(2), 127–134.

Lu, M. C., & Halfon, N. (2003). Disparities in birth outcomes: A life course perspective. *Maternal and Child Health Journal, 7*(1), 13–30.

Lu, M. C., Kotelchuck, M., Hogan, V., Jones, L., Wright, K., & Halfon, N. (2010). Closing the Black-White gap in birth outcomes: A life course approach. *Ethnicity & Disease, 20*(S2), s2–s7.

Marmot, D., & Allen, J. J. (2014). Social determinants of health equity. *American Journal of Public Health, 104*(S4), S517–S519.

Martin, J. (2013, August 21). After 25 years, "Just Do It" remains iconic tagline. *USA Today*. Retrieved from http://www.usatoday.com/story/sports/nba/2013/08/20/nike-just-do-it-turns-25/2679337

Matthew, D. B. (2015). *Just medicine: A cure for the racial inequality in American health care.* New York, NY: New York University Press.

Mathews, T. J., MacDorman, M. F., Thoma, M. E., & Division of Vital Statistics. (2015). Infant mortality statistics from the 2013 Period Linked Birth/Infant Death Data Set. *National Vital Statistics Reports, 64*(9).

Montagu, A. (1942). *Man's most dangerous myth: The fallacy of race.* New York, NY: Harper.

National Institute on Minority Health and Health Disparities. (n.d.). History. Retrieved from http://www.nimhd.nih.gov/about/overview/history

National League for Nursing. (2016). Achieving diversity and meaningful inclusion in nursing: A living document from the National League for Nursing. Retrieved from http://www.nln.org/docs/default-source/about/vision-statement-achieving-diversity.pdf?sfvrsn=2

Phrase Finder. (n.d.). Get over it. Retrieved from http://www.phrases.org.uk/meanings/get-over-it.html

Quinn, S. C. (2001). The National Negro Health Movement: Lessons for eliminating health disparities today. *Minority Health Today, 2*(3), 42–43.

Quinn, S. C., & Thomas, S. B. (2001). The National Negro Health Week: 1915 to 1951: A descriptive account. *Minority Health Today, 2*(3), 44–49.

Robert Wood Johnson. (2015). Health disparities. Retrieved from https://www.rwjf.org/en/our-focus-areas/topics/health-disparities.html

Ronald Reagan Presidential Foundation and Library. (2010). Just say no. Retrieved from http://www.reaganfoundation.org/details_f.aspx?p=RR1008NRHC&tx=6

Schulman, K. A., Berlin, J. A., Harless, W., Kerner, J. F., Sistrunk, S., Gersh, B. J., . . . Escarce, J. J. (1999). The effect of race and sex on physicians' recommendations for cardiac catheterization. *New England Journal of Medicine, 340*(8), 618–626.

Spong, C. Y., Iams, J., Goldenberg, R., Hauck, F. R., & Willinger, M. (2011). Disparities in perinatal medicine: Preterm birth, stillbirth, and infant mortality. *Obstetrics and Gynecology, 117*(4), 948–955.

Smedley, B. D., Stith, A. Y., & Nelson, A. R. (Eds.). (2003). *Unequal treatment: Confronting racial and ethnic disparities in health care.* Washington, DC: National Academies Press.

Stolberg, S. G. (2002, March 21). Race gap seen in health care of equally insured patients. *New York Times.* Retrieved from http://www.nytimes.com/2002/03/21/us/race-gap-seen-in-health-care-of-equally-insured-patients.html

Thomas, S. B., Quinn, S. C., Butler, J., Fryer, C. S., & Garza, M. A. (2011). Toward a fourth generation of disparities research to achieve health equity. *Annual Review of Public Health, 32*, 399–416.

Torres, G., & Milun, K. (1990). Translating "Yonnondio" by precedent and evidence: The Mashpee Indian case. In K. Crenshaw, N. Gotanda, N. Peller, & K. Thomas (Eds.), *Critical race theory: The key writings that formed the movement.* New York, NY: The New Press.

Tripp, S., & Grueber, M. (2011). Economic impact of the Human Genome Project: How a $3.8 billion investment drove $796 billion in economic impact, created 310,000 jobs, and launched the genomic revolution. Battelle Memorial Institute Technology Partnership and Practice. Retrieved from http://www.battelle.org/docs/default-document-library/economic_impact_of_the_human_genome_project.pdf

W. K. Kellogg Foundation. (2016). Kellogg Health Scholars: Connecting academe, community, and policy. Retrieved from http://www.kellogghealthscholars.org/

Whitehead, M., Dahlgren, G., & Gilson, L. (2001). Developing the policy response to inequities in Health: A global perspective. In T. Evans, M. Whitehead, F. Diderichsen, A. Bhuiya, & M. Wirth (Eds.), *Challenging inequities in health care: From ethics to action* (pp. 309–322). New York, NY: Oxford University Press.

Williams, D., & Mohammed, S. (2009). Discrimination and racial disparities in health: Evidence and needed research. *Journal of Behavioral Medicine, 32,* 20–47.

Wise, P. H. (2003). The anatomy of a disparity in infant mortality. *Annual Review of Public Health, 24,* 241–262.

Witt, W. P., Cheng, E. R., Wisk, L. E., Litzelman, K., Chatterjee, D., Mandell, K., & Wakeel, F. (2014). Maternal stressful life events prior to conception and the impact on infant birth weight in the United States. *American Journal of Public Health, 104*(S1), S81–S89.

IV

Select Nursing Models and Theories

Chapter 18

Models and Theories Focused on Nursing Goals and Functions

Kathleen Masters

INTRODUCTION

There are numerous perspectives from which nursing models and theories may be viewed and subsequently classified. This chapter examines nursing models and theories that may be categorized as focusing on goals and functions. From the standpoint of each model or theory, it will address the roles and functions of advanced practice nurses (APNs) and the goals of nursing care. Four of the most prominent nursing models and theories in this category include Florence Nightingale's environmental model of nursing, Virginia Henderson's 14 components of basic nursing care, Dorothy Johnson's behavioral system model, and Nola J. Pender's health promotion model.

While neither Nightingale nor Henderson defined her work as a theory of nursing, it is evident from the current vantage point that the work of these nursing pioneers provided the theoretical foundation for the practice discipline of nursing. Johnson was also a pioneer in the world of nursing theory. While influenced by the thinking of Nightingale, Johnson also incorporated theories from other disciplines and pushed theoretical thinking in nursing to a higher conceptual level with the development of the behavioral system model. While these three works were general in nature, more recently Pender has contributed to the theoretical basis for nursing practice with the introduction of a model that, while still allowing for generalization across populations, is specific to health promotion. In this chapter, the work of these nurse theorists will be presented in chronological order, beginning with background information and followed by a discussion of each theory.

THE ENVIRONMENTAL MODEL OF NURSING: FLORENCE NIGHTINGALE

Background

Florence Nightingale was born on May 12, 1820, in Florence, Italy, the second child of an affluent British family. As a youngster, she displayed exceptional intellectual ability and was well educated for a female in the Victorian era, having been tutored by her father in math, philosophy, languages, and religion. Nightingale was active in aristocratic society but believed that her life could be more useful. She was obsessed with the poverty, disease, and suffering of the masses; to the dismay of her family, she believed she was called by God to be a nurse (Woodham-Smith, 1951). At the age of 25, Nightingale expressed a desire to become a nurse, but her parents refused her request. Over the next 7 years, she continued her study of math, science, hospitals, and public health while she made repeated attempts to change the minds of her parents (Dietz & Lehozky, 1963).

During a trip to Egypt with family and friends in 1849, Nightingale spent time with the Sisters of Charity of St. Vincent de Paul, where her conviction to study nursing was reinforced (Tooley, 1910). The next year, Nightingale traveled to the Kaiserswerth Institute in Germany. She spent only 2 weeks at Kaiserswerth but vowed that she would return to study nursing. In 1851, Nightingale announced to her family that she planned to return to Germany to study nursing. Finally, at age 31, Nightingale was permitted to travel back to Kaiserswerth, where she learned about the care of the sick and the importance of discipline and commitment to God (Donahue, 1985).

In 1853, after receiving an endowment from her father, Nightingale moved to London, where she became superintendent of the Hospital for Invalid Gentlewomen, thereby realizing her goal of working as a nurse (Cook, 1913). During the Crimean War, Nightingale traveled to Üsküdar (called Scutari in Nightingale's era), Turkey, along with 38 other nurses. When they arrived, the women were faced with the prospect of overcrowded barracks and atrocious sanitary conditions. Nightingale focused her efforts on organizing nursing services and eliminating sanitation problems in the hospital; ultimately, she proved successful in decreasing the mortality rate in the Crimean War. Upon her return home to London, she eventually established the Nightingale School of Nursing at St. Thomas's Hospital, which was the beginning of professional nursing (Donahue, 1985).

Nightingale expressed her views about nursing in many formats. She wrote letters, pamphlets, and government reports. In addition, in 1859, Nightingale published *Notes on Nursing: What It Is, and What It Is Not*, a book that represented her first effort at putting her philosophy and description of nursing into one document (Reed & Zurakowski, 1989).

During the last 50 years of her life, although Nightingale suffered from poor health, she spent significant time writing letters, books, reports, and meeting with friends and colleagues from within the confines of her home. She died in London on August 13, 1910, at 91 years of age.

Nightingale's 13 Canons Central to the Environmental Model of Nursing

In her writings, Nightingale did not plan to develop a theory, but rather sought to describe nursing and delineate general rules for nursing practice, thereby making her model both descriptive and practical. Nursing care using Nightingale's model is centered on her 13 canons, which include the following precepts (Nightingale, 1860/1969):

1. *Ventilation and warmth:* The interventions subsumed in this canon include keeping the patient and the patient's room warm and keeping the patient's room well ventilated and free of odors. Specific instructions included to "keep the air within as pure as the air without" (p. 10).
2. *Health of houses:* This canon includes the five essentials of pure air, pure water, efficient drainage, cleanliness, and light.
3. *Petty management:* Continuity of care for the patient when the nurse is absent is the essence of this canon.
4. *Noise:* Instructions include the avoidance of sudden noises that startle or awaken patients and keeping noise in general to a minimum.
5. *Variety:* This canon refers to an attempt to provide variety in the patient's room in order to avoid boredom and depression.
6. *Food intake:* Interventions include the documentation of the amount of food and liquids that the patient ingested.
7. *Food:* Instructions include trying to include patient food preferences.
8. *Bed and bedding:* The interventions in this canon include comfort measures related to keeping the bed dry and wrinkle free.
9. *Light:* The instructions contained in this canon relate to adequate light in the patient's room.
10. *Cleanliness of rooms and walls:* This canon focuses on keeping the environment clean.
11. *Personal cleanliness:* This canon includes measures such as keeping the patient clean and dry.
12. *Chattering hopes and advice:* Instructions in this canon include the avoidance of talking without reason or giving advice that is not supported by fact.
13. *Observation of the sick:* This canon includes instructions related to making observations and documenting observations.

When they incorporate Nightingale's 13 canons into their caregiving, APNs include questioning and observation in their nursing assessments of patients. Questions the nurse asks relate to food preferences, as well as food and fluid intake. Nursing observations are focused on environmental influences on patients—for example, the effects of noise, light, and nutrition on patients. The Nightingale model involves nurses manipulating environmental

---

Box 18-1   Case Study Using Nightingale's Environmental Model

Mrs. Little, who is 78 years old and a Caucasian, visits your primary care clinic. She recently underwent coronary artery bypass graft surgery. This morning at the clinic, Mrs. Little complains that she has not been able to sleep since she was hospitalized. She lives with her daughter's family, which includes two teenagers. Mrs. Little has not eaten much recently.

   Nursing care for Mrs. Little using the Nightingale environmental model begins with an assessment of environmental factors that are impacting the patient; in this case, manipulation of the environment is needed to promote sleep and nutrition. This manipulation of the environment might include educating Mrs. Little and her daughter about eliminating noise and unnecessary light during the hours when Mrs. Little normally sleeps. Inquiry related to the patient's food preferences is conducted in the presence of Mrs. Little's daughter. In addition, teaching might include information about comfort and relaxation measures such as clean, wrinkle-free linens and maintenance of room temperature conducive to sleeping. Evaluation will be based on the quantity and quality of sleep and the nutritional intake of Mrs. Little, as well as her subsequent restoration of health.

---

factors that affect the patient's health status, including noise, light, cleanliness, bedding, and ventilation. Evaluation is based on the effect of changes in the environment on the patient's health. Observation is the primary method of data collection and evaluation of outcomes (Nightingale, 1860/1969). A case illustrating care and treatment administered by APNs using Nightingale's environmental model of nursing appears in **Box 18-1**.

The 13 canons are central to Nightingale's model, but they are not all-inclusive. Nightingale believed that nursing is a calling and that the recipients of nursing care are holistic individuals with a spiritual dimension; thus, under her model, the nurse is expected to care for the spiritual needs of patients in spiritual distress. (What are some ways that modern-day APNs might provide holistic care with a spiritual dimension?) Nightingale also believed that nurses should be involved in health promotion and health teaching both with patients who are sick and with those who are well (Bolton, 2006).

Major Concepts of the Environmental Model of Nursing According to Nightingale

Nightingale's environmental model of nursing represented a landmark in the development of nursing science and provided the foundation for the discipline's four metaparadigm concepts of (1) person, (2) environment, (3) health, and (4) nursing. Her model, however, focuses primarily on the patient and the environment. In other words, the primary function of the nurse in Nightingale's view is to manipulate the physical and social factors that affect health and illness in order to enhance patient recovery.

Person

While not specifically defined, the person in Nightingale's environmental model is quite simply the recipient of nursing care. The person is viewed in relation to the environment and the impact of the environment on the person's health status.

Environment

The physical environment was stressed in Nightingale's model, although she did acknowledge the potential impact of the social environment on the health of the patient. Components of the environment discussed by Nightingale include aspects of both the external environment (temperature, bedding, ventilation) and the internal environment (food, water, and medications).

Health

Nightingale did not specifically define the concept of health, but she believed that nature alone could cure disease. She described health as "not only to be well, but to be able to use well every power we have to use" (Nightingale, 1860/1969, p. 24).

Nursing

Nursing to Nightingale was, above all, "service to God in the relief of man" (Nightingale, 1858, p. 2). The nurse's function, according to Nightingale, is to alter or manage the environment to put patients in the best possible situation for the natural laws of health to act upon them (Johnson & Webber, 2010); thus the ultimate goal of nursing activities is patient health. Nightingale also believed that nurses should provide care for both healthy and ill people and discussed health promotion activities as part of the role of the nurse (Lobo, 2002).

Analysis of Nightingale's Environmental Model of Nursing

The analysis and critique of Nightingale's environmental model of nursing presented here will consist of an examination of assumptions and propositions, as well as the analysis of clarity, simplicity, generality, empirical precision, and derivable consequences of this model.

Assumptions of Nightingale's Environmental Model of Nursing

While Nightingale did not explicitly state any theoretical assumptions, numerous assumptions can be extracted from her work. Philosophical assumptions that can be extracted include the following: (1) nursing is a calling; (2) nursing is an art and a science; (3) persons can control the outcomes of their lives and, therefore, can pursue perfect health; (4) nursing requires a specific educational base; and (5) nursing is distinct and separate from medicine (Selanders, 1995). The following assumptions also may be inferred from Nightingale's work: (1) maintaining a clean room, bedding, and clothes aids in patient recovery; (2) noise can be harmful to patients; and (3) managing the environment improves the health of the patient (Johnson & Webber, 2010).

Propositions of Nightingale's Environmental Model of Nursing

The primary relationship statements that APNs can derive from the writings of Nightingale include (1) the person is desirous of health, so the nurse, nature, and the person will cooperate in order for all reparative processes to occur, and (2) the nurse's role is to prevent the reparative process from being interrupted and to provide conditions that optimize the reparative process (Pfettscher, 2010). The APN reader of this chapter might imagine scenarios where these two propositions are included in advanced practice.

Analysis: Clarity, Simplicity, Generality, Empirical Precision, and Derivable Consequences

The analysis of Nightingale's environmental model presented here is based on the theory evaluation criteria of clarity, simplicity, generality, empirical precision, and derivable consequences as suggested by Chinn and Kramer (2008).

Nightingale's model places an emphasis on relationships not regarded as revolutionary or complex by current standards. At the same time, it provides a broad framework for organizing observations about a large number of nursing phenomena, thereby making the model broad in scope and giving it generality (Reed & Zurakowski, 1989). The components of the model are clearly articulated. The model is a simple one, with only three major relationships specified—(1) environment to patient, (2) nurse to environment, and (3) nurse to patient—yet attempts to provide guidelines for all nurses in all situations. While some of the specific directives may no longer be applicable, the general concepts, including the relationships between the nurse, the patient, and the environment, remain highly relevant to modern-day practitioners (Pfettscher, 2010).

Nightingale's environmental model of nursing was developed inductively, with the proposed laws of health and nursing being derived from Nightingale's observations and many of the principles originating from the observations made during her wartime experiences (Pfettscher, 2010). The major concepts are clearly defined, and the relationships among the concepts flow logically based on the definitions of the concepts, giving the model internal consistency (Reed & Zurakowski, 1989). The concepts and relationships are presented as truths, rather than testable statements, however (Pfettscher, 2010).

Nightingale's writings remain important to the profession of nursing at all levels of nursing practice. The basic principles of environmental manipulation and psychological patient care are applied in modern nursing practice situations (Pfettscher, 2010).

Discussion

Nightingale probably would not have described her work as theoretical, but today it is recognized as a scholarly effort that continues to give credibility to basic ideas related to nursing theory. Nightingale's model was developed long ago in response to a need for environmental reform. Although some of Nightingale's rationales have been modified or disproved by advances in medicine and science, many of the concepts in her theory have not only endured, but they have been used as general guidelines for nurses for more than 150 years (Pfettscher, 2010). In particular, her work in relation to illness prevention and health restoration remains highly relevant to current nursing practice (Johnson & Webber, 2010) in both the acute care and community health settings, and in both the domestic and global healthcare arenas. In addition, Nightingale's example of commitment to healthcare advocacy and systems leadership to improve care is essential in contemporary advanced practice nursing (American Association of Colleges of Nursing [AACN], 2006).

FOURTEEN COMPONENTS OF BASIC NURSING CARE: VIRGINIA HENDERSON

Background

Virginia Avenel Henderson was born on March 19, 1897, in Kansas City, Missouri, and died on November 30, 1996, at 98 years of age. During her lifetime and over the course of her more than 60-year career as a nurse, teacher, author, and researcher, Henderson made such significant contributions to the discipline of nursing that she has been referred to by some as "the Florence Nightingale of the twentieth century" (Tomey, 2006).

Henderson's interest in nursing began during World War I and stemmed from her desire to help the sick and wounded in the military. Henderson graduated from the Army School of Nursing in 1921 and began practice at the Henry Street Visiting Nurse Service in New York City. In 1926, she returned to school at Columbia University Teachers College in New York City, where she would complete her bachelor of science and master of arts in nursing education. Henderson taught nursing at Teachers College and Yale University. In her faculty role, Henderson worked with Harmer on the revision of *Textbook of the Principles and Practice of Nursing* (1939). In the next edition, published in 1955, Henderson introduced her now famous definition of nursing. Some of Henderson's other scholarly endeavors included the *Nursing Studies Index Project* (four volumes) (1959–1971); *Basic Principles of Nursing Care* (1960, 1997), which was translated into more than 20 languages; *The Nature of Nursing* (1966); and *The Nature of Nursing: Reflections After 25 Years* (1991). At 75 years of age, Henderson began to focus on international teaching and speaking.

Henderson authored one of the most accurate definitions of nursing, promoted nursing research as the basis for nursing knowledge, advocated for humane and holistic care for patients internationally, and represented nursing with dignity, honor, and grace throughout her career, which spanned most of the 20th century. Henderson was awarded 12 honorary doctoral degrees, as well as the International Council of Nursing's prestigious Christiane Reimann Prize during her exemplary career (American Nurses Association, n.d.).

Henderson's 14 Components of Nursing Care

Henderson elaborated on her definition of nursing by identifying 14 basic needs on which nursing care is based. Eight of these needs pertain directly to bodily functions; the remaining six relate to safety and finding meaning in life (Shelly & Miller, 2006). It follows that the fundamentals of nursing (i.e., the 14 components of nursing care) include helping others provide for their 14 basic needs:

1. To breathe normally
2. To eat and drink adequately
3. To eliminate bodily wastes
4. To move and maintain desirable postures
5. To sleep and rest
6. To select suitable clothes; dress and undress
7. To maintain body temperature within normal range by adjusting clothing and modifying the environment
8. To keep the body clean and well groomed and protect the integument
9. To avoid dangers in the environment and avoid injuring others
10. To communicate with others in expressing emotions, needs, fears, or opinions
11. To worship according to one's faith
12. To work in such a way that there is a sense of accomplishment
13. To play or participate in various forms of recreation
14. To learn, discover, or satisfy the curiosity that leads to normal development and health and use the available health facilities (Henderson, 1966, 1991)

Nursing Care and Henderson's 14 Components of Nursing

Delivering nursing care based on the 14 basic needs and the corresponding 14 components of nursing care identified by Henderson is not difficult to conceptualize because Henderson and Nite used the 14 components as a framework for the 1978 edition of their textbook, *Principles and Practice of Nursing*. Advanced nursing practice and care using Henderson's theory revolves around meeting patient needs in the areas of respiration, nutrition, elimination, body mechanics, rest and sleep, keeping clean and well groomed, controlling the environment, communication, human relations, work, play, and worship.

Henderson and Nite (1978) offered specific details for administering nursing care. APNs can apply these same interventions in advanced nursing care. For example, meeting basic needs involving patient respiration includes caregiving related to the following areas:

- Pulmonary ventilation
- Diffusion and transport of gases
- Regulation of respiration
- Factors affecting normal respiration (i.e., smoking, age, obesity, emotions, environmental pollution, anesthesia, and surgery)

Providing advanced nursing care to meet basic needs involving nutrition will include caregiving related to these areas:

- Nutrition and quality of life
- Dietary essentials
- Fluid balance
- Food selection and the optimal diet
- Conditions that favor digestion and assimilation
- Diet in sickness
- Nursing measures in oral feedings

Advanced nursing care to meet basic needs involving elimination covers the following areas:

- Elimination of waste from the intestines
- Elimination of waste from the kidneys
- Elimination of waste by the skin and lungs
- Measuring and recording elimination

Meeting basic needs involving patient movement and posture focuses on the following areas:

- Body mechanics and posture
- Exercise in health and sickness
- Helping the sick and handicapped to move
- Transportation in illness and traveling with patients
- Prevention and treatment of pressure ulcers

Meeting basic needs involving patient rest and sleep requires that the APN focus on two areas:

- Rest in health and illness
- Inducing sleep

Providing advanced nursing care to meet a patient's basic needs involves educating caregivers about keeping the patient clean and well groomed and maintaining temperature. This education includes caregiving related to the following areas:

- Personal cleanliness and morning care (care of skin and nails; shaving; care of the mouth, teeth, and dentures; care of the nose; hygiene of the eyes; care of the hair; making the patient's bed)
- Providing the patient with suitable clothing and conditions to maintain body temperature

Advanced nursing practice involved in controlling the environment will meet the patient's basic needs related to the following issues:

- Lighting (natural light, artificial light, psychology of lighting)
- Atmospheric conditions (humidity, temperature, purity of air, air pressure, altitude)
- Water supply and waste disposal
- Aesthetics
- Controlling pests (insects and rodents)
- Preventing mechanical injury, burns, poisoning, and electric shock
- Providing and maintaining a sanitary environment
- Providing and maintaining a sanitary food service and maintaining a sanitary laundry service
- Disinfection and sterilization
- Preventing and controlling infection

Advanced nursing care involved in basic needs of communication, human relations, and learning includes factors associated with the following areas:

- Ways of communication (being as communication, use of the senses in communication, speech and language, nonlanguage communication, and communication technology)
- Communication: strengthening bonds and reducing barriers (mental states and sensory defects as barriers; language, culture, age-related, and gender-related communication bonds and barriers; and hospitalization and illness effects upon communication)
- Therapeutic communication and relationships (nurse–patient interaction; family and groups; communication through touch, music, art, role-playing, and reading and writing; and creating a therapeutic environment)
- Learning and perception through the life cycle
- Health goals (national and international health goals, individual health goals, health education for health promotion and prevention of illness) and health guidance or health teaching

Advanced nursing care also involves basic needs of work and play:

- The meaning and nature of work and leisure
- Retirement and leisure time
- Adult play and recreation
- Children's play
- The nurse's role in providing an opportunity for work and play

Providing advanced nursing care to meet basic needs involving worship will cover the following areas:

- The search for meaning in life
- Knowledge of major living religions
- Religious leaders as members of health teams
- Ways in which nurses help those they serve meet their spiritual needs

For the assessment phase of the nursing process using Henderson's theory, APNs will assess the needs of the patient based on the 14 basic needs. Specifically, the APN will assess the patient's respiratory status, nutritional status, elimination, movement, activities of daily living, sleep, maintenance of body temperature, hygiene, environment, ability to communicate, needs related to work, recreation and learning, and spiritual needs. Based on the assessment data and considering the strength, will, and knowledge of the patient, the APN will determine whether the patient requires assistance to meet his or her basic needs. If assistance is required in any area, a plan will be designed so that the necessary nursing care can be provided.

The goal of the planning phase of the nursing process is to design a plan to meet patient needs based on any deficits identified in the assessment phase of the process, while simultaneously helping the patient gain independence as rapidly as possible so that the nurse becomes dispensable rather than indispensable. The implementation phase focuses on assisting the patient with the performance of activities that contribute to the maintenance of health, recovery from illness, or peaceful death. Interventions in this phase of the nursing process are based on physiological principles, as well as individual characteristics such as age; culture; and physical, intellectual, and emotional capabilities. Evaluation is based on the ability of patients to meet their basic human needs without assistance from the nurse or with decreasing assistance.

Major Concepts of Nursing According to Henderson

Henderson did not consider her work to be a theory of nursing and did not explicitly define all of the domains of nursing. It is possible, however, to identify and describe the metaparadigm concepts of nursing from her publications (Furukawa & Howe, 2002).

Person

Henderson viewed the person as the patient who is composed of biological, psychological, sociological, and spiritual components (although these components are inseparable), but who requires assistance to achieve independence in relation to the 14 basic needs that correspond to the 14 identified components of nursing care. The patient and family are viewed as a unit (Henderson, 1964).

Environment

Henderson broadly defined environment as "the aggregate of all the external conditions and influences affecting the life and development of an organism," using a definition taken from the 1961 edition of *Webster's New Collegiate Dictionary* (Henderson & Nite, 1978). She considered the environment to be composed of three components—biological, physical, and behavioral. Biological components of the environment include all living things, such as plants, animals, and microorganisms. Physical components of the environment comprise sunlight, water, oxygen, carbon dioxide, organic compounds, and the nutrients used by plants for growth and provide a sphere "in which all living things operate" (Henderson & Nite, 1978, p. 829). According to Henderson, these biological and physical components come together to form an ecosystem characterized by a delicate balance; thus, an interdependent relationship exists between living organisms and their surroundings, such that changes in one component result in changes in other parts of the ecosystem.

A third environmental component also exists. This behavioral component comprises the way in which human beings are engaged in social interactions, customs, and economic, legal, political, and religious systems, all of which influence human health (Henderson & Nite, 1978).

Health

While Henderson did not explicitly state a definition of health, she implied that health is equivalent to independence. The level of health is directly related to the patient's ability to independently meet the 14 basic needs (Henderson & Nite, 1978).

Nursing

Henderson is perhaps best known for her definition of nursing, first published in 1955 (Harmer & Henderson, 1955), and presented again in 1966 with minor revisions. According to Henderson:

> The unique function of the nurse is to assist the individual, sick or well, in the performance of those activities contributing to health or its recovery (or to a peaceful death) that he would perform unaided if he had the necessary strength, will, or knowledge and to do this in such a way as to help him gain independence as rapidly as possible. (Henderson, 1966, p. 15)

While Henderson defined nursing in functional terms, she emphasized the art of nursing, as well as the need for empathetic understanding, stating that the nurse must "get inside the skin of each of her patients in order to know what he needs" (Henderson, 1964, p. 63). She believed that "the beauty of . . . nursing is the combination of your heart, your head and your hands and where you separate them, you diminish them" (McBride, 1997, as cited by Gordon, 2001).

Henderson (1991) went on to say,

> The nurse is, and should be an independent practitioner and able to make independent judgments as long as he, or she, is not diagnosing, prescribing treatment for disease, or making a prognosis, for these are the physician's functions. But the nurse is viewed as the authority on basic nursing care.

Over the last 40 years, however, advanced nursing practice has evolved to include many of the independent functions previously described by Henderson as functions reserved only for physicians. Today's APNs promote a comprehensive approach to health care, which includes making advanced practice judgments, diagnosing, prescribing, and emphasizing the overall health and wellness of their patients. Henderson's definition of nursing and her 14 components of nursing are completely viable for advanced nursing practice today.

Analysis of Henderson's Definition of Nursing and 14 Components of Nursing

The analysis and critique of Henderson's work presented here encompass an examination of her assumptions and propositions, as well as an analysis of the clarity, simplicity, generality, empirical precision, and derivable consequences of the definition of nursing and 14 components of nursing as proposed by Henderson.

Assumptions of Henderson's Definition and 14 Components of Nursing Care

Henderson did not explicitly state assumptions. Even so, it is possible to extrapolate 17 primary assumptions from her publications:

1. The nurse has a unique function to help well or sick persons.
2. The nurse functions as a member of the medical team, but independently of the physician.
3. The patient's needs are covered by the 14 components of nursing.
4. The 14 components of nursing care encompass all possible functions of nursing.
5. The nurse and patient are always working toward a goal, whether it is patient independence or a peaceful death.
6. Health promotion is an important goal of the nurse.
7. The patient and the family are a unit.
8. The mind and the body of the person are inseparable.
9. The patient requires assistance toward independence.

10. The person must maintain physiological and emotional balance.
11. Health is basic to human functioning.
12. Health requires independence and interdependence.
13. Persons will achieve or maintain health if they have the strength, will, and knowledge to do so.
14. Illness may interfere with the ability of persons to control their environment.
15. Nurses should protect persons from environmental injury.
16. Nurses should know about social customs and religious practices.
17. Professional practice is generated from research-based knowledge (Henderson, 1966, 1991; Runk & Muth Quillin, 1989; Tomey, 2002, p. 102).

Propositions of Henderson's Definition and 14 Components of Nursing Care

The primary relationship statements gleaned from Henderson's work are related to the nurse–patient relationship: (1) the nurse as a substitute for the patient, (2) the nurse as a helper to the patient, and (3) the nurse as a partner with the patient (Tomey, 2002). In times of serious illness, the nurse is seen as the substitute for what the patient is missing owing to lack of strength, will, or knowledge. Henderson reflected this view when she stated the following:

> [The nurse] is temporarily the consciousness of the unconscious, the love of life for the suicidal, the leg of the amputee, the eyes of the newly blind, a means of locomotion for the infant, knowledge and confidence for the young mother, and the mouthpiece for those too weak or withdrawn to speak and so on. (1966, p. 16; 1991, p. 22)

During the patient's convalescence, the nurse assists the patient in regaining his or her independence. Working as partners, the nurse and the patient together formulate the plan of care. Henderson asserts that the "nurse must get inside the skin" of each patient to know what the patient needs, and then the identified needs must be validated with the patient (Henderson, 1966, p. 16; 1991, p. 22; Tomey, 2002).

Analysis: Clarity, Simplicity, Generality, Empirical Precision, and Derivable Consequences

Henderson seems to have used deduction to develop her definition of nursing and 14 needs from physiological and psychological principles. The assumptions of Henderson's definition are logical and have a high level of agreement with literature and research conclusions of scientists in other fields. For example, the 14 basic needs correspond closely to Maslow's hierarchy of human needs, even though Henderson had no knowledge of Maslow's work at the time she identified these needs in her work (Tomey, 2002).

Henderson's definition of nursing and the basic needs are simply stated and clear, yet broad enough in scope to include the function of nurses at all levels of practice caring for all types of patients. Her work is of sufficient scope to affect nursing theory and practice. Moreover, Henderson's definition of nursing has the potential to include the whole person, even though the definition is derived primarily from the physiological perception (Runk & Muth Quillin, 1989).

The concept of nursing in Henderson's work contains many variables and relationships, and the 14 needs, although they appear simple, can become complex when an alteration in need occurs and all of the parameters relating to the need are considered. Even with this level of complexity, the conceptual definitions and relationships demonstrate internal consistency (Tomey, 2002).

Because Henderson did not intend to develop a theory of nursing, she did not develop the interrelated theoretical statements or operational definitions necessary to provide theory testability. As Tomey (2002) pointed out, however, this extension is possible. Henderson's work has been influential in nursing curriculum development, in clinical nursing practice, and in the promotion of clinical nursing research.

Discussion

Henderson's work is viewed as a philosophy of the purpose and function of nursing (Pokorny, 2010). Her textbook *Principles and Practice of Nursing*, in which the definition of nursing and 14 nursing functions were explicated, was widely used in schools of nursing for several decades; thus, her definition of nursing has significantly influenced the practice of multiple generations of nurses. Henderson's definition of nursing and 14 nursing functions were aimed at explaining the totality of nursing behavior rather than laying the foundation for the development of a nursing theory; however, her ideas have continued to be useful in promoting further conceptual development among nurse theorists. In addition, Henderson's philosophy that nursing care should be based on evidence rather than tradition, an idea that was novel at the time, is currently foundational to the discipline of nursing, and a hallmark of the APN prepared at the doctoral level (AACN, 2006).

THE BEHAVIORAL SYSTEM MODEL: DOROTHY JOHNSON

Background

Dorothy E. Johnson was born in 1919 in Savannah, Georgia. She graduated from nursing school in 1938, earned a bachelor of science in nursing from Vanderbilt University in 1942, and received a master of public health from Harvard University in 1948.

Johnson served as faculty at both Vanderbilt University School of Nursing and the University of California in Los Angeles. Over the course of her career, she published more than 30 articles, 4 books, and many reports, and she was presented with numerous honors. She died in 1999 at 80 years of age.

According to Johnson, her behavioral system model was in the process of development for nearly the entire course of her professional life (Johnson, 1990). Through a comprehensive analysis, Fawcett (2005) identified Johnson's behavioral system model as one of the seven conceptual models of nursing. The model's roots can be traced back to the work of behavioral scientists in psychology, sociology, and ethnology, with heavy reliance on systems theory (Loveland-Cherry & Wilkerson, 1989). Johnson's theory was also influenced by Nightingale's work—especially her belief that nursing's goal is to help individuals prevent or recover from disease or injury with a focus on the patient rather than the specific disease (Johnson, 1990). Johnson's initial work began with an effort to develop content for nursing courses in the basic curriculum by focusing on common human needs and using care and comfort as organizing principles, and then moved to stress tension reduction. Through reasoning, Johnson began to theorize that nursing's specific contribution to patient welfare was the fostering of efficient and effective behavioral functioning. That perspective led her to accept the theoretical view of the person as a behavioral system, similar to the way that physicians accept the person as a biological system (Fawcett, 2005; Johnson, 1990).

Johnson's Behavioral System Model

The goals of nursing in Johnson's behavioral system model are to maintain or restore behavioral system balance. Her model for nursing presents the patient as a living open system, comprising a collection of behavioral subsystems that interrelate to form a behavioral system. Because the subsystems are linked and open, a disturbance in one subsystem will likely have an effect on the other subsystems (Johnson, 1980). The seven subsystems of behavior proposed by Johnson include the (1) achievement, (2) affiliative, (3) aggressive, (4) dependence, (5) sexual, (6) eliminative, and (7) ingestive subsystems.

Subsystems include four structural components:

1. The drive or goal of the subsystem reflects the motivation or reasons for the behaviors of the subsystem. Motivational drives directing the activities or behaviors of the subsystems may vary from strong to weak and are constantly changing because of maturation, experience, and learning.
2. The set is the ordinary or normal behaviors that the patient prefers to use to meet the goal of a subsystem.
3. The choice represents the options that are available to patients to meet their subsystem goals. This structural component is influenced by variables such as gender, age, culture, socioeconomic status, and health status.
4. The action or behavior emanates as a consequence of the previous three structural components. The question of concern in relation to the structural component of behavior is whether the behavior is efficient and effective in relation to subsystem goal attainment. This is the only structural component that can be directly observed (Johnson, 1980).

Each of the seven subsystems has a function. The achievement subsystem functions to control or master an aspect of self or environment to achieve a standard. This subsystem encompasses intellectual, physical, creative, mechanical, and social skills. The affiliative or attachment subsystem forms the basis for social organization. Its consequences include social inclusion, intimacy, and the formation and maintenance of strong social bonds. The aggressive or protective subsystem functions to protect and preserve the system. The dependency subsystem promotes helping or nurturing behaviors. Its consequences include approval, recognition, and physical assistance. The sexual subsystem has the function of procreation and gratification and includes development of gender-role identity and gender-role behaviors. The eliminative subsystem addresses "when, how, and under what conditions we eliminate," whereas the ingestive subsystem "has to do with when, how, what, how much, and under what conditions we eat" (Johnson, 1980, p. 213).

Johnson asserted that each of these subsystems, as well as the system as a whole, has certain functional requirements that must be met through the effort of the individual or through outside assistance for continued growth, development, and viability. These functional requirements include (1) protection from noxious influences with which the system cannot cope, (2) nurturing through input of supplies from the environment (examples include food, friendship, and caring), and (3) stimulation by experiences, events, and behavior that would enhance growth and prevent stagnation (Johnson, 1980, p. 212).

The nursing process for the behavioral system model is Johnson's nursing diagnostic and treatment process. The components of this process include determination of the existence of a problem, diagnostic classification of problems, management of nursing problems, and evaluation of behavioral system balance and stability.

When nurses use Johnson's conceptual model as part of advanced practice, the focus of the assessment process is obtaining information to evaluate current behavior in terms of past patterns, determining the effects of the current illness on behavioral patterns, and establishing the maximum level of health. The assessment specifically focuses on gathering information related to the structure and function of the seven behavioral subsystems, as well as the environmental factors that influence the behavioral subsystems (Holaday, 2006). During the assessment phase, APNs obtain data about the nature of the behavioral functioning related to goal attainment—specifically, whether the patient's behavior is purposeful, orderly, and predictable. APNs need to interview the patient and family also to assess the condition of the subsystem structural components and evaluate the patient's behavior for behavioral system balance and stability. From the data collected, APNs make inferences and independent judgments related to the organization, interaction, and integration of the subsystems (Fawcett, 2005).

Within Johnson's conceptual model, problems may be classified as internal subsystem problems or intersystem problems. Internal subsystem problems include situations when functional requirements are not met, there is inconsistency or disharmony among components of the subsystem, or behavior is not appropriate for the culture. Intersystem problems include situations when the behavioral system is dominated by one or two subsystems or a conflict exists between two or more subsystems (Fawcett, 2005).

The goals of the management of nursing problems for APNs and other nurses are to restore, maintain, or attain the patient's behavioral system balance and stability and to help the patient achieve an optimal level of balance and functioning. The goals of management could be accomplished through the temporary imposition of external regulatory or control mechanisms, the repair of damaged subsystem structural components, or the fulfillment of subsystem functional requirements (Johnson, 1980). For example, APNs may temporarily impose external regulatory or control mechanisms by setting limits for behavior, inhibiting ineffective behavioral responses, assisting the patient to develop new responses, and reinforcing appropriate behaviors. Repair of damaged structural components includes interventions that modify the drive or motivation, or redirect goals. Interventions can also attempt to alter set behaviors through instruction or counseling and add choices through teaching new skills. In addition, the nurse can intervene to fulfill functional requirements by protecting the patient from overwhelming negative influences that exceed the patient's coping ability, by nurturing the patient through input of adequate essential supplies, and by providing stimulation to enhance growth and prevent stagnation (Fawcett, 2005; Johnson, 1980).

Evaluation is based on the attainment of the goal of balance in the identified subsystems. Evaluation of behavioral system balance and stability is accomplished as the APN compares the patient's behavior after treatment to indices of behavioral system balance and stability (Fawcett, 2005; Johnson, 1980). A case involving advanced nursing practice that illustrates the use of Johnson's behavioral system model appears in **Box 18-2**.

Major Concepts of Nursing According to Johnson

Person

Within the behavioral system model, the person is viewed as a behavioral being—that is, a behavioral system with seven subsystems of behavior. Under the original model, the role of medicine was to focus on the biological system and the role of nursing was to focus on the behavioral system. Today's APNs, however, focus on both biological and behavioral systems.

Environment

In the behavioral system model, the environment includes both the internal environment and the external environment; the latter is not a part of the individual's behavioral system,

Box 18-2   Case Study Using Johnson's Behavioral System Model

Mrs. Akins is the primary caregiver for her husband, who has been diagnosed with Alzheimer disease. Nursing care begins with the assessment phase of Johnson's nursing diagnostic and treatment process and includes an assessment of each of the subsystems.

Assessment of the aggressive or protective subsystem reveals that Mrs. Akins is frustrated and is struggling to cope with the increasing burden of caring for her husband, who often does not recognize her. Assessment of the dependency subsystem reveals that Mrs. Akins feels isolated socially and emotionally, because she has no time for socialization while caring for her husband; in addition, few friends or family members understand what is happening to Mr. Akins. Assessment of the achievement subsystem reveals that Mrs. Akins not only struggles with the question of why this is happening to her, but she is trying also to remain self-sufficient and thus has not asked friends and family members for help. Affiliative or attachment subsystem assessment reveals that Mrs. Akins's relationships with family and friends have been adversely affected because she has no time or energy left to socialize while constantly caring for Mr. Akins.

Assessment of the ingestive and eliminative subsystems reveals Mrs. Akins to be slightly overweight but with no bowel function abnormalities. She admits that she does not have time to cook as much as she did before Mr. Akins became sick. In response to sexual subsystem assessment, Mrs. Akins states that she is often tired, depressed, and overwhelmed with caring for her husband and finds intimacy difficult with a person who often cannot remember who she is.

Structural component assessment includes the assessment of drive, set, choice, and action. Next, the problems are diagnostically classified. Nursing management of the problems is then initiated.

Nursing management of Mrs. Akins's problems should include attention to the issues identified in the aggressive, dependency, affiliative, and achievement subsystems. The nurse encourages Mrs. Akins to express her feelings of frustration and to ask for assistance from family members. The nurse provides information related to professional services and community resources, including support groups and respite care services. The nurse facilitates education of family members and provides informational materials related to Alzheimer disease. Evaluation includes an assessment of behavioral system balance.

but it nevertheless influences the system. Strong environmental forces can disturb the balance of the behavioral system and threaten stability of the system (Loveland-Cherry & Wilkerson, 1989).

Health

Johnson referred to two types of health: physical health and social health (Johnson, 1980). According to Johnson, health is determined by the interaction of various psychological, social, biological, and physiological factors. Efficient and effective functioning of the system, which results in behavioral system balance and stability, is equivalent to a state of health. Illness can be defined then as behavioral system imbalance and instability.

Nursing

According to Johnson's behavioral system, nursing is an external regulatory force that acts to preserve the organization and integrity of the patient's behavior at an optimal level under those conditions in which the behavior constitutes a threat to physical or social health or in which illness is found. This force operates through the imposition of external regulatory or control mechanisms, through attempts to change structural units in desirable directions, or through the fulfillment of the functional requirements of the subsystems. Under Johnson's behavioral system, the purpose of nursing practice is "to facilitate restoration, maintenance, or attainment of behavioral system balance and stability" (Johnson, 1980, p. 214). These goals are accomplished through the use of Johnson's nursing diagnostic and treatment process, which is a pragmatic method for APNs. Today's APNs using Johnson's behavioral system model would consider the balance and stability of the biological system in attempting to accomplish these goals. During the nursing era when Johnson developed her behavioral system with her specifications and language, nurses did not take on these responsibilities; thus, she did not account for today's role of the APN. Even so, because of its relevance, her nursing diagnostic and treatment process can be translated easily to advanced practice.

Analysis of the Behavioral System Model

The analysis and critique presented here consist of an examination of assumptions and propositions, as well as an analysis of the clarity, simplicity, generality, empirical precision, and derivable consequences of the behavioral system model as proposed by Johnson.

Assumptions of the Behavioral System Model

Johnson based her theory on four explicit and implicit assumptions:

1. Behavior is the sum total of physical, biological, and social factors.
2. A person is a system of behavior characterized by repetitive, predictable, and goal-directed behaviors that always strive toward balance.
3. There are different levels of balance and stabilization, and levels are different during different time periods.
4. Persons expend large amounts of energy attempting to maintain or reestablish behavioral system balance in response to imbalance caused by persistent excessive forces (Holaday, 2010; Meleis, 2007, p. 281).

Propositions of the Health Behavior Model

Primary relationships are seen in the behavioral system model between the person and the environment; the person, health, and the environment; and the person, nursing, and health. Primary relationships of the behavioral system model include the following notions: (1) the behavioral system manages its relationship with the environment, which is self-maintaining as long as conditions remain orderly; (2) balance is essential for effective and efficient functions of the person, and a lack of balance in the structural or functional requirements of the subsystems leads to poor health; and (3) nursing is an external regulatory force that acts to restore balance to the behavioral system (Holaday, 2010; Johnson, 1980).

Analysis: Clarity, Simplicity, Generality, Empirical Precision, and Derivable Consequences

Johnson developed the behavioral system model using inductive reasoning that was based on her observations during many years of nursing practice, as well as on nursing literature and research. The model is fairly simple in terms of the number of concepts, and the concepts of nursing and behavioral system are described in detail. Johnson's model has nearly unlimited applicability with ill persons; however, it has not yet been used as extensively with well persons (Holaday, 2010). Regarding the criticism that her model did not allow for a focus on prevention, Johnson (1990) stated, "Preventive nursing is not possible until problems in the behavioral system are explicated. To the extent that any problem that might arise can be anticipated . . . preventive action is in order" (p. 31).

The concepts within the behavioral system model are clearly and consistently defined (Loveland-Cherry & Wilkerson, 1989), and the comprehensiveness of this conceptual model has proven to be adequate for providing direction for nursing research, education, administration, and practice (Fawcett, 2005). Some adaptations of Johnson's model have appeared in the literature as the model has been used by others, including the addition of an eighth subsystem dealing with restorative behavior and some alternative interpretations of the functions of subsystems (Fawcett, 2005). In response to these additions and alterations, Johnson (1990) stated, "These changes are such that they alter the fundamental nature of the behavioral system as originally proposed, and I do not agree with them" (p. 27).

Discussion

Johnson's behavioral system model makes an important contribution to nursing knowledge by directing attention to the person's behavior rather than the disease state. Johnson used that distinction to clarify the different foci of the disciplines of nursing and medicine (Fawcett, 2005). At the time when she undertook her work, there was no delineated theoretical framework for the discipline of nursing. Thus Johnson began her work in earnest related to the conceptualization of nursing and the other components of the behavioral system model; according to this pioneer, it was only when these elements were defined and specific goals were articulated that professionals would be able to begin to speak of a "science of nursing" (Johnson, 1959). Johnson's work is an excellent example of using scientific underpinnings for practice (AACN, 2006).

THE HEALTH PROMOTION MODEL: NOLA J. PENDER

Background

Nola J. Pender was born in 1941 in Lansing, Michigan. She graduated in 1962 with a diploma in nursing. In 1964, Pender completed a bachelor of science in nursing at Michigan State University. By 1969, she had completed a doctor of philosophy in psychology and education. During this time in her career, Pender began looking at health and nursing in a broad way, including defining the goal of nursing care as optimal health.

In 1975, Pender published a model for preventive health behavior; her health promotion model first appeared in the first edition of the text *Health Promotion in Nursing Practice* in 1982. Pender's health promotion model has its foundation in Albert Bandura's (1977) social learning theory (which postulates that cognitive processes affect behavior change) and is influenced by Fishbein's (1967) theory of reasoned action (which asserts that personal attitudes and social norms affect behavior).

Pender's Health Promotion Model

McCullagh (2009) labeled Pender's health promotion model as a middle-range integrative theory, and rightly so. Fawcett (2005) decisively presented the difference between a conceptual model for nursing and a model for middle-range theory. A model for middle-range theory is usually a graphic representation or schematic diagram of a middle-range theory. McCullagh's (2009) rationale for labeling Pender's model a middle-range integrative theory is that it portrays the multidimensionality of persons interacting with their interpersonal and physical environments as they pursue health while integrating constructs from expectancy-value theory and social cognitive theory with a nursing perspective of holistic human functioning (Pender, 1996). With the third edition of *Health Promotion in Nursing Practice* (1996), Pender revised the health promotion model significantly. This revised model is the subject of the discussion in this chapter.

Pender's health promotion model includes three major categories: (1) individual characteristics and experiences, (2) behavior-specific cognitions and affect, and (3) behavioral outcome. Each of these categories will be considered here separately.

The first category includes each person's unique personal characteristics and experiences, which affect that individual's actions. Significant components within this category are prior related behavior and personal factors. Prior related behavior is important in influencing future behavior. Pender proposed that prior behavior has both direct and indirect effects on the likelihood of engaging in health-promoting behaviors. In particular, past behavior has a direct effect on the current health-promoting behavior through habit formation: Habit strength increases each time a behavior occurs. Prior behavior is proposed to indirectly influence health-promoting behavior through perceptions of self-efficacy, benefits, barriers, and activity-related affect or emotions (Pender, Murdaugh, & Parsons, 2006). Personal factors include biological factors such as age, body mass index, pubertal status, menopausal status, aerobic capacity, strength, agility, or balance; psychological factors include self-esteem, self-motivation, and perceived health status; and sociocultural factors include race, ethnicity, acculturation, education, and socioeconomic status. Some personal factors are amenable to change, whereas others are immutable (Pender et al., 2006).

The second category encompasses behavior-specific cognitions and affect, which serve as behavior-specific variables within the health promotion model. Behavior-specific variables are considered to have motivational significance. In the health promotion model, nursing interventions target these variables because they are amenable to change. The behavior-specific cognitions and affect identified in the health promotion model include (1) perceived benefits of action, (2) perceived barriers to action, (3) perceived self-efficacy, and (4) activity-related affect. Other cognitions fall into the category of interpersonal influences and situational influences. Sources of interpersonal influences on health-promoting behaviors include family, peers, and healthcare providers. Interpersonal influences include norms, social support, and modeling; they shape the person's tendency to participate in health-promoting behaviors. Situational influences on health-promoting behavior include perceptions of available options, demand characteristics, and aesthetic features of the environment. Within Pender's model, nursing plans are tailored to meet the needs of diverse patients based on assessment of prior behavior, behavior-specific cognitions and affect, interpersonal factors, and situational factors (Pender et al., 2006, pp. 54–56).

The third category within Pender's model is the behavioral outcome. Commitment to a plan of action marks the beginning of a behavioral event. This commitment propels the person into the behavior unless that action is confounded by a competing demand that cannot be avoided or a competing preference that is not resisted. Interventions in the health promotion model focus on raising consciousness related to health-promoting behaviors, promoting self-efficacy, enhancing the benefits of change, controlling the environment to support behavior change, and managing the barriers to change. Health-promoting behavior, which is ultimately directed toward attaining positive health outcomes, is the product of the health promotion model (Pender et al., 2006, pp. 56–63).

Major Concepts of Nursing According to Pender

Person

The person in the health promotion model refers to the individual who is the primary focus of the model. In Pender's model, each person has unique personal characteristics and experiences that affect subsequent actions. It is recognized that individuals learn health behaviors within the context of the family and the community, which explains why the model for assessment includes components and interventions at the family and community levels, as well as the individual level (Pender, Murdaugh, & Parsons, 2002, 2006). This concept is taken a step further in the latest edition (Pender, Murdaugh, & Parsons, 2011), in which the term client refers to individuals, families, and communities who are all viewed as active participants in health promotion.

Environment

In the health promotion model, the environment encompasses the physical, interpersonal, and economic circumstances in which persons live. The quality of the environment depends on the absence of toxic substances, the availability of restorative experiences, and the accessibility of human and economic resources needed for healthful living. Socioeconomic conditions such as unemployment, poverty, crime, and prejudice have adverse effects on health, whereas environmental wellness is manifested by balance between human beings and their surroundings (Pender et al., 2006, p. 9; Pender et al., 2011, p. 8).

Health

Health is viewed as a positive high-level state. According to Pender, the person's definition of health for himself or herself is more important than any general definition of health (Pender et al., 2006; Sakraida, 2010). Health is viewed in the context of health promotion and disease prevention. Health promotion is behavior that is motivated by a desire to increase well-being and optimize human health potential, whereas disease prevention or health protection is behavior motivated by a desire to actively avoid illness, detect illness early, or maintain functioning within the constraints of illness (Pender et al., 2011, p. 5). Health promotion is viewed as a multidimensional concept that includes the dimensions of the individual, the family, the community, socioeconomic status, cultural factors, and environmental factors (Pender et al., 2011, pp. 6–8).

Nursing

The role of the nurse in the health promotion model revolves around raising consciousness related to health-promoting behaviors, promoting self-efficacy, enhancing the benefits of change, controlling the environment to support behavior change, and managing the barriers to change (Pender et al., 2006, pp. 57–63). A major function of the APN role is the focus on health promotion. This model serves as a significantly pragmatic process for APNs to use to encourage health-promoting behaviors by patients and to address the benefits of change.

Analysis of the Health Promotion Model

The analysis and critique presented here comprise an examination of assumptions and propositions, as well as the analysis of clarity, simplicity, generality, empirical precision, and derivable consequences of Pender's health promotion model.

Assumptions of the Health Promotion Model

Assumptions of the health promotion model reflect both nursing and behavioral science perspectives. The seven major assumptions emphasize the active role of the patient in shaping and maintaining health behaviors and in modifying the environmental context for health behaviors:

1. Persons seek to create conditions of living through which they can express their unique human potential.
2. Persons have the capacity for reflective self-awareness, including assessment of their own competencies.
3. Persons value growth in directions viewed as positive and attempt to achieve a personally acceptable balance between change and stability.
4. Persons seek to actively regulate their own behavior.
5. Persons in all their biopsychosocial complexity interact with the environment, both progressively transforming the environment and being transformed over time.
6. Health professionals constitute a part of the interpersonal environment, which influences persons throughout their life span.
7. Self-initiated reconfiguration of person–environment interactive patterns is essential for behavior change (Pender et al., 2002, p. 63).

Propositions of the Health Promotion Model

The health promotion model is based upon 14 theoretical propositions. These theoretical relationship statements provide a basis for research related to health behaviors:

1. Prior behavior and inherited and acquired characteristics influence health beliefs, affect, and enactment of health-promoting behavior.
2. Persons commit to engaging in behaviors from which they anticipate deriving personally valued benefits.
3. Perceived barriers can constrain commitment to action (a mediator of behavior), as well as actual behavior.
4. Perceived competence or self-efficacy to execute a given behavior increases the likelihood of commitment to action and actual performance of behavior.

5. Greater perceived self-efficacy results in fewer perceived barriers to a specific health behavior.

6. Positive affect toward a behavior results in greater perceived self-efficacy, which can, in turn, result in increased positive affect.

7. When positive emotions or affect are associated with a behavior, the probability of commitment and action are increased.

8. Persons are more likely to commit to and engage in health-promoting behaviors when significant others model the behavior, expect the behavior to occur, and provide assistance and support to enable the behavior.

9. Family, peers, and healthcare providers are important sources of interpersonal influence who can increase or decrease commitment to and engagement in health-promoting behavior.

10. Situational influences in the external environment can increase or decrease commitment to or participation in health-promoting behavior.

11. The greater the commitment to a specific plan of action, the more likely health-promoting behaviors will be maintained over time.

12. Commitment to a plan of action is less likely to result in the desired behavior when competing demands over which persons have little control require immediate attention.

13. Commitment to a plan of action is less likely to result in the desired behavior when other actions are more attractive and thus preferred over the target behavior.

14. Persons can modify cognitions, affect, and the interpersonal and physical environments to create incentives for health actions (Pender et al., 2002, pp. 63–64).

Analysis: Clarity, Simplicity, Generality, Empirical Precision, and Derivable Consequences

Pender's health promotion model was formulated using inductive reasoning with existing research, which is a common approach to the building of middle-range theories. The research used to derive the model was based on adult samples that included male, female, young, old, well, and ill populations; this design allows the model to be generalized easily to adult populations (Sakraida, 2010).

The health promotion model is simple to understand, because it uses language familiar to nurses. The concept of health promotion is also popular in nursing practice and, therefore, is a practical principle for APNs' use. The relationships among the factors are linked, and relationships are identified and consistently defined. Considering all of these factors, it is not difficult to see why Pender's model is popular with practicing nurses and is frequently used as a tool in research. Nevertheless, it has not been used extensively in nursing education, where the emphasis is on illness care in acute care settings (Sakraida, 2010).

Discussion

Pender identified health promotion as a key global goal for the 21st century (Pender et al., 2011) and, through development of the health promotion model, has assisted in the delineation of the role of nursing in meeting that goal. The Health Promotion Model provides a framework for APNs to focus on clinical prevention and population health (AACN, 2006). Although Pender has now retired, her work on the health promotion model continues. Pender views the nurse's role in health promotion as more important than ever considering existing health disparities and the challenges of our current healthcare system (Pender et al., 2011). The current scenario of increasing costs for health care associated with episodic illness treatment, increases in chronic, preventable conditions within the population, and the focus on managing healthcare costs provide ample incentive to further explore the concepts of the health promotion model as APNs strive to improve health outcomes in patient populations.

SUMMARY

Although the four nursing models described in this chapter were conceived by four very different nurses whose careers spanned more than a century, they share a common thread: All place emphasis on the function of nursing practice in relation to health outcomes. For Nightingale, the function of nursing is to alter the environment to allow for action on the person by natural laws of health; for Henderson, the function of nursing is to assist the person to perform activities to gain independence; for Johnson, the function of the nurse is to impose external regulatory mechanisms in order to facilitate restoration of system balance; and for Pender, the nurse functions to raise consciousness, promote self-efficacy, and control the environment to allow for behavior change resulting in high-level health. All four of these nursing models also conceptualize the goal of nursing care as a restoration of the health of the patient, however differently the concept of health—or, for that matter, the concept of the patient—may be defined in their respective theories.

DISCUSSION QUESTIONS

1. Nightingale and Henderson considered the discipline of nursing to be both an art and a science. Aesthetic patterns of knowing and empirical patterns of knowing both constitute complex yet divergent ways of thinking. How can the APN perform simultaneously from an aesthetic perspective and a perspective based on empiricism?

2. Johnson's behavioral system model has been used in practice and research; as a result, multiple adaptations of this model have appeared in the literature. In response to these additions and alterations, Johnson (1990) stated, "These changes are such that they alter the fundamental nature of the behavioral system as originally proposed, and

I do not agree with them" (p. 27). Does a theory belong to the nurse theorist or to the discipline of nursing? Who has the right to add to or alter a theory? Should a theory be altered based on research evidence even if the original nurse theorist is not in agreement, or should the theory be maintained intact as a historical record?

3. Considering a patient scenario from advanced nursing practice and using a middle-range theory such as the health promotion model, demonstrate the connection and reciprocal relationship between theory, practice, and research.

4. The four theorists discussed in this chapter viewed nursing from various perspectives, yet they fundamentally agreed on the concepts of interest to the nursing profession, thereby influencing the evolution of nursing as a discipline and framing nursing knowledge. How has the development of these and other nursing theories helped to frame knowledge and shape the role of the APN?

REFERENCES

American Association of Colleges of Nursing. (2006, October). The essentials of doctoral education for advanced nursing practice. Retrieved from http://www.aacn.nche.edu/dnp/Essentials.pdf

American Nurses Association. (n.d.). Hall of fame: Virginia A. Henderson (1897–1996) 1996 inductee. Retrieved from http://www.nursingworld.org/FunctionalMenuCategories/AboutANA/Honoring -Nurses/HallofFame/19962000Inductees/hendva5545.aspx

Bandura, A. (1977). *Social learning theory.* Englewood Cliffs, NJ: Prentice Hall.

Bolton, K. (2006). Nightingale's philosophy in nursing practice. In M. R. Alligood & A. M. Tomey (Eds.), *Nursing theory: Utilization and application* (3rd ed., pp. 89–102). St. Louis, MO: Mosby.

Chinn, P. L., & Kramer, M. K. (2008). *Integrated knowledge development in nursing* (7th ed.). St. Louis, MO: Elsevier-Mosby.

Cook, E. (1913). *The life of Florence Nightingale* (Vols. 1 and 2). London, UK: Macmillan.

Dietz, D. D., & Lehozky, A. R. (1963). *History and modern nursing.* Philadelphia, PA: F. A. Davis.

Donahue, M. P. (1985). *Nursing: The finest art.* St. Louis, MO: Mosby.

Fawcett, J. (2005). *Contemporary nursing knowledge: Analysis and evaluation of nursing models and theories* (2nd ed.). Philadelphia, PA: F. A. Davis.

Fishbein, M. (1967). *Readings in attitude theory and measurement.* New York, NY: Wiley.

Furukawa, C. Y., & Howe, J. S. (2002). Definition and components of nursing: Virginia Henderson. In J. B. George (Ed.), *Nursing theories: The base for professional nursing practice* (5th ed., pp. 83–109). Upper Saddle River, NJ: Prentice Hall.

Gordon, S. C. (2001). Virginia Avenel Henderson: Definition of nursing. In M. Parker (Ed.), *Nursing theories and nursing practice* (pp. 143–1 49). Philadelphia, PA: F. A. Davis.

Harmer, B., & Henderson, V. (1939). *Textbook of the principles and practice of nursing* (4th ed.). New York, NY: Macmillan.

Harmer, B., & Henderson, V. (1955). *Textbook of the principles and practice of nursing* (5th ed.). New York, NY: Macmillan.

Henderson, V. (1964). The nature of nursing. *American Journal of Nursing, 64,* 62–68.

Henderson, V. (1966). *The nature of nursing: A definition and its implications for practice, research, and education*. New York, NY: Macmillan.

Henderson, V. (1991). *The nature of nursing: Reflections after 25 years*. New York, NY: National League for Nursing Press.

Henderson, V., & Nite, G. (1978). *Principles and practice of nursing* (6th ed.). New York, NY: Macmillan.

Holaday, B. (2006). Johnson's behavioral system model in nursing practice. In M. R. Alligood & A. M. Tomey (Eds.), *Nursing theory: Utilization and application* (3rd ed., pp. 157–180). St. Louis, MO: Mosby.

Holaday, B. (2010). Dorothy Johnson: Behavioral system model. In A. M. Tomey & M. R. Alligood (Eds.), *Nursing theorists and their work* (7th ed., pp. 366–390). St. Louis, MO: Mosby.

Johnson, B. M., & Webber, P. B. (2010). *An introduction to theory and reasoning in nursing* (3rd ed.). Philadelphia, PA: Lippincott Williams & Wilkins.

Johnson, D. E. (1959). The nature and science of nursing. *Nursing Outlook, 7*(5), 291–294.

Johnson, D. E. (1980). The behavioral system model for nursing. In J. Riehl & C. Roy (Eds.), *Conceptual models for nursing practice* (2nd ed., pp. 207–216). New York, NY: Appleton-Century-Crofts.

Johnson, D. E. (1990). The behavioral system model for nursing. In M. E. Parker (Ed.), *Nursing theories in practice* (pp. 23–32). New York, NY: National League for Nursing.

Lobo, M. L. (2002). Environmental model: Florence Nightingale. In J. B. George (Ed.), *Nursing theories: The base for professional nursing practice* (5th ed., pp. 155–188). Upper Saddle River, NJ: Prentice Hall.

Loveland-Cherry, C. J., & Wilkerson, S. A. (1989). Dorothy Johnson's behavioral system model. In J. J. Fitzpatrick & A. L. Whall (Eds.), *Conceptual models of nursing* (2nd ed., pp. 147–163). Englewood Cliffs, NJ: Prentice Hall.

McCullagh, M. C. (2009). Health promotion. In S. J. Peterson & T. S. Bredow (Eds.), *Middle range theories: Application to nursing research* (2nd ed., pp. 290–303). Philadelphia, PA: Wolters Kluwer Health/Lippincott Williams & Wilkins.

Meleis, A. I. (2007). *Theoretical nursing: Development and progress* (4th ed.). Philadelphia, PA: Lippincott Williams & Wilkins.

Nightingale, F. (1858). *Subsidiary notes as to the introduction of female nursing into military hospitals in peace and war*. London, UK: Harrison and Sons.

Nightingale, F. (1860/1969). *Notes on nursing: What it is, and what it is not*. New York, NY: Dover.

Pender, N. J. (1982). *Health promotion in nursing practice*. Norwalk, CT: Appleton-Century-Crofts.

Pender, N. J. (1996). *Health promotion in nursing practice* (3rd ed.). Stamford, CT: Appleton & Lange.

Pender, N. J., Murdaugh, C. L., & Parsons, M. A. (2002). *Health promotion in nursing practice* (4th ed.). Upper Saddle River, NJ: Prentice Hall.

Pender, N. J., Murdaugh, C. L., & Parsons, M. A. (2006). *Health promotion in nursing practice* (5th ed.). Upper Saddle River, NJ: Prentice Hall.

Pender, N. J., Murdaugh, C. L., & Parsons, M. A. (2011). *Health promotion in nursing practice* (6th ed.). Upper Saddle River, NJ: Pearson.

Pfettscher, S. A. (2010). Florence Nightingale: Modern nursing. In A. M. Tomey & M. R. Alligood (Eds.), *Nursing theorists and their work* (7th ed., pp. 71–90). St. Louis, MO: Mosby.

Pokorny, M. E. (2010). Nursing theorists of historical significance. In A. M. Tomey & M. R. Alligood (Eds.), *Nursing theorists and their work* (7th ed., pp. 54–68). St. Louis, MO: Mosby.

Reed, P. G., & Zurakowski, T. L. (1989). Nightingale revisited: A visionary model for nursing. In J. J. Fitzpatrick & A. L. Whall (Eds.), *Conceptual models of nursing: Analysis and application* (2nd ed., pp. 33–47). Norwalk, CT: Appleton & Lange.

Runk, J. A., & Muth Quillin, S. I. (1989). Henderson's comprehensive definition of nursing. In J. J. Fitzpatrick & A. L. Whall (Eds.), *Conceptual models of nursing: Analysis and application* (2nd ed., pp. 109–121). Norwalk, CT: Appleton & Lange.

Sakraida, T. J. (2010). The health promotion model. In A. M. Tomey & M. R. Alligood (Eds.), *Nursing theorists and their work* (7th ed., pp. 434–453). St. Louis, MO: Mosby.

Selanders, L. C. (1995). Life and times of Florence Nightingale. In C. M. McQuiston & A. A. Webb (Eds.), *Foundations of nursing theory: Contributions of 12 key theorists* (pp. 421–431). Thousand Oaks, CA: Sage.

Shelly, J. A., & Miller, A. B. (2006). *Called to care: A Christian worldview for nursing* (2nd ed.). Downers Grove, IL: InterVarsity Press.

Tomey, A. M. (2002). Virginia Henderson: Definition of nursing. In A. M. Tomey & M. R. Alligood (Eds.), *Nursing theorists and their work* (5th ed., pp. 98–111). St. Louis, MO: Mosby.

Tomey, A. M. (2006). Nursing theorists of historical significance. In A. M. Tomey & M. R. Alligood (Eds.), *Nursing theorists and their work* (6th ed., pp. 54–67). St. Louis, MO: Mosby.

Tooley, S. A. (1910). *The life of Florence Nightingale*. London, UK: Cassell.

Woodham-Smith, C. (1951). *Florence Nightingale*. New York, NY: McGraw-Hill.

Chapter 19

Models and Theories Focused on a Systems Approach

Martha V. Whetsell
Yolanda M. Gonzalez
María Elisa Moreno-Fergusson

INTRODUCTION

Nursing professionals use theories in their practice to describe, explain, predict, and prescribe. The development and use of theories also is a way to generate and disseminate new knowledge in nursing. The application of nursing theory in practice depends on nurses' knowledge of theories, as well as their understanding of how philosophies, models, and theories relate to one another (Alligood, 2002). Using conceptual models as an overarching model for practice, research, education, and administration keeps nursing theory at the forefront of the profession and, ideally, leads advanced practice nurses (APNs) to become proficient in testing and generating theory. With the use of conceptual models and theory in clinical practice, nurses create new ways of thinking and introduce new and expanded ways of delivering health care.

This chapter focuses on three conceptual nursing models that are all based on the systems perspective—the Roy adaptation model, King's conceptual system, and the Neuman systems model. Systems science is an interdisciplinary field of physical, chemical, and psychological structures for nature and society. A system can be a single organism, an object, an organization, or a society.

GENERAL SYSTEMS THEORY

General systems theory grew from thermodynamics—a branch of physics, chemistry, and engineering. This theory is grounded in the premise that the world is composed of systems that are interconnected and influenced by one another. The two main assumptions of this theory are as follows: (1) energy is needed to maintain an organizational state, and (2) a dysfunction in one system has an effect on other systems (Boulding, 1956). The origin of systems theory dates back at least to the 1920s, when theorists sought to explain the interrelatedness of organisms in ecosystems. In 1928, the biologist Ludwig von Bertalanffy became the first person to propose that a system is characterized by the interactions of its components and that the interactions are nonlinear. It was not until 1951, however, that von Bertalanffy extended the theory to include biological systems (McNeill & Freiberger, 1994). In 1968, he published the influential book *General System Theory*.

It might be said that Florence Nightingale introduced systems theory in nursing when she stated that nursing laws would be defined (Riehl & Roy, 1974). King (1964) presented the foundation for the general systems framework in her article titled "Nursing Theory: Problems and Prospect." It was not until 1970, however, that Roy published the first article and implemented her systems model—known as the Roy adaptation model—as the basis of a nursing curriculum at Mount St. Mary's College in Los Angeles, California (Roy, 2009). Neuman introduced the Neuman systems model in 1970 at the University of California, Los Angeles, and in 1972 Neuman and Young published an article about the model.

The nursing systems models are based on a framework of organized complexity and an interaction among all of the models' components. Such models are dynamic in that they can be used to investigate the client's continuous relationship with the environment. According to Fawcett (2005), the use of systems thinking demands flexibility, which in turn demands the use of creativity to meet the challenges associated with the complex societal changes occurring in this century. This consideration is particularly significant given Fawcett's (2009) assertion that only a strong link between theory and research will advance nursing knowledge; this link supports the building of conceptual–theoretical–empirical (C-T-E) structures for research. Fawcett (2009) described two methods of C-T-E: one for theory-generating research and the other for theory-testing research (p. 21).

THE ROY ADAPTATION MODEL

The History

Sister Callista Roy recalled that the origins of her adaptation model date back to 1964, when she was a master's-level student at Mount St. Mary's College in Los Angeles. In 1970, she published the basic ideas of her conceptual model in an article titled "Adaptation: A Conceptual Framework for Nursing" in *Nursing Outlook*. In 1971 and 1973, two additional articles were published and the model was further explained in a chapter of Riehl and Roy's (1974) book, *Conceptual Models for Nursing Practice*. A more comprehensive explanation of the model can be found in Roy's (1976) book, *Introduction to Nursing: An Adaptation Model*. Further refinements of the model were published in the second edition of that book (Roy, 1984). Roy's clinical experiences in pediatric nursing and neurological nursing were important influences in the development of her model (Roy, 2009).

The primary influencers for defining the key aspects of Roy's adaptation model included the systems theory described by von Bertalanffy (1968) and the work of physiological psychologist Harry Helson (1964), who developed adaptation-level theory. Helson proposed that adaptation involves both psychological and physical processes when an individual faces environmental stimuli. He described three kinds of stimuli—focal, contextual, and residual—that come together and result in a pooled effect. On the basis of those principles, Roy described how adaptation could help people conserve the energy needed to heal and to cope with new life experiences (Roy & Whetsell, personal communication, 2005).

The Philosophy and Assumptions

Roy's (2009) model was based on two underlying philosophical assumptions—humanism and veritivity. *Humanism* is the "broad movement in philosophy and psychology that recognizes the individual and subjective dimensions of human experiences as central to knowing and valuing" (p. 28). In 1988, Roy introduced the concept of *veritivity*—"a principle of human nature that affirms a common purposefulness of human existence" (Roy, 1988, as cited in Roy, 2009, p. 27). She described living systems as totalities made of parts that are unified by a purpose, not simply by cause–effect relationships. The veritivity principle is related to four aspects of human society: (1) human existence's purpose, (2) humankind's shared purpose, (3) activity and creativity for the common good, and (4) value and meaning of life (Roy & Andrews, 1999).

Roy acknowledged that her spiritual orientation was a meaningful philosophical influence for development of her model. She also became interested in Teilhard de Chardin's work in 1955, largely because of its characteristic reconciliation of science and spirituality. According to Roy, nurses assume the responsibility of believing in each person's life purpose (Roy, 2009). People share a common destiny and find meaning in mutual relationships established with other persons, the world, and God. Roy emphasized the commonality that underlies people's unity and diversity (Roy, 2006). Activity and creativity for the common good are involved in veritivity, and each single human being is different from each other human being; that is, each individual has a unique identity (Roy, 2009). The principle of veritivity allows the nurse to meet the social mandate to help change the system by contributing to the common good through the application of knowledge in practice (Roy & Whetsell, personal conversation, 2005). Roy's last assumption about veritivity is the value and meaning of life; thus the person is the main domain of interest (Roy, 1996). Similarly, Maritain (1966) viewed a person's life as having a higher value than mere social utility.

The Model

Roy's first three books—published in 1976, 1984, and 1991—highlighted the many colleagues and students who were involved in her work. In 1987, nursing scholars calculated that more than 10,000 nurses were taught by nursing faculty or had graduated from schools that used Roy's model as a curricular framework (Roy, 1996).

Roy developed the Roy adaptation model while maintaining a unique focus on the changes that occur in the human adaptive system and in the environment. The model's central feature is adaptation. According to this model, problems in adaptation materialize when the adaptive systems of a person are unable to respond to stimuli from internal or external environments (Roy & Andrews, 1999).

Major Elements

Roy did not define the metaparadigm concepts as human beings (person), health, environment, and nursing. Instead, Roy labeled the major elements as adaptation, person, environment, health, and goal of nursing.

Adaptation

Adaptation is the process and outcome in which individuals and groups become integrated with their environment through conscious choices (Roy, 2009). Adaptive responses promote integrity in terms of human beings' goals, which are survival, growth, reproduction, mastery, and personal and environmental transformation. All responses that do not contribute to the integrity of the goals of the human system are recognized as ineffective responses.

Person

Early in the development of her model, Roy defined the *person* as an adaptive system with internal processes that act to maintain the integrity of the person (Roy & Andrews, 1999, p. 18). An expansion of the concept of person along with the addition of *groups* was incorporated in the 1990s as part of the model, in the adaptation systems. Described as totality made of parts behaving purposefully, the person uses innate and acquired mechanisms for biological, psychological, and social adaptation. These internal processes include the regulator and cognator subsystems for individuals and the stabilizer and innovator subsystems for people in groups (Roy, 2009).

Environment

Environment is defined as all conditions, circumstance, and influences surrounding and affecting the development and behavior of humans as adaptive systems, with particular consideration of human and earth resources (Roy, 2009, p. 26). The environment includes all focal, contextual, and residual stimuli (see the definitions in the subsection "Stimulus").

Health

Over time, the concepts of Roy's model were expanded, with health being one of the main foci. In 1964, Roy described *health* as an inherent dimension of a person's life and noted how the health–sickness continuum may vary from severe illness to maximum well-being. More recently, Roy has described health as a "state and a process of being and becoming an integrated and whole person" (Roy, 2009, p. 48). The concept of health is unidimensional, whereas the concept of nursing is represented by science and art. In Roy's systems theory, the scientific assumptions of the model link the adaptation-level theory described by Helson (1964) with the main concepts of her model. Individuals are regarded as holistic, adaptive systems that are more than the sum of their parts and that function as a whole in constant interaction with the environment (Roy & Andrews, 1999). Similar to how a system has inputs, processes, and outputs, people have stimulus inputs and an adaptation level.

Goal of Nursing

According to Roy and Andrews (1999), nursing is "the protection, promotion, and optimization of health and abilities, prevention of illness and injury, alleviation of suffering through the diagnosis and treatment of human response, and advocacy in the care of individuals, families, communities, and populations" (p. 6). The *goal of nursing* is "to promote the health of individuals and societies" (Roy, 2009, p. 54). In pursuing this goal, nurses integrate specialized knowledge from the applied sciences to formulate health promotion and illness management strategies for people. Nursing knowledge is focused on how people—sick or well—interact with their environments to enhance well-being and flourishing.

Adaptive Systems

Adaptive systems include stimuli, adaptation level, and behavior. They are holistic systems that are defined in terms of human beings.

Stimulus

A *stimulus* is the trigger that provokes a response; it can be viewed as the point of interaction between the human system and the environment (Roy, 2009). The constructs of stimuli in Roy's model are based on Helson's work relating to focal, contextual, and residual concepts. The focal stimulus evokes a primary internal or external awareness by the individual or the group, contextual stimuli are additional environmental factors that operate from within or outside the individual, and residual stimuli are other environmental factors that generate effects that may not be readily apparent in a given situation (Roy, 2009). Stimuli can change rapidly and often do so constantly because of the interactions between people and their environment.

Adaptation Level

Adaptation level includes three conditions of the human adaptive system: (1) integrated, (2) compensatory, and (3) compromised. As Roy stated, "The level of adaptation conveys that the human adaptive system is not passive in relation to the environment and that the person and the environment are in constant interaction with each other" (Roy, 2009, p. 37). The integrated level means that the structures and functions of the life processes work as one whole to meet the needs of humans. The compensatory level is where the cognator and regulator subsystems for individuals have been activated; or for groups, it is where the stabilizer and innovator subsystems have been activated and are working to meet needs. The compromised level is initiated in response to the system's diminishing adaptation because the integrated and the compensatory levels are no longer working.

Behavior

Behavior is defined as internal or external actions and reactions that occur under specific circumstances (Roy, 2009). Behavior is sometimes objectively observed and measured or subjectively reported by individuals or people in groups. Output behavior indicates how well a system can adapt while interacting with the environment; this relationship is the target of nursing interventions.

The behavioral response is evident in the coping process, but it remains independent of this process. The processes involving the human being as an adaptive system underscore the various ways in which people deal with the demands of their environment. These processes specifically focus on those behaviors that meet the goals for adaptation; they relate to responses that promote the integrity of the human system in terms of adaptation goals (Roy & Andrews, 1999). Put simply, the behavioral response can be either adaptive or ineffective, as described in the previous section on model elements.

Coping Processes

Coping processes are "innate or acquired ways of interacting with—that is, responding to and influencing—the changing environment" (Roy & Andrews, 1999, p. 41). The coping processes include the coping capacity, cognator and regulator subsystems for coping processes, and stabilizer and innovator subsystems for control processes.

Coping Capacity

Coping capacity is viewed as an important stimulus to enhance adaptation. One's coping ability as an adaptive system serves as a significant internal input for the person; output, in contrast, relates to the actual behavior. Coping involves the four dimensions already mentioned: regulator and cognator coping subsystems for individuals, and stabilizer and innovator control subsystems for groups.

Cognator and Regulator Coping Processes

The *cognator subsystem* for individuals is a coping process that interacts primarily with the four adaptive modes. This system includes four cognitive–emotive channels: (1) perceptual and information processing, (2) learning, (3) judgment, and (4) emotion.

The *regulator subsystem* for individuals constitutes a major coping process that includes an extremely linked physiological mode. The neurochemical and endocrine systems respond unconsciously to stimuli through neural, chemical, and endocrine coping channels; thus, they affect the fluid, electrolyte, and acid–base balance, as well as the endocrine system. These responses are interrelated and act in concert with one another, rather than in isolation, to maintain the equilibrium of the systems.

Stabilizer and Innovator Control Processes

The *stabilizer subsystem* for groups is a control process associated with systems maintenance involving structures, values, and daily activities to fulfill the purpose of the social system. The *innovator subsystem* is a control process related to individuals in groups; it encompasses structures and processes associated with change and growth within social systems.

Adaptive Modes

The coping process responses constitute the outputs of the human adaptive system. These responses are reflected in behaviors, which are interrelated *adaptive modes*. As such, adaptation is evident in four adaptive modes for individuals: (1) physiological, (2) self-concept, (3) role function, and (4) interdependence. For groups, the four adaptive modes are (1) physical, (2) identity, (3) role function, and (4) interdependence. Thus "behavior in one mode may have an effect on or act as stimulus for one or all the other modes" (Roy & Andrews, 1999, p. 51).

Physiological/Physical Mode

The *physiological mode* reflects the way that individuals as physical beings interact with the environment. The physiological mode pertains to the individual. In this mode, persons manifest the physical processes and activities of living organisms (Roy, 2009). The behavior in this mode represents the physiological manifestations of a person's cells, organs, and systems. This mode has nine components: five basic needs (oxygenation, nutrition, elimination, activity and rest, and protection) and four processes (senses, fluid and electrolyte balance, neurological function, and endocrine function). The basic need of the physiological mode is physiologic integrity.

By comparison, the *physical mode* relates to "the way the human adaptive system of the group manifests adaptation relative to basic operating resources, that is, participants, physical facilities and fiscal resources" (Roy, 2009, p. 43). The fundamental need of the physical mode is resource adequacy.

The Self-Concept/Group Identity Mode

The *self-concept mode* reflects personal aspects of individuals related to behavior. A self-concept is "the composite of beliefs and feelings that an individual holds about him or herself at a given time" (Roy, 2009, p. 44). The basic need for the self is psychic and spiritual integrity—that is, the need to know who one is so that the person can live with a sense of unity and purposefulness in the universe (Roy, 2009). Self-concept includes three components: (1) physical self (body image and body sensations), (2) personal self (self-consistency, self-ideal), and (3) the moral–ethical–spiritual self.

The *group identity mode* reflects group aspects of behavior. It comprises four subdimensions: (1) interpersonal relationships, (2) group self-image, (3) social milieu, and (4) group culture. The basic need underlying this mode is identity integrity of the group.

The Role Function Mode

Focusing on the roles that the person has in society, the basic needs underlying the *role function mode* have been identified as social integrity, role clarity, and the need to know who one is in relation to others so that one can act. This mode relates to the function or responsibility that an individual or group has in society.

The individual has three types of roles:

1. A *primary role*, which is unchangeable because it is based on age, gender, and developmental stage.
2. A *secondary role*, which is related to the expectations of the individual and the primary role. This role is an important one because it relates to the life project of each individual.
3. A *tertiary role*, which is temporary, is linked to the first two roles. In general, the tertiary role can change and is derived from the secondary and primary roles. Tertiary roles are freely chosen and often relate to small tasks undertaken in the course of a person's life.

In relation to groups, Roy (2009) established that the role's functions are "the vehicle through which the goals of the social system are actually accomplished" (p. 44)—relating to their mission or the tasks associated with the functions of the group. The role function mode for nursing groups includes the function of administrators and staff, the management of information, and systems for decision making and maintaining order.

The Interdependence Mode

The *interdependence mode* is the category of behavior related to relationships that individuals and groups establish with others. For individuals, this mode focuses on those interactions through which the individual receives and gives love, respect, and value. The basic need of this mode is nurturing relationships. For groups, this category reflects the group's social context.

The adaptive modes reflect the responses of the coping processes of the individual or group to the focal, contextual, and residual stimuli. These modes are interrelated, such that a response in one mode affects the responses in the other three modes and is expressed in an individual's behavior. Roy's adaptation model is a *systems* model, and also it has elements of an "interactional" model. It was developed specifically to be used in caring for individual clients, but it has been further developed for use with families and communities.

The Nursing Process

When implementing the nursing process according to the Roy adaptation model, human experiences and responses are approached in a nontraditional way. An individual or a group of individuals is viewed as a holistic adaptive system. Stimuli from the internal and external environments trigger the coping processes manifested by the four adaptive modes. The nurse assesses the behavior of the person or group and the influence of the stimuli on behavior; on the basis of this assessment, the nurse then formulates nursing diagnoses.

Roy (2009) viewed the nursing process as relating to human beings as adaptive systems. This process includes six steps:

1. Assessment of behavior
2. Assessment of stimuli
3. Nursing diagnosis
4. Goal setting
5. Intervention
6. Evaluation

Assessment of Behavior

The first step involves gathering behavioral data. During the assessment, the nurse systematically examines responses in each adaptive mode, uses observational skills, and compares current measurements to preestablished measurements. Effective communication and caring take precedence—an approach that contributes to the effectiveness of nurse–patient interactions.

Assessment of Stimuli

The second step of the nursing process is an extension of the first and encompasses the identification of internal and external stimuli affecting particular behaviors. In completing this assessment, the nurse utilizes skills similar to those applied in the first step. Identifying the behavior that threatens the integrity of the system is the primary concern. During the identification process, the nurse pinpoints the focal, contextual, and residual stimuli that influence the response, as well as the adaptation level that contributes to adaptive or ineffective behavior.

Nursing Diagnosis

Nursing diagnosis, according to Roy, is a judgment process that confirms the adaptation status of the person or the group. In formulating a diagnosis, the nurse primarily uses critical thinking. The nursing diagnosis includes behaviors with the most relevant influencing stimuli (Roy, 2009, p. 68).

Goal Setting

Goal setting entails the establishment of clear statements vis-à-vis the outcomes of nursing care, as well as the time frame for the expected attainment of the goal. Goal setting is established following the nurse's assessment. The statement of a goal helps it to materialize and ensures that the behavior of the person or the group becomes the focus.

Nursing Intervention

The nursing intervention step requires that the nurse work with the person or group to choose nursing interventions that promote the adaptation process. After the selection of nursing-appropriate interventions, nurses develop an approach to initiate the steps needed to change the focal stimuli and enhance coping abilities.

Evaluation

Evaluation is the last step of the nursing process; it involves an assessment of the effectiveness of the nursing intervention based on the previously established goals. This step could be the last one in the process, but it might also serve as a change agent to begin a new intervention if the previous goal was not achieved.

The most valuable feature of this process is the collaboration between the person or group and the nurse in every step of the nursing process. Under the auspices of the Roy adaptation model, the effectiveness of the intervention depends on the nurse's knowledge of the situation and the way in which the nurse obtains collaboration from the person or persons involved.

Application of the Model to Education, Research, and Practice

The use of the Roy adaptation model for nursing education is well documented. This model is used not only in the United States, but also in Asia, Europe, South America, Central America, and Mexico. One of the benefits of using the Roy adaptation model in education is that it provides students with a solid structure for thinking in a holistic manner and developing critical thinking skills. Indeed, the benefit of using this model as a framework for nursing practice has been demonstrated throughout the world, although the level of integration of the model into practice varies among hospitals and countries. Roy's model generally is found to be useful in focusing, organizing, and directing nurses' thoughts and actions regarding client care, resulting in a perception that the quality of nursing and client outcomes are improved. An example is easing the patient into a state of adaptability to care. The nursing role in this adaptation process is pivotal in maintaining adaptive responses and converting ineffective responses to adaptive ones to achieve health.

Research indicates that the Roy adaptation model is a conceptual model of nursing being used in nursing practice in the United States, Japan, Brazil, Colombia, Mexico, Panama, and Peru. Collectively, the studies in these countries demonstrate that using the model leads to better adaptability to care by patients and improved healthcare outcomes (Moreno & Alvarado, 2009).

Literature has shown that the Roy adaptation model is most useful as a tool when used in nursing research. Numerous quantitative and qualitative research studies have been conducted using Roy's model as a conceptual framework, and several research instruments have been derived from it (Fawcett, 2005). Many middle-range theories have been created and derived from Roy's conceptual system. A review of the literature revealed that the model has been used in descriptive studies of personal responses to environmental stimuli and correlations between the modes, manifestations of the stimuli, and effects of nursing interventions that are linked to propositions of the model.

THE KING CONCEPTUAL SYSTEM AND THEORY OF GOAL ATTAINMENT

The History

Imogene King was the first nurse theorist to develop a nursing framework and a middle-range theory related to it (Sieloff & Frey, 2007). Born in 1923, King graduated with a diploma in nursing from St. John's Hospital in St. Louis, Missouri, in 1945, a bachelor's degree in nursing education from St. Louis University in 1948, a master's degree in nursing from St. Louis University in 1957, and a doctorate of education from Teachers College, Columbia University, in New York City in 1961. Two decades later, in 1980, she was conferred an honorary doctorate from Southern Illinois University. King began her academic career at St. Louis University, then taught at Loyola University in Chicago, and ultimately moved to the University of South Florida, where, after a distinguished career, she became professor emeritus. In 1964, King was one of the pioneers who urged nursing professionals to focus on the organization of nursing knowledge, arguing that a theoretical body of knowledge was necessary for the advancement of nursing.

In her 1968 article titled "A Conceptual Frame of Reference for Nursing," King presented the concepts of social systems, health, interpersonal relationships, and perceptions as being universal to the discipline of nursing (King, 1968, 1995). In 1971, in her book *Toward a Theory for Nursing*, she began to refine the *conceptual system*. She further refined the conceptual system when she introduced the theory of goal attainment as part of her model in *A Theory for Nursing: Systems, Concepts, Process* (1981a). It is in this book that she presented the concepts of environment and person, suggested that fewer dichotomies exist between health and illness, changed the terminology in her theory from "adaptation" to "adjustment," and distinguished a person as a human being or individual rather than as "man."

The Philosophy

King's philosophical worldview is a systems and interactional approach, as evidenced by her admonition that her framework should be read "from the perspective of General System Theory and a science of wholeness" (King, 1990, p. 74). King validated her philosophy as driven by Greek philosophy and grounded in the Aristotelian–Thomistic perspective, which includes that of individuals striving for the end goal of happiness and flourishing. Persons must be motivated and guided to understand the necessity of using new and consistent behaviors to facilitate the process of goal attainment.

The Models

The Conceptual System

The core of King's conceptual system is the notion that human beings are open systems interacting constantly with the environment (King, 1989). King's conceptual model incorporates three interacting systems: *personal*, *interpersonal*, and *social*. She discovered these three systems when she began categorizing health issues by way of a systems approach, which was shaped by von Bertalanffy's (1968) general systems theory and interaction theory.

King's (1989) model reflects the metaparadigm concepts of person, environment, health, and nursing as systems. The concept of person is represented by the three systems (personal system, interpersonal system, and social system); a set of concepts for each system provides a method for nurses to organize their knowledge, skills, and values. Client goals are met through the transaction between the nurse and client. This interaction, which occurs over time, constitutes a transaction, such that eventually the person's goal is met (King, 1997, 2001).

Personal System

The hub of the personal system is the individual (person), whether healthy or ill, who gathers and uses information to assist him or her in understanding another individual or group (King, 1975, 1995). The composition of the seven concepts—perception, self, growth and development, body image, time, personal space, and learning—form the whole, complex personal system. Human beings are open systems responding to and coping with stimuli on the basis of their expectations, other people, events, and objects. The personal system is influenced by variables—namely, age, habits, situations, place in the family, and roles—that lead to the performance of the function.

Interpersonal System

In King's (1981a) framework, interpersonal systems are groups (small or large) of people. Interpersonal systems enclose six concepts—communication, interaction, roles, stress, coping, and transaction—all of which transpire at some point during the nursing process. Perceptions shape the person-to-person and person-to-environment interactions, but communication is the mode through which individuals make transactions, such as setting goals, choosing the strategies for attaining the goals, and attempting to maintain their health.

Social System

The social system is an "organized boundary system of social roles, behaviors and practices developed to maintain values and the mechanisms to regulate the practices and rules" (King, 1981a, p. 115). The social system addresses the needs of individuals and of the subgroups that are formed by certain commonalities, such as age, patterns of behavior, roles, and status. The concepts that make up the social system include authority, decision making, organization, power, and status.

Other Concepts

Other concepts that King included in the conceptual system are authority, body image, communication, decision making, growth and development, interaction, organization, perception, power, role, self, space, status, time, and transaction. These complex concepts are interrelated in the interactions of human beings with their environment. The metaparadigm concepts used by King are environment, health, nursing, and person. (Refer to the personal system for an explanation of person.)

According to King (1981a), the environment is holistic and transformative because individuals continually adjust their internal environment to transform energy in order to adjust to the continuous changes of the external environment. Although King did not explicitly define *internal environment* and *external environment*, she recognized the environment as functioning to bring harmony to the internal and external interactions.

King's (1981a) view of health is "a process of human growth and development and relates to the way individuals deal with stress of growth and development while functioning within the cultural pattern in which they were born and to which they attempt to conform" (p. 4). With this thought in mind, individuals undergo constant dynamic change in their state of health; they require continuous adjustment to stress to achieve physiological stability. King (1981a) did not identify health and illness on a linear continuum because she chose not to address certain abstract, and required, concepts, particularly wellness; rather, King saw illness as an imbalance in the person's physiological or psychological makeup, constituting a disturbance in the dynamic state of the person.

The focus of nursing is the human being and human acts. Nursing is an observable behavior found in a society's many healthcare systems. It is a process of action, reaction, and interaction, whereby a nurse and client share information about their perceptions in the nursing situation (King, 1995). King (1971, 1991) based her framework on the assumption that nursing's focus is on interactions between individuals and their environment to promote, maintain, and restore their health. The nurse–client transactions, which are different in each situation, comprise a sequence of behaviors that establish expectations, mutual goals, and interdependent roles. Each nursing action and its effectiveness vary with each transaction, depending on the extent to which goals are realistic and nursing judgments are valid.

According to Sieloff and Frey (2007), the following propositions were included in early publications by King (1981a):

- The nursing process is conducted within a social system that includes five dimensions: (1) the nursing process, (2) the individuals involved in the nursing process, (3) the individuals involved in the environment within which the nursing process is activated, (4) the social organization within which the nursing process is activated, and (5) the community within which the social organization functions.
- The nursing process will differ, depending on the individual nurse and each recipient of nursing services.
- The nursing process will differ relative to all individuals in the environment.
- The nursing process will differ relative to the social organization in which the nursing process takes place.
- The relationship among the dimensions affects the nursing process.
- Nursing includes specific components: (1) nursing judgment, (2) nursing action, (3) communication, (4) evaluation, and (5) coordination.
- The nursing judgment will vary relative to each nursing action.
- The effectiveness of nursing action will vary in the extent to which it is communicated to those responsible for its implementation.
- Nursing action is more effective if the goals are communicated and standards of nursing performance have been established.

- Nursing action is based on facts, which may change; thus nursing judgments and actions are evaluated and revised as the situation changes.
- Nursing is a component of health care; thus, health care is affected by the coordination of nursing with health services. (pp. 401–402)

Theory of Goal Attainment

King's theory of goal attainment, which was derived from her conceptual framework, focuses on holism and includes nursing as a process that is interactional in nature. These interactions lead to the critical transactions that result in goal attainment (King, 1992; Sieloff Evans, 1991). Emphasis is placed on interpersonal systems and the phenomena of process and outcomes (goals). These goals become criteria for measuring the effectiveness of nursing care.

Assumptions

King's theory of goal attainment is based on the following assumptions:

- Individuals are social beings.
- Individuals are sentient beings.
- Individuals are rational beings.
- Individuals are reacting beings.
- Individuals are perceiving beings.
- Individuals are controlling beings.
- Individuals are purposeful beings.
- Individuals are action-oriented beings.
- Individuals are time-oriented beings.
- Perceptions of nurse and of client influence the interaction process.
- Goals, needs, and values of nurse and client influence the interaction process.
- Individuals have a right to knowledge about themselves.
- Individuals have a right to participate in decisions that influence their life, their health, and community services.
- Health professionals have a responsibility to share information that helps individuals make informed decisions about their health care.
- Individuals have a right to accept or reject health care.
- Goals of health professionals and goals of recipients of health care may be incongruent. (King, 1981b, pp. 143–144)

The major concepts of goal attainment include communication, growth and development, interaction, perception, role, space, stress, time, and transaction (King, 1981b). Decision making is a shared collaborative process where the nurse and client share information for the purpose of setting and attaining goals.

Propositions

According to King (1981b), the major concepts mentioned in the last section are embedded in the following propositions of the theory of goal attainment:

1. If perceptual accuracy is present in the nurse–client interaction, transaction will occur.
2. If the nurse and the client make transactions, goals will be attained.
3. If goals are attained, satisfaction will occur.
4. If goals are attained, effective nursing care will occur.
5. If transactions are made in the nurse–client interaction, growth and development will be enhanced.
6. If role expectations and role performance as perceived by the nurse and the client are congruent, transaction will occur.
7. If role conflict is experienced by the nurse, the client, or both, stress in nurse–client interactions will occur.
8. If nurses with special knowledge and skills communicate appropriate information to clients, mutual goal setting and goal attainment will occur.

Hypothesis

King (1981b) developed the following hypothesis from the theory of goal attainment:

1. Perceptual accuracy in nurse–client interactions increases mutual goal setting.
2. Communication increases mutual goal setting between nurses and clients and leads to satisfaction.
3. Satisfaction in nurses and clients increases the likelihood of goal attainment.
4. Goal attainment decreases stress and anxiety in nursing situations.
5. Goal attainment increases client learning and coping ability in nursing situations.
6. Role conflict experienced by clients, nurses, or both decreases transactions in nurse–client interactions.
7. Congruence in role expectations and role performance increases transactions in nurse–client interactions. (p. 156)

Nursing Application of King's Conceptual System and Theory of Goal Attainment

King's conceptual framework, both the conceptual system and the theory of goal attainment, are applicable to nursing practice, education, research, and administration. The discipline of nursing and nursing knowledge continue to be advanced by King's work on the nursing process, systems, and goal attainment. Many researchers and theorists have accelerated the progress made on King's work.

Fawcett (2005) emphasized that conceptual models, such as King's conceptual system, or grand theories, can serve as an overarching frame of reference for nursing and the phenomena of interest in nursing practice, but they cannot be applied directly to practice. Instead, middle-range theories must serve as theories for direct practice applicability, and the concepts within the middle-range theories must be consistent with the nurse's (or institution's) adopted conceptual model. Many nurses have aligned their frame of reference with King's systems framework in their practice, education, or administration.

King formulated her middle-range theory of goal attainment from her conceptual system. The theory of goal attainment provides a meaningful application for nurses. Nurses have long been interacting with clients and making goal-setting transactions with patients. Although the social systems concept was not a definite system in her theory of goal attainment, as it was in her conceptual system, the other two systems—personal and interpersonal—were clearly linked.

THE NEUMAN SYSTEMS MODEL

Betty Neuman described the Neuman systems model as "a unique systems-based perspective that provides a unifying focus for approaching a wide range of nursing concerns" (Neuman, 2002a, p. 3). This model is a comprehensive guide for nursing practice, research, education, and administration and has the potential for unifying health-related theories through the examination of the relationships between nursing intervention and patient response to stressors. The wellness, multidimensionality, and wholistic systemic perspective of the Neuman systems model has demonstrated its relevance and reliability in various clinical and educational settings in the United States and abroad (Neuman, 2002a).

The Evolution of the Neuman Systems Model

Neuman was born in 1924 in Lowell, Ohio. In 1947, she received a registered nurse diploma from People's Hospital School of Nursing in Akron, Ohio. She later moved to California, where she gained experience as a hospital staff nurse, school nurse, industrial nurse, and clinical instructor in medical–surgical, critical care, and communicable disease nursing. In 1957, Neuman received a bachelor's degree from the University of California at Los Angeles (UCLA) with a double major in psychology and public health. In 1966, she received a master's degree in nursing from UCLA; she received a doctor of philosophy degree in clinical psychology from Pacific Western University in 1985.

Neuman was a pioneer in the community mental health movement in the late 1960s. In mid-1970, she introduced the Neuman systems model for nursing education and practice. A refinement of the model was published in the first edition of Riehl and Roy's 1974 book,

Conceptual Models for Nursing Practice. Further refinements were presented in 1982 in the first edition of Neuman's own book, titled *The Neuman Systems Model: Application to Nursing Education and Practice* (Neuman, 1982).

Neuman's conceptual model has undergone many changes since its inception in 1970. Today the Neuman systems model provides nursing with a comprehensive, flexible, wholistic, and systems-based guide that focuses (1) on the response of the client systems to actual or potential environmental stressors and (2) on the use of primary, secondary, and tertiary nursing prevention interventions for retention, attainment, and maintenance of optimal client wellness (Neuman, 1996).

The Philosophy

Neuman's philosophy is based on wholism, reality, and wellness, along with her assumptions about interactions of four metaparadigm concepts—person, environment, health, and nursing. She derived the term *wholism* from the holistic systems concept introduced by de Chardin (1955), a Catholic priest, scientist, and philosopher who believed in the wholeness of life as being the interconnectedness of the human spirit and mind. Neuman (1996) recognized her systems model as a wholistic conceptual framework for guiding nursing interactions with clients. A focal point in the Neuman model is nurses' insight and involvement in the response of the client system to actual or potential environmental stressors.

Neuman's notion about *reality* mirrors gestalt theory in three ways:

1. Emphasis on the perceived
2. Awareness of *what is* and not *what should be*
3. Completely understanding the patterns and structures in unity, or the whole situation in a perceptual field

Encasing the client system is a perceptual field in dynamic equilibrium, where all parts or variables work together as a whole. Reality is based on the client's perspective. Neuman (2002a) described the wholeness of the perceptual field as "the total organization of the field" (p. 12), or nurses "taking into consideration the simultaneous effects of the interacting variables—physiological, psychological, sociocultural, developmental, and spiritual" (p. 13).

Neuman (1995) classified her systems model as a wellness model—that is, as a model of retaining wellness and ensuring optimal wellness attainment. *Wellness* is generally described by degrees. From Neuman's (1995) perspective, optimal wellness "represents the greatest possible degree of system stability at a given point in time" (p. 25). Clients perceive their own degree of wellness and health, but the definition of health encompasses a broader perspective than just each client's perception of health. According to Neuman, wellness needs to be defined and negotiated between the client and the nurse because of the interrelationship between the systems energy, the environment, and the nurse's perception of the client's health.

The Model

The metaparadigm concepts within the Neuman systems model are human beings, environment, health, and nursing. This systems-based model includes two major components: stress and systematic feedback loops (Neuman, 1995). The client is considered an open system in which continual cycles of input, process, output, and feedback make up an active organizational pattern. The client is simultaneously an individual as well as part of a group, a family, or a community. Neuman considered all variables affecting a client's response to environmental stressors and explains that knowing something about one part of a system enables us to know something about another part. As systems become more complex, the internal conditions of regulation become more intricate. Even so, the nursing goal is to obtain wellness through retention and attainment of client system stability. Neuman (2002a) also stated that the interaction with the environment is mutual—meaning that the client and the environment could each have a positive or negative effect on the other.

The Neuman systems model reflects a wholistic orientation to wellness (Neuman, 1995). It is similar to gestalt theory in stating that each system is surrounded by a perceptual field that is in dynamic equilibrium (Edelson, 1970). The Neuman model also reflects Lazarus's (1999) and Selye's (1946) theories of stress, and Caplan's (1964) conceptual model of levels of prevention (Harris, Hermiz, Meininger, & Steinkeler, 1994). Moreover, Neuman suggested that in understanding the systems model from a wholistic point of view, we must consider five variables of the person: (1) physiological, (2) psychological, (3) sociocultural, (4) developmental, and (5) spiritual. Particular awareness of these variables must be exercised, though they are connected only with reference to the whole (Neuman, 2002a). In effect, the system has a core structure comprising basic survival factors that are common to species (George, 1996)—namely, system variables, genetic features, and the strengths and weaknesses of the system parts. Examples in the healthcare setting include hair, body temperature regulation ability, the homeostatic functioning of body systems, cognitive ability, physical strength, and factors that are encircled by concentric rings of barriers (the flexible line of defense, the normal line of defense, and the lines of resistance), which act as boundaries to provide protection to the system (Fawcett, 2005; Neuman, 2002a).

Structure of the Model

The Neuman systems model is an open systems model that provides nursing with a unifying focus (Neuman, 2002a). The client system expands the perspective of nursing by taking into account all variables that will affect a client's response to stressors. In doing so, it explains how stability is obtained in relation to the stressors imposed on the client by the environment (Fawcett, 2005).

The basic structure is related to system variables, as well as to unique person variables. The model adopts a wholistic approach that views the client as an open system, the environment as both internal and external, and the interplay of human and environment as a process of interaction of matter and energy (Harris et al., 1994).

In Neuman's model, the total system interacts with the environment. The system relating to the client is affected by five variables—that is, five characteristics of the person (Harris et al., 1994). The basic structure is a combination of all the variables applicable to human survival and those variables unique to each individual. Homeostasis occurs when available energy exceeds the amount being used by the system. In this interaction process, matter, energy, and information are exchanged by a system and its environment through feedback from the process of intake and output. The goal is an equalization of energy gain and loss at a desired level to produce homeostasis. The variables reside within the basic structure because they are part of the flexible line of defense (Neuman, 2002a).

The Flexible Line of Defense

The *flexible line of defense* forms the outer barrier to (or, put another way, cushions) the normal line of defense of the client system. This mechanism serves as a protective buffer system for the client's normal or stable state. The flexible line of defense is dynamic and can be altered in a relatively short period of time. If all possible defenses prevent the invasion of the stressors and keep the system free of symptomatology, then this line of defense acts like an accordion—expanding away from the normal line of defense and providing protection as it draws closer. When flexible lines of defense fail, the normal line of defense is activated (Neuman, 2002b).

The Normal Line of Defense

The *normal line of defense* denotes what the client has overcome because it acts as a protective buffer system for the client's stable state. The normal line of defense is used also as a baseline from which to measure health deviation (Neuman, 2002b). Each line of defense is made up of similar protective elements related to the five variables; in other words, it keeps the system free from stressor reactions. The function of the normal line of defense is dynamic, rather than stable, and can be changed over a short period of time (Neuman, 2002b). Its expansion reflects an enhanced wellness state (Fawcett, 2005). When the flexible line of defense is no longer capable of protecting the client or fails to provide protection to the normal line of defense, however, the lines of resistance become activated.

The normal line of defense represents system stability over time; it is the solid boundary line that encircles the broken internal lines of resistance. Because it represents what each client has become over time, this line of defense can be used as a standard against which to measure wellness level or health deviation. The interrelationships of the five client systems variables with environmental stressors help to determine the extent to which a client is stable (Neuman, 2002a).

Lines of Resistance

The *lines of resistance* serve as a protective mechanism whose function is to stabilize the client system and return it to the normal wellness level (Neuman, 2002b). Graphically, these lines of resistance may be depicted as a series of concentric broken circles surrounding and protecting the basic structure. They become activated when environmental stressors invade the normal line of defense—for example, as in the activation of the platelets in response to a laceration. If the lines of resistance are effective, the system can reconstitute its defenses; if the lines of resistance are not effective, the resulting energy depletion can result in death.

Stressors

Stressors are forces that disrupt and can operate within the system (Neuman, 2002b). They comprise environmental tension forces that cause system instability; these forces can each have a positive or negative effect on the system. The outcome of the effect depends on the system perception and ability to negotiate its effect. According to gestalt theory, stressors influence the reaction to all other stressors (Lazarus, 1999).

Stressors include three dimensions:

1. *Intrapersonal:* occur within the person or family relationships (e.g., emotions)
2. *Interpersonal:* occur between individuals or between the individual and the community (e.g., role expectations or family relationships)
3. *Extrapersonal:* occur outside the individual, such as community groups (e.g., healthcare policies)

The reaction of the client to any stressor will influence the treatment of the symptoms. The nurse can predict the client's adjustment on the basis of past coping behavior, which in turn depends on the strength of the lines of resistance and defense. The nurse may also attempt to restore stability to the system by means of primary, secondary, and tertiary interventions. According to Lazarus (1999), cognitive appraisal determines the degree of stress felt, whereas coping functions mediate the reaction.

Prevention as Intervention

According to Neuman, the point of entry to the healthcare system is the *primary prevention* level. Before a reaction occurs, it strengthens the clients and helps them to deal with stressors; at the same time, it influences the environment to reduce the stressors. It strengthens the flexible lines of defense through health promotion and maintenance of wellness (Neuman, 2002b). For example, doing exercise every day for 30 to 40 minutes benefits all body systems; teaching people to wash their hands before eating helps to prevent *E. coli* infection. In a community setting such as a daycare center for elderly people, the primary prevention could be a vaccination journey against pneumococcal and influenza infection.

Secondary prevention occurs after the client has reacted to a stressor. The goal of secondary prevention is not only to identify the stress point of entry, but also to protect the basic core structures. This level of prevention focuses on the types of interventions that could be used alone or simultaneously to prevent damage to the central core by strengthening the internal lines of resistance and/or removing the stressor. The notion of secondary prevention as intervention is related to the treatment of symptoms that follows the reaction of the stressors (Neuman, 2002a). Examples of secondary interventions include the treatment of pressure ulcers in a bedridden patient and the nursing care that a community needs after an earthquake.

Tertiary prevention follows after the system has been treated through secondary prevention. This level supports the client by adding or reducing energy so that the system can be reconstituted (Neuman, 2002a). An example of a tertiary prevention is the nursing care provided for a person who recently had a car accident and had a leg amputated. In this situation, the nurse is prompted to focus on the patient's actual symptoms, and later, to plan for the patient's achievement of long-term goals aimed at prevention of secondary complications.

Neuman's Perception of Nursing

The Neuman systems model nursing process was designed specifically for the implementation of the model and has been developed to address three issues in this regard:

1. *Nursing diagnosis:* obtained through assessment and consideration of the five variables in three stressor areas
2. *Nursing goals:* negotiated with the client and taking into account both the client's and the nurse's perceptions
3. *Nursing outcomes:* considered in relation to five variables and achieved through primary, secondary, and tertiary interventions

According to Neuman, the major concern of nursing is to obtain significant and comprehensive client data in order to make a comprehensive objective diagnosis (Fawcett, 2005). The data synthesized in this way provide a rationale for future nursing action. A unique feature of the Neuman systems model nursing process is the determination of the perceptions held by the client and the nurse.

Neuman (1995) perceived health as energy that produces the finest system stability at any point in time. Thus health is a continuum with a wellness condition, marked by the highest available energy, at one extreme and death, which signifies total energy absence, at the other extreme. In using this model, the nurse focuses his or her practice on promoting system stability through attainment, retention, and maintenance of optimal wellness and wholeness. The concept of prevention as intervention facilitates the use of the nursing process in persons as individuals or groups with the goal of achieving client system stability and maintaining protective barriers. With primary prevention as intervention, nursing knowledge is applied to assessment and nursing intervention for the purposes of identification and reduction of risk factors associated with environmental stressors to prevent reaction. Primary prevention encompasses the goal of health. Secondary prevention involves treatment actions based on client symptomatology after system reaction. The goal in this circumstance is to provide correct treatment to obtain optimal client system stability. Secondary prevention is provided when primary prevention is not effective. Tertiary prevention involves actions that promote wellness after treatment. According to Neuman (2002b), if nurses are to keep a system stable, they must create a connection between the client, the environment, health, and nursing.

In the first step of the nursing process, the nurse acquires significant and comprehensive data related to the impact of the environmental stressors. Analysis of these data provides the rationale for nursing action (Neuman, 2002c). The nursing diagnostic statement should reflect the entire client condition.

Outcome Identification and Planning

Outcome identification and planning involve negotiation between the caregiver and the client or recipient of care. The overall goal of the caregiver is to guide the client to conserve energy and to use energy as a force to move beyond the present (Neuman, 2002c).

Nursing Goals

Neuman's goals for nursing are based on the synthesis of a comprehensive database about the client and the theory appropriate to the client's and the caregiver's perceptions and possibilities for functional competence in the environment. A unique feature of Neuman's systems model is the mutual determination of any interventions in order to formulate goals. During this step, the evaluation confirms that the anticipated or prescribed change has (or has not) occurred. Immediate- and long-range goals are structured in relation to the short-term goals (Neuman, 2002c).

Evaluation

Neuman's evaluation component in the nursing process involves evaluating outcomes. Nurses evaluate the effectiveness of their interventions on the basis of the degree to which clients met their goals. With evaluation, nurses determine the client's status in the health–illness continuum so that changes can be made as needed in the planning and implementation of care (Neuman, 2002c).

Education

Neuman compels students to use logic, deduction, and induction in developing their nursing care plans. Most importantly, the model reveals to students that client perceptions are an integral part of the nursing process and should be included in the data collection and client outcome development steps (Neuman, 1995).

Newman, Neuman, and Fawcett (2002) offered some valuable guidelines for education:

- The curriculum focuses on the client system's reaction to environmental stressors.
- The curriculum content encompasses all of the concepts in the model.
- Education can occur in educational and technical programs.
- Students must critically think.
- Teaching–learning strategies must foster critical thinking and independent learning.

Practice

The Neuman systems model provides APNs and other nurses with a different frame of reference for addressing health conditions within distinctive settings. In the literature describing the use of the Neuman systems model in practice, the reader can appreciate how the model guides wholistic approaches to client care. International research, for example, has revealed broad use of this model (Engberg, 1995; Vaughan & Gough, 1995). The Neuman systems model also supports the use of clinical tools that are practical and that guide wholistic assessment and prevention for individuals, families, communities, and organizations; these tools help to guide the practitioner's clinical practice.

The model has been used in several areas of practice. In the United States, the model has made a significant contribution in a neglected area of health care: postpartum mood disorders (PPMDs). Kendall-Tackett (1993) contributed significantly to the prevention of health problems in young childbearing families by describing primary, secondary, and tertiary interventions for PPMDs.

The following guidelines are delineated for practice (Freese, Neuman, & Fawcett, 2002):

- The purpose is to assist clients to retain, attain, or maintain optimal system stability.
- Practice problems include actual or potential reactions to stressors.
- Practice takes place in any healthcare setting.
- The participants are persons, families, and communities who are faced with stressors.
- The practice process of the model consists of three components: diagnosis, goals, and outcomes.

Along with these guidelines, other precepts exist for administration of healthcare systems (Shambaugh, Neuman, & Fawcett, 2002):

- The focus is the client system.
- The purpose is to facilitate the delivery of the primary, secondary, and tertiary prevention interventions directed toward maintaining optimal stability.
- Administrators and healthcare personnel must have knowledge of the content of the Neuman systems model to facilitate its implementation.
- Healthcare services are located in appropriate settings where primary, secondary, and tertiary prevention can be delivered.
- The management strategies focus on achieving optimal client stability.

Research

The Neuman systems model has been the basis for a wide range of studies, from descriptions of the Neuman phenomena to experiments testing the effects of prevention intervention on multiple system outcomes (Fawcett, 2002). The following guidelines for research, which were based on the Neuman systems model, were extrapolated by Louis, Neuman, and Fawcett (2002) from several studies.

- The purpose of the model is to predict the effects of primary, secondary, and tertiary prevention interventions on retention, attainment, and maintenance of client stability, and to determine the cost–benefit trade-off and utility of prevention interventions.
- The phenomena of interest include physiological, psychological, sociocultural, developmental, and spiritual variables.
- The problems to be studied deal with the impact of stressors on the client's stability.
- The research methods include inductive and deductive research using quantitative and qualitative research.
- Study participants may include clients, families, groups, and communities.
- The model-based research contributes to the understanding of the influence of prevention on the relationship between stressors and client stability.

Contributions to Nursing

According to Fawcett, the primary contribution of the Neuman systems model has been pragmatic, in that the model can be used as a guide for nursing education and practice, it can be translated to other cultures, and it has the potential to facilitate resolution of universal nursing concerns (Fawcett, 2005). The Neuman systems model portrays the interest of the profession in seeing people as a wholistic system. This comprehensive system guides nursing practice, research, education, and administration; it helps nurses to organize their practice within a broad perspective. Neuman places substantial emphasis on wellness and the central role that clients play in setting goals and identifying prevention interventions. Her model also has the potential to unify other health professions through the clarification of the commonalities that exist in different disciplines.

A nursing process format and an assessment intervention tool are available that were designed to facilitate implementation of the Neuman systems model. The Neuman systems model is a good fit for approaches that emphasize the interrelationships among the body, mind, and spirit of the client in a constantly changing environment and society.

ANALYSIS OF THE MODELS

In their models, Roy, King, and Neuman depicted nursing logically as a science, yet in their explanation of the connections between mind and intuition, they described nursing as an art. According to Fawcett (2005), these theorists and their models brought to light the diverse factors that constitute professional nursing. Nurses and nursing scholars began to see the profession's complexities that arose from the quick expansion of nursing knowledge development during this time period.

In 1964, King published discussions of nursing as a science rather than an occupation; she initiated the discourse about theory development related to nursing. During the early 1970s, Neuman's systems model was introduced for nursing education and practice; at approximately the same time, Roy developed her adaptation model for nursing education, nursing administration, and nursing research.

Conceptual models (or grand theories), according to Fawcett (2005), provide an overarching model for clinical practice, education, administration, methodology, and discipline inquiry, but they cannot be applied directly to practice. Instead, middle-range theories must serve as theories for direct practice applicability, and the concepts within the middle-range theories must be consistent with the nurse's (or institution's) adopted conceptual model.

These three theorists—Roy, King, and Neuman—all integrated their systems' concepts with nursing phenomena, thereby clarifying and defining nursing knowledge in relation to the science. Organized in a unique manner, the models focus on a solution for the complex needs of the client. Adopting a conceptual model brings a certain reality and arrangement of the concepts to advanced practice. In this reality, APNs then process, integrate, and synthesize information through the cognitive, psychomotor, and affective domains to shape their clinical practice. Characteristics of the three models are summarized here:

1. The models represent the evolution of nursing as a profession (Silva & Rothbart, 1983), starting from the development of nursing knowledge based on the observation of human experience as it relates to the maintenance of health, to using the nursing process, which remains congruent with social expectations regarding nursing practice. The value of the models is not just that they promote the exploration of the effectiveness of new nursing interventions, theory testing, and development, but that they provoke

deeper questions about how nurses can contribute to the well-being of humanity as a whole (Roy, 2009).
2. The models provide structure, process, function, resources, and goals for nursing as a discipline and a profession, leading to creative approaches for human care by defining the person, the environment, and health (Fawcett, 2005). These nursing models provide nurses with a framework for describing human phenomena and the tools needed to predict and control clinical outcomes in order to achieve better health outcomes for clients.
3. The models were derived from research, serve as the basis for researching phenomena that affect client stability, and serve as a basis for the development of new nursing strategies that will influence client recuperation and well-being (Fawcett, 2005).
4. These models provide a certain reality or conceptual arrangement to the phenomena of interest and the concepts involved. As APNs begin to understand and explain concepts and potential relationships within their chosen conceptual model, they can create and refine nursing interventions designed to diminish stress and enhance life patterns.

SUMMARY

This chapter was a review of three conceptual models and one middle-range theory based on a systems approach—the Roy adaptation model, King's conceptual system, King's theory of goal attainment, and the Neuman systems model. The models are useful for viewing nursing from different perspectives, such as health promotion, primary prevention, secondary prevention, and tertiary prevention. Roy's model is focused on adaptation and coping. King provided a conceptual system of interactions and transactions between nurses and clients within three systems—personal, interpersonal, and group. King's theory of goal attainment—namely an emphasis on mutual goal setting between the nurse and the client—was derived from her conceptual system. Neuman's model is focused on the wellness of the client in terms of environmental stressors and the client's reactions to those stressors. The three models are conceptual models, as defined by Fawcett (2005), and they provide nurses with a purposive reality and conceptual arrangement for nursing.

DISCUSSION QUESTIONS

1. Explore one research instrument or questionnaire that you could use to measure King's concept of goal setting from her theory of goal attainment.
2. What are the common propositions of each of the three conceptual models? How do they differ from one another?
3. Choose one of the three conceptual models described in this chapter. Search databases to find at least one middle-range theory (except King's theory of goal attainment) that was derived from the chosen model. Explain how the concepts of the conceptual model and the middle-range theory are consistent and are linked.

REFERENCES

Alligood, M. (2002). Practice made perfect: Higher level aspirations for practice nurses. *Journal of Advanced Nursing, 40*(1), 122.

Boulding, K. E. (1956). General systems theory: The skeleton of science. *Management Science, 2*(3), 197–208.

Caplan, G. (1964). *Principles of prevention psychiatry.* Oxford, England: Basic Books.

de Chardin, P. T. (1955). *The phenomenon of man.* London, UK: Collins.

Edelson, M. (1970). *Sociotherapy and psychotherapy.* Chicago, IL: University of Chicago Press.

Engberg, I. B. (1995). Brief abstracts: Use of the Neuman systems model in Sweden. In B. Neuman (Ed.), *The Neuman systems model* (3rd ed., pp. 653–656). Norwalk, CT: Appleton & Lange.

Fawcett, J. (2002). *Analysis and evaluation of contemporary nursing knowledge, nursing models and theories.* Philadelphia, PA: F. A. Davis.

Fawcett, J. (2005). *Contemporary nursing knowledge: Analysis and evaluation of nursing models and theories* (2nd ed.). Philadelphia, PA: F. A. Davis.

Fawcett, J. (2009). *Analysis and evaluation of conceptual models of nursing.* Philadelphia, PA: F. A. Davis.

Freese, B. T., Neuman, B., & Fawcett, J. (2002). Guidelines for Neuman systems model-based clinical practice. In B. Neuman & J. Fawcett (Eds.), *The Neuman systems model* (4th ed., pp. 37–42). Upper Saddle River, NJ: Prentice Hall.

George, G. B. (1996). Betty Neuman. In J. B. George (Ed.), *Nursing theories: The base for professional nursing practice* (4th ed., pp. 252–279). Norwalk, CT: Appleton & Lange.

Harris, S. M., Hermiz, M. E., Meininger, M., & Steinkeler, S. E. (1994). Betty Neuman: Systems model. In A. Marriner-Tomey (Ed.). *Nursing theorists and their work* (3rd ed.). St. Louis, MO: Mosby.

Helson, H. (1964). *Adaptation level theory.* New York, NY: Harper & Row.

Kendall-Tackett, K. (1993). *Post-partum depression: A comprehensive approach for nurses.* Newbury Park, CA: Sage.

King, I. M. (1964). Nursing theory: Problems and prospect. *Nursing Science, 2,* 394–403.

King, I. M. (1968). A conceptual frame of reference for nursing. *Nursing Research, 17,* 27–31.

King, I. M. (1971). *Toward a theory for nursing: General concepts of human behavior.* New York, NY: Wiley.

King, I. M. (1975). A conceptual frame of reference for nursing. *Nursing Research, 17,* 27–31.

King, I. M. (1981a). *A theory for nursing: Systems, concepts, process.* New York, NY: Wiley.

King, I. M. (1981b). *A theory of goal attainment: General concepts of human behavior.* New York, NY: Wiley.

King, I. M. (1989). King's general systems framework and theory. In J. P. Riehl-Sisca (Ed.), *Conceptual models for nursing practice* (3rd ed., pp. 149–158). Norwalk, CT: Appleton & Lange.

King, I. M. (1990). Health as the goal for nursing. *Nursing Science Quarterly, 3,* 123–128.

King, I. M. (1991). Nursing theory 25 years later. *Nursing Science Quarterly, 4,* 94–95.

King, I. M. (1992). King's theory of goal attainment. *Nursing Science Quarterly, 5,* 19–26.

King, I. M. (1995). A systems framework for nursing. In M. A. Frey & C. L. Sieloff (Eds.), *Advancing King's systems framework and theory of nursing* (pp. 14–22). Thousand Oaks, CA: Sage.

King, I. M. (1997). King's theory of goal attainment. *Nursing Science Quarterly, 10,* 180–185.

King, I. M. (2001). Theory of goal attainment. In M. Parker (Ed.), *Nursing theories and nursing practice* (pp. 275–286). Philadelphia, PA: F. A. Davis.

King, I.M. (2007). King's structure, process, and outcome in the twenty-first century. In C. Sieloff & M.A. Frey (Eds.), *Middle range theory development using King's conceptual system*. New York, NY: Springer.

Lazarus, R. (1999). *Stress and emotion: A new synthesis*. New York, NY: Springer.

Louis, M., Neuman, B., & Fawcett, J. (2002). Guidelines for Neuman systems model-based nursing research. In B. Neuman and J. Fawcett (Eds.), *The Neuman systems model* (4th ed., pp. 113–149). Upper Saddle River, NJ: Prentice Hall.

Maritain, J. (1966). *The person and the common good* (J. J. Fitzgerald, Trans.). Notre Dame, IN: University of Notre Dame Press.

McNeill, D., & Freiberger, P. (1994). *Fuzzy logic: The revolutionary computer technology that is changing our world*. New York, NY: Simon & Schuster.

Moreno, M. E., & Alvarado, A. (2009). Aplicación del modelo de adaptación de Callista Roy en Latinoamérica. *Aquichan, 9*, 62–72.

Neuman, B. (1982). *The Neuman systems model: Application to nursing education and practice*. Norwalk, CT: Appleton-Century-Crofts.

Neuman, B. (1995). *The Neuman systems model* (3rd ed.). Norwalk, CT: Appleton & Lange.

Neuman, B. (1996). The Neuman systems model in research and practice. *Nursing Science Quarterly, 9*, 67–70.

Neuman, B. (2002a). The Neuman systems model. In B. Neuman & J. Fawcett (Eds.), *The Neuman systems model* (4th ed., pp. 3–33). Upper Saddle River, NJ: Prentice Hall.

Neuman, B. (2002b). The future and the Neuman systems model. In B. Neuman & J. Fawcett (Eds.), *The Neuman systems model* (4th ed., pp. 319–321). Upper Saddle River, NJ: Prentice Hall.

Neuman, B. (2002c). Assessment and intervention based on the Neuman systems model. In B. Neuman & J. Fawcett (Eds.), *The Neuman systems model* (4th ed., pp. 347–359). Upper Saddle River, NJ: Prentice Hall.

Newman, M., Neuman, B., & Fawcett, J. (2002). Guidelines for Neuman systems model-based education for the health professions. In *The Neuman systems model* (4th ed., pp. 191–215). Upper Saddle River, NJ: Prentice Hall.

Riehl, J. P., & Roy, C. (1974). *Conceptual models for nursing practice*, New York, NY: Appleton-Century-Crofts.

Roy, C. (1970). Adaptation: A conceptual framework for nursing. *Nursing Outlook, 18*(3), 18–23.

Roy, C. (1971). Adaptation: A basis for nursing practice. *Nursing Outlook, 19*(4), 254–257.

Roy, C. (1973). Adaptation: Implication for curriculum change. *Nursing Outlook, 21*(3), 163–168.

Roy, C. (1976). *Introduction to nursing: An adaptation model*. Englewood Cliffs, NJ: Prentice Hall.

Roy, C. (1984). *Introduction to nursing: An introduction model* (2nd ed.). Englewood Cliffs, NJ: Prentice Hall.

Roy, C. (1988). An explication of the philosophical assumptions of the adaptation model. *Nursing Science Quarterly, 1*(1), 26–34.

Roy, C. (1991). *An adaptation model*. Thousand Oaks, CA: Sage.

Roy, C. (1996). Domain primacy: Use of a theoretical framework to guide the selection of subject matter for theory development and methods of inquiry. In the University of Rhode Island College of Nursing Conference Proceedings, *Building a cumulative knowledge base from fragmentation to congruence of philosophy, theory, method of inquiry and practice* (pp. 69–75). Proceedings of the 4th and 5th Symposia of the Knowledge Development Series. Kingston, RI: University of Rhode Island College of Nursing.

Roy, C. (2006). *The Roy adaptation model: Relevance to theory-based education, practice, and research*. Conference presentation. Roy Adaptation Association. Los Angeles, CA.

Roy, C. (2009). *The Roy adaptation model* (3rd ed., pp. 2–54). Upper Saddle River, NJ: Pearson Education.

Roy, C., & Andrews, H. A. (1999). *The adaptation model* (2nd ed.). Norwalk, CT: Appleton & Lange.

Selye, H. (1946). The general adaptation syndrome. *Journal of Clinical Endocrinology, 6*(2), 117–230.

Shambaugh, B. F., Neuman, B., & Fawcett, J. (2002). Guidelines for Neuman systems model-based administration of health care services. In *The Neuman systems model* (4th ed., pp. 265–270). Upper Saddle River, NJ: Prentice Hall.

Sieloff Evans, C. (1991). *Imogene King: A conceptual framework for nursing*. Newbury Park, CA: Sage.

Silva, M., & Rothbart, D. (1983). *An analysis of changing trends in philosophies of science*. New York, NY: Wiley.

Vaughan, B., & Gough, P. (1995). Use of the Neuman systems model in England: Abstracts. In B. Neuman, *The Neuman systems model* (3rd ed., pp. 599–605). Norwalk, CT: Appleton & Lange.

von Bertalanffy, L. (1968). *General system theory*. New York, NY: George Braziller.

Chapter 20

Models and Theories Focused on Human Existence and Universal Energy

Violet M. Malinski

INTRODUCTION

Undoubtedly the nursing figure most associated with the focus on energy in nursing is Martha E. Rogers (1914–1994), who posited a radically different view of both the human being and the environment. Rogers is best remembered for having introduced a new worldview in nursing with her revolutionary, future-oriented, basic nursing science, known as the science of unitary human beings. Although Rogers made descriptions of this worldview available throughout the 1970s on class handouts, the first formal publications of this perspective did not appear until 1986 (Madrid & Winstead-Fry, 1986; Malinski, 1986). Rogers (1992) included the final version in her seminal article in *Nursing Science Quarterly*. Briefly, she described shifts from an older to a newer worldview in a variety of areas—for example, from cell theory to field theory, from homeostasis to homeodynamics, from three-dimensionality to pandimensionality, from an entropic to a negentropic universe, from causation and adaptation to mutual process, and from person and environment as separate to unitary.

Initially, Rogers was the only theorist whose work fit this new worldview in nursing, but she was soon joined by Margaret Newman, with her theory of health as expanding consciousness (HEC), and by Rosemarie Rizzo Parse, with her theory of humanbecoming. Both of the later theorists offer a view of human transformation and emphasize the centrality of the nurse–person relationship via true presence (for Parse) and transforming presence (for Newman). Elizabeth Barrett, following the Rogerian assumption that change is ongoing, diverse, creative, and unpredictable, derived her theory of power as knowing participation in change from Rogerian nursing science. All of these perspectives describe nursing as having roots outside of the biomedical model, offering an alternative vision of nursing knowledge, practice, and research.

ROGERS'S SCIENCE OF UNITARY HUMAN BEINGS

Rogers (1970, 1990, 1992) was an early advocate for nursing as both science and art, as well as a learned profession in need of an organized body of nursing-specific knowledge. Her view of humans as irreducible wholes integrated with their environments in "a pan-dimensional universe of open systems, points to a new paradigm, and initiates the identity of nursing as a science. The purpose of nurses is to promote health and well-being for all persons wherever they are. The art of nursing, then, is the creative use of the science of nursing for human betterment" (Rogers, 1992, p. 28). Rogers's science of unitary human beings encompasses four postulates, three principles, and a range of theories derived initially by Rogers herself and later by other Rogerian theorists.

The four postulates—energy fields, openness, pattern, and pandimensionality—together express reality as described in this nursing science. Change that is predictable, resulting from a cause–effect sequence, yields to change that is unpredictable, diverse, and innovative. Starting with the idea that the infinite, continuously flowing energy field is fundamental to all life means that humans and environments are irreducible, pandimensional energy fields, distinct but not separate, engaging in a continuous mutual process where change occurs simultaneously for both. In an open universe of energy fields, there are no divisions or boundaries; thus, energy flows continuously through human and environmental fields in an unbroken wave, characterized by patterning.

Todaro-Franceschi's (1999) philosophical study of energy from multiple perspectives, including Rogerian nursing science, highlighted the communal, transformative nature of energy, an ongoing process of becoming that is, by nature, unpredictable. We cannot bring about change; "We can only participate in the inherent, communal process of energy transformation" (p. 111).

Pattern refers to the ever-flowing motion of the energy field; it is described by Rogers (1992) as continuously changing while revealing itself through manifestations of the unitary human–environmental field mutual process. Pattern manifestations reveal increasing diversity of field patterning in characteristics such as lesser and greater diversity; longer, shorter, and seemingly continuous rhythms; slower, faster, and seemingly continuous motion; time experienced as slower, faster, and timelessness; pragmatic, imaginative, and visionary awareness; and longer sleeping, longer waking, and beyond waking experiences (Rogers, 1992).

Pandimensionality refers to "a nonlinear domain without spatial or temporal attributes" (Rogers, 1992, p. 29), thus transcending traditional ideas about space and time, with perceived boundaries not necessarily matching tangible ones. Pandimensional awareness, for example, encompasses phenomena commonly labeled paranormal, which in Rogerian nursing science are manifestations of a changing diversity of field patterning.

As part of her new worldview shift away from older ideas such as homeostasis, equilibrium, and adaptation, Rogers chose *homeodynamics* as the concept that her principles exemplified, in acknowledgment of the ever-changing nature of life and the world. The principles underlying homeodynamics are resonancy, helicy, and integrality (Rogers, 1992). Together they describe the nature and process of continuous change within the human–environmental field.

Resonancy is the "continuous change from lower to higher frequency wave patterns in human and environmental fields" (Rogers, 1992, p. 31). The principle of resonancy describes the way change occurs, fluctuating throughout lower- and higher-frequency wave patterns—sometimes one, sometimes the other. Rogers (1990) clarified that persons can "experience lesser diversity and greater diversity [and] time as slower, faster, or unmoving. Individuals are sometimes pragmatic, sometimes imaginative, and sometimes visionary" (p. 10). One manifestation is not valued more highly than the other; rather, both lower- and higher-frequency awareness are integral to the wholeness of the rhythmical pattern. As Phillips (1994) noted, "When the rhythmicities of lower–higher frequencies work together, they yield innovative diverse patterns" (p. 15).

Helicy is the "continuous, innovative, unpredictable, increasing diversity of human and environmental field patterns" (Rogers, 1992, p. 31). The principle of helicy describes the nature of change in field patterning as ongoing, creative, and diverse. According to Phillips (2010a), this is a "becoming diversity of pattern that is innovative, creative, and unpredictable" (p. 57). *Integrality* is the "continuous mutual human and environmental field process" (Rogers, 1992, p. 31). It specifies that change occurs simultaneously for human and environment because they constitute a unitary whole that cannot be divided into two separate fields.

Taken together, the three principles of homeodynamics describe the mutual patterning process of human and environmental fields as one that changes continuously, innovatively, and unpredictably, fluctuating throughout lower and higher frequencies. Rogers (1990) believed these principles would serve as a guide for practice and research flowing from her nursing science.

Rogers (1992) identified three theories, but she encouraged others to identify additional theories in the belief that multiple theories could be derived from her nursing science. First, the theory of accelerating change (originally accelerating evolution) suggests that change is accelerating in human–environment field patterning, offering the possibility of "new norms with a wider range of distribution of differences among individuals" (p. 32). Indeed, perhaps the only norm is accelerating change. Aging provides an example, with Rogers suggesting that rather than a process of inevitable decline, aging of the human field is a creative process with increasing diversity in field manifestations such as sleeping, waking, dreaming, and perception of time passing.

Second, the theory of the emergence of paranormal phenomena suggests that experiences commonly labeled paranormal are actually manifestations of innovative field patterning and pandimensional awareness. For example, health patterning modalities such as imagery, meditation, and Therapeutic Touch transcend traditionally perceived limitations of time, space, and physical boundaries, opening the door to new, creative opportunities for healing and well-being.

There is an expanding view of living and dying. Rogers (1970) postulated that both dying and birthing are a creative transforming of energy. This idea is captured in a song written, sung, and recorded by Maura Kennedy in 2008 based on a dream she had. In her song "Breathe," she wondered if birth is really a kind of dying and death a kind of birth. Todaro-Franceschi (2006) identified the occurrence of synchronicities in the experiences of bereaved persons grieving the loss of a spouse, finding that such experiences helped them relate to their deceased loved ones in new, meaningful ways and showing that dying is a transition rather than an end. Malinski (2012) synthesized the unitary rhythm of dying–grieving, also illustrative of Rogers's (1970) belief that dying is a process at once creative and transforming, with no real beginning or ending. As stated by Malinski (2012), "Dying–grieving is a process of kaleidoscopic patterning flowing now swiftly, now gently, spiraling creatively through shifting rhythms of now-elsewhen-elsewhere, becoming in solitude and silence alone—all one, timeless, boundaryless" (p. 242).

Rogers's third theory, manifestations of field patterning in unitary human beings (formerly the correlates of pattern), was discussed earlier as the nonlinear, creative, unpredictable process of change in human–environmental field patterning. Rogers offered some manifestations of this relative diversity as examples, including rhythmical fluctuations of motion, time experience, and sleeping–waking, but she encouraged others to identify additional ones.

Rogers (1992) believed that her science "identifies nursing's uniqueness and signifies the potential of nurses to fulfill their social responsibility in human service" (p. 33). She adamantly maintained that "autonomous nursing practice directed by nurses holding valid baccalaureate and higher degrees with an upper division major in nursing science is central to the future" (p. 33). Her vision encompassed individualized, community-based services, including development of nursing centers and practice incorporating noninvasive therapeutic modalities such as Therapeutic Touch, imagery, meditation, humor, laughter, music, and movement. Although she believed that unconditional love and hope can facilitate healing and well-being, Rogers did not view caring as unique to nursing. Rather, she saw caring as a way of using knowledge—specifically, in terms of how nurses might use Rogerian nursing science for the betterment of humankind (Rogers, 1992).

Rogers called for an emphasis on human rights, client decision making, and noncompliance in the belief that clients know themselves best and have the right to make informed choices about health care. This belief, joined with her great sense of humor, was in evidence some years ago when Rogers had pencils printed up with the statement, "Be noncompliant, you'll live longer." She noted that her basic assumption of increasing diversity calls for the provision of healthcare services that are individualized to a greater degree than ever before—a feat that cannot be achieved with standardized tools or a normative approach to patient care.

Theory derivation from the science of unitary human beings continues today. Rogers noted that her science calls for nurses to envision creative new ways to describe and understand unitary phenomena within a pandimensional view of people and their world (Malinski, 2006). Selected examples of this ongoing work include Reed's (1991, 2003) theory of self-transcendence, Hills and Hanchett's (2001) theory of enlightenment, Butcher's (1993) theory of kaleidoscoping in life's turbulence, Bultemeier's (1997) theory of perceived dissonance, Alligood and McGuire's (2000) theory of aging, and Butcher's (2003) theory of aging as emerging brilliance, among others.

Although Rogers died in 1994, the science of unitary human beings lives on in the community of Rogerians who continue to use and refine it in their own conceptualizations, practice, and research. One noteworthy Rogerian scholar is Phillips (2010b), who recently proposed and elaborated on the ideas of "energyspirit" and "Homo pandimensionalis" in an exploration of expanding "pandimensional relative present awareness" (p. 8). *Energyspirit* is the key to all life, all that is, and *Homo pandimensionalis* represents the unanticipated, creative, transformational changes taking place in the human–environment mutual process, in keeping with the basic ideas of Rogerian nursing science. Phillips (2016) is developing a new theory, the theory of pandimensional awareness–integral presence, which he suggests is a combination of Rogers's theories of accelerating change and the paranormal. This theory "opens perception–experience of visible–invisible phenomena of the universe energyspirit for living and transcending" (p. 44). He noted, "The idea is to help people participate in broadening their pandimensional awareness–integral presence for wellbecoming" (p. 44) and offered beginning ideas for creation of an instrument to measure diversity of awareness–presence.

Barrett's Power as Knowing Participation in Change

A prime example of early and continuing theory development is Barrett's (1986, 1990, 1998, 2010) theory of power as knowing participation in change, which she first described in her 1983 dissertation, the culmination of her study with Rogers at New York University. Picking up on Rogers's (1970) assumption that change is continuous and humans can participate knowingly in change, Barrett identified this knowing participation in change as power. She developed a theory, power tool, and practice method, which Rogerians have been using for some 30 years.

The discussion in this section is based on the content of Barrett's interactive website, www.drelizabethbarrett.com (redesigned in late 2009), and her 2015 chapter in *Nursing Theories and Nursing Practice*. Barrett differentiates between *power-as-freedom*, represented by her theory, and the traditional view of *power-as-control*, both of which manifest in the world in multiple forms. Power-as-freedom represents a spiritual worldview, whereas power-as-control represents a material worldview. Four inseparable dimensions character-ize power, encapsulated in the following statement: "Power is being **aware** of what one is **choosing** to do, **feeling free** to do it and **doing it intentionally**" (emphasis in the original) (Barrett, 2009a). Power enhancement is represented by the acronym POWER, where P = possibilities, O = openness, W = will, E = energy, and R = reversing. As stated by Barrett (2009b), "Power is openness to possibilities using the energy of the will to change through the principle of reversing."

Barrett described the four observable dimensions of power as inseparable and continu-ously fluctuating. They are measured with the Power as Knowing Participation in Change Tool (PKPCT), also known as the Power Meter. This instrument consists of 52 items in a semantic differential format that assess the four dimensions of power. Taken together, they yield a person's or group's power profile, which identifies areas of greater and lesser power. Because change is a given in Rogerian science, this profile changes as the human–environmental mutual process changes, whether with individuals, families, or groups. The PKPCT is widely used in both research and practice.

Numerous studies have been conducted in several countries using the PKPCT. This tool has been translated into Danish, Swedish, Japanese, Korean, French, German, Haitian, and Portuguese. Caroselli and Barrett (1998) published a review of 39 studies conducted as of 1993. Kim (2009) conducted a review of 46 studies carried out since 1983, including 27 studies reviewed by Caroselli and Barrett and another 18 completed since their 1998 publi-cation. Significant positive correlations have been noted between power or a power subscale and such variables as human field motion, life satisfaction, feminism, well-being, purpose, transformational leadership style, imagination, empathy, hope, spirituality, and perceived health. Significant negative correlations have been noted with such variables as chronic pain, distress, anxiety, hopelessness, alcohol dependence, and transactional leadership style.

Practice is conducted via Barrett's health patterning methodology, which takes into account both pattern manifestation knowing and voluntary mutual patterning. The first process consists of discovering what is going on and what the person wants. Indeed, her first question is, "What do you want?" (Barrett, 2015, p. 500). In the second process, the nurse assists the person to "freely choose with awareness ways to participate to make happen the changes they want to happen and to enhance their well-being by focusing on intention, aim, and direction with no attachment to outcome" (Barrett, 2009c). Another early ques-tion is, "Where do you see yourself in your life right now?" (Barrett, 2015, p. 500). The two processes occur simultaneously, and both nurse and client jointly participate in them. Health patterning modalities, such as Therapeutic Touch, imagery, music, and movement, provide ways to facilitate a client's knowing participation in creating change and can serve as a framework for individualized power prescriptions.

The power profile, which identifies areas of greater and lesser power, assists the nurse in designing the power prescription—that is, the plan the client can follow to enhance awareness, choices, freedom, and involvement. The power profile varies as human–environmental field patterning changes. The changes tell us something about the nature of awareness, the type of choice being made, the degree to which a person feels free to act intentionally, and the manner in which a person is involved in creating change (Barrett, 1986, 2010). In living power-as-freedom, Barrett (2010) notes that people make and act on choices that promote health, consistent with what health means to them. We "can participate knowingly in changing any situation in our lives" (p. 52). Barrett suggests that people ask themselves questions such as, "What am I aware of?" and "What choices am I making" followed by questions such as, "Do the changes I intend to create interfere with anyone else's freedom?" and "Do the changes I intend to create attempt to control, dominate, manipulate or bring harm to anyone?" (p. 52). Readers are referred to both the website and the 2015 chapter for practice examples.

Other Rogerian-Based Practice Examples

Other Rogerians have met Rogers's challenge to develop innovative practice methods consistent with Rogerian nursing science. Cowling (1993, 1997), for example, offered a pattern appreciation method, consistent with Barrett's health patterning therapy, suggesting 10 constituents characteristic of Rogerian practice:

1. Field pattern manifestations are the focus.
2. The client's experiences, perceptions, and expressions are taken as manifestations of pattern and a focus for pattern appreciation.
3. Information about pattern in all forms, from sensory to lab data to feelings, is sought.
4. The nurse uses all forms of awareness—from sensory to intuition to tacit knowing—to cultivate pandimensional awareness in appreciating pattern information.
5. The nurse then engages in both synthesis and synopsis to view the information as manifestations of a unitary whole interpreted within a unitary perspective.
6. The nurse constructs a pattern profile that unites the client's experiences, perceptions, and expressions in a meaningful narrative or art form such as a picture, metaphor, or photograph.
7. This pattern profile is shared with and verified by the client, and the nurse and the client engage in mutual discussion of options, goals, and patterning strategies.
8. Health patterning is based on knowing participation in change.
9. The health patterning approaches are determined by the client.
10. Knowledge derived from pattern appreciation reflects the unique human–environmental field pattern of the client.

Butcher (Butcher, 2006; Butcher & Malinski, 2015) synthesized the work of Barrett and Cowling in a comprehensive practice model, the unitary pattern-based practice (praxis) method. He identified the focus of nursing care as "recognizing manifestations of patterning through pattern manifestation knowing and appreciation and by facilitating the client's ability to participate knowingly in change, harmonizing person/environmental integrality, and promoting healing potentialities and well-being through voluntary mutual patterning" (Butcher, 2006, p. 170).

Rogerian Research

Research in the science of unitary human beings "enables one to understand better the nature of human evolution and its multiple, unpredictable potentialities. Description, explanation, and vision strengthen a nurse's ability to practice according to the level and scope of preparation and knowledge in the science of nursing" (Rogers, 1992, p. 33). Vision replaces prediction given the focus on diverse, unpredictable potentialities in this nursing science. Rogers maintained that quantitative and qualitative methodologies might potentially be appropriate for conducting such research, depending on the nature of the research question, but she also called for the development of new methods and tools (Malinski, 2008).

Not surprisingly, early research in Rogerian nursing science focused on tool development, primarily tied to the proposed manifestations of change. Ference (1986) explored motion (slower/faster/seems continuous) as the focus for her Human Field Motion Test, in which the concepts "my motor is running" and "my field expansion" are rated using a semantic differential format. Time (slower/faster/timelessness) provided the focus for Paletta's (1990) Temporal Experience Scale, which consists of three subscales rating the three experiences of time passing using metaphors. Hastings-Tolsma (Watson, Barrett, Hastings-Tolsma, Johnston, & Gueldner, 1997) explored lesser diversity/greater diversity in creating the Diversity of Human Field Pattern Scale, which assesses change occurring in the human–environmental field process using a 16-item Likert scale. Watson (Watson et al., 1997) identified dreaming as a beyond-waking manifestation in the manifestation of longer sleeping/longer waking/beyond waking, creating a 20-item Likert scale to assess diversity of dream experience. Gueldner (Gueldner, 1996; Watson et al., 1997) developed a picture tool composed of 18 pairs of black and white drawings designed to represent low- and high-frequency descriptors of concepts in her Index of Human Field Energy. This tool was later modified to become the Well-Being Picture Scale (Gueldner et al., 2005). Applications of this tool include validating it as a measure of mood (Johnston, Guadron, Verchot, & Gueldner, 2011) and using it to appraise well-being in pregnancy (Reis & Alligood, 2008). Anderson and Ashman (2011) found that the tool correlated with presenting symptom distress, as measured by the Brief Symptom Inventory-18 (BSI-18), in a group of patients with cancer undergoing radiation therapy. The Well-Being Picture Scale was also easier for nurses and patients to use than the BSI-18. Terwillinger, Gueldner, and Bronstein (2012) evaluated a children's version of the Well-Being Picture Scale.

Recognizing that concepts such as self-esteem and body image are not appropriate in Rogerian nursing science, Johnston (Johnston, 1994; Watson et al., 1997) used Phillips's (1990) idea of human field image and designed the Human Field Image Metaphor Test. Composed of 25 metaphors, this Likert-type tool is designed to measure the two domains of human field image, perceived potential and integrality, with human field image defined as "individual awareness of the infinite wholeness of the human field" (Watson et al., 1997, p. 94).

Carboni (Barrett, Cowling, Carboni, & Butcher, 1997; Carboni, 1992) argued that in the unitary view nurses could not intervene and, therefore, could not conduct research designed to quantitatively test hypotheses without violating basic assumptions of Rogerian nursing science. She developed a qualitative measure, the Mutual Exploration of the Healing Human Field–Environmental Field Relationship, "designed to capture changing configurations of energy field patterns" (Carboni, 1992, p. 137). Nurse and client complete this instrument together to understand their mutual healing process. Carboni's tool taps into descriptions of experiences and expressions of those experiences—for example, via metaphor and picture.

As indicated earlier, Rogers identified the need for new research methods as key to conducting research related to her proposed worldview. It is interesting to note that the three developed to date—the Rogerian process of inquiry, the unitary field pattern portrait research method, and unitary case inquiry—employ qualitative rather than quantitative methods, reflecting the debate in Rogerian circles over the appropriate methodology for research in Rogerian nursing science (Barrett et al., 1997).

Carboni (1995) developed a Rogerian process of inquiry designed "to investigate the enfolding–unfolding change of human field–environmental field energy field patterns in order to understand the nature of human evolution and its multiple, unpredictable potentialities" (p. 36). She identified 16 characteristics of this process of inquiry, starting with *a priori* nursing theory, grounded in the science of unitary human beings and theories derived from it, that guide the flow of Rogerian inquiry, which proceeds in the following way. First, the Rogerian researcher envisions multiple potentialities for change as field patterning flows in lower- or higher-frequency wave patterns, revealing configurations of lesser or greater diversity. This, in turn, yields visionary insights into such potentialities. Next, the Rogerian researcher maintains an explicit focus on energy fields because field patterns reflect the whole, which "is the only valid concern of Rogerian research" (p. 25), and the only source of unitary meaning. Manifestations of field patterning are identified and explored, even as the researcher remains open to the possibility that new manifestations might emerge and be identified.

The Rogerian researcher conducts the process of inquiry in the pandimensional field enfolding researcher, participants, and the natural setting; observer and observed are integral to this investigation. Observations and shared descriptions are processed by the researcher and participants through mutual exploration and discovery, and the researcher uses unitary instruments such as the healing human field–environmental field relationship qualitative measure to generate shared descriptions of field patterns. All data are synthesized inductively and deductively to identify unitary constructs, which are then interpreted within Rogerian nursing science and explored for their potential to generate new insights and perhaps the synthesis of new theories. Carboni also developed a pandimensional unitary process report to present the study, its processes, and conclusions, along with special criteria for trustworthiness of the research in the form of credibility, unitary integrity, and auditability.

Butcher (1994, 1998, 2005) developed the unitary field pattern portrait method to create a unitary understanding of pattern manifestations with a focus on well-being and human betterment. Butcher identified eight aspects to be addressed:

1. Initial engagement
2. *A priori* nursing science
3. Immersion
4. Manifestation of knowing and appreciation
5. The unitary field pattern profile
6. The mutually constructed unitary field pattern profile
7. The unitary field pattern portrait
8. Theoretical unitary field pattern portrait

In addition, Butcher identified three processes: (1) creative pattern synthesis, (2) immersion and crystallization, and (3) evolutionary interpretation (Butcher & Malinski, 2015). The criteria of trustworthiness and authenticity are used to ensure rigor (Butcher, 1998, 2005). Butcher (2006) used his method to study dispiritedness in later life, synthesizing a description of the experiences, perceptions, and expressions of dispiritedness that can be used to enhance nurses' understanding and appreciation of this phenomenon. He noted that sharing the pattern profile with clients can potentially enhance their knowing participation in change, perhaps inspiring clients as they work with nurses to enhance active involvement, intensify connectedness with persons and nature, and facilitate hope.

Cowling (1998) developed unitary case inquiry and identified unitary appreciative inquiry for use with individuals, groups, or communities to explore a phenomenon, concern, or situation from a unitary perspective (Cowling, 2001). With this approach, researcher and participants engage in a shared, mutual process where all experiences, perceptions, and expressions are viewed together as reflections of wholeness and field pattern and used to construct a pattern profile. This profile can be constructed jointly or by either researcher or participant. It may then be shared in the form of story, poetry, or art—whatever is most meaningful for the persons involved. Cowling's major focus in research and practice has been the experience of despair.

Applications in Advanced Practice Nursing: Science of Unitary Human Beings

Healthcare consumer Mandl (1997) issued a plea to educate the public about Rogerian nursing science following her experience with Rogerian nursing at a major medical center. Unexpectedly hospitalized following a pancreatitis attack, she found herself no longer in the role of a competent businessperson, but rather she became a patient who was frightened and confused, emotionally distraught, and feeling like a victim. Healthcare providers came and went, all talking to one another but rarely to her. At 11:00 p.m., a nurse practitioner entered her room and sat with her. They talked and shared stories of their experiences. As Mandl reported,

> I didn't realize just how angry and scared I was until we started talking. She massaged my body, held my hand, stroked my head, adjusted the pillows and the tubes, all the while soothing me with words and touch. . . . I felt calmed, I felt understood, I received compassion and healing. (p. 237)

Once discharged, Mandl began reading Rogers's work and sought out health patterning with Barrett. She offered ways to bring Rogers into the mainstream, noting that people could find different ways to approach health issues once they discover their power to change their expectations.

Madrid (1990), the advanced practice nurse mentioned in Mandl's vignette, described her Rogerian practice with Roger, a patient who was hospitalized with AIDS and a gastrointestinal bleed. When he told her that nothing seemed to help him, including his medications, and that his skin felt on fire, Madrid began Therapeutic Touch, which she continued for 30 minutes. Roger relaxed and told her he felt great. She then taught him relaxation techniques and helped him focus on relaxing his muscles, after which he was able to sleep. When he awoke, he shared the story of his life.

When his body next contracted in pain, Madrid learned that the only way Roger could urinate was to strain and force out short bursts of urine, an extremely painful process for him in which all his muscles contracted, increasing his pain. She led him through deep breathing and relaxation by first having him synchronize his breathing with hers, after which he was able gently to release a stream of urine. After she washed his hair, Roger took interest in his appearance and had the energy to shave and trim his mustache.

Next, Madrid enlisted Roger's participation in a more aesthetic arrangement of the flowers in his room. He listened to music, noticing that it was like he was hearing favorite pieces for the first time, feeling "boundless in nature . . . as if he had lost all physical, spatial attributes and was infinite with the universe" (Madrid, 1990, p. 98). When he mentioned sadly that he would probably never have the chance to spend another evening on the beach, Madrid led Roger through an imagery exercise so that, once again, he could sit on the beach and enjoy the sunset, which moved him deeply. He died the next day. As Madrid (1990) explained,

> It was not sophisticated technology that made such a difference that evening. It was the art of nursing . . . the caring and application of knowledge to human betterment . . . generated from the principles of resonancy, helicy, and integrality. (p. 99)

Several years after this experience, Madrid (1994) described her use of Barrett's health patterning methodology with another hospitalized dying patient. She noted the need for continuing pattern appraisal to guide practice strategies because pattern manifestations were continuously changing. Storytelling, massage, Therapeutic Touch, and affirmations were among the uniquely nursing practices that Madrid brought to her patient's care, along with the standard care provided to a person with leukemia experiencing a blast crisis.

Gold (1997), an advanced practice certified holistic nurse, called for nurses to understand and identify what is unique to nursing; this knowledge, she suggested, should guide their vision in the practice of nursing and support nurses in finding meaning, value, and satisfaction in their practice. She provided examples of her work with patients, including her experiences with an 82-year-old man hospitalized with sepsis, atrial fibrillation, and pemphigus who spoke no English. Rather than concentrating on his medical diagnoses, she focused on behavioral manifestations of his energy field, which she described as a pattern of independence and passion. Using silence, active listening, caring facial expressions, and Therapeutic Touch, Gold and her patient accessed a place beyond words where each touched the other's heart. In recounting her experiences with this patient, Gold (1997) stated, "I continue to feel his pandimensional presence in my life" (p. 253).

NEWMAN'S THEORY OF HEALTH AS EXPANDING CONSCIOUSNESS

Two pivotal experiences in the development of Newman's theory were her experiences as primary caregiver for her mother, who had amyotrophic lateral sclerosis (Lou Gehrig disease), and her doctoral work at New York University with Martha Rogers (Newman, 2008). Through her interactions with her mother, Newman came to know her mother as a whole person, rather than as a patient defined by her disease, and she recognized how the restrictions her mother experienced in time, space, and movement became her restrictions as well. Movement, time, and space remained foundational concepts for Newman as she studied rehabilitation nursing and embarked on her doctoral dissertation exploring the relationship between time and movement. Consciousness emerged as another important concept once she realized how study subjects were compensating for imposed alterations of natural movement.

Newman was challenged to come up with her own view of health by Rogers's view of health and illness as aspects of the life process, rather than as a unique focus for nursing. Her major premise is that health is expanding consciousness: "Health encompasses disease and non-disease and is a manifestation of the underlying pattern of person–environment" (Newman, 1994, p. 11).

Newman (2008) credits Rogers's (1970) emphasis on mutual process as introducing a new focus—albeit one not immediately recognized or appreciated—on relational process, or the mutuality of the nurse–client relationship in research and practice rather than the traditional observer–observed focus prevalent at the time. As she transitioned from quantitative methods to an appreciation for qualitative methods as more appropriate for use with her theory, Newman realized that research is practice. As a consequence, she suggested that one cannot study a person, family, group, or community. Rather, the Newman nurse engages with the client in a unitary process that simultaneously contains the theory. This praxis is presented as theory–research–practice (Newman, 2008), a unitary whole. Once again, as in the more recently developed Rogerian research methods, the researcher is the instrument of data collection.

Another early influence on Newman was Bentov's (1977) idea that life is a process of expanding consciousness, which he defined as the informational capacity of the system as it interacts with the environment. Newman also found support for her theory in physicist David Bohm's (1980) formulation of the implicate and explicate orders of reality. The *implicate* is the underlying pattern of all that is, unbounded by space and time. In contrast, all that is observed and accepted as "real" serves as *explication* of this unseen reality, unfolding in perceived time and space. All observable manifestations, then, including disease, are manifestations of the underlying pattern of the whole.

Chemist Ilya Prigogine's theory of dissipative structures (Prigogine & Stengers, 1984) pointed to disorder as a path to higher consciousness. When disorder occurs in a previously ordered system, he suggested, the system moves in self-organizing but seemingly random ways toward a higher level of organization. Finally, Arthur Young (1976) described stages in expanding consciousness, using the downward–upward motion of a "V" or rhythmic wave format to indicate the descending and ascending shift from potential to absolute freedom. It is at the downward point that a choice point exists. The old ways are no longer working, there is a loss of freedom, and, for the system to evolve, a shift must occur with a choice that allows increasing freedom and higher consciousness.

For Newman (2008), all this translated into consciousness as the information of the system, a dynamic pattern. She suggested that the appropriate focus for nursing is the person, who serves as the pattern of the evolving whole, continually transforming throughout unpredictable and often seemingly chaotic processes.

Like Rogers, who described the older and newer worldviews in nursing, with the latter laying the groundwork for her nursing science, Newman (2008) recognized that her theoretical ideas, along with those of scientists whose work supported her ideas, necessitated a paradigm shift, one characterized by dynamic order and unity, where "order is revealed in the relationships that emerge" (p. 13). The focus, then, becomes the nurse–client relationship, whether the client is an individual, family, group, or community. This relationship, Newman suggested, must be allowed to unfold naturally.

Earlier, Newman, Sime, and Corcoran-Perry (1991) had described three philosophical perspectives that could help nurses understand differences in research and knowledge development in nursing. The first word in each pair of terms represents how phenomena are viewed, the second the nature of change that occurs (Newman, 2008). In the *particulate–deterministic* view, phenomena are seen as isolated and can be manipulated in experimental designs, with causal inferences being made and tested. In the *interactive–integrative* view, phenomena interact and cannot be isolated; multiple variables need to be considered, and change is probabilistic rather than predictable. In the *unitary–transformative* view, the focus is on the evolving pattern of the whole, and change represents a transformation in this patterning. This last pair describes a participatory view that necessitates a move to what Newman (2008) identified as *compassionate consciousness*, following through on the definition of nursing as caring in the human health experience identified earlier by Newman, Sime, and Corcoran-Perry (1991). Inherent values reflect "wholeness (health), caring, evolving pattern, mutual process, and transformation. The phenomenon of nursing is a dynamic nurse–client relationship viewed within a unitary perspective of health" (Newman, 2008, p. 19). Health is the pattern of the whole and reflects the chaos of transformation, which takes the participant to another phase of becoming and connectedness. According to Newman (2005), "The thing that makes a difference in practice is the caring, creative presence of the nurse in recognizing the pattern of the whole" (p. 9).

The paradigm shift initiated by Rogers and continued by Newman (1994, 2008) encompasses a move from treating symptoms to searching for pattern, from viewing pain and disease as negative to seeing them as important sources of pattern information, from disease as entity to disease as process, and from the body as a machine to be repaired to the human as a dynamic energy field continuous with the larger environmental field (see **Box 20-1**).

Newman (2008) synthesized three basic assumptions of her theory of HEC:

1. Health is an evolving *unitary pattern* of the whole, including patterns of disease.
2. Consciousness is the *informational capacity* of the whole and is revealed in the evolving pattern.
3. Pattern identifies the human–environmental process and is characterized by *meaning*. (p. 6; emphasis in the original)

The manifestations of expanding consciousness are found in Newman's (1994) concepts of time and timing, integration via movement, expansion of space-time, choice point and beyond, and beyond space-time. Patterning of space, time, and movement is rhythmical and individualized. Preferred patterns of the individual, group, family, or community may be in or out of synchrony with the patterns of other people, healthcare settings, and events occurring around them, with such experiences of disorganization presenting opportunities for growth. In nurse–client relationships, as in all healthcare settings, it is important to sense readiness for connecting and relating so that timing is mutual and comfortable for all participants. In a classic article, Newman, Lamb, and Michaels (1991) highlighted the value of nurses being free to connect with clients in the community when the latter were ready, rather than by setting arbitrary appointments. Describing the practice at Carondelet

---

Box 20-1 Pattern Formation: Human as Dynamic Energy Field

Newman (2008) cites the example of a friend with medically uncontrolled hyperthyroidism treated by Dora Kunz, who, along with Dolores Krieger, developed Therapeutic Touch. Kunz described a pattern of diffused energy. On reflection, Newman realized that her friend did, indeed, expend energy in many ways, through commitments to family, friends, and work, and that she neither ate regularly nor got enough sleep to refresh and energize her. Although her friend's thyroid was working hard to keep up with her fast-paced life, telling her to cut back on activities was working against her pattern, not with it. The friend followed Kunz's advice and made sure to increase sources of energy, thereby gaining pattern insight. Ultimately, this knowledge enabled her to decrease her intake of medication and avoid surgery. According to Newman (2008), "Her disease was a manifestation of the whole, not a separate entity to be attacked as though it were alien to the person" (p. xvi).

Pharris (cited in Newman, 2008) offered the example of a man who made repeated visits to the emergency department (ED) for chest pain, resulting in multiple tests and admissions to rule out heart attack, but nothing helped him. On yet another visit to the ED, after provision of the initial care, Pharris sat and talked with him. During the conversation, she noted, "Your heart seems to be hurting" (p. 97). The patient told her that his wife had left him and that he had a disability, which contributed to his feeling stuck emotionally and physically. They talked through what this experience meant to him and how he could get on with his life, including referral to a public health nurse. The man did not return to the ED. In this case, the focus on a meaningful life event revealed a pattern and ways for transformative change.

To offer an example from my personal experience, a friend was experiencing severe shoulder and upper back pain. As we talked, we both came to the same realization: My friend felt as if she was carrying the weight of the world on her shoulders. She immediately began making changes in her life, including giving herself permission to say no.

Providing a relational, caring presence while focusing on pattern recognition enables the Newman nurse and client to learn about experiences, meaning, and transformative change together. Both health and illness become important sources of pattern information.

St. Mary's Hospital and Health Center in Tucson, Arizona, where nurses were freed from the usual bureaucratic time constraints, these authors noted that nurses recognized the importance of timing in their relationships with clients and the rhythm of when to connect and when to separate, describing it as "a crucial dimension of authenticity in the nurse–client relationship" (Newman, Lamb, et al., 1991, p. 406).

HEC can be diagrammed along a "V" parallel to Young's (1976; cited in Newman, 1994) depiction of the evolution toward freedom and choice. For Young, the top left point of the V represented potential freedom, with steps moving down the left arm representing binding and centering, the move from loss of individuality to sense of self; coming to the choice point at the bottom of the V, a new awareness as one seeks to learn the laws governing life; initiating a move up the right arm of the V into decentering and unbinding, involving transcendence and awareness of greater purpose and meaning; and culminating in real freedom at the top of the right arm of the V. Newman (1994) used the V to represent potential consciousness at the top left point, moving down through space and time to the choice point and beyond at the base, and then up through infinite space and timelessness to absolute consciousness. All persons experience this rhythmic up-and-down flowing of evolving consciousness throughout our lives.

Movement is a basic expression of life and reflects, via rhythmical patterning of tempo, personal organization and environmental integration. Consciousness is expressed in movement, persons interact with the environment via movement, and communication reflects this rhythmic tempo (Newman, 1994). Restricted movement—such as is often experienced in situations involving illness, trauma, bed rest, and so forth—involves changing perceptions of time and space. This dynamic situation offers opportunities for reflection and evolving new patterns of relating, as the old ones no longer work, propelling one "into a realm beyond space-time" (Newman, 1994, p. 60). For example, Jonsdottir (1998) explored the life patterns of 10 people with chronic obstructive pulmonary disease, finding a common theme of isolation and being closed in as they experienced activity restrictions and difficulties in expressing themselves and relating to others. This theme was manifested in different life pattern configurations. Notably, Jonsdottir found indications that some of these patients were beginning to glimpse the choice point—that is, the turning point of pattern recognition.

When persons encounter a disorganized, disruptive pattern characterized by fluctuation, the opportunity for creative change emerges, with the potential for transformation. Through this evolution, the individual transcends the usual experiences of space and time, entering experiences beyond space and time that are potentially transforming not only for the person but for all their relationships.

It is at the choice point and beyond that a turning point in evolving consciousness can occur, as people reflect on the pattern of their lives and relationships in their lives, seeking new rules for themselves as consciousness evolves beyond space-time. Here lie opportunities for experiencing and appreciating a new reality or consciousness, one that lifts people out of themselves and incorporates others in a more loving, compassionate way.

Neill (2005) explored life patterns of seven women living with either multiple sclerosis (MS) or rheumatoid arthritis (RA). She distinguished choice points from turning points at the stage of movement, the downward point of the "V" discussed earlier, and identified four new ways of living that could help nurses recognize where clients are in stages of expanding consciousness. The four ways of living occurred during transcendent stages of expanding consciousness, representing both change and transformation (ascending arm of the V), and were drawn by Neill from narratives reflecting boundarylessness and timelessness. After reaching a choice point, the women found meaning that restored harmony in their lives, despite the failure to cure either MS or RA. For example, all seven women spoke of finding simple pleasures, unique to each. All focused on being positive, and most developed optimistic philosophies that enabled them to preserve their quality of life. The women with MS described gaining self-control and a sense of wholeness, captured by Neill as self-differentiation. Neill suggested that nurses can "harmonize their caring with individual person–environment interaction patterns" (p. 341). For example, when an individual is in early stages of time or space (the descending arm of the V), it is too soon to focus on self-transcendent activities. For someone who is progressing beyond the choice point and beginning to focus on strategies for finding simple pleasures, being positive, gaining self-control, and experiencing self-differentiation can assist in finding new ways of living.

Patterns connect; they identify relationships with people and the environment. As nurse and client come together in an interference pattern of resonating waves, a new pattern is formed. Resonance is the way nurses gain patterning information. As Pharris (2015) noted, resonance "is a way to sense into the whole," enabling nurses "to tap into the pattern of the whole" (p. 286). Pharris also noted that nurses must be open, able to free the self of any preconceived ideas, expectations, judgments, or cultural beliefs and values, in order to resonate with patients. As they come together and then move apart, there is the potential for recognition of patterning, insight, choice, and transformation for both parties if the nurse is fully present with the client in a shared experience of the present. Then their meeting "forms a new rhythmic pattern of the combined fields" (Newman, 2008, p. 55). The process of pattern recognition focuses on meaning—that is, what is meaningful in the life of the person—and is elicited through story or narrative and reflected back by the nurse. Although relationships unfold unpredictably, the potential always exists for greater freedom, connectedness, and caring within relationships. Thus, Newman (1994, 2008) sees pattern recognition as a form of knowing from within, sensing into the pattern, and a form of caring.

Newman Praxis

Praxis involves establishing the mutuality of an encounter, eliciting the story or narrative of meaningful events and people in a person's life, developing the narrative as segments over time to depict the emerging pattern, diagramming that pattern, sharing and verifying this understanding with the client, and applying the theory of HEC. Nurses provide a presence that is transforming, integrating, and healing. As they engage in praxis, they are also developing meaningful nursing knowledge.

When engaging in research, the Newman nurse expands on the previously described activities by seeking institutional review board approval as appropriate and obtaining informed consent from participants. The process of informed consent takes on new meaning within the theory of HEC. According to Hayes (2005), it is unethical to approach everyone in the same way; rather, patterning configurations must be taken into account when engaging with others. For example, restrictions in movement affect a person's sense of time and timing, so the nurse must be aware of and sensitive to these differences, striving for synchrony with the person in the sharing of information and asking the person to make a choice about whether to participate in research.

The dialogue between nurse and client is usually audio recorded when used for research purposes. The phases described here, which were first outlined by Newman (2008), fit both research and practice. Specifically, the nurse practitioner/researcher (PR) begins with an *a priori* theory, being grounded in HEC. The first phase is engaging with the client/participant (CP), where the PR's intention is to be fully present with the CP. The PR asks for a description of the most meaningful persons and events in the CP's life. This phase 1 interview comprises a nondirective process, guided by the CP, with the nurse PR engaging in active listening, general prompting if necessary, clarifying, and using intuitive hunches to guide his or her participation in the dialogue. Because this is a mutual process, the PR is free to share a personal story, if appropriate. It is meaning— rather than data or information—that is key in this phase, which ends with a natural pause or a feeling of closure.

In phase 2, development of the narrative, the PR identifies the statements considered most important by the CP and arranges them in a chronology depicting a narrative of the most significant relationships. This information can then be depicted pictorially using a flowing up and down trajectory in lines and rhythmic swirls with descriptions and/or metaphors representing person–environment patterns of relatedness.

In one or more follow-up meetings (phase 3), the PR and the CP review the data and the pictorial pattern together, with the CP adding or modifying data as appropriate and the PR asking for clarification as needed. Insight may occur as both parties reflect together, indicating signs of pattern recognition. According to Newman (2008), most researchers state at least three such follow-up meetings are necessary. If no pattern recognition occurs, this finding is considered equally meaningful: It may reflect the absence of an observable pattern.

The fourth phase reflects HEC theory application. Although the PR began with theory and reflected on it throughout the process, more intense examination of the theory occurs during phase 4, including possible comparisons to other theories that are compatible with HEC theory. The PR notes any transformational changes that took place, both for the CP and for the nurse. Again, this is a mutual process.

During the course of this four-phase process, reciprocal patterns of family and community may become evident, which the PR can subsequently turn into dialogue with family and/ or community. An excellent example of this evolution is provided by Pharris (2005), who identified a community troubled by a rising rate of youth homicide and then used the HEC praxis, first with 12 young men incarcerated for murder, to explore this issue. She noted that her purpose was to find out what was meaningful for the youths, rather than which factors led them to murder someone. Her purpose was not to discover how the community should change; instead, Pharris trusted that meaningful insights would emerge through dialogue. Her intention was not to empower the community because she recognized that power was already embedded within the community; as a consequence, she believed, answers would emerge along with actions to be taken as the praxis unfolded.

What emerged from Pharris's series of dialogues with the young men were themes such as never being asked or asking themselves similar questions before and now finding an intensified quest for personal meaning and new conceptualizations of how they might get on with their lives while in prison. Pharris (2005) identified "not a common pattern of pathologically disturbed youth, but rather a common pattern of interaction with the community that surrounded them" (p. 88) that had failed to protect and engage them, characterized by abuse and/or separation, stigmatizing events between ages 9 to 12 years with no adult to help them, truancy, casual sex, use of drugs and alcohol, feeling alienated, and easy access to guns. She then took the patterns and stories to 16 community agencies and groups, where all concerned experienced "ah-ha" moments as they discerned ways to "reweave their presence in young people's lives and in the lives of their families" (p. 89).

MacNeil (2012) described Newman's research praxis as an "interactive unity," as researcher and participant come together for the wholeness of the pattern to emerge in dialogue (p. 262). In her study of the complexity of living with hepatitis C in a group of adults, MacNeil identified the main theme of "the experience of struggling to overcome" (p. 263). Several participants discussed how difficult it was to find healthcare professionals who understood hepatitis C, what it meant to the person, and who was willing to work with them, highlighting the potential value of understanding the experience from the person's perspective in order to provide effective nursing care.

Rosa (2016) conducted an integrative review on the use of Newman's praxis with those living with chronic illnesses, adults and families, finding that it "led to patient-centered, comprehensive, compassionate, and safe care" (p. 216). For an integrative review of research based in Newman's theory, see Smith's 2011 article "Integrative Review of Research Related to Margaret Newman's Theory of Health as Expanding Consciousness."

Applications in Advanced Practice Nursing: Health as Expanding Consciousness

The advanced practice nurse following Newman's theory of HEC can make a difference in people's lives through transforming presence, or being fully present in the relationship (Newman, 2008). As an example, Newman cites Falkenstern's doctoral research exploring the nursing relationship with families of children having special care needs: "One does not practice nursing using this theory. . . . One embodies the theory; the theory becomes a 'way of being' in presencing with the client" (Falkenstern, 2003, p. 213; Falkenstern, Gueldner, & Newman, 2009).

Jones (Clarke & Jones, 2011) emphasized the difference between the medical model, with its focus on fixing, removing, and curing quickly, and Newman's assertion that symptoms are an expression of the whole, not the diseased/malfunctioning part. Symptoms may be cured, but the underlying pattern persists and may manifest again. This is a process that occurs over time, not at some fixed point in time. As stated by Jones, "The nurse's goal is to be with persons, to be aware and intentionally present so the patients can look at their own patterns" (Clarke & Jones, 2011, p. 224).

Noveletsky-Rosenthal and Solomon (2005) used a model of structured reflection with advanced practice nursing students to foster a nursing identity and help them develop a way to sense pattern. Although this experience was in an entry-level program, presenting unique challenges in the socialization process as professional nurses, these authors' points apply to other graduate programs where the educational focus is heavily biomedical. In Newman's theory, pattern evolves over time; pattern discovery is accomplished through examinations of multiple interactions over time to identify recurring themes. In Noveletsky-Rosenthal and Solomon's work, students from primary and ambulatory care settings used advanced practice clinical seminars as a forum for engaging in individual and collective reflection on practice and theory. The students came to understand that it was their connectedness with patients that separated their practice from that of other healthcare providers and that what was left unspoken was as meaningful as what was spoken. Students gained insight into their own patterns, as well as the patterns of clients, reevaluating personal beliefs and ways of interacting and recognizing self-imposed barriers to connecting with clients (Noveletsky-Rosenthal & Solomon, 2005). Ongoing reflection is necessary if the nurse is to continue growing and changing, using insights that emerge to make informed choices.

Imagine the vistas opening for creative change if advanced practice nurses embodied the theory of HEC in every encounter with an individual, family, group, or community. Opportunities to enhance healing and well-being would expand exponentially, transcending specific roles, settings, and patient populations. Newman's praxis process has helped nurses and clients understand patterning and achieve insights into the potential for transformative change among people living with such diverse conditions as cancer, cardiac disease, diabetes, MS, RA, dementia, chronic obstructive pulmonary disease, and chronic skin wounds. For example, Rosa (2006) used the praxis methodology to gain understanding of 18 men and women, ages 49 to 98 years, who were living with chronic skin wounds. She discovered a new way to look at the experience of physical threat and to consider how that state is integrated into patterning over time. Rosa's findings informed practice through the model of wholistic healing that she developed, which focuses on healing the whole person: "The *closing the gap: process model of wholistic healing and personal transformation* describes participants' healing journey when guided by the nurse through phases of self-awareness, deepening awareness, appreciating meaning, and transformation" (emphasis in the original) (p. 357). Rosa noted that this mutual partnership supports recognition of problems and facilitates both lifestyle choices and personal healing. Specific clinical outcomes included increases in self-awareness, body image, openness to support, commitment to change, well-being, and satisfaction with nursing care, along with improved wound healing. Rosa (2006) concluded that "the findings in this research study offer evidence that an advanced practice nurse–patient relationship focused on understanding a person's pattern encouraged personal lifestyle changes to improve chronic wound healing" (p. 357).

Pierre-Louis, Akoh, White, and Pharris (2011) engaged in Newman-theory guided community-based collaborative action research to understand the experience of African American women living with type 2 diabetes. This process provided a holistic view of health problems and disparities while facilitating insights leading to action. The authors reported, "Through dialogue, women come to understand the patterns of their lives and realize their own potential for action using their own wisdom to guide meaningful transformations" (Pierre-Louis et al., 2011, p. 235).

MacLeod (2011) explored the experiences of spousal caregivers whose spouses had been discharged home following coronary artery bypass graft surgery. Recommendations included reevaluating the current discharge education provided, recognizing the importance of early interaction with the caregiving dyad, and improving strategies to understand the experience and better facilitate the "caregiver's ability to deal with the ensuing chaos and uncertainty found in the assumption of this role" (MacLeod, 2011, p. 255).

Pharris (2015) offered a practice exemplar involving an adult nurse practitioner and a patient with diabetes and hypertension in a community clinic. She showed how experiences with this patient and with others in the community with similar situations broadened the focus to that of the community's pattern of health and associated meanings.

ROSEMARIE RIZZO PARSE'S HUMANBECOMING SCHOOL OF THOUGHT

Parse first introduced her theory of "man–living–health" in 1981; she has made significant changes to the theory over the ensuing years (see Parse, 1998, 2007, 2014, 2015). Parse originally drew on ideas from Rogers (principles and postulates), along with existential phenomenology (tenets of intentionality and human subjectivity along with concepts of coconstitution, coexistence, and situated freedom). Her original synthesis of these ideas produced nine philosophical assumptions that were synthesized into three assumptions reflecting her major themes of meaning, rhythmicity, and transcendence (Parse, 1998), but her work continues to evolve.

One difference is the evolution from the original theory into a school of thought, a knowledge tradition shared by a community of scholars with a specific ontology represented by the assumptions and principles, an epistemology identifying the focus of inquiry, and appropriate methodology for practice and research (Parse, 1998). This school of thought evolved into the humanbecoming paradigm, with Parse (2014, 2015) identifying three paradigms in nursing—totality, simultaneity, and humanbecoming. She identifies the latter as going beyond the metaparadigm and all other paradigms identified in nursing. In the humanbecoming paradigm, the focus of study is "universal *living* experiences," research is qualitative, and "living the art of humanbecoming is in true presence with illuminating meaning, shifting rhythms, and inspiring transcendence" (Parse, 2015, p. 265). (Parse [2015] does not use the term nursing practice, noting that practice is usually defined in dictionaries as habit, doing over, to drill, etc., and so does not fit with living the art of humanbecoming.) Key to humanbecoming is the idea that change is ongoing, moving through a rhythmic flow of apparent opposites or paradoxes that are natural rhythmical shiftings expressed as pattern preferences (Parse, 2014). As she envisioned the humanbecoming school of thought in the year 2050, Parse (2007) clarified important features of her theory. She highlighted the meaning of indivisible cocreation by merging terms to make both *humanbecoming* and *humanuniverse* one word. She explicitly identified four postulates that had been embedded in the ontology of her theory and that permeate the three principles: (1) illimitability, (2) paradox, (3) freedom, and (4) mystery. Humans structure personal meanings (first principle), configure rhythmical patterns of relating (second principle), and cotranscend with the possibles (third principle) in "cocreating reality illimitably with paradoxical rhythms" and with "inherent freedom in the impenetrable mystery of being human" (Parse, 2007, p. 309).

Parse's vision for 2050 identifies nurses as living their art in all settings imaginable. In these environments, they focus on enhancing quality living as defined by persons, families, and communities rather than carrying out orders or actions determined by members of other healthcare disciplines. Humanbecoming sciencing, according to Parse, will focus on relevant living experiences changing over time as people and communities change. The values of human freedom and dignity will be a consistent focus for humanbecoming nurses, who will be "the preeminent *professional* healthcare presence" (emphasis in the original) (p. 309).

According to principle 1, "Structuring meaning is the imaging and valuing of languaging" (Parse, 2014, p. 35). The paradoxical rhythms of reflective–prereflective and explicit–tacit knowing of imaging, confirming–not confirming of valuing, and speaking–being silent and moving–being still of languaging are inherent to this principle. Rather than confronting some independent, external reality, humans construct reality through the significance they give situations throughout the "was," "is," and "will be" all experienced simultaneously. Imaging or picturing our world involves comparing the new within the whole of one's personal framework or worldview. Personal beliefs are reflected in the choosing–not choosing among imaged options. Meaning changes continuously as the individual explores new beliefs and diverse options.

Parse's (2014) second principle describes rhythmical patterning of humanuniverse: "Configuring rhythmical patterns is the revealing–concealing and enabling–limiting of connecting–separating" (p. 35). Disclosing, not disclosing; living opportunities and restrictions simultaneously; choosing to be with or to be apart from others—these rhythms are present as we cocreate patterns of relating in the process of humanbecoming.

The third principle highlights the process of ongoing change: "Cotranscending with possibles is the powering and originating of transforming" (Parse, 2014, p. 35). Humanbecoming is moving beyond what is to what might be (hopes and dreams) while pushing–resisting (powering) new ways of viewing both the familiar and the new. Originating helps people identify personal uniqueness as they create new ways of conforming–not conforming in the certainty–incertainty of living (Parse, 1998). Each human shares commonalities with others while remaining distinct. Choices are unpredictable, so there is no certainty of outcomes, only creative imaginings of what might be as people are continuously transforming. Meaning, rhythmicity, and transcendence are the heart of the three principles.

Current developments in the humanbecoming school of thought include delineation of the humanbecoming leading–following model (Parse, 2008a, 2014), the humanbecoming mentoring model (Parse, 2008b, 2014), and the humanbecoming teaching–learning model (Parse, 2004, 2014). In addition, Parse (2009, 2014) described her humanbecoming family model as an alternative to traditional views of family. Community has been conceptualized from the humanbecoming perspective, with specific community change concepts and processes identified (Parse, 2003, 2012, 2014) and creative sciencing within the humanbecoming community model described.

Parse (2010) identified human dignity as a humanbecoming ethical phenomenon, identifying the fundamental tenets of reverence, awe, betrayal, and shame. She suggested ways of sciencing these tenets while simultaneously living them.

Humanbecoming Research

The process of inquiry in the humanbecoming school of thought is termed *sciencing* (White, 1938) to denote that it is an ongoing process. The focus is understanding humanuniverse living experiences. Two types of basic research appropriate to humanbecoming theory have been identified—the phenomenological–hermeneutic research method introduced by Parse and the humanbecoming hermeneutic method pioneered by Cody to study the meaning of lived experiences through print and art forms. The applied research method is the qualitative descriptive preproject–process–postproject method, which is used to evaluate what happens in settings that use humanbecoming theory to guide practice (Parse, 1998, 2001, 2015).

The focus of the Parse method is universal living experiences such as joy, hope, grieving, and suffering, described by participants in a variety of ways, including words, metaphors, poetry, photography, and music. Information is gathered in dialogue, different from an interview, where the researcher engages in true presence with participants. Once the research has been approved and informed consent has been obtained, the researcher enters into dialogical engagement with the participant. After an opening such as, "Please tell me about your experience of . . ." (Parse, 2014, p. 62), the researcher follows the lead of the participant, not asking questions but encouraging the person to expand or clarify. The dialogue is audio and video recorded if possible. In extraction–synthesis the researcher moves from essences extracted from the data provided by participants in their own language to higher levels of abstraction as the researcher first synthesizes essences in his or her theory language and then identifies propositions, core concepts, and finally the structure of the living experience that provided the focus for the study. This heuristic interpretation links findings back to the principles of humanbecoming theory while moving forward through creative sciencing into future perspectives. Thus the three processes of this method are dialogical engagement, extraction–synthesis, and heuristic interpretation.

Examples of humanbecoming sciencing include the lived experiences of feeling disappointed (participants from a community health center's foot care clinic; Bunkers, 2012), feeling stronger (community-dwelling adults; Doucet, 2012), feeling unsure (community-dwelling adults; Maillard-Struby, 2012), doing the right thing (community-dwelling adults; Smith, 2012), feeling bored (elders either residing in a long-term care facility or affiliated with a church outreach program; Baumann, 2013), and the living experience of difficulty telling the truth (nurses and a physician) (Baumann, 2015).

One example of international use of the Parse method is provided in a book edited by Parse (1999) that describes 13 studies conducted in nine countries (United States, Australia, Canada, Finland, Italy, Japan, Sweden, Taiwan, and the United Kingdom), whose participants ranged from individuals living in a leprosarium to families living with coronary disease to children and elders. All researchers explored the question, "What is the structure of the lived experience of hope?" (Parse, 1999, p. 6). Examples of core concepts that emerged included "expectancy among the arduous," "enduring with vitality," "benevolent affiliations," "creating anew with cherished priorities," "transfiguring enlightenment," "liberation and arduous restriction," "contentment of desired accomplishments," "resolute perseverance," "formidable ambiguity," and "trusting in potentiality" (pp. 291–292). In Bunkers and Daly's (1999) Australian study of hope in families living with coronary disease, the structure of hope was defined as "anticipating possibilities amid anguish, while enduring with vitality in intimate affiliations" (p. 57). Taken together, the findings from the 13 studies deepen understanding of the living experience of hope.

In the humanbecoming hermeneutic method, the researcher selects a literary or art form to ponder. He or she notes any insights and ideas that emerge from this source, records them, contemplates them, and remains open to new insights. The focus is discovering "emergent meanings of universal living experiences" (Parse, 2014, p. 78). Cody (2001), for example, applied this method to multiple readings of Tennessee Williams' play *Cat on a Hot Tin Roof* and multiple viewings of the film version of this work. He identified the meaning of mendacity as the refusal to bear witness—a "turning-away-from" and an "unloving, judgmental way of being/becoming . . . that serves to alienate others and engender mistrust" (pp. 215–216). He noted how the importance of bearing witness has emerged in both nursing and non-nursing literature as a critical factor in affirming personhood and common humanity. Therefore, the refusal to bear witness "clearly contributes dangerously to experiences of devastation, horror, and misery in individuals, families, and communities" (p. 219).

The final research method employed in conjunction with Parse's humanbecoming school of thought is the qualitative descriptive preproject–process–postproject method, which is used in settings that have chosen humanbecoming theory as a framework for practice. Information is gathered before initiation of the project, midway through the project, and at the end. Once the initial information has been gathered, teaching–learning sessions on humanbecoming theory are provided for nurses and other healthcare providers. Once the midway information has been gathered, the teaching–learning sessions continue. Once the postproject information has been gathered, the researcher applies the process of analysis–synthesis to identify and synthesize themes from all information sources, ending in theory-based thematic conceptualizations.

Bournes (2002) looked at six such studies across a variety of settings and synthesized three themes reflecting changes in nurses' beliefs and practices. Transforming intent represented a shift in purpose, with nurses "becoming available, honoring the person's knowing, and shifting patterns of practice" (p. 191). Unburdening joy represented more meaningful, rewarding practice. Struggling with change captured the difficulties of living the theory in practice. Patients and families appreciated the attention and caring; many said that nurses made a difference in their lives and as a result they found care more meaningful and open. From these studies, Bournes synthesized a set of universal values for knowledge development in nursing—namely, being accountable to the people served; listening to what people say, regarding their input as important for health and honoring their opinions; and respecting the right to self-determination.

Living the Art of Humanbecoming

As part of his or her humanbecoming practice, the nurse invites the person, group, family, or community to discuss the meaning of a situation, moving with the flow in a dialogue reflecting ups and downs, joys and struggles, reaching toward hopes and dreams, and moving beyond what is to what might be. The goal "is true presence in bearing witness and being with others in their changing patterns of living quality" (no longer quality of life) (Parse, 2015, p. 269). True presence is possible in face-to-face dialogues, silent immersions, and lingering presence. Dialogues may involve discussion or other forms of expression such as interpretations of stories, movies, art, music, and photography. Silent immersion is being without words, a silent bearing witness that is still fully present with the other. Lingering presence is the remembered presence, whether explicitly or tacitly recalled. As stated by Parse (2015), "True presence is lived nurse with person, family, and community in illuminating meaning, synchronizing rhythms, and mobilizing transcendence" (p. 270).

Individuals have the choice to transcend to the possibles as they change value priorities in true presence with the nurse. Parse notes that this kind of decision making may occur during the course of such processes as creative imagining, affirming personal becoming, and glimpsing the paradoxical. Imagining what life or a situation might be like if lived in a different way and uncovering personal patterns of preferences and deciding which to change help create the opportunity to do so. Looking at incongruence sheds light on conflict and can help change one's view.

Documentation involves, first, living quality as conveyed by the person or group as they describe the meaning of a situation, patterns with others, and hopes and wishes. Second are rhythms of becoming, paradoxical themes articulated in living humanbecoming. Third are intents and priorities in humanbecoming as articulated by the person or group. Fourth are descriptions of experiences, how patterns are changing, again from the perspective of the person or group (Parse, 2014).

Applications in Advanced Practice Nursing: Humanbecoming Theory

Cody (2003) described how the Charlotte Rainbow PRISM Model of community health nursing services delivery, affiliated with the Family and Community Nursing Department at the University of North Carolina at Charlotte, was derived from humanbecoming theory along with community-based and community health nursing. The term *Rainbow* in the model's name was chosen to express commitment to respect for diversity; PRISM is an acronym for *p*resence, *r*espect, *i*nformation, *s*ervices, and *m*ovement:

- *Presence* is being with, face-to-face, attending to, and staying with the community over time.
- *Respect* is honoring dignity and persons' rights and responsibilities to make choices, with nursing activities guided by the community's values, hopes, and dreams.
- *Information* is about and for clients. The nurse listens, is mindful that clients make their own choices, and makes information available that clients say they want to support decision making. Thus the teaching–learning process consists of client-directed education.
- *Services* are helpful acts that clients see as desirable and meaningful. They are provided by registered nurses (including undergraduate nursing students), advanced practice registered nurses (faculty, family nurse practitioners, graduate students), and advanced practice community health nurses (faculty and graduate students).
- *Movement* is change in desired directions, with nurses following the lead of people served. According to Cody (2003), "Nurses encourage, support, and coparticipate in movement as determined by the community" (p. 52).

For nurse practitioners and nurse practitioner students, the usual care expectations are met, such as physical assessments, but all care is provided in a manner consistent with the PRISM model. For example, given the focus on constituents' desires and values, no smoking cessation programs were offered as part of this program because cigarette smoking provided comfort to the women, who voiced no desire to stop. What one group of women did desire was an evening discussion and support group, so one was established. Although not all the nurses accepted bearing witness in true presence as the essence of practice, all learned about it and other elements of Parse's theory via orientation and periodic seminars (Cody, 2003).

Bunkers (2003) has described the Health Action Model for Partnership in Community (HAMPIC), developed in Sioux Falls, South Dakota, in 1997; formation of this model was guided by Parse's theory as well. In HAMPIC, community is defined as a process of living in relationships and advanced practice community nurses focus on the connections–disconnections within the community. As Bunkers (2003) explained, "In creating health action plans the nurses work with the community in exploring hopes and fears for changing patterns of health, thus changing the community's quality of life" (p. 74). The three integral components of this model are advanced practice nurses, the steering committee, and site communities. As explained by Bunkers, "The intent of advanced community nursing in the HAMPIC 'is to connect in true presence with persons and communities and to understand their health experiences with connections–disconnections and their hopes for changing patterns of health'" (Bunkers, Nelson, Leuning, Crane, & Josephson, 1999, p. 96, as cited in Bunkers, 2003, p. 78). The nurses participate in an ongoing study of Parse's humanbecoming theory. The steering committee is composed of community agency personnel and persons served by the HAMPIC program who meet regularly to make sure the voices of those served are heard. Site communities are partners in the model and vary widely, from soup kitchens to residential housing for the homeless to community health centers.

Josephson (2000), an advanced practice nurse at HAMPIC, described her work with a group that included Native American women at a drop-in center for women and families needing a safe place. More than 100 women met over the years to focus on quality of life issues and serve as family for one another. They began with a women's club to discuss issues of common interest and then chose to develop a group health description and health action plan. The group named itself Women of Hope-Tiospaye, a Native American Dakota word meaning "kinship within an extended family." Letcher (2000) described living the humanbecoming theory at one of the HAMPIC community health centers, sharing the evolving story of John, a Sudanese immigrant, through paradoxical rhythms that emerged and his living the person–community relationship and experiencing community interconnectedness within the HAMPIC program.

Williamson (2000), a client, movingly recounted her personal relationship with an advanced practice nurse living the humanbecoming theory and the changes she experienced through that relationship. Feeling worthless; being depressed; enduring antipsychotic drugs, shock treatments, and hospitalization at a state institution; ending up homeless and living in her car, Williamson encountered Diane, the humanbecoming nurse, as she did her laundry at the local HAMPIC drop-in center. Diane invited her to attend the on-site women's group. Food was served, so Williamson went. As Williamson (2000) reported, "The curious thing about the situation was that the group decided what health issues they wanted to learn about. . . . Although it was hard to believe, Diane's attentions were always focused on each individual as each person spoke" (p. 126). Williamson discussed the gradual evolution of her relationship with Diane and its effects on her life: "Because of the true presence that Dr. Parse's theory teaches, and the way Diane lives it, I have become more of who I really am" (p. 126).

Over time, Williamson became part of the steering committee for the drop-in center. She attended and met Parse at a theory conference. Eventually, Williamson became a participant in and a recruiter for a Parse research study. She participated in cocreating her Personal Health Descriptions and Health Action Plan. In addition, she expressed herself in poetry. Notably, she rephrased a personally meaningful sentence from Ecclesiastes 3:2–8 as follows: "The possibles of the not-yet will become explicit" (p. 128).

Williamson's journey from feeling devalued and unimportant throughout her life to feeling important and being honored as a person is a powerful illustration of the value of true presence. Regardless of the specific advanced practice role and specialty focus, a hallmark of nursing practice is engaging in relationships with clients. That nursing self can be nurtured and honored through cultivation of true presence in living humanbecoming theory, whether the task at hand is physical assessment, pharmacological management, or teaching.

Karnick (2005) acknowledged that living humanbecoming can be a challenge for a nurse practitioner, especially in the current healthcare system. She gave a beautiful illustration of living humanbecoming with children, noting that colleagues who find this approach too time consuming still notice the qualitative difference in her practice and are intrigued by her way of relating with children and the closeness of the relationships she forms.

Kim, Lee, and Baumann (2011) illuminated the experiences of three North Korean refugee families living in South Korea from the perspective of the humanbecoming family model, noting the importance of working with families who have lived through extreme hardships without judging or being critical of the painful decisions they had to make. As Kim et al. (2011) explained, "The humanbecoming family model provides a framework for nursing that focuses on honoring the dignity and creative potential of persons and families without needing to label them or pathologize their behaviors" (p. 277).

Doucet and Maillard-Struby (2009) described practice scenarios showing how nurses in hospital, community, and school settings lived the humanbecoming leading–following model. Parse (2014) offered an example of a family situation involving parents and two adolescent children.

SUMMARY

It is nursing theory-based practice that differentiates nurses from other healthcare providers and that resonates so meaningfully with the persons, groups, families, and communities served by nurses. Examples abound in the literature to assist advanced practice nurses who are interested in pursuing nursing theory-based practice. One cannot practice or live what one does not know. The first step, therefore, is immersing oneself in a chosen theory and finding like-minded colleagues to continue knowingly participating in personal and professional change. It is a journey worth making!

DISCUSSION QUESTIONS

1. What is meant by the concept of pattern for each theorist discussed in this chapter? What is the importance of pattern for advanced practice nurses?
2. How can advanced practice nurses live HEC, humanbecoming, or Rogerian nursing science in fast-paced settings where much of the work to be done is medically based?

REFERENCES

Alligood, M. R., & McGuire, S. L. (2000). Perception of time, sleep patterns and activity in senior citizens: A test of a Rogerian theory of aging. *Visions: The Journal of Rogerian Nursing Science, 8*, 6–14.

Anderson, F. R., & Ashman, J. (2011). Establishing the correlation between well-being and presenting symptomatology in persons who are seriously ill. *Visions: The Journal of Rogerian Nursing Science, 18*, 41–46.

Barrett, E. A. M. (1986). Investigation of the principle of helicy: The relationship of human field motion and power. In V. M. Malinski (Ed.), *Explorations on Martha Rogers' science of unitary human beings* (pp. 173–184). Norwalk, CT: Appleton-Century-Crofts.

Barrett, E. A. M. (1990). Rogers' science-based nursing practice. In E. A. M. Barrett (Ed.), *Visions of Rogers' science-based nursing* (pp. 31–44). New York, NY: National League for Nursing.

Barrett, E. A. M. (1998). A Rogerian practice methodology for health patterning. *Nursing Science Quarterly, 11*, 136–138.

Barrett, E. A. M. (2009a). Become your own powerhouse. Retrieved from http://www.drelizabeth barrett.com

Barrett, E. A. M. (2009b). The power as knowing participation in change theory. Retrieved from http://www.drelizabethbarrett.com/background/power-knowing-participation-change-theory

Barrett, E. A. M. (2009c). Health patterning modalities. Retrieved from http://www.drelizabeth barrett.com/what-i-do/health-patterning-modalities

Barrett, E. A. M. (2010). Power as knowing participation in change: What's new and what's next. *Nursing Science Quarterly, 23*, 47–54.

Barrett, E. A. M. (2015). Barrett's theory of power as knowing participation in change. In M. C. Smith & M. E. Parker (Eds.), *Nursing theories and nursing practice* (4th ed., pp. 495–508). Philadelphia, PA: Davis.

Barrett, E. A. M., Cowling, W. R., Carboni, J. T., & Butcher, H. K. (1997). Unitary perspectives on methodological practices. In M. Madrid (Ed.), *Patterns of Rogerian knowing* (pp. 47–62). New York, NY: National League for Nursing.

Baumann, S. L. (2013). Feeling bored: A Parse research method study with older adults. *Nursing Science Quarterly, 26*, 42–52.

Baumann, S. L. (2015). The lived experience of difficulty telling the truth: A Parse method study. *Nursing Science Quarterly, 28*, 49–56.

Bentov, I. (1977). *Stalking the wild pendulum.* New York, NY: Dutton.

Bohm, D. (1980). *Wholeness and the implicate order.* London, UK: Routledge & Kegan Paul.

Bournes, D. A. (2002). Research evaluating human becoming in practice. *Nursing Science Quarterly, 15*, 190–195.

Bultemeier, K. (1997). Rogers' science of unitary human beings in nursing practice. In M. R. Alligood & A. Marriner-Tomey (Eds.), *Nursing theory: Utilization and practice* (pp. 153–174). St. Louis, MO: Mosby.

Bunkers, S. S. (2003). Community: An emerging mosaic of human becoming. In R. R. Parse (Ed.), *Community: A human becoming perspective* (pp. 73–95). Sudbury, MA: Jones & Bartlett Publishers.

Bunkers, S. S. (2012). The lived experience of feeling disappointed: A Parse research method study. *Nursing Science Quarterly, 25*, 53–61.

Bunkers, S. S., & Daly, J. (1999). The lived experience of hope for Australian families living with coronary disease. In R. R. Parse (Ed.), *Hope: An international human becoming perspective* (pp. 45–61). New York, NY: National League for Nursing.

Bunkers, S. S., Nelson, M., Leuning, C., Crane, J., & Josephson, D. (1999). The health action model: Academia's partnership with the community. In E. Cohen & V. DeBack (Eds.), *The outcomes mandate: Case management in health care today* (pp. 92–100). St. Louis, MO: Mosby.

Butcher, H. K. (1993). Kaleidoscoping in life's turbulence: From Seurat's art to Rogers' nursing science. In M. E. Parker (Ed.), *Patterns of nursing theories in practice* (pp. 183–198). New York, NY: National League for Nursing.

Butcher, H. K. (1994). The unitary field pattern portrait method: Development of a research method within Rogers' science of unitary human beings. In M. Madrid & E. A. M. Barrett (Eds.), *Rogers' scientific art of nursing practice* (pp. 397–429). New York, NY: National League for Nursing.

Butcher, H. K. (1998). Crystallizing the processes of the unitary field pattern portrait research method. *Visions: The Journal of Rogerian Nursing Science, 6*, 13–26.

Butcher, H. K. (2003). Aging as emerging brilliance: Advancing Rogers' unitary theory of aging. *Visions: The Journal of Rogerian Nursing Science, 11*, 55–66.

Butcher, H. K. (2005). The unitary field pattern portrait research method: Facets, processes, and findings. *Nursing Science Quarterly, 18*, 293–297.

Butcher, H. K. (2006). Unitary pattern-based praxis: A nexus of Rogerian cosmology, philosophy, and science. *Visions: The Journal of Rogerian Nursing Science, 14*(2), 8–33.

Butcher, H. K., & Malinski, V. M. (2015). Martha E. Rogers' science of unitary human beings. In M. E. Parker & M. Smith (Eds.), *Nursing theories and nursing practice* (4th ed., pp. 237–261). Philadelphia, PA: F. A. Davis.

Carboni, J. T. (1992). Instrument development and the measurement of unitary constructs. *Nursing Science Quarterly, 5*, 134–142.

Carboni, J. T. (1995). A Rogerian process of inquiry. *Nursing Science Quarterly, 8*, 22–37.

Caroselli, C., & Barrett, E. A. M. (1998). A review of the power as knowing participation in change literature. *Nursing Science Quarterly, 11*, 9–16.

Clarke, P. N., & Jones, D. A. (2011). Expanding consciousness in nursing education and practice. *Nursing Science Quarterly, 24*, 223–226.

Cody, W. K. (2001). "Mendacity" as the refusal to bear witness: A human becoming hermeneutic study of a theme from Tennessee Williams' "Cat on a Hot Tin Roof." In R. R. Parse (Ed.), *Qualitative inquiry: The path of sciencing* (pp. 205–220). Sudbury, MA: Jones & Bartlett Publishers.

Cody, W. K. (2003). Human becoming: Community change concepts in an academic nursing practice setting. In R. R. Parse (Ed.), *Community: A human becoming perspective* (pp. 49–71). Sudbury, MA: Jones & Bartlett Publishers.

Cowling, W. R. (1993). Unitary practice: Revisionary assumptions. In M. E. Parker (Ed.), *Patterns of nursing theories in practice* (pp. 199–212). New York, NY: National League for Nursing.

Cowling, W. R. (1997). Pattern appreciation: The unitary science/practice of reaching essence. In M. Madrid (Ed.), *Patterns of Rogerian knowing* (pp. 129–142). New York, NY: National League for Nursing.

Cowling, W. R. (1998). Unitary case inquiry. *Nursing Science Quarterly, 11*, 139–141.

Cowling, W. R. (2001). Unitary appreciative inquiry. *Advances in Nursing Science, 23*(4), 32–48.

Doucet, T. J. (2012). Feeling strong: A Parse research method study. *Nursing Science Quarterly, 25*, 62–71.

Doucet, T. J., & Maillard-Struby, F. (2009). The humanbecoming leading–following model in practice. *Nursing Science Quarterly, 22*, 333–338.

Falkenstern, S. (2003). *Nursing facilitation of health as expanding consciousness in families who have a child with special health care needs.* Unpublished PhD dissertation, Pennsylvania State University, University Park, PA.

Falkenstern, S. K., Gueldner, S. H., & Newman, S. H. (2009). Health as expanding consciousness with families with a child with special healthcare needs. *Nursing Science Quarterly, 22*, 267–279.

Ference, H. M. (1986). The relationship of time experience, creativity traits, differentiation, and human field motion. In V. M. Malinski (Ed.), *Explorations on Martha Rogers' science of unitary human beings* (pp. 95–105). Norwalk, CT: Appleton-Century-Crofts.

Gold, J. (1997). The practice of nursing from a unitary perspective. In M. Madrid (Ed.), *Patterns of Rogerian knowing* (pp. 249–256). New York, NY: National League for Nursing.

Gueldner, S. H. (1996). Index of field energy. *Rogerian Nursing Science News, 8*(4), 6.

Gueldner, S. H., Michel, Y., Bramlett, M. H., Liu, C. F., Johnston, L. W., Endo, E., . . . Carlyle, M. S. (2005). The Well-Being Picture Scale: A revision of the index of field energy. *Nursing Science Quarterly, 18*, 42–50.

Hayes, C. (2005). Linking Newman's theory of health as expanding consciousness to ethics and caring. In C. Picard & D. Jones (Eds.), *Giving voice to what we know: Margaret Newman's theory of health as expanding consciousness in nursing practice, research, and education* (pp. 27–39). Sudbury, MA: Jones & Bartlett Publishers.

Hills, R. G., & Hanchett, E. (2001). Human change and individuation in pivotal life situations: Developing and testing the theory of enlightenment. *Visions: The Journal of Rogerian Nursing Science, 9*, 6–19.

Johnston, L. W. (1994). Psychometric analysis of Johnston's Human Field Image Metaphor Scale. *Visions: The Journal of Rogerian Nursing Science, 2*, 7–11.

Johnston, N., Guadron, M., Verchot, C., & Gueldner, S. (2011). Validation of the Well-Being Picture Scale (WPS) as a measure of mood. *Visions: The Journal of Rogerian Nursing Science, 18*, 8–21.

Jonsdottir, H. (1998). Life patterns of people with chronic obstructive pulmonary disease: Isolation and being closed in. *Nursing Science Quarterly, 11*, 160–166.

Josephson, D. K. (2000). Women of Hope-Tiospaye. *Nursing Science Quarterly, 13*, 300–302.

Karnick, P. M. (2005). Human becoming theory with children. *Nursing Science Quarterly, 18*, 221–226.

Kim, H. K., Lee, O. J., & Baumann, S. L. (2011). Nursing practice with families without a country. *Nursing Science Quarterly, 24*, 273–278.

Kim, T. S. (2009). The theory of power as knowing participation in change: A literature review update. *Visions: The Journal of Rogerian Nursing Science, 16*(1), 19–39.

Letcher, D. C. (2000). Buying your life. *Nursing Science Quarterly, 13*, 303–305.

MacLeod, C. E. (2011). Understanding experiences of spousal caregivers with health as expanding consciousness. *Nursing Science Quarterly, 24*, 245–255.

MacNeil, J. M. (2012). The complexity of living with hepatitis C: A Newman perspective. *Nursing Science Quarterly, 25*, 261–266.

Madrid, M. (1990). The participating process of human field patterning in an acute-care environment. In E. A. M. Barrett (Ed.), *Visions of Rogers' science-based nursing* (pp. 93–104). New York, NY: National League for Nursing.

Madrid, M. (1994). Participating in the process of dying. In M. Madrid & E. A. M. Barrett (Eds.), *Rogers' scientific art of nursing practice* (pp. 91–100). New York, NY: National League for Nursing.

Madrid, M., & Winstead-Fry, P. (1986). Rogers' conceptual model. In P. Winstead-Fry (Ed.), *Case studies in nursing theory* (pp. 73–102). New York, NY: National League for Nursing.

Maillard-Struby, F. (2012). Feeling unsure: A lived experience of humanbecoming. *Nursing Science Quarterly, 25*, 72–81.

Malinski, V. M. (1986). Further ideas from Martha Rogers. In V. M. Malinski (Ed.), *Explorations on Martha Rogers' science of unitary human beings* (pp. 9–14). Norwalk, CT: Appleton-Century-Crofts.

Malinski, V. M. (2006). Rogerian science-based nursing theories. *Nursing Science Quarterly, 19*, 7–12.

Malinski, V. M. (2008). Research diversity from the perspective of the science of unitary human beings. *Nursing Science Quarterly, 21*, 291–293.

Malinski, V. M. (2012). Meditations on the unitary rhythm of dying-grieving. *Nursing Science Quarterly, 25*, 239–244.

Mandl, A. (1997). A plea to educate the public about Martha Rogers' science of unitary human beings. In M. Madrid (Ed.), *Patterns of Rogerian nursing* (pp. 236–238). New York, NY: National League for Nursing.

Neill, J. (2005). Health as expanding consciousness: Seven women living with multiple sclerosis or rheumatoid arthritis. *Nursing Science Quarterly, 18*, 334–343.

Newman, M. A. (1994). *Health as expanding consciousness* (2nd ed.). New York, NY: National League for Nursing.

Newman, M. A. (2005). Caring in the human health experience. In C. Picard & D. Jones (Eds.), *Giving voice to what we know: Margaret Newman's theory of health as expanding consciousness in nursing practice, research, and education* (pp. 3–10). Sudbury, MA: Jones & Bartlett Publishers. Reprinted from the *International Journal of Human Caring, 6*(2), 2002.

Newman, M. A. (2008). *Transforming presence: The difference that nursing makes.* Philadelphia, PA: F. A. Davis.

Newman, M., Lamb, G. S., & Michaels, C. (1991). Nurse case management: The coming together of theory and practice. *Nursing and Health Care, 12*(8), 404–408.

Newman, M. A., Sime, A. M., & Corcoran-Perry, S. A. (1991). The focus of the discipline of nursing. *Advances in Nursing Science, 14*(1), 1–6.

Noveletsky-Rosenthal, H., & Solomon, K. (2005). Cultivating a way to sense pattern with advanced practice nursing students. In C. Picard & D. Jones (Eds.), *Giving voice to what we know: Margaret Newman's theory of health as expanding consciousness in nursing practice, research, and education* (pp. 179–186). Sudbury, MA: Jones & Bartlett Publishers.

Paletta, J. L. (1990). The relationship of temporal experience to human time. In E. A. M. Barrett (Ed.), *Visions of Rogers' science-based nursing* (pp. 239–253). New York, NY: National League for Nursing.

Parse, R. R. (1998). *The human becoming school of thought: A perspective for nurses and other health professionals*. Thousand Oaks, CA: Sage.

Parse, R. R. (Ed.). (1999). *Hope: An international human becoming perspective*. New York, NY: National League for Nursing.

Parse, R. R. (Ed.). (2001). *Qualitative inquiry: The path of sciencing*. Sudbury, MA: Jones & Bartlett Publishers.

Parse, R. R. (Ed.). (2003). *Community: A human becoming perspective*. Sudbury, MA: Jones & Bartlett Publishers.

Parse, R. R. (2004). A humanbecoming teaching-learning model. *Nursing Science Quarterly, 17*, 33–35.

Parse, R. R. (2007). The humanbecoming school of thought in 2050. *Nursing Science Quarterly, 20*, 308–310.

Parse, R. R. (2008a). The humanbecoming leading–following model. *Nursing Science Quarterly, 21*, 369–375.

Parse, R. R. (2008b). A humanbecoming mentoring model. *Nursing Science Quarterly, 21*, 195–198.

Parse, R. R. (2009). The humanbecoming family model. *Nursing Science Quarterly, 22*, 305–309.

Parse, R. R. (2010). Rosemarie Rizzo Parse's humanbecoming school of thought. In M. E. Parker & M. C. Smith (Eds.). *Nursing theories and nursing practice* (3rd ed., pp. 277–289). Philadelphia, PA: F. A. Davis.

Parse, R. R. (2012). New humanbecoming conceptualizations and the humanbecoming community model: Expansions with sciencing and living the art. *Nursing Science Quarterly, 25*, 44–52.

Parse, R. R. (2014). *The humanbecoming paradigm: A transformational worldview*. Pittsburgh, PA: Discovery International.

Parse, R. R. (2015). Rosemarie Rizzo Parse's humanbecoming paradigm. In M. C. Smith & M. E. Parker (Eds.), *Nursing theory and nursing practice* (4th ed., pp. 263–278).

Pharris, M. D. (2005). Engaging with communities in a pattern recognition process. In C. Picard & D. Jones (Eds.), *Giving voice to what we know: Margaret Newman's theory of health as expanding consciousness in nursing practice, research, and education* (pp. 83–94). Sudbury, MA: Jones & Bartlett Publishers.

Pharris, M. D. (2015). Margaret Newman's theory of health as expanding consciousness. In M. E. Parker & M. C. Smith (Eds.), *Nursing theories and nursing practice* (4th ed., 279–300). Philadelphia, PA: F. A. Davis.

Phillips, J. R. (1990). Research and the riddle of change. *Nursing Science Quarterly, 3*, 55–56.

Phillips, J. R. (1994). The open-ended nature of the science of unitary human beings. In M. Madrid & E. A. M. Barrett (Eds.), *Rogers' scientific art of nursing practice* (pp. 11–25). New York, NY: National League for Nursing.

Phillips, J. R. (2010a). The universality of Rogers' science of unitary human beings. *Nursing Science Quarterly, 23,* 55–59.

Phillips, J. R. (2010b). Perspectives of Rogers' relative present. *Visions: The Journal of Rogerian Nursing Science, 17,* 8–18.

Phillips, J. R. (2016). Rogers' science of unitary human beings: Beyond the frontier of science. *Nursing Science Quarterly, 29,* 38–46.

Pierre-Louis, B., Akoh, V., White, P., & Pharris, M. D. (2011). Patterns in the lives of African American women with diabetes. *Nursing Science Quarterly, 24,* 227–236.

Prigogine, I., & Stengers, I. (1984). *Order out of chaos: Man's new dialogue with nature.* Boulder, CO: Shambhala.

Reed, P. G. (1991). Toward a theory of self-transcendence: Deductive reformulation using developmental theory. *Advances in Nursing Science, 13*(4), 64–77.

Reed, P. G. (2003). The theory of self-transcendence. In M. J. Smith & P. R. Liehr (Eds.), *Middle range theory for nursing* (pp. 145–166). New York, NY: Springer.

Reis, P. J., & Alligood, M. R. (2008). Well-being in pregnancy: A pilot study using the Well-Being Picture Scale. *Visions: The Journal of Rogerian Nursing Science, 15,* 8–17.

Rogers, M. E. (1970). *An introduction to the theoretical basis of nursing.* Philadelphia, PA: F. A. Davis.

Rogers, M. E. (1990). Nursing: Science of unitary, irreducible human beings: Update 1990. In E. A. M. Barrett (Ed.), *Visions of Rogers' science-based nursing* (pp. 5–11). New York, NY: National League for Nursing.

Rogers, M. E. (1992). Nursing and the space age. *Nursing Science Quarterly, 5,* 27–34.

Rosa, K. C. (2006). A process model of healing and personal transformation in persons with chronic skin wounds. *Nursing Science Quarterly, 19,* 349–358.

Rosa, K. C. (2016). Integrative review on the use of Newman praxis relationship in chronic illness. *Nursing Science Quarterly, 29,* 211–218.

Smith, M. C. (2011). Integrative review of research related to Margaret Newman's theory of health as expanding consciousness. *Nursing Science Quarterly, 24,* 256–272.

Smith, S. M. (2012). The lived experience of doing the right thing: A Parse method study. *Nursing Science Quarterly, 25,* 82–89.

Terwilliger, S. H., Gueldner, S. H., & Bronstein, L. (2012). A preliminary evaluation of the Well-Being Picture Scale-Children's Version (WPS-CV) in a sample of fourth and fifth graders. *Nursing Science Quarterly, 25,* 155–159.

Todaro-Franceschi, V. (1999). *The enigma of energy: Where science and religion converge.* New York, NY: Crossroad.

Todaro-Franceschi, V. (2006). Synchronicity related to dead loved ones: A natural healing modality. *Spirituality and Health International, 7,* 151–161.

Watson, J., Barrett, E. A. M., Hastings-Tolsma, M., Johnston, L., & Gueldner, S. (1997). Measurement in Rogerian science: A review of selected instruments. In M. Madrid (Ed.), *Patterns of Rogerian knowing* (pp. 87–99). New York, NY: National League for Nursing.

White, L. (1938). Science is sciencing. *Philosophy of Science, 5*(4), 369–389.

Williamson, G. J. (2000). The test of a nursing theory: A personal view. *Nursing Science Quarterly, 13,* 124–128.

Young, A. (1976). *The reflexive universe: Evolution of consciousness.* San Francisco, CA: Briggs.

Chapter 21

Models and Theories Focused on Competencies and Skills

Mary W. Stewart

INTRODUCTION

Consider your earliest days of nursing school. What do you recall? What experiences first come to mind? Regardless of our entry level into nursing practice, our educational journeys began in similar ways. Initially, we learned the competencies and skills to be a nurse. We primarily focused on concrete skills and anticipated opportunities to stick someone with a needle or insert a tube into an orifice. Competencies, by comparison, were vague aspirations to which our instructors referred. Faithfully, the educational process moved us beyond our initial triumphs to a deeper understanding and greater appreciation of the expertise of nursing. Often to our own amazement, our toolbox filled with more resources, and our place in nursing emerged. Our ability to care for patients became multidimensional and grounded in theory, knowledge, experience, and intuition. This chapter focuses on three theoretical approaches that underpin competency and skills approaches to nursing care, with specific attention to theoretical contributions at the advanced practice level.

Nursing science is rooted in philosophies and theories that shape the discipline. A dynamic construct, nursing knowledge evolves from diverse ways of knowing. Knowledge development provides the path to relevant and effective nursing practice. As practitioners who aim to use best evidence, we need to understand how knowledge develops through various theoretical lenses. Furthermore, we are challenged to value diverse contexts in which knowing matures (Chinn & Kramer, 2015). As we explore these theories of competencies and skills, we want to identify their potential contributions to how we view nursing science, knowledge, and practice on a global scale.

When discussing theoretical pillars of nursing, we must recognize nursing's moral obligation as a discipline and science. Nursing is aimed at contributing to the health of individuals and the health of society (Grace, 2006). Regardless of the political climate, nursing has been unwavering in the principle of health as a human good. Advanced practice nurses (APNs) are responsible for sounding nursing's voice. Evaluating theoretical support for the principle of individual and societal health plays a substantial role in determining the relevance and applicability of theoretical tenets of nursing practice.

FROM NOVICE TO EXPERT

Based on Dreyfus and Dreyfus's model of skill acquisition and skill development, Benner developed one of the most useful models for professional advancement in nursing. Benner (1984) distinguished five levels of nursing practice: novice, advanced beginner, competent, proficient, and expert. Additionally, Benner identified two aspects that discriminate among these levels: (1) Clinicians live in different worlds depending on their level of practice, and (2) clinicians develop *agency*, or a sense of responsibility toward their patients (Mitre, Alexander, & Keller, 1998). In their unique worlds, clinicians utilize different guides for taking action.

Benner's (1984) model of skill acquisition provides three general aspects of changes across these skilled competency levels:

1. Movement from reliance on abstract principles (novice) to experiences (expert) to view and guide practice
2. Movement from seeing all pieces of a situation as equally relevant (novice) to seeing the whole with varying degrees of relevant pieces (expert)
3. Movement from the detached observer (novice) to the engaged doer (expert)

Using Heideggerian principles of text interpretation, context, and holistic inquiry, Benner (1984) synthesized interviews to describe nursing knowledge as embedded in nursing practice. She referred to this approach as a "hybrid of theory and experience" (p. 41). Although the explication of interpretive phenomenology is beyond the scope of this chapter, it is important to note that Benner (1994) used this approach to find *meaning* in her research:

> The goal of studying persons, events, and practices in their own terms is to understand world, self, and other. The interpreter moves back and forth between the foreground and background, between situations, and between the practical worlds of the participants. (pp. 99–100).

This to-and-fro movement is central to understanding the participants' stories. At the same time, one assumption of this process is that the world can never be fully known (1994). According to Benner (1994), her research aim was "to uncover meanings and knowledge embedded in skilled practice. By bringing these meanings, skills, and knowledge into public discourse, new knowledge and understanding are constituted" (p. 218).

The logical development of Benner's theory is appealing. She identified expert competencies, which were then classified into seven domains of nursing practice: the helping role, the teaching–coaching function, the diagnostic and patient-monitoring function, effective management of rapidly changing situation, administering and monitoring therapeutic interventions and regimens, monitoring and ensuring the quality of healthcare practices, and organizational and work-role competencies (Benner, 1984).

Although depicted two-dimensionally, the domains and competencies have no specific beginning or ending. The nurse moves in and out of the relationship with the patient at whatever place best meets the patient's need. Call to mind the "to and fro" movement in the model's development. Unlike a linear model that lists tasks in sequential order, Benner's theory is both situation based and interpretive (Benner, 1984). The *embodiment* of nursing expertise (i.e., the nurse's body) takes over the clinical skill, allowing the nurse to know with feelings, senses, and thinking (Brykczynski, 2006). This knowing guides the nurse to undertake the right action. APNs have developed expertise through their interactions with patients in various settings over time; this investment is a resource that positions the APN in the expert role.

As a practice discipline, nursing extends beyond the science that guides it and examines research findings in the clinical setting. Practice provides the arena for working out relationships. Nurses' narratives indicate understanding that a list of tasks and analytical supports to direct practice alone are insufficient in achieving best practices; ethical principles and aesthetic knowing are also essential.

The APN recognizes the value of past experiences, clinical guidelines, and procedural aids. At the same time, the APN gives careful attention to his or her intuition that supersedes these rudimentary practices. Because of this developed sense of knowing, APNs pay attention to detail, recognize potential outcomes, and take action to prevent deleterious events. In a crisis, the APN evolves as a leader, directing the actions needed and managing multiple interventions simultaneously. The expert nurse recognizes that science is vital, but insufficient when applied in the absence of the nurse's knowing.

Clinical forethought is another contribution of APNs. Even when the nurse is wrong about the outcome of a patient situation, forethought allows for pausing, questioning, and contemplating. APNs listen to patients and respond accordingly. They prioritize interventions on the basis of patient needs and recognize that absolute certainty is impossible. It is possible, however, to stay ahead of a situation through diligent observation, common sense, and quick action (Benner, Hooper-Kyriakidis, & Stannard, 1999).

Caring dominates nursing. While the APN's competencies, domains, assumptions, and development influence decision making, the primacy of nursing is caring (Benner & Wrubel, 1989). As defined by Benner and Wrubel (1989), caring "means that persons, events, projects, and things matter to people" (p. 1). Care represents connection of thought, feeling, and action in ways of knowing and being. Without caring, nursing does not exist.

Because caring makes involvement possible, caring is essential for coping. According to Benner and Wrubel (1989), "Coping cannot cure or abolish loss and pain. Coping can help one manage those experiences, but coping based on caring also allows for the possibility of joy, the satisfactions of attachment" (p. 3).

Caring is specific and relational. The nurse's understanding of illness allows for joining of the patient's experience and the illness. When a nurse is able to be with a patient, through the sharing of presence, recognition of their common humanity ensues. This awareness defines caring as the basis for nursing practice (Benner & Wrubel, 1989). The APN is in the best position to see and seize these moments, to lead others by example, and to enrich the stories of the patients and families who trust in the nurse's care.

Benner's work on caring as central to nursing practice emphasizes the key role of human morality in this interplay. The context of the human situation served as a critical component of her identification of nursing domains and competencies. Based in research and derived from real-world practice experiences, Benner's work enjoys wide acceptance (Brykczynski, 2006).

As experts, APNs can be more sensitive and responsive to the insecurities of the novice or advanced beginner nurse. Likewise, the APN can deal with the tension between the educational setting and the clinical expectations. The beginner relies on abstract principles, models, and theories to perform safely. In contrast, the expert deviates from this basis to engage in a deeper level of questioning in clinical situations. In addition to past experiences, the expert has a matured level of perception that goes beyond facts, concepts, and theories. As such, according to Benner (1984), "The theoretician must always depend on the practitioner for clinical knowledge development and for finding puzzles and questions that current theorizing does not predict or cover" (p. 187).

The relational aspect of Benner's (1984) work is paramount: "Nursing is relational and therefore cannot be adequately described by strategies that leave out content, context, and function" (p. 42). Nursing is holistic, nonprocedural, and relationship dependent. As a result of their extensive experiences, APNs inherently possess a knowing that cannot be explicated with words; they have a developed sense of intuition that moves them beyond knowing facts to knowing how to meet the patient in a relationship.

Relationships based on mutual respect and caring lead to healing. The envelopment of genuinely caring for patients provides nurses with a unique power that is both modest and wise. Benner (1984) identified six qualities of powers associated with nurses' caring: transformative power, integrative caring, advocacy, healing power, participative/affirmative power, and problem solving. Nurses' humility concerning this power may cause them to mute their voices, especially as novices and advanced beginners. In contrast, APNs have a matured sense of power, with accompanying opportunities to utilize that influence in ways that benefit the individual patient and society as a whole.

Benner's contributions have been subjected to critiques and inspired debate. Altmann (2007) proposed that Benner's work best represents a philosophy, rather than a testable theory. She referred to it as "seminal qualitative research which lays the foundation for understanding nursing expertise and skill acquisition" (p. 122). Quick to acknowledge the value of Benner's work, Altmann aimed to put the model into its place as a support for nursing, education, practice, and research.

In a lengthy debate, English (1993), Darbyshire (1994), and Paley (1996) presented their perspectives on the value of Benner's model. First, English (1993) questioned Benner's definition of intuition and what he perceived as the ambiguity of the expert role. He proposed that intuition be redefined in cognitive terms—using cognitive psychology models of memory to give clearer explanations. English questioned the claim that not all nurses could be experts and called for ways to test Benner's claims.

In a response, Darbyshire (1994) criticized English for an apparent ignorance of the interpretive phenomenological method. Defending Benner vigorously, Darbyshire addressed several of English's comments, including the notion that Benner's work was "denigrating to nurses." Arguing the contrary position, Darbyshire cited evidence of empowerment and guidance for nurses in various fields.

In 1996, Paley replied to the previous opinions and focused on the rift between positivist science and interpretive phenomenology. He advised releasing both absolutist views and moving beyond the divisive rhetoric. According to Paley (1996), attention should be given instead to the study and understanding of contemporary philosophy; we should learn about "recent philosophy of science and put that to work" (p. 671).

Application of the Novice-to-Expert Model

Benner's work finds relevance in a multitude of situations. Robert, Tilley, and Petersen (2014) espoused Benner's model as context for developing a concept analysis on nursing intuition. They looked at the power of intuition in decision making, particularly among novice nurses (2014).

The novice-to-expert model is frequently used in the development of mentorship programs (Dracup & Bryan-Brown, 2004; Nedd, Galindo-Ciocon, & Belgrave, 2006; Wolak, McCann, & Madigan, 2008). As collaborations between academia and practice partners expand, the framework has been used to guide preceptor workshops (Clipper & Cherry, 2015; Schaubhut & Gentry, 2010) and specialty training (Gregory, Bolling, & Langston, 2014). Agencies adopted this model to develop career ladders and guide practice in field settings (Marble, 2009; Murphy, 2005) and to inform technology in the implementation of clinical decision support systems in nursing practice (Courtney, Alexander, & Demiris, 2008). Others have applied Benner's learning paradigm in evaluating simulation learning, an exploding area of nursing education and practice, in specialty nursing areas (Inch, 2013; Thomas, 2015).

Benner's work has also been used to develop new understanding of what constitutes advanced nursing practice (Christensen, 2011). Integrating pattern recognition, a focus of

Benner for the expert, to the traditional *knowing-how and knowing-that* framework, posits an alternate way to better define advanced nursing knowledge (Christensen, 2011). As nurse practitioner specialties expand and area-specific competencies are required, Benner has given specialty organizations a meaningful way to describe and detail the categories of expertise development (Cates et al., 2015; Quallich, Bumpus, & Lajiness, 2015).

Most recently, Benner partnered with researchers from the Department of Veterans Affairs to describe needs of wounded service members from the Iraq and Afghanistan wars (Kelley, Kenny, Gordon, & Benner, 2016). They used interpretive and relational research methods espoused throughout Benner's impressive career. Different kinds of injuries, battlefield intervention, rapid transport, and technology in contemporary military conflicts have given rise to a new patient population requiring new nursing knowledge and care. Consequently, the role of the nurse case manager has evolved to effectively and holistically meet the needs of wounded service members, including assistance with reentry to civilian living, life coaching, and family support (Kelley et al., 2016).

Nursing education has weaved Benner's work into curriculum development, faculty evaluation, faculty mentorship, clinical reasoning and decision making, and APN preparation (Carlson, Crawford, & Contrades, 1989; Field, 1987; Hawkins & Fontenot, 2009; Koharchik, Caputi, Robb, & Culleiton, 2015). Latham and Fahey (2006) used the model for APN role self-assessment. Through activities of reflection, APN students were guided to identify their point of view about where they were on the novice-to-expert continuum. Students recognized that some characteristics of the novice were dominant as they "began again" in preparation for their new APN role. Faculty used the students' baseline as a place of understanding and mapped their plan for growth. Furthermore, faculty emphasized the emotional feelings and educational needs of the APN students at each level of competency. In response to the rise in doctor of nursing practice (DNP) programs, competency development has been a major aspect of supporting master's-prepared nurses to transition into their new roles (Purdue & Roberts, 2014).

THE AMERICAN ASSOCIATION OF CRITICAL-CARE NURSES SYNERGY MODEL FOR PATIENT CARE

A second model for understanding and guiding practice, specifically in the critical care area, is the American Association of Critical-Care Nurses (AACN) Synergy Model for Patient Care. The AACN aimed to identify patient and family characteristics that drive the competencies nurses bring to the bedside. The model suggests that when nurse competencies match patient needs, the nurse and patient co-create synergy and foster optimal practice outcomes (AACN, n.d.). For example, a patient with complex needs requires a highly competent nurse. When that pairing exists, the best patient outcomes become possible.

The process started with the AACN's assumptions that critical care nurses bring a unique skill set to the bedside and that the whole of critical care nursing is greater than the sum of its parts (i.e., critical care tasks). Hardin (2013) described the timeline for this model's development as beginning in the 1990s with AACN's goal to find a model that moved the nurse beyond a task list. By 2000, five assumptions of the model were realized, followed by four additional assumptions in 2003. Currently, nine assumptions underlie the Synergy Model (Becker, Kaplow, Muenzen, & Hartigan, 2006):

1. A patient is a holistic entity who is at a particular developmental stage and must be considered as a whole (body, mind, spirit) being.
2. The patient, family, and community provide a context for the nurse–patient relationship.
3. Patients can be described by a variety of characteristics, which are connected and contribute to one another; they cannot be looked at in isolation.
4. Nurses can be described on a number of dimensions. The interrelated dimensions paint a profile of the nurse.
5. A goal of nursing is to restore each patient to an optimal level of wellness as defined by the patient. Death can be an acceptable outcome, where the nurse helps move a patient toward a peaceful end-of-life experience.
6. Nurses create the care environment, and the environment affects what a nurse can do.
7. Impact areas are interrelated, and the nature of that interrelatedness may change as a function of experience, situation, or setting changes.
8. Nurses may work to optimize outcomes for patients, their families, healthcare providers, and the healthcare system.
9. Nurses bring their background to each situation, including their education/knowledge and skills/experience.

Early in the model's development, a think tank identified six quality outcomes related to nursing: patient and family satisfaction, rate of adverse incidents, complication rate, adherence to discharge plan, mortality rate, and length of stay (Hardin, 2013). Outcomes derived from the patients include functional changes, behavioral changes, trust, satisfaction, comfort, and quality of life. Those derived from nursing include physiological changes, complications, and the extent to which treatment objectives were met. Finally, outcomes from the healthcare system include readmission rate, length of stay, and cost utilization per case (Curley, 1998). The Synergy Model was found to be congruent with these patient, nursing, and system outcomes (Hardin & Kaplow, 2005).

The AACN Synergy Model includes 16 concepts: 8 nurse characteristics and 8 patient characteristics (Hardin, 2013). The nurse characteristics are delineated into levels of expertise ranging from novice (1) to expert (5). Similarly, the patient characteristics range from the worst patient state (1) to the best patient state (5). Definitions for levels 2 and 4 remain undetermined. (See **Table 21-1** and **Table 21-2**.)

The AACN Synergy Model for Patient Care is relationship focused. For example, nurses construct the patient and nurse relationship by identifying patient needs and matching them

Table 21-1   Characteristics of Patients in the AACN Synergy Model for Patient Care

Characteristic	Definition	Levels
Resiliency	Capacity to return to restorative level of functioning using compensatory or coping mechanisms	1. *Minimal:* unable to mount a response, failure of compensatory/coping mechanisms, minimal reserves, brittle 3. *Moderate:* able to mount a moderate response, able to initiate some degree of compensation, moderate reserves 5. *High:* able to mount and maintain a response, intact compensatory/coping mechanisms, strong reserves, endurance
Vulnerability	Susceptibility to actual or potential stressors that may adversely affect patient outcomes	1. *High:* susceptible; unprotected, fragile 3. *Moderate:* somewhat susceptible; somewhat protected 5. *Minimal:* safe; out of the woods; protect fragile others
Stability	Ability to maintain a steady-state equilibrium	1. *Minimal:* labile; unstable; unresponsive to therapies; high risk of death 3. *Moderate:* able to maintain steady state for limited period of time; some responsiveness to therapies 5. *High:* constant; responsive to therapies; low risk of death
Complexity	Intricate entanglement of two or more systems	1. *High:* intricate; complex patient/family dynamics; ambiguous/vague; atypical presentation 3. *Moderate:* moderately involved patient/family dynamics 5. *Minimal:* straightforward; routine patient/family dynamics; simple/clear cut; typical presentation
Resource availability	Extent of resource that the patient, family, and community bring to the situation	1. *Few resources:* necessary knowledge, skills, financial support not available; minimal personal/psychological supportive resources; few social systems resources 3. *Moderate resources:* limited knowledge, skills, financial support available; limited personal/psychological supportive resources; limited social systems resources

Table 21-1   Characteristics of Patients in the AACN Synergy Model for Patient Care (*Continued*)

Characteristic	Definition	Levels
		5. *Many resources:* extensive knowledge and skills available and accessible; financial resources readily available; strong personal/psychological supportive resources; strong social systems resources
Participation in care	Extent to which the patient and family engage in aspects of care	1. *No participation:* patient and family unable or unwilling to participate in care 3. *Moderate level of participation:* patient and family need assistance in care 5. *Full participation:* patient and family fully able to participate in care
Participation in decision making	Extent to which the patient and family engage in decision making	1. *No participation:* patient and family have no capacity for decision-making; requires surrogacy 3. *Moderate level of participation:* patient and family have limited capacity; seeks input/advice from others in decision-making 5. *Full participation:* patient and family have capacity, and makes decision for self
Predictability	Characteristic that allows one to expect a certain course of events or course of illness	1. *Not predictable:* uncertain; uncommon patient population/illness; unusual or unexpected course; does not follow critical pathway, or no critical pathway developed 3. *Moderate:* wavering; occasionally noted patient population or illness 5. *High:* certain; common patient population/illness; usual and expected course; follows critical pathway

Reproduced from http://www.aacn.org/WD/Certifications/Content/synmodel.pcms. Reprinted by permission of American Association of Colleges of Nursing.

with nursing competencies. The relationships between nurses are also important. A healthy connection allows for improved teamwork and maximized use of personnel to enhance patient safety. Finally, the nurse and healthcare system relationship allows for analysis of the political, economic, and financial realities of health care. The synergy created from these relationships positions the patient, nurse, and healthcare system for optimal clinical outcomes.

Table 21-2 Characteristics of Nurses in the AACN Synergy Model for Patient Care

Characteristic	Definition	Level 1 (Novice)	Level 3 (Competent)	Level 5 (Expert)
Clinical Judgment	Clinical reasoning, which includes clinical decision making, critical thinking, and a global grasp of the situation, coupled with nursing skills acquired through a process of integrating formal and informal experiential knowledge and evidence-based guidelines	Collects basic-level data; follows algorithms, decision trees, and protocols with all populations and is uncomfortable deviating from them; matches formal knowledge with clinical event to make decisions; questions the limits of one's ability to make clinical decisions and delegates the decision making to other clinicians; includes extraneous detail	Collects and interprets complex patient data; makes clinical judgments on the basis of an immediate grasp of the whole picture for common or routine patient populations; recognizes patterns and trends that may predict the direction of illness; recognizes limits and seeks appropriate help; focuses on key elements of case while sorting out extraneous details	Synthesizes and interprets multiple, sometimes conflicting, sources of data; makes judgment on the basis of an immediate grasp of the whole picture, unless working with new patient populations; uses past experiences to anticipate problems; helps patient and family see the *big picture*; recognizes the limits of clinical judgment and seeks multidisciplinary collaboration and consultation with comfort; recognizes and responds to the dynamic situation
Advocacy and Moral Agency	Working on another's behalf and representing the concerns of the patient/family and nursing staff; serving as a moral agent in identifying and helping to resolve ethical and clinical concerns within and outside the clinical setting	Works on behalf of patient; self-assesses personal values; aware of ethical conflicts/issues that may surface in clinical setting; makes ethical/moral decisions on the basis of rules; represents patient when the patient cannot represent self; aware of patients' rights	Works on behalf of patient and family; considers patient values and incorporates in care, even when differing from personal values; supports colleagues in ethical and clinical issues; moral decision making can deviate from rules; demonstrates give and take with patient's family,	Works on behalf of patient, family, and community; advocates from patient/family perspective, whether similar to or different from personal values; advocates ethical conflict and issues from patient/family perspective; suspends rules—patient and family drive moral decision making; empowers

		allowing them to speak/represent themselves when possible; aware of patient and family rights	the patient and family to speak for/represent themselves; achieves mutuality within patient/professional relationships
Caring Practices	Nursing activities that create a compassionate, supportive, and therapeutic environment for patients and staff, with the aim of promoting comfort and healing and preventing unnecessary suffering. Includes, but is not limited to, vigilance, engagement, and responsiveness of caregivers, including family and healthcare personnel	Focuses on the usual and customary needs of the patient; no anticipation of future needs; bases care on standards and protocols; maintains a safe physical environment; acknowledges death as a potential outcome	Responds to subtle patient and family changes; engages with the patient as a unique patient in a compassionate manner; recognizes and tailors caring practices to the individuality of patient and family; domesticates the patient's and family's environment; recognizes that death may be an acceptable outcome	Has astute awareness and anticipates patient and family changes and needs; fully engaged with and sensing how to stand alongside the patient, family, and community; caring practices follow the patient and family lead; anticipates hazards and avoids them, and promotes safety throughout patient's and family's transitions along the healthcare continuum; orchestrates the process that ensures the patient's and family's comfort and concerns surrounding issues of death and dying are met

(Continues)

Table 21-2 Characteristics of Nurses in the AACN Synergy Model for Patient Care (Continued)

Characteristic	Definition	Level 1 (Novice)	Level 3 (Competent)	Level 5 (Expert)
Collaboration	Working with others in a way that promotes/ encourages each person's contributions toward achieving optimal/ realistic patient/family goals. Involves intra- and interdisciplinary work with colleagues and community	Willing to be taught, coached, and/or mentored; participates in team meetings and discussions regarding patient care and/ or practice issues; open to various team members' contributions	Seeks opportunities to be taught, coached, and/or mentored; elicits others' advice and perspectives; initiates and participates in team meetings and discussions regarding patient care and/or practice issues; recognizes and suggests various team members' participation	Seeks opportunities to teach, coach, and mentor and to be taught, coached, and mentored; facilitates active involvement and complementary contributions of others in team meetings and discussions regarding patient care and/or practice issues; involves/recruits diverse resources when appropriate to optimize patient outcomes
Systems Thinking	Body of knowledge and tools that allow the nurse to manage whatever environmental and system resources exist for the patient/family and staff, within or across healthcare and non-healthcare systems	Uses a limited array of strategies; limited outlook—sees the pieces or components; does not recognize negotiation as an alternative; sees patient and family within the isolated environment of the unit; sees self as key resource	Develops strategies on the basis of needs and strengths of patient/ family; able to make connections within components; sees opportunity to negotiate but may not have strategies; developing a view of the patient/ family transition process; recognizes how to obtain resources beyond self	Develops, integrates, and applies a variety of strategies that are driven by the needs and strengths of the patient/family; global or holistic outlook—sees the whole rather than the pieces; knows when and how to negotiate and navigate through the system on behalf of patients and families; anticipates needs of patients and families as they move through the healthcare system; utilizes untapped and alternative resources as necessary

Response to Diversity	Sensitivity to recognize, appreciate, and incorporate differences into the provision of care. Differences may include, but are not limited to, cultural differences, spiritual beliefs, gender, race, ethnicity, lifestyle, socioeconomic status, wage, and values	Assesses cultural diversity; provides care on the basis of own belief system; learns the culture of the healthcare environment	Inquires about cultural differences and considers their impact on care; accommodates personal and professional differences in the plan of care; helps patient/family understand the culture of the healthcare system	Responds to, anticipates, and integrates cultural differences into patient/family care; appreciates and incorporates differences, including alternative therapies, into care; tailors healthcare culture, to the extent possible, to meet the diverse needs and strengths of the patient/family
Facilitation of Learning	Ability to facilitate learning for patients/families, nursing staff, other members of the healthcare team, and community. Includes both formal and informal facilitation of learning	Follows planned educational programs; sees patient/family education as a separate task from delivery of care; provides data without seeking to assess patient's readiness or understanding; has limited knowledge of the totality of the educational needs; focuses on a nurse's perspective; sees the patient as a passive recipient	Adapts planned educational programs; begins to recognize and integrate different ways of teaching into delivery of care; incorporates patient's understanding into practice; sees the overlapping of educational plans from different healthcare providers' perspectives; begins to see the patient as having input into goals; begins to see individualism	Creatively modifies or develops patient/family education programs; integrates patient/family education throughout delivery of care; evaluates patient's understanding by observing behavior changes related to learning; is able to collaborate and incorporate all healthcare providers' and educational plans into the patient/family educational program; sets patient-driven goals for education; sees patient/family as having choices and consequences that are negotiated in relation to education

Reproduced from http://www.aacn.org/WD/Certifications/Content/synmodel.pcms. Reprinted by permission of American Association of Colleges of Nursing.

Application of the AACN Synergy Model

Since its inception, the AACN Synergy Model has been widely used in critical care areas. Becker and colleagues (2006), for example, surveyed acute care nurse practitioners (NPs) and clinical nurse specialists (CNSs) using an instrument based on the Synergy Model and found distinct contributions by each group to critical care nursing. CNS participants were more evenly engaged in clinical judgment, caring practices, facilitation of learning, and clinical inquiry. By comparison, the NP participants concentrated the majority of their activities on clinical judgment and advocacy actions (Becker et al., 2006).

Wysong and Driver (2009) used the AACN Synergy Model to assess patients' perceptions of nurses' skill. Patients' comments regarding nurses' skill fit well with seven of the eight nurse characteristics/competencies delineated in the Synergy Model. Clinical inquiry was not recognized by any of the patients. In contrast, nurses' caring practices were identified as the most important trait of a skilled nurse; all patients identified this factor as important. In the words of Wysong and Driver (2009), "Friendly nurses seem like they know everything" (p. 34).

Vulnerability, including hearing loss, of older adults has been the focus of scholarly work (Hardin, 2012, 2015). One of the eight patient characteristics in the AACN Synergy Model, vulnerability refers to one's susceptibility to stressors that may negatively impact patient outcomes. Older adults, a growing population, experience greater vulnerability in critical care units. The Synergy Model provides guidance for nurses caring for these individuals (Hardin, 2012, 2015).

Other uses of the model include development of a nursing productivity system in critical care units (Kohr, Hickey, & Curley, 2012). Also, critical care preceptor/orientation programs based on the competencies and measured by nursing satisfaction have been effective (Welch & Austin, 2008). Patient satisfaction, likewise, was studied through direct and indirect connections of the nurse and patient characteristics (Tejero, 2012). Nurse–patient bonding played a mediating role in relations between patient predictability and patient satisfaction, as well as nurse facilitation of learning and patient satisfaction (2012). Brewer and colleagues (2007) tested a case report form based on the model in a population of adult and pediatric patients. Results showed that the form was internally consistent, and nurses who were unskilled in use of the tool were able to use it to assess patients without difficulty (2007). Kelleher (2006) applied the AACN Synergy Model to patient care assessment and the critical care nurse's personal reflection of the assessment.

In the critical care unit, Smith (2006) applied the AACN Synergy Model to address spirituality. One underlying assumption of the model is that the patient is a holistic being, including a spiritual dimension. Smith identified four areas of the model related to spiritual character: two patient characteristics—resiliency and resources; and two nurse characteristics—caring practices and response to diversity. Smith suggested the model could be used to organize and guide five nursing interventions:

1. *Caring practices:* Accurately identify spiritual needs.
2. *Response to diversity:* Make congruent matches.
3. *Support resiliency:* Make appropriate referrals.
4. *Support resiliency:* Make space and time for group and individual religious rituals and spiritual practices.
5. *Support resource availability:* Make connections between patients and their spiritual support systems (p. 45).

Smith concluded that more research on spiritual care, particularly the frequency and monitoring of spiritual assessments, is needed. Furthermore, the AACN Synergy Model provides a basis for that examination (Smith, 2006).

The AACN model has also been examined outside the critical care setting. Medical-surgical nurses care for many highly complex patients. Carter and Burnette (2011) developed assessment tools for nursing competence and patient acuity based on the Synergy Model, with positive results. Cox and Galante (2003) incorporated the AACN Synergy Model in a masters-level curriculum preparing critical care nurse specialists. Cox (2003) described its use by CNSs to care for victims of intimate-partner violence. In an outpatient congestive heart failure (CHF) clinic, Hardin and Hussey (2003) reviewed the model's applicability to a CHF patient case study. These researchers looked at the patient characteristics as existing along a continuum, just as the nursing competencies can be placed on a continuum. Because the patient characteristics change with the patient's condition, the nurse recognizes that nursing competencies must change to maintain synergy and optimal patient outcomes. Hardin and Hussey (2003) commented that critical care patients are often cared for outside hospital walls, and the model's flexibility allows it to be appropriately applied with various patient populations in nontraditional settings.

Other applications of the model have drawn on the patient and nurse characteristics as a discussion guide in nursing rounds (Mullen, 2002). Swickard, Swickard, Reimer, Lindell, and Winkelman (2014) used the AACN Synergy Model as theoretical support in the development of a new tool to facilitate transfer of patients between hospitals. To optimize safe and effective transfers, the instrument is used to match nurse competencies with specific patient needs during critical care transport (Swickard et al., 2014). Curley (1998) is credited with a classic report on the AACN Synergy Model for Patient Care and its use in optimizing patient outcomes. In Curley's foundational work, the characteristics and competencies are amply described. Case studies and questions for certification examination review are also included. Curley outlined the model's contribution of providing defined nurse characteristics/competencies and patient characteristics/needs and explained how the *best fit* of these characteristics can lead to the best possible patient outcomes. As the fundamental principle, the patient's needs drive the nurse's competencies. Thus, the AACN Synergy Model holds the promise of opening new dialogue across many settings and disciplines (Curley, 1998; Pope, 2002).

RELATIONSHIP-BASED CARE: A MODEL FOR TRANSFORMING PRACTICE

As in the two models previously discussed, Koloroutis (2004) posited that relationships are central to optimal nursing care. The Relationship-Based Care (RBC) Model consists of six core components: leadership, teamwork, professional nursing practice, patient care delivery system, resources, and outcomes measurement. The patient and family are at the center of all of the components.

Three crucial relationships make up the RBC Model: (1) the care provider's relationship with patients/families, (2) the care provider's relationship with self, and (3) the care provider's relationship with colleagues. The nurse patient relationship is the bond that forms the core of the healing environment. The second relationship, nurse to self, is often overlooked but remains critical to the nurse's ability to form a relationship with the patient. Caring for oneself may be seen as selfish, and by strict definition, it is. However, selfishness or a focus on self, is a "health-full" endeavor that cannot be foregone. Restoring oneself is a precursor to aiding in the restoration of others. The third relationship is between the nurse and the healthcare system. This broader community operates best when the first two relationships are strong and vital. The interdependence of all three relationships propels us toward optimal healthcare outcomes. A caring and healing environment is the context for these relationships and the way in which RBC thrives. (See **Table 21-3**.)

We experience the essence of care in the moment when one human being connects to another. When compassion and care are conveyed through touch, through a kind act, through competent clinical interventions, or through listening and seeking to understand the other's experience, a healing relationship is created. This is the heart of RBC (Koloroutis, 2004, p. 5)

In the preface to Koloroutis's book, Jean Watson identified three requirements for transformation: leaders committed to change, an organization's adoption of a way to change, and clear communication of goals (Koloroutis, 2004, p. vii). Watson went on to say that these three things combine with the 12 basic value assumptions of the model (see **Table 21-4**) to guide the transformative process. Together, they change what is current into something new.

Koloroutis (2004) defined four elements for transforming the patient care delivery environment: I_1 = inspiration, I_2 = infrastructure, E_1 = education, and E_2 = evidence. When these elements work in sync, as evidenced by the formula (I_2E_2), they simplify the process of engaging people to enjoy success while continuing to change the care environment.

Table 21-3   Key Elements of the Relationship-Based Care Model

Key Element	Description
Leadership	Leaders exist at all levels of an organization. Leaders create caring cultures that are healing. Leaders know the vision, model it, take action toward it, and support others to fulfill it. Leaders solve problems.
Outcomes measurement	RBC has a positive impact on patient outcomes. Data are meaningful and motivational. Achieving outcomes requires planning, periodic assessment of measured outcomes, and perseverance.
Resources	Nursing staff and managers share responsibility for resources—their acquisition, judicious use, and appropriate management. Effective use of resources requires critical and creative thinking. The resources needed for practice are determined by the nurse–patient relationship.
Patient care delivery	The system provides support for caregivers in collegial relationships. Professional development is encouraged and supported. Patient care delivery is organized and driven by the nurse–patient relationship.
Professional nursing	The nurse–patient relationship is sacred and the basis for professional nursing. The nurse has a social responsibility and is accountable for working within the scope of practice. The nurse has six practice roles—sentry, guide, healer, collaborator, teacher, and leader. Effective nursing practice requires an understanding of the human condition. Caring is the essence of professional nursing.
Teamwork	Teamwork is a predictor of quality patient care. Diverse interdisciplinary members share a common purpose and work toward that aim. All members contribute. Group energy and interdependence lead to excellent patient care delivery and outcomes.

Reproduced from Koloroutis, M. (Ed.). (2004). *Relationship-based care: A model for transforming practice.* Minneapolis, MN: Creative Health Care Management. Used with permission. © Creative Health Care Management. www.chcm.com.

Table 21-4 Twelve Basic Value Assumptions of the Relationship-Based Care Model

1. The meaning and essence of care are experienced in the moment when one human being connects with another.
2. Feeling connected to one another creates harmony and healing; feeling isolated destroys spirit.
3. Each and every member of an organization, in all disciplines and departments, has a valuable contribution to make.
4. The relationship between patients and their families and members of the clinical team belongs at the heart of care delivery.
5. Care providers' knowledge of self and self-care are fundamental requirements for quality care and healthy interpersonal relationships.
6. Healthy relationships among members of the healthcare team lead to the delivery of quality care and result in high levels of patient, physician, and staff satisfaction.
7. People are most satisfied when their roles and daily work practices are in alignment with their personal and professional values—when they know they are making a positive difference for patients, families, and their colleagues.
8. The value of relationships in patient care must be understood, valued, and agreed to by all members of the healthcare organization.
9. A therapeutic relationship between a patient/family and a professional nurse is essential to quality patient care.
10. Patient experiences improve measurably when staff members "own" their practice and know that they are valued for their contributions.
11. People willingly change when they are inspired and share a common vision, when an infrastructure is implemented to support the new ways of working, when relevant education is provided for personal and professional development, and when they see evidence of the success of the new plan.
12. Transformational change happens one relationship at a time.

Reproduced from Koloroutis, M. (Ed.). (2004). *Relationship-based care: A model for transforming practice.* Minneapolis, MN: Creative Health Care Management. Used with permission. © Creative Health Care Management. www.chcm.com.

- *Inspiration* promotes movement, a "drawing forth" within an organization. People are valued and consequently inspired. Patient-centered care inspires others.
- *Infrastructure* refers to the practices, systems, and processes through which vision is achieved. It is the foundation that allows change to occur.
- *Education* promotes competence, confidence, and personal commitment. An assumption is made that people want to do a good job. Personal growth and professional development are inseparable.
- *Evidence* indicates that change has happened and is viable within the organization. Evidence then links back to inspiration: Seeing results inspires further investment in the transformation process.

Leaders, such as APNs, need to know and follow the five conditions for I_2E_2 to work. Specifically, they need to meet the following criteria: (1) clarity, know where they are going; (2) competence, know expectations and have support to acquire the skills needed to meet those expectations; (3) confidence, believe that one possesses necessary knowledge and skills; (4) collaboration, work together toward a common goal; and (5) commitment, each person makes contributions, takes ownership, and collaborates with others. When leaders ensure the existence of these five conditions, goals are achieved. In this way, RBC provides the chance to clarify roles, responsibilities, authority, and accountability in APNs' work. This model includes individual and collective proficiency, clinical skills, critical/creative thinking, and interpersonal skills. It is the "essence of leadership at the point of care" (Dingman, 2005, p. 136).

A founder of the movement toward primary care nursing, Marie Manthey discussed her view of RBC in a 2006 interview (Manthey & Lewis-Hunstiger, 2006). Manthey viewed RBC as a return to nursing's roots in primary care. Using the start of the first Nightingale schools in 1873 as a beginning point, she noted that nurses did not work in hospitals for the first 60 years of nursing's existence. Instead, student nurses worked in hospitals with a registered nurse as director of both the nursing school and the nursing service. Citing the 1920 census, Manthey explained that during that time, 80% of registered nurses worked as independent practitioners (fee-for-service caregivers in homes), 10% ran hospitals, and 10% were in public health. During the Great Depression, however, nurses needed work and exchanged their services for room and board in hospitals. That pattern continued until 1968, with the advent of professional primary care nursing based on the nurse–patient relationship.

In the 1990s, economic pressures replaced primary nursing with "team" nursing. Manthey and Lewis-Hunstiger (2006) referred to this approach as "FRED—Frantically Running Every Day" (p. 7). In contrast, RBC is a hopeful response to FRED. RBC calls APNs back to the concepts of responsibility, accountability, and authority. These principles of decentralized nursing departments must also apply to APNs' personal lives. Being in the right relationship with ourselves includes the knowledge that we have the choice to think, feel, and act in certain ways.

Three kinds of thinking are inherent in RBC (Manthey & Koloroutis, 2004):

1. *Critical thinking:* systematic; multidimensional; sees what is there and what is not; includes critical feeling; involves humility in choosing what to do
2. *Creative thinking:* questions what the day will look like; encourages tolerance of ambiguity
3. *Reflective thinking:* time and space to pause; silence for reflection and to rejuvenate

To date, critical thinking has garnered the most significant attention and inspired the most debate. Creative thinking, by comparison, has remained largely out of the spotlight. Critics claim that creative thinking takes too much time, when in truth, sitting at the bedside with a patient to discuss how the patient envisions the day takes only a moment. Reflective thinking, although desirable and pursued, is difficult to do in most work environments. Places of calm, quiet, and solemnity do not exist for most nurses in the workplace. Traveling to and from work provides some opportunity for reflection but is often jumbled with thoughts of tasks—to do, done, and left undone (Manthey & Koloroutis, 2004).

RBC provides a systems framework where one cares for patients, self, and others. In this setting, positive outcomes (e.g., clinical safety, clinical quality, satisfaction, recruitment and retention, high morale, and achievement of goals) become possible. The potential for these outcomes has led to the adoption of RBC as a model of nursing care (Beaty, 2006).

Application of the Relationship-Based Care Model

Patient engagement starts with RBC; consequently, discussions about patient engagement and satisfaction are critical in our changing healthcare system and evolving compensation standards (Guglielmi, 2014). Focused on caring, the RBC Model has been the framework to support a plethora of introspective actions by nursing groups across the country (Carabetta, Lombardo, & Kline, 2013; Winsett & Hauck, 2011; Woolley et al., 2012). RBC is a natural fit to support the Magnet journey (Guanci, 2016).

Maklebust and Suchy (2007) implemented the RBC Model in a comprehensive cancer center and used it in practical ways. Job descriptions were rewritten to reflect caring behaviors. Nurses sat with patients to identify mutual goals. Staff names and goals were written on whiteboards in patient rooms. Shift report began to include communication of patient goals and preferences. Around the center, posters with pictures of staff demonstrating RBC actions were displayed. Weekly continuing education offerings were conducted to inform and inspire the staff. Authors reported wide acceptance of the model with improved patient and nurse satisfaction (Maklebust & Suchy, 2007).

RBC has also been used as an intervention of caring. An instructional intervention was developed from the RBC Model to improve work environment and caring (Nelson, Tinker, & Smith, 2013). Another unique application of this primary nursing care model was in a pediatric hematology and oncology unit. After evaluation of the current care model, the importance of care continuity and meaningful nurse–patient relationships were of highest value (Nadeau, Pinner, Murphy, & Belderson, 2016).

Notably, staffing patterns, reduced lengths of patient stays, and technology-saturated systems may threaten the continuity of the nurse–patient relationship that is central to RBC. To overcome these obstacles, we must remember as nurses that being present with the patient is not necessarily a time-intensive activity. As we perform tasks, we can connect with the patient. We can exchange ideas. We can listen to the patient's perspective (Manthey & Lewis-Hunstiger, 2006).

Nurse educators are challenged to move beyond the mere teaching of time assessment and management. In the past, we have focused on thinking critically but have largely ignored the need to articulate that thinking to others. Now, however, we must recognize that we need to teach students to prioritize and to articulate their rationale for prioritizing and meeting needs.

The reality of practice is that the nurse's time must be balanced between needs, priorities, and resources. The two factors that drive nursing's work are orders and patient acuity. We do not have time to do everything. Inexperienced nurses do not prioritize and may let things fall off the list; whereas, experienced nurses prioritize and manage detailed responsibilities (Benner, 1984; Manthey & Lewis-Hunstiger, 2006). Nurses need to find a way to reconcile not getting everything done. We have to release the tendency to see ourselves as victims and begin to espouse a long-term perspective. The RBC culture represents a step in that direction. In adopting its tenets, it would behoove APNs to remember that nursing is licensed by society to make prioritization judgments.

SUMMARY

Each model described in this chapter guides us back to a fundamental of nursing: the relationship between nurse and patient. The rare trust this connection embodies began with the inception of nursing and thrives today in all settings and populations. Our professional and personal responsibility is to invest in that relationship, using a variety of skills and competencies (see **Box 21-1**). When promoting house sales, realtors often say the most critical factors are "Location, location, location." In the sacred profession of nursing, our cornerstone is "Relationships, relationships, relationships." Let us guard that prize with all of our being.

Box 21-1   APN Skills and Competencies Undergirding Trust in the Nurse–Patient Relationship
• APNs have expertise owing to their numerous interactions with patients in various settings over time. The continuum of the expert (Benner, 1984) can serve as a guide for the roles and responsibilities of the APN.   • APNs have the opportunity and responsibility to guide neophyte nurses in clinical teaching.   • APNs need to read about and understand the debates related to models of practice. At the same time, they must avoid becoming so engaged in the weeds (rhetoric) that they lose the view from the trees (holistic perspective).   • APNs are leaders in the establishment and growth of nurse–patient relationships.   • APNs strengthen nurse–nurse relationships by responsible use of personnel.   • APNs are expected to engage in politics and the economics of the nurse–system relationship.   • Leading by example, APNs model friendliness and a sense of competence that reassures their patients, colleagues, and society.

DISCUSSION QUESTIONS

1. Using Benner's novice-to-expert model, how would you, as an APN, respond to a nurse with limited clinical experience who comes to you for professional guidance?
2. As an APN, which practice areas do you see as favorable for adoption of the AACN Synergy Model? How would you lead in that effort?
3. Describe what Relationship-Based Care (RBC) would look like in your area of advanced nursing practice. In that setting, how would you measure outcomes at the nurse-to-patient, nurse-to-nurse, and nurse-to-system levels?

REFERENCES

Altmann, T. K. (2007). An evaluation of the seminal work of Patricia Benner: Theory or philosophy? *Contemporary Nurse, 25*(1–2), 114–123.

American Association of Critical-Care Nurses. (n.d). The AACN Synergy Model for Patient Care. Retrieved from http://www.aacn.org/WD/Certifications/Content/synmodel.pcms

Beaty, B. (2006). Relationship-based care: A true evolution of primary nursing. *Creative Nursing, 12*(1), 3.

Becker, D., Kaplow, R., Muenzen, P. M., & Hartigan, C. (2006). Activities performed by acute and critical care advanced practice nurses: American Association of Critical-Care Nurses study of practice. *American Journal of Critical Care, 15*, 130–148.

Benner, P. (1984). *From novice to expert: Excellence and power in clinical nursing practice.* Menlo Park, CA: Addison-Wesley.

Benner, P. (1994). The tradition and skill of interpretive phenomenology in studying health, illness, and caring practices. In P. Benner (Ed.), *Interpretive phenomenology: Embodiment, caring, and ethics in health and illness* (pp. 99–127). Thousand Oaks, CA: Sage.

Benner, P., Hooper-Kyriakidis, P., & Stannard, D. (1999). *Clinical wisdom and interventions in critical care: A thinking-in-action approach.* Philadelphia, PA: Saunders.

Benner, P., & Wrubel, J. (1989). *The primacy of caring: Stress and coping in health and illness.* Menlo Park, CA: Addison-Wesley.

Brewer, B., Wojner-Alexandrov, A. W., Triola, N., Pacini, C., Cline, M., Rust, J. E., & Kerfoot, K. (2007). AACN Synergy Model's characteristics of patients: Psychometric analyses in a tertiary care health system. *American Journal of Critical Care, 16*, 158–167.

Brykczynski, K. A. (2006). Benner's philosophy in nursing practice. In M. R. Alligood & A. M. Tomey (Eds.), *Nursing theory: Utilization and application* (3rd ed., pp. 131–156). St. Louis, MO: Mosby-Elsevier.

Carabetta, M., Lombardo, K., & Kline, N. (2013). Implementing primary care in the perianesthesia setting using a Relationship-Based Care Model. *Journal of PeriAnesthesia Nursing, 28*, 16–20.

Carlson, L., Crawford, N., & Contrades, S. (1989). Nursing student novice to expert: Benner's research applied to education. *Journal of Nursing Education, 28*, 188–190.

Carter, K. F., & Burnette, H. D. (2011). Creating patient–nurse synergy on a medical-surgical unit. *MEDSURG Nursing, 20*, 249–254.

Cates, L. A., Bishop, S., Armentrout, D., Verklan, T., Arnold, J., & Doughty, C. (2015). Initial development of C.A.T.E.S.: A simulation-based competency assessment instrument for neonatal nurse practitioners. *Neonatal Network, 34,* 329–342.

Chinn, P. L., & Kramer, M. K. (2015). *Knowledge development in nursing* (9th ed.). St. Louis, MO: Elsevier-Mosby

Christensen, M. (2011). Advancing nursing practice: Redefining the theoretical and practical integration of knowledge. *Journal of Clinical Nursing, 20,* 873–881.

Clipper, B., & Cherry, B. (2015). From transition shock to competent practice: Developing preceptors to support new nurse transition. *Journal of Continuing Education in Nursing, 46,* 448–454.

Courtney, K. L., Alexander, G. L., & Demiris, G. (2008). Information technology from novice to expert: Implementation implications. *Journal of Nursing Management, 16,* 692–699.

Cox, C. W., & Galante, C. M. (2003). An MSN curriculum in preparation of CCNSs: A model for consideration. *Critical Care Nurse, 23*(6), 74–80.

Cox, E. (2003). Synergy in practice: Caring for victims of intimate partner violence. *Critical Care Nursing Quarterly, 26,* 323–330.

Curley, M. (1998). Patient–nurse synergy: Optimizing patients' outcomes. *American Journal of Critical Care, 7*(1), 64–72.

Darbyshire, P. (1994). Skilled expert practice: Is it "all in the mind"? A response to English's critique of Benner's novice to expert model. *Journal of Advanced Nursing, 19,* 755–761.

Dingman, S. (2005). A dialogue on relationship-based care: Reflection on practice. *International Journal for Human Caring, 9,* 136.

Dracup, K., & Bryan-Brown, C. W. (2004). From novice to expert to mentor: Shaping the future. *American Journal of Critical Care, 13,* 448–450.

English, I. (1993). Intuition as a function of the expert nurse: A critique of Benner's novice to expert model. *Journal of Advanced Nursing, 18,* 387–393.

Field, P. A. (1987). The impact of nursing theory on the clinical decision making process. *Journal of Advanced Nursing, 12,* 563–571.

Grace, P. J. (2006). Philosophies, models, and theories: Moral obligations. In M. R. Alligood & A. M. Tomey (Eds.), *Nursing theory: Utilization and application* (3rd ed., pp. 67–85). St. Louis, MO: Mosby-Elsevier.

Gregory, S., Bolling, D. R., & Langston, N. F. (2014). Partnerships and new learning models to create the future perioperative nursing workforce. *AORN Journal, 99,* 96–105.

Guanci, G. (2016). How relationship-based care supports the Magnet journey. *Nursing Management, 47*(1), 9–12.

Guglielmi, C. L. (2014). The growing role of patient engagement: Relationship-based care in a changing health care system. *AORN Journal, 99,* 517–528.

Hardin, S. R. (2012). Hearing loss in older critical care patients: Participation in decision making. *Critical Care Nurse, 32*(6), 43–50.

Hardin, S. R. (2013). The AACN Synergy Model. In S. J. Peterson & T. S. Bredow (Eds.), *Middle range theories: Application to nursing research* (3rd ed., pp. 294–305). Philadelphia, PA: Wolters Kluwer/Lippincott Williams & Wilkins.

Hardin, S. R. (2015). Vulnerability of older patients in critical care. *Critical Care Nurse, 35*(3), 55–61.

Hardin, S. R., & Hussey, L. (2003). AACN Synergy Model for Patient Care: Case study of a CHF patient. *Critical Care Nurse, 23*(1), 73–76.

Hardin, S. R., & Kaplow, R. (2005). *Synergy for clinical excellence: The AACN Synergy Model for Patient Care.* Sudbury, MA: Jones and Bartlett Publishers.

Hawkins, J. W., & Fontenot, H. (2009). What do you mean you want me to teach, do research, engage in service, and clinical practice? Views from the trenches: The novice and expert. *Journal of the American Academy of Nurse Practitioners, 21,* 358–361.

Inch, J. (2013). Perioperative simulation learning and post-registration development. *British Journal of Nursing, 22,* 1166–1172.

Kelleher, S. (2006). Providing patient-centered care in an intensive care unit. *Nursing Standard, 21*(13), 35–40.

Kelley, P. W., Kenny, D. J., Gordon, D. R., & Benner, P. (2015). The evolution of case management for service members injured in Iraq and Afghanistan. *Qualitative Health Research, 25,* 426–439.

Koharchik, L., Caputi, L., Robb, M., & Culleiton, A. L. (2015). Fostering clinical reasoning in nursing students. *American Journal of Nursing, 115,* 58–61.

Kohr, L. M., Hickey, P. A., & Curley, M. A. Q. (2012). Building a nursing productivity measure based on the Synergy Model: First steps. *American Journal of Critical Care, 21,* 420–431.

Koloroutis, M. (Ed.). (2004). *Relationship-based care: A model for transforming practice.* Minneapolis, MN: Creative Health Care Management.

Latham, C. L., & Fahey, L. J. (2006). Novice to expert advanced practice nurse role transition: Guided student self-reflection. *Journal of Nursing Education, 45*(1), 46–48.

Maklebust, J., & Suchy, S. (2007). Implementing relationship-based care in a comprehensive cancer center [Abstract]. *Oncology Nursing Forum, 34,* 571.

Manthey, M., & Koloroutis, M. (2004). Resource driven practice. In M. Koloroutis (Ed.), *Relationship-based care: A model for transforming practice* (pp. 183–214). Minneapolis, MN: Creative Health Care Management.

Manthey, M., & Lewis-Hunstiger, M. (2006). Relationship-based care: Customized primary nursing. *Creative Nursing, 12*(1), 4–11.

Marble, S. G. (2009). Five-step model of professional excellence. *Clinical Journal of Oncology Nursing, 13,* 310–315.

Mitre, J. C., Alexander, J. E., & Keller, S. L. (1998). Patricia Benner: From novice to expert: Excellence and power in clinical nursing practice. In A. M. Tomey & M. R. Alligood (Eds.), *Nursing theorists and their work* (4th ed., pp. 157–172). St. Louis, MO: Mosby.

Mullen, J. E. (2002). The Synergy Model in practice: The Synergy Model as a framework for nursing rounds. *Critical Care Nurse, 22*(6), 66–68.

Murphy, F. (2005). Preparing for the field: Developing competence as an ethnographic field worker. *Nurse Researcher, 12*(3), 52–60.

Nadeau, K., Pinner, K., Murphy, K., & Belderson, K. M. (2016). Perceptions of a primary nursing care model in a pediatric hematology/oncology unit. *Journal of Pediatric Oncology Nursing.* doi:1043454216631472

Nedd, N., Galindo-Ciocon, D., & Belgrave, G. (2006). Guided growth intervention: From novice to expert through a mentoring program. *Journal of Nursing Care Quality, 21*(1), 20–23.

Nelson, J., Tinker, A., & Smith, S. (2013). Relationship-based care as an intervention of caring for vulnerable adults in home care. *International Journal for Human Caring, 17*(2), 59–66.

Paley, J. (1996). Intuition and expertise: Comments on the Benner debate. *Journal of Advanced Nursing, 23,* 665–671.

Peterson, S., & Bredow, T. (2013). *Middle range theories: Application to nursing research* (3rd ed.). Philadelphia, PA: Lippincott, Williams, & Wilkins.

Pope, B. (2002). Working together to meet patient and family needs. *Nursing, 32*(7), 6–7.

Purdue, G., & Roberts, B. (2014). The doctor of nursing practice and role assimilation: Strategies for success. *Clinical Scholars Review, 7,* 109–113.

Quallich, S. A., Bumpus, S. M., & Lajiness, S. (2015). Competencies for the nurse practitioner working with adult urology patients. *Urologic Nursing, 35,* 221–230.

Robert, R. R., Tilley, D. S., & Petersen, S. (2014). A power in clinical nursing practice: Concept analysis on nursing intuition. *MEDSURG Nursing, 23,* 343–349.

Schaubhut, R. M., & Gentry, J. A. (2010). Nursing preceptor workshops: Partnership and collaboration between academia and practice. *The Journal of Continuing Education in Nursing, 41,* 155–160.

Smith, A. R. (2006). Using the Synergy Model to provide spiritual nursing care in critical care settings. *Critical Care Nurse, 26*(4), 41–47.

Swickard, S., Swickard, W., Reimer, A., Lindell, D., & Winkelman, C. (2014). Adaptation of the AACN Synergy Model for Patient Care to critical care transport. *Critical Care Nurse, 34,* 16–29.

Tejero, L. M. S. (2012). The mediating role of the nurse–patient dyad bonding in bringing about patient satisfaction. *Journal of Advanced Nursing, 68,* 994–1002.

Thomas, C. M. (2015). Developing a theory-based simulation educator resource. *Nursing Education Perspectives, 36,* 340–342.

Welch, S., & Austin, C. (2008). Development of an ICU preceptor program based on the AACN Synergy Model for Patient Care [Abstract]. *Critical Care Nurse, 28*(2), e6.

Winsett, R. P., & Hauck, S. (2011). Implementing relationship-based care. *The Journal of Nursing Administration, 41,* 285–290.

Wolak, E. S., McCann, M. F., & Madigan, C. K. (2008). Bridging the gap between the novice and expert nurse: The development of a mentoring program [Abstract]. *Critical Care Nurse, 28*(2), e23.

Woolley, J., Perkins, R., Laird, P., Palmer, J., Schitter, M. B., Tarter, K., & Woolsey, M. (2012). Relationship-based care: Implementing a caring, healing environment. *MEDSURG Nursing, 21,* 179–184.

Wysong, P. R., & Driver, R. (2009). Patients' perceptions of nurses' skill. *Critical Care Nurse, 29*(4), 24–37.

Chapter 22

Theories Focused on Caring

Joanne R. Duffy

INTRODUCTION

Caring is an evolving human science (Watson, 2012), a relational process (Duffy, 2013), a "nurturing way to relate to a valued other" (Swanson, 2016), and a way of being human (Roach, 1987) that enhances personhood (Boykin & Schoenhofer, 2001a). According to Duffy (2009, 2013), when practiced authentically, caring relationships lead to feeling "cared for," an antecedent to optimal patient, nurse, and system outcomes. It has been the subject of much focus in nursing for the last 30 years, having formerly been described as the "moral ideal of nursing" (Watson, 1985, p. 29) and used by many to guide research, design measurement tools, lead, educate, and practice professional nursing. Some have contended that caring is the essence of nursing (Leininger, 1984; Watson, 1979, 1985), while others have asserted that caring is not solely the purview of nursing (Boykin & Schoenhofer, 2015). Within the disciplinary interpretation of nursing, however, caring has been a central tenet not only for theorists, but also for students and nursing educators, and is deeply reflected in the American Nurses Association's *Code for Nurses With Interpretive Statements* (Boykin & Schoenhofer, 2015). Duffy (2013) contends that in the larger context of healthcare systems, when relationships among patients, families, nurses, and the entire healthcare team are of a caring nature, intermediate consequences occur, enabling forward progress or advancement.

Caring is a universal phenomenon that occurs in all societies and cultures (Leininger, 1978, 1991). In fact, Watson (2012) views human caring as a process that is "connected to universal human struggles and human tasks" (p. x). It is manifested most noticeably in many families. For example, in the parent–child relationship, parents can be observed delivering physical, emotional, and educative actions that enhance safety, promote physical growth, and encourage emotional and cognitive development in their children. According to Mayerhoff (1970), caring is essential for the attainment of such human goals. Thus, caring relationships are transforming in that they facilitate human change, growth, and forward movement, adding significantly to the evolution of human life. In the parent–child relationship, parental caring actions are founded on a loving bond or connection between parent and child that assumes expanded potentials and future advancement in the children. In the patient–nurse relationship, caring actions are founded on disciplinary values and the use of relational strategies that provide the context for specific nursing interventions that ultimately engender advancement (in terms of improving health outcomes) in recipients.

In the context of health care, the vulnerability of persons of all ages and backgrounds creates an unusual dependency on healthcare providers (in this case, professional nurses) for behaviors, skills, and attitudes that help protect patients from harm, enable the delivery of high-quality services, preserve human dignity, instill confidence, enable participation in care processes and decisions, promote comfort, uphold hope, and advance general well-being. As patients and families try to negotiate the complex healthcare system and discover the meaning of their illness experience, professional nurses who cultivate and sustain caring relationships with them enable the positive emotion of *feeling cared for* (Duffy, 2013). It is this optimistic emotion that often energizes patients and families to participate, learn, follow through, interact, and persist in meeting their health goals. Furthermore, nurses also benefit from caring relationships with patients and families in that such relationships provide the needed feedback about the important work they do, affording meaning that may, in fact, facilitate increased work satisfaction. Caring in this instance is not viewed as simply kind words or courteous acts, but rather a cohesive blending of disciplinary values, knowledge-based actions, skilled approaches, and affirmative attitudes that, taken together, guide the human-to-human patient–provider relationship. *It is within this caring relationship that the uniqueness of the patient becomes known to the nurse and the meaning of the illness experience can be fully appreciated by the patient.* Caring relationships, therefore, are the medium for healthcare decisions, interventions, and, ultimately, healing and health.

Since caring, along with its explicit knowledge, specialized skills, and attitudes, provides the conduit for healthcare delivery, health services grounded in caring are vital in the delivery of safe, high-quality services. Such services are the basis for ongoing interactions, accurate gathering and reporting of pertinent assessment data, establishment of relevant diagnoses, provision of effective interventions, and continuous improvement. Numerous frameworks have advanced the knowledge of how caring contributes to health and healing (for both the care provider and the care recipient). To better appreciate the phenomenon of caring, four theories are presented in this chapter: (1) the Nursing as Caring Theory, (2) the Theory of Human Caring Science, (3) the Theory of Caring and Healing, and (4) the Quality–Caring Model.

THE NURSING AS CARING THEORY (ANNE BOYKIN AND SAVINA SCHOENHOFER)

The Nursing as Caring Theory is considered a grand theory (Boykin & Schoenhofer, 1993) and was heavily influenced by Mayerhoff's (1970) and Gaut's (1984) philosophical and theoretical discussions of caring, Roach's (1987) five C's (compassion, competence, confidence, conscience, and commitment), and Paterson and Zderad's (1988) humanistic views of nursing. While considering the curricular infrastructure at Florida Atlantic University, Boykin and Schoenhofer (1990, 1993) carefully analyzed existing work on caring using an organizing framework that helped identify common themes and unique stances among several caring scholars. Their resulting theory was intended to be a practice theory that honors the special nature of all persons as caring. The central assumption of the theory—that all persons are caring by virtue of their humanness—underlies its major concepts: personhood, the nursing situation, calls for nursing, and nursing as caring.

Personhood is "a process of living grounded in caring" (Schoenhofer & Boykin, 1993, p. 83) and is enhanced in "nurturing relationships with caring others" (p. 83). The *nursing situation* is the lived experience between a patient and a nurse that affects one's personhood. Each nursing situation is unique and dynamic. In this situation, the nurse brings his or her caring self and comes to know the other person as a caring human. In this nursing situation, *calls for nursing* that request specific forms of caring can be heard by the nurse. As the nurse responds to these calls, the other's unique experience and personal growth can be enhanced. In this theory, the focus of nursing is living caring and growing in caring. As such, caring is the body of knowledge from which professional nurses uniquely respond through specific expressions of caring nurturance (Boykin & Schoenhofer, 2015). Finally, *intentionality* of the nurse, defined as "consistently choosing personhood as a way of life and the aim of nursing" (Schoenhofer, 2002, p. 39), generates commitment and fuels resulting nursing actions.

The major assumptions of the Nursing as Caring Theory are summarized here:

- Persons are caring by virtue of their humanness.
- Persons are caring from moment to moment.
- Persons are whole or complete in the moment.
- Personhood is a way of living grounded in caring.
- Personhood is enhanced through participating in nurturing relationships with caring others.
- Nursing is both a discipline and a profession. (Boykin & Schoenhofer, 2015)

Boykin and Schoenhofer (2015) do not view caring as the unique province of nursing, but rather as a central value that focuses the profession. Boykin, Schoenhofer, Smith, St. Jean, and Aleman's (2003) view of all persons as whole or complete just as they are does not incorporate the nursing process because it assumes some modification or change in persons is needed. Rather, these authors see nursing as "coming to know persons as caring" (Aleman, 2003, p. 224) and creating caring responses that advance personhood. They view nursing as both a discipline and a profession, with practice guided by the theory entailing intention, formal study, and reflection on experience. The use of storytelling of the nursing situation as a form of evidence of nursing as caring as well as other methodologies, such as interpretive phenomenology, have characterized their approach to the study of caring (Schoenhofer, 2002).

The Nursing as Caring Theory has been applied both in curricular design and in various implementation and research projects. For example, Boykin, Schoenhofer, Smith, Jean, & Aleman (2003), together with hospital-based investigators, reported the results of a project in which an 18-bed telemetry unit in a 350-bed for-profit hospital implemented the theory. Through the use of dialogue and specific practice strategies, patient and nurse satisfaction in this unit improved. A lesson learned through this project included that returning to fundamental nursing values created transformation. Another innovative application of the theory is detailed by Bulfin (2005). A partnership between a university (Florida Atlantic University) and a community hospital (Boca Raton Community Hospital) used the Nursing as Caring Theory to frame a professional practice model. Through four phases (education, understanding self, storytelling, and specific practice strategies), the model was evaluated using pre- and postintervention patient satisfaction measures. Postsatisfaction scores improved, although significance testing was not described. Qualitative approaches, such as patient letters, were also used in the evaluation of the project.

Another acute care unit project was evaluated after implementation of the Nursing as Caring Theory (Dyess, Boykin, & Bulfin, 2013). In this participatory action project, nurses clearly expressed a commitment to caring. In a systems implementation of the model (Pross, Hilton, Boykin, & Thomas, 2011), the process of transforming ways of relating was described as an important foundation for sustained change. Likewise, integrating caring theory into education and practice was explained through an academic service partnership where faculty members, staff, and students were exposed to and expected to practice caring together (Dyess, Boykin, & Riggs, 2010). Thus, the Nursing as Caring Theory has been applied by nurses, nurse educators, and nurse leaders in a variety of settings. The authors' most recent text, *Health Care System Transformation for Nursing and Health Care Leaders: Implementing a Culture of Caring* (Boykin, Schoenhofer, & Valentine, 2014), challenges current health system practices and offers a person-centered, caring framework upon which to transform health care.

Although progress is being made in terms of showcasing Nursing as Caring practice and gathering evidence related to the value of the theory, more systematic evaluation of its benefits to both patients and nurses is warranted. Future research using multiple methods will aid in this effort. For example, specific qualitative methods might elicit richer descriptions of caring situations and their consequences from both nurses' and patients' perspectives. Descriptive studies examining relationships between patients who receive nursing care on the basis of the theory and nursing-sensitive outcomes are needed as well. Finally, developing and testing specific nursing interventions grounded in the theory in varying populations would provide further validation.

THE THEORY OF HUMAN CARING SCIENCE (JEAN WATSON)

From a strong foundation in educational counseling and psychology, Jean Watson first developed the Theory of Human Caring while designing an integrated baccalaureate curriculum in a large school of nursing (Watson, 1979). Watson's goal was to present nursing as a distinct entity, a profession, a discipline and science in its own right, separate from, but complementary to, medicine.

The Theory of Human Caring was more formally articulated in 1985, when Watson authored the book *Nursing: Human Science and Human Care*. In this text, Watson elaborated on the caring occasion, the transpersonal nature of caring, the 10 carative factors, phenomenal fields, the influence of time (past, present, and future), and human growth—all of which are major concepts in the theory. In this theory, all persons are considered to be unique and to have a life history, social norms, and experiences that generate a subjective reality or phenomenal field. A *caring occasion* occurs whenever the nurse and another person come together with their unique subjective realities, seeking to connect to each other in the present. During this moment, with the *carative factors* authentically present, the interaction is considered to be transpersonal (unified body, mind, and spirit; collective consciousness; one with the universe). This *transpersonal caring relationship* conveys deep connections to the spirit of another that transcend time, space, and physicality, ultimately affecting the consciousness field as a whole, generating endless possibilities, facilitating human growth, learning, and development. Thus, both the care provider and the one being cared for evolve from the encounter (Watson, 1985).

Later, more spiritual and energy-related aspects of caring were incorporated in the theory, with heightened awareness of the nurse's intentionality and own personal evolution (Watson, 1999). Likewise, a more sacred dimension of nursing's work with a philosophical–ethical–moral dimension was presented in Watson's (2006) book *Caring Science as Sacred Science*. Moreover, Watson has showcased her evolving views on caring resulting from personal experiences, fresh perspectives on the convergence of transpersonal caring and unitary science theories (Watson & Smith, 2002), and metaphysical orientations. In doing so, Watson has suggested that caring is a foundational framework of caring–healing professions and laid the groundwork for a revised edition of her first book, *Nursing: The Philosophy and Science of Caring, Revised Edition* (Watson, 2008*)*. In this revised text, Watson first presents *caritas nursing* as the more mature perspective of nursing and transitioned the 10 carative factors to 10 *caritas processes*.

In 2012, Watson authored *Human Caring Science: A Theory of Nursing*. This text includes a more expanded worldview of universal cosmology (human connectedness) that affirms human caring science as the "disciplinary foundation for the nursing profession" (Watson, 2012, p. xi). It showcases a more unitary-transformative grand theory of evolving consciousness that includes a global worldview of connectedness to all. In this revision Watson clarifies the 10 *caritas processes*.

Caritas comes from the Greek word meaning "to cherish"; it connotes something that is very precious. Watson's evolving path to this way of thinking highlights the connections between caring, spirituality, and human love. The connectedness of caring and love allows for deeper transpersonal and healing relationships, enriching for both the patient and the nurse (Watson, 2015). Working within this expanded caring consciousness allows deeper connections between the human condition and universal love. Related to this evolving theoretical stance on caring, Watson (2015) posits that this direction becomes a "converging paradigm for nursing's future" (p. 325).

A major concept in this evolved theory is the *caritas field*, which is described as a conscious healing presence founded on caring and love that profoundly changes the relational experience for nurses and patients alike (Watson, 2012). Thus, the more evolved clinical caritas processes reflect spirituality and love for others.

The evolution of Watson's Theory of Human Caring Science is a valuable example of the practical side of theory development. Changing worldviews, new insights and experiences, and emerging evidence provided the background for new or revised concepts and relationships over the course of the theory's development. In an effort to expand the study of caring, Watson collated and critiqued 22 instruments for assessing and measuring the concept (Watson, 2003, 2009) and participated in the development of the Watson Caritas Patient Score (Brewer & Watson, 2015). Many of these instruments have been subsequently used to evaluate how nurses and patients perceive caring, how caring relates to other health concepts (e.g., patient experiences), nurses' perspectives of manager caring, caring in nursing education, and multisite benchmarking studies.

Numerous health systems have incorporated the theory into their professional practice models as they prepare for Magnet recognition. For example, using Watson's model as the foundation, some health systems have integrated the theory into various patient care delivery systems (Watson & Foster, 2003), while others have demonstrated their commitment to the theory through documentation systems (Rosenberg, 2006), creating healing spaces for nurse time-outs, instilling centering practices into nursing workflow, and performing caring-based rounds (Watson, 2015). Furthermore, schools of nursing have used the model for curricular planning, teaching–learning strategies, and course content (Beck, 2001; Cook & Cullen, 2003), while others have studied caring within a broader educational context (Sitzman, 2015, 2016). Some have tested interventions on the basis of the caring theory or used the theory as the study's conceptual foundation (Arslan-Özkan, Okumuş, & Buldukoğlu, 2014; Erci, 2003; Smith, Kemp, Hemphill, & Vojir, 2002; Suliman, Welman, Thomas, & Omer, 2009), albeit the Theory of Human Caring Science as it was originally conceptualized. According to Watson (2006), research in caring embraces inquiries that are both reflective and subjective, as well as objective–empirical.

Watson's Theory of Human Caring Science has played a major role in helping professional nurses honor their unique and distinct values and has influenced the scholarship of countless others, including the theorists reviewed in this chapter. Boyd (2008) contended that the theory is especially useful for those with mental illness (p. 71); however, Frisch and Frisch (2011) cautioned that some patients (on the basis of their illness) may not easily enter this form of mutuality. The theory, with its current "caritas consciousness" concept, represents an authenticity of person that transcends the biomedical and bureaucratic nature of most health systems, sometimes presenting practical challenges for nurses' work in the acute care environments. That being said, many U.S. acute care hospitals have embraced Watson's theory as a component of their professional practice models!

In 2007, Watson established the Watson Caring Science Institute, a nonprofit that was recently transitioned to the University of Colorado as the Watson Caring Science Center (University of Colorado, n.d.). In this newly developed center, human caring knowledge, ethics, and clinical practice are advanced through educational programs (including a focused caring science PhD track), partnerships, research, and international collaboration. Watson has made extraordinary contributions to the discipline of nursing over the last four decades and continues her work guiding health professionals in this transforming and evolving human caring science. Ongoing evaluation of the theory in terms of its measurement, authentic application, and potential value to patients, families, health professionals, and the larger health system are warranted.

THE THEORY OF CARING AND HEALING (KRISTEN SWANSON)

Kristen Swanson's middle-range theory of caring was developed through inductive methods while studying three groups of women. In this theory, caring is defined as "a nurturing way of relating to a valued other toward whom one feels a personal sense of commitment and responsibility" (Swanson, 1991, p. 162). Using data from women who miscarried, neonatal intensive care unit caregivers (both parents and professionals), and at-risk mothers, five caring processes—maintaining belief, knowing, being with, doing for, and enabling—were described. Swanson maintains that while caring is not unique to nursing, it informs those relationships central to nursing.

Maintaining belief demonstrates faith in the capacity of others and provides nurses with the foundation for the commitment to serve (both society in general and individual patients). *Knowing* refers to understanding how others' lives have meaning; it avoids assumptions and focuses on the one being cared for in order to better comprehend the client's lived reality. *Being with* incorporates emotional presence. It conveys to clients that they matter and assures them that their reality is appreciated. It includes physical presence as well as ongoing availability. *Doing for* involves nursing behaviors that preserve another's wholeness. It includes comforting, anticipating, protecting, maintaining confidentiality and dignity, interpersonal listening, teaching, coaching, referring, supporting and guiding, providing feedback, and validating the other's reality. *Enabling* implies facilitating another's capacity through providing information, being present and sharing, and assisting behaviors.

In 1993, Swanson structured these processes such that they were ordered to influence the intended outcome—namely, client well-being. Later, Swanson completed a meta-analysis of the state of caring research. In this review, although 130 empirical studies were identified, 18 of those provided evidence of the consequences of caring and noncaring both for nurses and for patients. More importantly, she highlighted the clear significance of caring knowledge to current nursing practice and identified its implications for the nursing practice of the future (Swanson, 1999).

Using knowledge of caring and the inductively developed theory of caring, Swanson set out on a program of research that focused on responses to miscarriage and interventions to promote healing subsequent to early pregnancy loss. After completion of the meta-analysis, Swanson tested an intervention in a study of 242 women who had miscarried (Swanson, 1999). Using a caring-based counseling intervention, she conducted a randomized trial with a Solomon four-group design to test the intervention on several outcomes. Findings revealed that the caring intervention had a positive effect on disturbed mood, anger, and level of depression. In addition, a majority of the patients reported satisfaction with the caring intervention. Monitoring caring as delivered in the miscarriage study involved both qualitative and quantitative (including the development of the Caring Professional Scale [Swanson, 2002]) methods. Items on this instrument were derived from the five caring processes, and preliminary psychometric properties were evaluated.

A follow-up intervention-focused study using 341 couples compared three types of couples-focused interventions to no treatment, with the goal being to identify strategies to help men and women resolve depression and grief during the first year after a miscarriage (Swanson, Chen, Graham, Wojnar, & Petras, 2009). Through this rigorous experimental design, findings revealed that overall, while participation in any of the three intervention arms accelerated women's grief resolution, their resolution of depression was best enhanced by the three nurse-led and caring-based counseling sessions. Women who received three nurse counseling sessions were three to eight times more likely to see a faster decline in their symptoms of depression than were women who received similar but limited help or no such help.

Despite the limitations imposed by the predominantly White and heterosexual samples, Swanson was able to demonstrate the benefits of caring interventions in terms of decreased depression, improved mood, decreased anger, and intervention satisfaction for persons who had experienced a pregnancy loss. Swanson and her students followed up with a conceptual model of miscarriage (Wojner, Swanson, & Adolfsson, 2011), a secondary analysis (Huffman, Schwartz, & Swanson, 2015), and development of the meaning of miscarriage scale (Huffman, Swanson, & Lynn, 2014). Further and extended evidence of her work is found in the empirical literature related to parents' experiences with children undergoing congenital heart surgery (Wei Roscigno, Hanson, & Swanson, 2015; Wei et al., 2016).

Recently, Swanson supplemented her theory by presenting a connection between caring and healing (Swanson, 2015), maintaining that "when a provider takes the time to know, be with, do, enable, and maintain belief in the other, the recipient feels a sense of wholeness" (p. 530). While some would classify Swanson's Theory of Caring and Healing as a practice or situational theory (since it was developed as an outcome of studying a limited patient population), others have used it beyond pregnancy loss to guide professional practice and curricula. For example, the theory was implemented in a large health system in the Southeast, and improvements were noted in patient and nurse satisfaction levels, patient pain, and response to call lights (Tonges & Ray, 2011). Swanson continues to work with students and faculty members in her role as Dean at the University of Seattle and with health systems as they implement cultures of caring. Swanson's persistence in observing, applying, validating, and refining the Caring and Healing Theory provides an exemplary model of the relationship between theory and research.

THE QUALITY–CARING MODEL (JOANNE R. DUFFY)

Developed to fill a perceived practice and research void in the late 1980s, the Quality–Caring Model was initially informed by Duffy's involvement in quality improvement and clinical experiences with acute hospitalized patients who, when asked about their dissatisfaction with care, verbalized, "no one cares." In these encounters with acutely ill hospitalized adults, Duffy observed that the fundamental patient–nurse caring relationship (a deeply held disciplinary value) was frequently marginalized from the often routine task-oriented nature of nursing work. This incongruity between professional values and work behaviors was considered serious because, as Duffy began to investigate, nurses linked it to work dissatisfaction and patients linked it to poorer health outcomes, both important indicators of healthcare quality.

Corroborated by the consequences of noncaring as reported in the literature (Reiman, 1986), Duffy first set out to narrow the gap between disciplinary values and behaviors and current professional practice by studying the linkage between nurse caring relationships and quality, with the ultimate intention of demonstrating how nurse caring contributes to improved patient outcomes. After developing the Caring Assessment Tool (CAT) to measure patients' perceptions of caring, Duffy used this instrument to conduct the original study that significantly associated nurse caring to patient satisfaction (1990, 1992). The CAT was later adapted to assess student nurses' perceptions of faculty caring (via the CAT-edu) and staff nurses' perceptions of nurse managers' caring (via the CAT-adm); findings demonstrated a positive relationship between nurse manager caring behaviors and staff nurse satisfaction (Duffy, 1993, 2008). Continued development and evaluation of the CAT instruments are ongoing. For example, an exploratory factor analysis of the CAT in 2007 and again in 2010 pointed to a one-factor solution and assisted with item reduction (Duffy, Brewer, & Weaver, 2010; Duffy, Hoskins, & Seifert, 2007). A factor analysis of the CAT-adm was recently completed, and new instruments, namely, patient perceptions of team caring, the caring intention scale, and the caring capacity scale, are presently under development or evaluation. Graduate students, individual researchers, nursing faculty members, and health systems throughout the world routinely use these instruments for assessment of caring relationships in varying contexts.

With valid and reliable instruments now available, Duffy continued her program of research but was struck by the lack of attention in the literature to the quality–caring link. In collaboration with Lois Hoskins, she developed the Quality–Caring Model in 2003. The model is considered middle range and deductive, drawing heavily on the works of Watson (1979, 1985, 1999); King (1981); Donabedian (1966); Mitchell, Ferketich, and Jennings (1998); and Irvine, Sidani, and Hall (1998). It supports the connections between nurse caring and quality health outcomes, "exposing the hidden value of nursing" (Duffy & Hoskins, 2003, p. 78)

Originally, the model depicted a linear process, but due to the complex, evolving, and interdependent nature of health systems, Duffy revised the model in 2009 (Duffy, 2009) and again in 2013 (Duffy, 2013), incorporating aspects of complexity theory (Holland, 1992, 1999). Assumptions and propositions of the model are available in these texts and in the later revision (2013). Some components of the model are reworded and presented in the larger context of health systems. The revised model identifies four evolving complex relationships that humans experience as they live and encounter the health system: relationships with self, community, patients and families, and other health professionals. In this way of thinking, relationships are central to human progress, including the improvement of health; when enacted in caring ways, relationships naturally lead to advancement or forward movement, even in challenging conditions. This overarching concept, *humans in relationships*, refers to the multidimensional relational nature of humans as they exist in society. The *relationship with self* includes embracing the thoughts, feelings, and experiences one holds, especially as they relate to nursing work. Regular attention to such emotions allows for accessing the inner wisdom drawn from practice and using this guidance to know and value the self as a prerequisite for engaging in caring interactions with others. *Caring relationships within larger communities* (such as neighborhoods or practice groups) raises the capacity of citizens and employees to address challenges and contribute to the welfare and development of members, including nurses themselves. When nurses are involved professionally in their broader communities, not only do communities benefit greatly, but nurses themselves express added meaning from their work.

Relationship-centered professional encounters include those independent relationships that nurses enjoy with patients and families as well as the interdependent collaborative relationships they establish with members of the entire healthcare team. During healthcare encounters, nurses' relationships with patients and families are considered to be primary and independent, delivered autonomously, and for which nurses are solely held accountable. Using caring behaviors, nurses cultivate mutually reciprocal human caring interactions with patients and families that inform future interactions and contribute to health outcomes. It is also theorized that caring relationships with patients and families benefit nurses in terms of the latter's professional growth, ongoing motivation, engagement, and work satisfaction. Collaborative relationships, in contrast, are multidisciplinary in nature and include those activities and responsibilities that nurses share with other members of the healthcare team. Collaborative relationships are enhanced when mutual caring relationships exist among the various professionals and are focused on the best interests of patients and their families. Such relationships are considered essential to the revised model, given that high-quality outcomes are enhanced when multiple healthcare providers work together as cohesive teams (Brandt, Lutfiyya, King, & Chioreso, 2014). In this way, continuity is enhanced and patients and families, as well as team members, feel cared for.

According to Duffy, caring relationships are grounded in specific behaviors and attitudes labeled caring behaviors. The *caring behaviors*—namely, mutual problem solving, attentive reassurance, human respect, encouraging manner, healing environment, appreciation of unique meanings, affiliation needs, and basic human needs—are fundamental to the concept of relationship-centered professional encounters because they are the visible, perceptible, quantifiable evidence of caring interactions that recipients can recognize, identify, and distinguish. Caring behaviors require specialized knowledge, attitudes, and behaviors that are directed toward health and healing. The behaviors, when applied expertly and over time, result in the recipient "feeling cared for" (Duffy, 2009, p. 196).

"Feeling cared for" is an important, positive emotion that is associated with contentment, met needs, acceptance, and validation (Duffy & Hoskins, 2003). As individuals perceive being cared for by their healthcare providers, they experience ease, understanding and connection, enhanced self-confidence, an awareness of being valued, comfort, and an optimistic outlook. In this affirmative state, "a sense of security develops that makes it easier to learn new things, change behaviors, take risks, and follow guidelines" (Duffy & Hoskins, 2003, p. 83). The feeling of being cared for is considered an antecedent to advancement, particularly related to nursing-sensitive patient outcomes such as increased knowledge, safety, decreased self-reported pain, decreased anxiety, maintenance of human dignity, increased participation (engagement), and positive experiences of care.

Self-advancing systems, defined as dynamic positive progress that enhances a system's well-being (Duffy, 2009, p. 196), is closely related to quality or value because this concept is dynamic and indicates some benefit or advantage. As caring relationships are cultivated with others over time, small changes or differences begin to emerge that can grow exponentially into longer-term positive outcomes that transform. Self-advancement is manifested individually, among groups, or even in large health systems as behavior changes, improvements, higher levels of health, maturation, learning, gains, or expansions.

Consideration of quality health outcomes as a consequence of the unique caring relationships central to daily nursing practice represents a practical, contemporary approach that showcases nursing's contribution and provides a useful way to generate evidence of its value. The model emphasizes the centrality of caring relationships, shifting the primary focus of professional nursing work to the more relational aspects of the practice.

The Quality–Caring Model has been adopted as a disciplinary framework for numerous U.S. health systems' professional practice models; used to ground experiential learning activities, including a graduate-level relationship-centered caring course and a relationship-centered leadership course; and used to provide the theoretical foundation for research projects, dissertations, scholarly projects, and theses. Additionally, it was used in the following efforts:

- To develop and evaluate the effect of a caring-based intervention on heart failure patients' quality of life and 30-day readmission rates (Duffy, Hoskins, & Dudley-Brown, 2005)
- To assess caring competencies of graduating seniors (Duffy et al., 2005)
- To evaluate its influence on patient, nurse, and system outcomes in two national demonstration projects conducted by the Health Resources and Services Administration (Relationship-Centered Caring in Acute Care, and Advancing Safety and Quality in Vulnerable Acute Care Patients Through Interprofessional Collaborative Practice)
- To generate valid and reliable measurements (previously cited)
- To pilot-test hospitalized older adults' electronic participation in assessing patient-centeredness (Duffy, 2013)
- To create the enabling conditions for an academic–service partnership that increased research productivity at year 1 (Duffy, Culp, Sand-Jecklin, Stroupe, & Lucke-Wold, 2015a; Duffy, Culp, Sand-Jecklin, Stroupe, & Yarberry, 2015b)
- To assess the feasibility of measuring patient perceptions of caring in a multisite collaboration study (Duffy & Brewer, 2011)

In the context of advanced nursing practice, the Quality–Caring Model accounts for the complexity of healthcare systems and honors the vital role that caring relationships play in advancing patient-centeredness and creating value in health systems. These characteristics offer a strong basis for practice that can assist in the development of relevant organizational processes and procedures. The doctor of nursing practice graduate may be involved in translating model concepts into clinical practice, use the model to guide clinical decision making, generate and evaluate evidence of the model's value (in terms of patient outcomes), implement clinical innovations (derived from the model) that change practice, and work with others in caring ways (use the caring behaviors) to alter individual and team behavior or impact organizational-level change. For example, advanced practice nurses may create an innovative method for improving patient engagement (drawing on model concepts) that could be evaluated for its success in reducing 30-day readmission rates and improving adherence.

The Quality–Caring Model, on the basis of its unique concepts and propositions, could also be used in advanced practice as the foundation for research or evaluation projects. For example, using the CAT (Duffy, Brewer, & Weaver, 2010), advanced practice nurses might correlate its scores with nursing-sensitive outcome indicators in their institutions, or the longitudinal success of Quality–Caring-based professional practice models, even benchmarking their organizations with others to improve performance. Considering that the CAT was piloted successfully with hospitalized older adults (Duffy, Kooken, Wolverton, & Weaver, 2012), using this method to assess caring relationships in real time might accelerate more actionable patient-centered practice changes. In fact, this measure could easily be incorporated into user-friendly information systems to promote rapid improvement activities.

In the direct care role, a nurse with advanced education may use the Quality–Caring Model to role-model self-caring; complete systematic and holistic assessments of individuals, communities, or systems; cultivate and sustain caring relationships with patients, families, and health team members; help problem solve with patients and families; make clinical decisions on the basis of evidence; and advance professional nursing practice. The model provides a guide for self-caring that includes remaining more aware (or mindful) as a particularly healthy way to work that deepens a nurse's ability to be present for patients, families, and team members. In fact, health professionals need to acknowledge and allow themselves to experience the feelings associated with their work, including suffering. Duffy asserts that this form of self-caring may be a necessary antecedent to caring for others. When role-modeled by advanced practice nurses, others may begin to incorporate such practices of their own.

Despite the success of the Quality–Caring Model as a foundation for professional practice, and on the basis of national consultations, Duffy has recently observed varying levels of "uptake" of professional practice models, which recently led to the authorship of *Professional Practice Models in Nursing: Successful Health System Integration* (2016). In this text, Duffy asserts that the benefits of such models may not yet be realized due to limited system integration. The text emphasizes a systematic process of system integration and dissemination so that the full impact of professional practice models (and nursing's contribution to health care) can be more fully appreciated.

Duffy continues her research on caring relationships, most recently designing an intervention to improve the delivery of patient-centered care in hospitalized older adults through real-time data and group reflection. Duffy's consultation work, particularly at the executive and board levels in health systems throughout the United States, continues to advance patient-centeredness and inspire quality–caring work cultures. More research on the benefits of the Quality–Caring Model is needed in diverse populations with larger multisite samples.

SUMMARY

No one universal theoretical approach to caring in nursing exists. In fact, two of the theories presented in this chapter use a philosophical/ethical approach (Boykin and Schoenhofer; Watson), one was developed inductively (Swanson), and one was developed deductively (Duffy). Each of these theories incorporates unique worldviews and concepts, yet all share commonalities to some extent. Specifically, the relational nature of caring, patient well-being or healing, nurses' ability to connect with others, and a disciplinary focus for nursing are features found in all of the theories reviewed in this chapter.

Professional practice models founded on caring theories are now incorporated on a widespread basis, albeit in varying degrees, and healthcare professionals at all levels are being exposed to them. Advanced practice nurses are now in positions where they can evaluate the consequences of these disciplinary perspectives (in terms of creating value for patients, families, and health systems). Assessments of barriers and facilitators to their implementation, as well as cost–benefit analysis, and evaluation of specific approaches that can accelerate, change, improve, and sustain the use of caring theories are also needed. Practicing nurses, educators, other health professionals, and those in leadership and policy positions are beginning to appreciate the relational aspect of health care and are demanding approaches that incorporate caring relationships to advance high-value health outcomes. Advanced practice nurses are key to crafting this future!

DISCUSSION QUESTIONS

1. Reflect on the vital nature of caring in health care. What are your thoughts?
2. Which sorts of knowledge, skills, and attitudes are required for caring professional practice?
3. How does the concept of personhood as used in the Nursing as Caring Theory (Boykin) relate to nurses?
4. Describe the evolution of the carative factors to clinical caritas processes (Watson).
5. Describe the systematic empirical process used in the development and validation of the Theory of Caring and Healing (Swanson).
6. Which theoretical contributions were used in the development of the Quality–Caring Model?
7. Reflect on the many interdependent relationships that exist in complex health systems. How do they shape these systems?
8. Describe a situation in which you cultivated a caring interprofessional relationship. What happened? What was your role? What did you learn from this experience?
9. As a nurse, how do you come to know the patient and his or her unique experience of illness?
10. As an advanced practice nurse, how do you role-model self-caring?

11. How would you advise professional nurses to better incorporate caring relationships in their practice? Which strengths can you bring to help address the importance of caring relationships? How would you evaluate this effort?
12. How does a new graduate experience caring relationships at your institution? How does this affect caring professional practice?
13. Which continuing education activities at your institution promote quality caring?
14. Develop three research or evaluation questions on the basis of one of the models presented in this chapter. What will you do with these questions?
15. As an advanced practice nurse, how does the study of caring theories inform your practice?

REFERENCES

American Nurses Association. (2015). *Code of ethics for nurses with interpretive statements.* Silver Spring, MD: Author.

Arslan-Özkan Okumuş, H., & Buldukoğlu, K. (2014). A randomized controlled trial of the effects of nursing care based on Watson's Theory of Human Caring on distress, self-efficacy and adjustment in infertile women. *Journal of Advanced Nursing, 70*(8), 1801–1812.

Beck, C. T. (2001). Caring within nursing education: A metasynthesis. *Journal of Nursing Education, 40,* 101–109.

Bevis, E. O., & Watson, J. (1989). *Toward a caring curriculum: A new pedagogy for nursing* (pp. iii–xix, 1–394). Washington, DC: National League for Nursing Publication.

Boyd, M.A. (2006). *Psychiatric nursing contemporary practice* (4th ed.). Philadelphia, PA: Lippincott Williams & Wilkins.

Boykin, A., & Schoenhofer, S. O. (1990). Caring in nursing: Analysis of extant theory. *Nursing Science Quarterly, 4,* 149–155.

Boykin, A., & Schoenhofer, S. O. (1993). *Nursing as Caring: A model for transforming practice.* New York, NY: National League for Nursing.

Boykin, A., & Schenhofer, S. O. (2001a). *Nursing as Caring: A model for transforming practice* (rev. ed.). Sudbury, MA: Jones & Bartlett Publishers.

Boykin, A., & Schoenhofer, S. O. (2001b). The role of nursing leadership in creating caring environments in health care delivery systems. *Nursing Administration Quarterly, 25*(3), 1–7.

Boykin, A., & Schoenhofer, S. O. (2015). Theory of Nursing as Caring. In M. C. Smith & M. E. Parker (Eds.), *Nursing theory and nursing practice.* Philadelphia, PA: F. A. Davis.

Boykin, A., Schoenhofer, S. O., Smith, N., St. Jean, J., & Aleman, D. (2003). Transforming practice using a caring-based nursing model. *Nursing Administration Quarterly, 27,* 223–230.

Boykin, A., Schoenhofer, S., & Valentine, K. (2013). *Health care system transformation for nursing and health care leaders: Implementing a culture of caring.* New York, NY: Springer Publishing.

Brandt, B., Lutfiyya, M. N., King, J. A., & Chioreso, C. (2014). A scoping review of interprofessional collaborative practice and education using the lens of the Triple Aim. *Journal of Interprofessional Care, 28*(5), 393–399.

Brewer, B. B., & Watson, J. (2015). Evaluation of authentic human caring professional practices. *Journal of Nursing Administration, 45*(12), 1–6.

Bulfin, S. (2005). Nursing as Caring Theory: Living caring in practice. *Nursing Science Quarterly, 18*(4), 313–319.

Cook, P. R., & Cullen, J. A. (2003). Caring as an imperative for nursing education. *Nursing Education Perspectives, 24*(4), 192–197.

Donabedian, A. (1966). Evaluating the quality of medical care. *Milbank Memorial Fund Quarterly, 44*(Part 2), 166–203.

Duffy, J. (1990). The relationship between nurse caring behaviors and selected outcomes of care among hospitalized medical-surgical patients. Doctoral Dissertation. The Catholic University of America. Ann Arbor, MI. University Microfilm 1992137361.

Duffy, J. (1992). The impact of nurse caring on patient outcomes. In D. Gaut (Ed.), *The presence of caring in nursing* (pp. 113–136). New York, NY: National League for Nursing Press.

Duffy, J. (1993). Caring behaviors of nurse managers: Relationships to staff nurse satisfaction and retention. In D. Gaut (Ed.), *Caring: A global agenda* (pp. 365–377). New York, NY: National League for Nursing Press.

Duffy, J. (2008). Caring Assessment Tool—administrative version. In J. Watson (Ed.), *Assessing and measuring caring in nursing and health science* (pp. 131–145). New York, NY: Springer.

Duffy, J. (2009). *Quality caring in nursing: Applying theory to clinical practice, education, and leadership*. New York, NY: Springer.

Duffy, J. (2013). *Quality caring in nursing and health systems: Applying theory to clinical practice, education, and leadership* (2nd ed.). New York, NY: Springer.

Duffy, J. (2016). *Professional practice models in nursing: Successful health system integration*. New York, NY: Springer.

Duffy, J., & Brewer, B. (2011). Feasibility of a Multi-institution Collaborative to Improve Patient–Nurse Relationship Quality. *Journal of Nursing Administration, 41*(2), 78–83.

Duffy, J., Brewer, B., & Weaver, M. (2010). Revision and psychometric properties of the Caring Assessment Tool. *Clinical Nursing Research*. doi:10.1177/1054773810369827

Duffy, J., Culp, S., Sand-Jecklin, K., Stroupe, L., & Lucke-Wold, N. (2015a). Nurses' research capacity, use of evidence, and research productivity in acute care: Year one findings from a partnership study. *Journal of Nursing Administration, 46*(1), 12–17.

Duffy, J., Culp, S., Sand-Jecklin, K., Stroupe, L., & Yarberry, C. (2015b). Nurses' research capacity and use of evidence in acute care: Baseline findings from a partnership study. *Journal of Nursing Administration, 45*(3), 158–164.

Duffy, J., & Hoskins, L. (2003). The Quality–Caring Model: Blending dual paradigms. *Advances in Nursing Science, 26*(1), 77–88.

Duffy, J., Hoskins, L., & Dudley-Brown, S. (2005). Development and testing of a caring-based intervention for older adults with heart failure. *Journal of Cardiovascular Nursing, 20*(3), 1–9.

Duffy, J., Hoskins, L. M., & Dudley-Brown, S. (2010). Improving outcomes for older adults with heart failure: A randomized trial using a theory-guided nursing intervention. *Journal of Nursing Care Quality, 25*(1), 56–64.

Duffy, J., Hoskins, L. M., & Seifert, R. F. (2007). Dimensions of caring: Psychometric properties of the Caring Assessment Tool. *Advances in Nursing Science, 30*(3), 235–245.

Duffy, J., Kooken, W., Wolverton, C., & Weaver, M. T. (2012). Evaluating patient-centered care: Feasibility of electronic data collection in hospitalized older adults. *Journal of Nursing Care Quality, 27*(4), 307–315.

Dyess, S. M., Boykin, A., & Bulfin, M. J. (2013). Hearing the voice of nurses in practice: A process of practice environment transformation linked to caring theory. *Nursing Science Quarterly, 26*(2), 167–173.

Dyess, S., Boykin, A., & Riggs, C. (2010). Integrating caring theory with nursing practice and education: Connecting with what matters. *Journal of Nursing Administration, 40*(11), 498–503.

Erci, B. (2003). The effectiveness of Watson's caring model on the quality of life and blood pressure of patients with hypertension. *Journal of Advanced Nursing, 41*(2), 1–10.

Frisch, N.C., & Frisch, LD. (2011). *Psychiatric mental health nursing* (4th ed.). Boston, MA: Delmar Cengage Learning.

Gaut, D. (1984). A theoretic description of caring as action. In M. Leininger (Ed.), *Care: The essence of nursing and health* (pp. 27–44). Thorofare, NJ: Charles B. Slack.

Holland, J. H. (1992). *Adaptation in natural and artificial systems: An introductory analysis with applications to biology, control, and artificial intelligence.* Cambridge, MA: MIT Press.

Holland, J. H. (1999). *Emergence: From chaos to order.* Reading, MA: Perseus Books.

Huffman, C. S., Schwartz, T. S., & Swanson, K. M (2015). Couples and miscarriage: The influence of gender and reproductive factors on the impact of miscarriage. *Women's Health Issues, 25*(5), 570–578.

Huffman, C. S., Swanson, K. M., & Lynn, M. R. (2014). Measuring the meaning of miscarriage: Revision of the Impact of Miscarriage Scale. *Journal of Nursing Measurement, 22*(1), 29–45.

King, I. M. (1981). *A theory of nursing: Systems, concepts, process.* New York, NY: Wiley.

Irvine, D. M., Sidani, S., & Hall, L. M. (1998). Linking outcomes to nurses' roles in health care. *Nursing Economics, 16*(2), 58–64.

Leininger, M. (1978). *Transcultural nursing: Concepts, theories, practices.* New York, NY: Wiley.

Leininger, M. M. (1984). Caring is nursing: Understanding the meaning, importance, and issues. In M. M. Leininger (Ed.), *Care: The essence of nursing and health* (pp. 83–93). Thorofare, NJ: Charles B. Slack.

Leininger, M. M. (1991). *Culture care diversity and universality: A theory of nursing.* New York, NY: National League for Nursing Press.

Mayerhoff, M. (1970). *On caring.* New York, NY: Harper & Row.

Mitchell, P., Ferketich, S., & Jennings, B. M. (1998). American Academy of Nursing Expert Panel on Quality Health Care: Quality health outcomes model. *Journal of Nursing Scholarship, 30*(1), 43–46.

Paterson, J., & Zderad, L. (1988). *Humanistic nursing* (2nd ed.). New York, NY: National League for Nursing.

Pross, E., Hilton, N., Boykin, A., & Thomas, C. (2011). The dance of caring persons. *Nursing Management, 42*(10), 25–30.

Reiman, C. (1986). Noncaring and caring in the clinical setting: Patients descriptions. *Topics in Clinical Nursing, 8*(2), 30–36.

Roach, S. (1987). *The human act of caring.* Ottawa, Canada: Canadian Hospital Association.

Rosenberg, S. (2006). Utilizing the language of Jean Watson's caring theory within a computerized clinical documentation system. *Computers, Informatics, Nursing, 24* (1), 53–56.

Schoenhofer, S. O. (2002). Choosing personhood: Intentionality and choosing nursing as caring. *Holistic Nursing Practice, 14*(4), 36–40.

Schoenhofer, S., & Boykin, A. (1993). Nursing as Caring: An emerging general theory of nursing. In M. E. Parker (Ed.), *Patterns of nursing theories in practice* (pp. 83–102). New York, NY: National League for Nursing.

Sitzman, K. (2015). Sense, connect, facilitate: Nurse educator experiences of caring online through Watson's lens. *International Journal of Human Caring, 19*(3), 25–29.

Sitzman, K. (2016). Mindful communication for caring online. *Advances in Nursing Science, 39*(1), 38–47.

Smith, M. C., Kemp, J., Hemphill, L., & Vojir, C. (2002). Outcomes of massage therapy for cancer patients. *Journal of Nursing Scholarship, 34*(3), 257–262.

Suliman, W., Welman, E., Thomas, L., & Omer, T. (2009). Applying Watson's nursing theory to assess patient perception of being cared for in a multicultural environment. *Journal of Nursing Research, 17*(4), 293–300.

Swanson, K. (1991). Empirical development of a middle range theory of caring. *Nursing Research, 40*(3), 161–166.

Swanson, K. (1993). Nursing as informed caring for the well-being of others. *Image: The Journal of Nursing Scholarship, 25*(4), 352–357.

Swanson, K. (1999). Effects of caring, measurement, and time on miscarriage impact and women's well-being. *Nursing Research, 48*(6), 288–298.

Swanson, K. M. (1999). What's known about caring in nursing science: A literary meta-analysis. In A. S. Hinshaw, S. Feetham, & J. Shaver (Eds.), *Handbook of clinical nursing research*. Thousand Oaks, CA: Sage.

Swanson, K. M. (2002). Caring Professional Scale. In J. Watson (Ed.), *Assessing and measuring caring in nursing and health science* (pp. 203–206). New York, NY: Springer.

Swanson, K. M. (2015). Kristen Swanson's Theory of Caring. In M. C. Smith & M. E. Parker (Eds.), *Nursing theory and nursing practice*. Philadelphia, PA: F. A. Davis.

Swanson, K. M. (2016). Dean's welcome. Seattle University, College of Nursing. Retrieved from https://www.seattleu.edu/nursing/about/deans-welcome

Swanson, K. M., Chen, H. T., Graham, J. C., Wojnar, D. M., & Petras, A. (2009). Resolution of depression and grief during the first year after miscarriage: A randomized controlled clinical trial of couples-focused interventions. *Journal of Women's Health, 18*(8), 1245–1257.

Tonges, M., & Ray, J. (2011). Translating caring theory into practice: The Carolina Care Model. *Journal of Nursing Administration, 41*(9), 374–381.

University of Colorado. (n.d.). Watson Caring Science Center. University of Colorado, College of Nursing Retrieved from http://www.ucdenver.edu/academics/colleges/nursing/programs-admissions/doctoral-programs/doctor-philosophy/caringscience/Pages/Main-Page-WCSC.aspx

Watson, J. (1979). *Nursing: The philosophy and science of caring*. Boston, MA: Little, Brown.

Watson, J. (1985). *Nursing: Human science and human care*. Norwalk, CT: Appleton-Century.

Watson, J. (1999). *Postmodern nursing and beyond*. Toronto, Canada: Churchill Livingstone.

Watson, J. (2003). *Instruments for assessing and measuring caring in nursing and health sciences*. New York, NY: Springer.

Watson, J. (2006). *Caring science as sacred science*. Philadelphia, PA: F. A. Davis.

Watson, J. (2008). *Nursing: The philosophy and science of caring* (rev. ed.). Denver, CO: Colorado University Press.

Watson, J. (2009). *Assessing and measuring caring in nursing and health science* (2nd ed.). New York, NY: Springer.

Watson, J. (2012). *Human caring science: A theory of nursing*. Burlington, MA: Jones & Bartlett Learning.

Watson, J. (2015). Jean Watson's Theory of Human Caring. In M. C. Smith & M. E. Parker (Eds.), *Nursing theories and nursing practice*. Philadelphia, PA: F. A. Davis

Watson, J., & Foster, R. (2003). The attending nurse caring model: Integrating theory, evidence and advanced caring–healing therapeutics for transforming professional practice. *Journal of Clinical Nursing, 12*, 360–365.

Watson, J., & Smith, M. (2002). Transpersonal caring science and the science of unitary human beings: A transtheoretical discourse for nursing knowledge development. *International Journal of Advanced Nursing, 37*(5), 452–461.

Wei, H., Roscigno, C., Hanson, C. C., & Swanson, K. M. (2015). Families of children with congenital heart disease: A literature review. *Heart and Lung: The Journal of Acute and Critical Care, 44*(6), 494–511.

Wei, H., Roscigno, C. I., Swanson, K. M., Black, B. P., Hudson-Barr, D., & Hanson, C. C. (2016). Parents' experiences of having a child undergoing congenital heart surgery: An emotional rollercoaster from shocking to blessing. *Heart and Lung: The Journal of Acute and Critical Care, 45*(2), 154–160.

Wojnar, D. M., Swanson, K. M., & Adolfsson, A. S. (2011). Confronting the inevitable: A conceptual model of miscarriage for use in clinical practice and research. *Death Studies, 35*(6), 536–558.

Chapter 23

Models and Theories Focused on Culture

Larry Purnell

INTRODUCTION

This chapter provides an overview of selected cultural models and theories commonly used in nursing practice, education, administration, and research. Although the main focus of this chapter is the Purnell model for cultural competence, other models and theories are briefly described. Some of these cultural models are not intended for research, but they have value when used in education, practice, and administration. Advanced practice nurses (APNs) have preparation in all of these areas and use cultural models, theories, and approaches accordingly. Exemplars are provided for cultural models and theories that have been used in nursing and healthcare research.

OVERVIEW OF CULTURAL MODELS AND THEORIES

Many differing definitions and meanings of theory exist, both within and outside of the nursing profession. Theory is not reality; it is abstract and complex and must be so that research can be generated to guide practice. According to Fawcett and DeSanto-Madeya (2012), theory is one or more relatively concrete and abstract concepts that are derived from a conceptual model, the propositions that describe those concepts, and the propositions that state specific relationships between two or more of the concepts. A theory can be grand or middle range, depending on its level and scope. Moreover, a theory must have (1) a purpose; (2) concepts that are systematically linked and defined and that interconnect the ideas of the theory; and (3) explicit and implicit assumptions. Nursing theory, of which there are four levels—metatheory, grand theory, middle-range theory, and practice theory—comprises either one or a combination of the following four types:

1. *Descriptive theory* identifies properties and components of a discipline, identifies meaning and observations, and describes which elements exist.
2. *Explanatory theory* identifies how the properties and components relate to one another and accounts for the functions of the discipline.
3. *Predictive theory* conjectures the relationships between the components of a phenomenon and predicts under which conditions the phenomena will occur.
4. *Prescriptive theory* addresses therapeutics and consequences of interventions (Fawcett & DeSanto-Madeya, 2012).

Because there is no agreement in the scientific community regarding the definitions of a conceptual model, conceptual framework, theoretical model, and theoretical framework, these terms are used interchangeably in this chapter. A *conceptual model* can be represented by words, diagrams, or pictures. Each theoretical/conceptual model or theory is evaluated on the basis of its clarity, simplicity, generality, empirical precision, and derivable consequences. Clarity is concerned with the logical and adequate arrangements of constructs and concepts. Simplicity is concerned with the number and complexity of concepts in the model. Generality is concerned with how the model or theory can be useful to APNs. Empirical precision is concerned with the ability of the model or theory to hold up over time. Derivable consequences refer to how practical and useful the theory or model is in relation to achieving important health outcomes (Purnell, 2000; StudyBlue, 2016).

Given the increasing complexity of culture in the United States, faculty in continuing education and schools of nursing are frequently looking for resources for teaching culture along with evidence-based materials. A few resources are the Jeffreys textbook *Teaching Cultural Competence in Nursing and Health Care: Inquiry, Action, and Innovation* (2010); the American Association of Colleges of Nursing's (AACN's) Toolkit for Cultural Competence in Master's and Doctoral Nursing Education (2011); and the Purnell textbook websites. In addition, the American Academy of Nursing, along with members of the Transcultural Nursing Society, established a task force to develop Guidelines for Implementing Culturally Competent Nursing Care (Douglas et al., 2014).

The content of this chapter is not focused on the numerous simplistic approaches that use acronyms as a guide for cultural assessment. Although some of these simplistic techniques can be used for collecting initial interview data, they do not work well with all ethnic and cultural groups, nor are they comprehensive. Two examples of acronymic approaches are BATHE and LEARN. The LEARN approach includes the following guidelines: **L**isten to your patients from their perspectives; **E**xplain your concerns and your reasons for asking for personal information; **A**cknowledge your patients' concerns; **R**ecommend a course of action; and **N**egotiate a plan of care that considers cultural norms and personal lifestyles (Berlin & Fowkes, 1983). The BATHE acronym stands for **B**ackground information, **A**ffect [sic] the problem has on the patient, **T**rouble the problem causes for the patient, **H**andling of the problem by the patient, and **E**mpathy conveyed by the healthcare provider (U.S. Department of Health and Human Services, n.d.).

ESSENTIAL TERMINOLOGY RELATED TO CULTURE

Many different definitions exist for culturally related terms. The definitions used in this chapter are adapted from the American Nurses Association's *Nursing: Scope and Standards of Practice*, Standard 8 (2015); the Expert Panel on Cultural Competence of the American Academy of Nursing (Giger et al., 2007); and Guidelines for Implementing Culturally Competent Nursing Care (Douglas et al., 2014). These definitions were developed in an attempt to reach a standard worldwide consensus and thereby decrease confusion related to the inconsistent definitions of culture-related terms. The confusion arises because a variety of terms and definitions that describe cultural awareness, cultural sensitivity, and cultural competence are used interchangeably in the literature. They have been presented in several international conferences. A few of these definitions are listed here:

- *Cultural awareness* is being knowledgeable about one's own thoughts, feelings, and sensations and having an appreciation of diversity in terms of the objective (material) culture, such as arts, clothing, foods, and other external signs of diversity.
- *Cultural sensitivity* is experienced when neutral language, both verbal and nonverbal, is used in a way that reflects sensitivity and appreciation for the diversity of another. Cultural sensitivity is conveyed through words, phrases, and categorizations that are intentionally avoided, especially when referring to an individual who may interpret them as impolite or offensive.
- *Cultural imposition* intrusively applies the majority cultural view to individuals and families. For example, prescribing a special diet without regard to a person's culture and limiting visitors to immediate family border on cultural imposition. In this context, healthcare providers must be careful in expressing their cultural values too strongly until cultural issues are more fully understood.
- *Cultural imperialism* is the practice of extending the policies and procedure of one organization—usually the dominant one—to disenfranchised and minority groups. Proponents of cultural imperialism appeal to universal human rights values and standards. Opponents posit that universal standards are a guise under which the dominant culture seeks to destroy or eradicate traditional cultures by setting worldwide public policy.
- *Cultural relativism* is the belief that behaviors and practices of people should be judged only in the context of their cultural system. Proponents argue that issues such as abortion,

euthanasia, female circumcision, and physical punishment in childrearing should be accepted as cultural values without judgment from the outside world. Opponents argue that cultural relativism may undermine condemnation of human rights violations and that family violence cannot be justified or excused on a cultural basis.

- *Ethnocentrism* is a universal tendency to believe that one's own worldview is superior to another's worldview. It is often experienced in the healthcare arena, in particular when the healthcare provider's own culture or ethnic group is considered superior to another.
- A *stereotype* is a simplified and standardized conception, opinion, or belief about a person or group. A healthcare provider who fails to recognize individuality within a group is jumping to conclusions about the individual or family.
- *Generalization* begins with assumptions about the individual or family within an ethno-cultural group but leads to further information seeking about the individual or family.
- *Race* is a viable term that relates to biology but also has sociological implications. Members of a particular race share distinguishing physical features such as skin color, bone structure, or blood group. Race as a social construct can limit or increase opportunities, depending on the setting.
- *Racism* refers to feelings of prejudice against persons of another race or group of people. Racist practices lead to interpersonal tension, isolation, discrimination, and overt anger.
- An *ethnic group* is a group of people whose members have different experiences and backgrounds from the dominant culture in terms of status, background, residence, religion, education, or other factors that functionally unify the group and act collectively in their effects.
- *Stigma* is a characteristic or trait that puts a strain on or reproaches a group's or individual's reputation or being.
- *Culture* is a learned, patterned behavioral response acquired over time that includes implicit versus explicit beliefs, attitudes, values, customs, norms, taboos, arts, and life ways accepted by a community of individuals. Culture is primarily learned and transmitted through the family and other social organizations, is shared by the majority of the group, includes an individualized worldview, guides decision making, and influences self-worth and self-esteem.

CULTURAL SELF-AWARENESS

Culture has a powerful unconscious impact on both patients and health professionals (Purnell, 2013). Each clinical encounter with an APN adds a unique dimension to the complexity of providing culturally competent care. The way APNs perceive themselves as competent is often reflected in the way they communicate with clients. Thus, it is essential for APNs to take time to think about themselves, their behaviors, and their communication styles in relation to their perceptions of different cultures.

Before addressing the multicultural backgrounds and unique individual perspectives of their patients, APNs must first address their own personal and professional knowledge, values, beliefs, ethics, and life experiences in a manner that optimizes assessment of and interactions with clients who come from cultures different from those of the APN. Self-awareness in cultural competence is a deliberate and conscious cognitive and emotional process of getting to know oneself; one's own personality, values, beliefs, professional knowledge, standards, and ethics; and the effects of these factors on the various roles one plays when interacting with individuals who are different from oneself. The ability to understand oneself sets the stage for integrating new knowledge related to cultural differences into the APN's knowledge base and perceptions of health interventions (Purnell, 2013).

SELECTED CULTURAL MODELS AND THEORIES

The limited space available here does not permit an exhaustive description of the numerous models and theories centered on culture. A brief description of the models most commonly used in practice, education, administration, and research follows. A more thorough description of the Purnell model for cultural competence is described in detail in the next section.

The Campinha-Bacote Model

The Campinha-Bacote model is a practice model that was originally developed in 1991. It has been revised several times since then. It focuses on the process of cultural competence in the delivery of healthcare services. This model, which is currently referred to as a *volcano model* (Campinha-Bacote, 2015), is used primarily in practice and education; it does not have an accompanying organizational framework. Included is a Biblically based model of Cultural Competence in the Provision of Health Care Services. A literature review did not reveal any research using the Campinha-Bacote model.

According to Campinha-Bacote (2015), individuals, as well as organizations and institutions, begin the journey to cultural competence by first demonstrating an intrinsic motivation to engage in the process of cultural competence. The five concepts in this model are described as follows:

1. *Cultural awareness:* The nurse becomes sensitive to the values, beliefs, lifestyle, and practices of the patient, and explores his or her own values, biases, and prejudices. Unless nurses go through this process in a conscious, deliberate, and reflective manner, there is always the risk of nurses imposing their own cultural values during the encounter.
2. *Cultural knowledge:* Cultural knowledge is the process through which nurses find out more about other cultures and the different worldviews held by people from other cultures. Understanding the values, beliefs, practices, and problem-solving strategies of culturally/ ethnically diverse groups enables nurses to gain confidence in their cultural encounters.

3. *Cultural skill:* Cultural skill as a process is concerned with carrying out a cultural assessment. On the basis of cultural knowledge, nurses are able to conduct an assessment in partnership with patients.
4. *Cultural encounter:* Cultural encounter is the process that provides the primary and experiential exposure to cross-cultural interactions with people who are culturally/ ethnically diverse from oneself.
5. *Cultural desire:* Cultural desire is a self-motivational aspect of individuals and organizations that encourages them to want to engage in the process of cultural competence.

Campinha-Bacote has emphasized that a cultural assessment is needed for every client because every person has values, beliefs, and practices that must be considered when the nurse is delivering healthcare services. Therefore, cultural assessments should not be limited to specific ethnic groups, but rather conducted with each patient (Campinha-Bacote, 2015). Although this model does not have an assessment guide, it does meet the criteria for simplicity, clarity, generality, and empirical precision. A graphical display and additional information about the Campinha-Bacote model can be found at the Transcultural C.A.R.E. Associates website (http://transculturalcare .net/a-biblically-based-model-of-cultural-competence/).

The Giger and Davidhizar Model

The transcultural assessment model developed by Giger and Davidhizar (Giger, 2012) focuses on assessment and intervention from a transcultural nursing perspective. In this model, each person is seen as a unique cultural being influenced by culture, ethnicity, and religion. The model has been used in education, practice, administration, and research. The six areas of human diversity and variation in the model are described as follows:

1. *Communication:* The factors that influence communication are universal, but they vary among culture-specific groups in terms of language spoken, voice quality, pronunciation, and use of nonverbal communication, including silence.
2. *Space:* People perceive physical and personal space through their biological senses. The cultural aspect of space reflects the degree of comfort one feels in proximity to others, in body movement, and in perception of personal, intimate, and public space.
3. *Social orientation:* Components of social organization vary by culture, with differences observed in what constitutes one's understanding of culture, race, ethnicity, family role and function, work, leisure, church, and friends in day-to-day life.
4. *Time:* Time is perceived, measured, and valued differently across cultures. Time is conceptualized in reference to the life span in terms of growth and development, perception of time in relation to duration of events, and time as an external entity outside of an individual's control.

5. *Environmental control:* Environment is more than just the place where one lives; it involves systems and processes that influence, and are influenced by, individuals and groups. Culture influences the understanding of how individuals and groups shape their environments and how environments constrain or enable individual health behaviors.

6. *Biological variations:* Biological variations include dimensions such as body structure, body weight, skin color, and internal biological mechanisms such as genetic and enzymatic predisposition to certain diseases, drug interactions, and metabolism.

The Giger and Davidhizar model proposes a framework that facilitates assessment of the individual. A set of questions is constructed under each of the six areas to generate information useful in planning care that is congruent with an individual's cultural orientation and needs. The model also represents a learning tool that can be used to explore issues about any of the six broad areas in practice. For nurses, flexibility and the involvement of the patient as an equal partner in the cultural assessment of needs are encouraged. The Giger and Davidhizar model can be used to elicit general explanatory models of health and illness. It meets the criteria for clarity, simplicity, generality, empirical precision, and derivable consequences (Giger, 2012).

The Papadopoulos, Tilki, and Taylor Model

The Papadopoulos, Tilki, and Taylor model—which focuses on the process of cultural competence in the delivery of healthcare services—was first published in 1998 and is used in education, practice, and administration. This model does not have an assessment guide or organizing framework. The four main components of this model are described as follows (Intercultural Education of Nurses in Europe, 2016):

1. *Cultural awareness:* Cultural awareness represents the first step toward cultural competence. It incorporates self-awareness, cultural identity, cultural adherence, ethnocentricity, stereotyping, and ethnohistory.

2. *Cultural knowledge:* Cultural knowledge is the second step toward cultural competence. It includes health beliefs and behaviors; anthropological, sociopolitical, and biological understanding; similarities and differences among cultures; and health inequities.

3. *Cultural competence:* Cultural competence includes assessment skills, diagnostic skills, and challenging and addressing prejudice, discrimination, and inequalities.

4. *Cultural sensitivity:* Cultural sensitivity includes empathy, interpersonal communication skills, trust and respect, acceptance, appropriateness, and barriers to cultural sensitivity.

This model meets the criteria for clarity, simplicity, generality, and empirical precision. A graphical display of this model can be found through the Leonardo da Vinci Partnership

Project website (2012; http://www.ieneproject.eu/download/Outputs/intercultural%20 model.pdf).

Leininger's Cultural Care Diversity and Universality Theory and Model

Leininger's cultural care diversity and universality theory and the sunrise model that depicts her theory are perhaps the most well known in nursing literature on culture and health (McFarland & Wehbe-Alamah, 2015). The theory draws from anthropological observations and studies of culture and cultural values, beliefs, and practices. The theory of transcultural nursing promotes understanding of both the universally held and common understandings of care among humans and the culture-specific caring beliefs and behaviors that define any particular caring context or interaction. According to Leininger, this theory is intended to be holistic: Culture is the specific pattern of behavior that distinguishes any society from others and gives meaning to human expressions of care (McFarland & Wehbe-Alamah, 2015).

The theory of cultural care diversity and universality is heavily used in education and research. It incorporates the following assumptions about care and caring as they relate to cultural competence (McFarland & Wehbe-Alamah, 2015):

- Care (caring) is essential to curing and healing, for there can be no curing without caring.
- Every human culture has generic, folk, or indigenous care knowledge and practices and usually some professional care knowledge and practices that vary transculturally.
- Culture care values, beliefs, and practices are influenced by and tend to be embedded in the worldview, language, philosophy, religion and spirituality, kinship, social, political, legal, educational, economic, technological, ethno-historical, and environmental contexts of cultures.
- A client who experiences nursing care that fails to be reasonably congruent with his or her beliefs, values, and caring life ways will show signs of cultural conflict, noncompliance, stress, and ethical or moral concern.
- Within a cultural care diversity and universality framework, nurses may take any or all of three culturally congruent action modes: (1) cultural preservation/maintenance, (2) cultural care accommodation/negotiation, and (3) cultural care repatterning/restructuring.

According to Leininger, *cultural care preservation/maintenance* refers to assistive, supportive, facilitative, or enabling professional actions and decisions that help individuals, families, and communities of a particular culture retain and preserve care values so that they can maintain well-being, recover from illness, or face possible handicap or death. *Cultural care accommodation/negotiation* refers to assistive, supportive, facilitative, or enabling professional actions and potential decisions that help individuals, families, and communities of a particular culture adapt to or negotiate with others for satisfying healthcare outcomes with professional caregivers. *Cultural care repatterning/restructuring* refers to the assistive, supportive, facilitative, and enabling roles filled by nurses and other healthcare providers to promote actions and decisions that may help the person, family, or community change or modify behaviors affecting their life ways, thereby achieving a new and different health pattern (McFarland & Wehbe-Alamah, 2015). These three action modes are sometimes used with other cultural theories and models.

Leininger recognized the comparative aspects of caring within and between cultures—hence the theory's acknowledgment of similarities as much as differences in caring in diverse cultures. Her transcultural model has implications for how nurses assess, plan, implement, and evaluate care of people from diverse cultural backgrounds. The sunrise model and theory have clarity, but they are complex. The model has generality for nursing, empirical precision, and derivable consequences. It can be found on the Transcultural Nursing Society's website (http://www.tcns.org/Theories.html).

Spector's HEALTH Traditions Model

Spector's health traditions model incorporates three main components: heritage consistency, HEALTH traditions, and Giger and Davidhizar's theory (Giger, 2012) about the cultural phenomena affecting health. *Heritage consistency* originally described the extent to which a person's lifestyle reflected his or her tribal culture but has since been expanded to study a person's traditional cultural background, such as European, Asian, African, or Hispanic. The values indicating heritage consistency exist on a continuum.

The HEALTH traditions model is based on the concept of holistic health and explores what people do to maintain, protect, or restore health. This model emphasizes the interrelationship between physical, mental, and spiritual health with personal methods of maintaining, protecting, and restoring health. To maintain physical health, for example, an individual may use traditional foods and clothing that have proven effective within the culture in the past. Protection of one's mental health may be achieved by receiving emotional and social support from family members and the community. Religious rituals may be performed, with the belief that they will assist in restoring health (Spector, 2013).

Spector also provides a Heritage Assessment Tool to determine the degree to which people or families adhere to their traditions. A traditional person observes his or her cultural traditions more closely. A more acculturated individual's practice is less observant of traditional practices (Spector, 2013). The model has clarity, simplicity, generality, and empirical precision.

THE PURNELL MODEL FOR CULTURAL COMPETENCE

The Purnell model for cultural competence has been classified as a grand, holographic, and complexity theory (StudyBlue, 2016) originated from education and practice.

In 1989, Purnell took third-year nursing students to a community hospital that was not accustomed to having students. Soon after the clinical experience began, it became obvious that the students and staff needed additional knowledge concerning culture. The students primarily came from White families of middle socioeconomic and upper-middle socioeconomic classes, but most of the patients and staff came from lower socioeconomic backgrounds or had a heritage rooted in Appalachia. As part of postconferences, Purnell began having sessions with students and staff that centered on patients', staffs', and students' cultures.

The next semester, Purnell had senior nursing students in five different emergency departments. Again, it became obvious that both students and staff could benefit from a cultural assessment guide, as well as from greater knowledge about the specific cultural groups to whom they were providing care.

The first step in formalizing the cultural educational experience was to develop a comprehensive organizing framework that was usable by both staff and students. The more APNs know about a specific ethnic or cultural group, the better their assessment of patients, which helps ensure culturally congruent care. For example, if APNs are not aware of the various traditional healthcare practitioners used by many Hispanic or Latino people (e.g., *curanderos, sobadores, masajistas, y(j)erberos, espiritistas, sacerdotes*), they will not know to ask about them (Purnell, 2013).

Over the next few years, Purnell further developed the organizing framework and expanded the model to include holographic and complexity theory. *Holographic* simply means that the theory is not confined to one discipline, but rather has applicability across health-related disciplines. In *complexity theory*, there is usually an accompanying organizing framework to simplify the theory. Complexity theory, similar to chaos theory, is characterized by large numbers of similar but independent domains; continuous change in the phenomena of interest, leading to adaptation to the environment to ensure survival; and self-organization over time. The system never reaches equilibrium because societal events necessitate ongoing change in beliefs and values (Rickles, Hawe, & Shiell, 2007).

This model has been used (1) in multiple practice sites; (2) in education as a guide to incorporate culture into baccalaureate, master's, and doctoral programs; (3) in research in Australia, Brazil, Canada, Chile, China, the Czech Republic, Ethiopia, Korea, Spain, Turkey, the United Kingdom, and the United States; and (4) in administration. It also has been used by non-nursing disciplines, such as physical therapy (Black-Lattanzi & Purnell, 2006), medicine (Braithwaite, 2003; Crandall, George, Marion, & Davis, 2003; Purnell, 2003a, 2003b), and occupational therapy (Nayar & Tse, 2006). In addition, the model has been translated into Arabic, Czech, Flemish, German, Italian, Korean, Portuguese, Spanish, Swedish, and Turkish, testifying to its use on a worldwide basis. Purnell has also consulted and made presentations about cultural competence in nursing and health care at numerous universities and healthcare organizations in Australia, Belize, Belgium,

China, Colombia, Costa Rica, Denmark, England, Hungary, Italy, Korea, Mexico, Panama, Portugal, Scotland, Spain, Sweden, Turkey, and the United States, testifying to its utility on an international scale.

Assumptions of the Purnell Model

The explicit assumptions upon which the model is based include the following:

1. All healthcare professions need similar information about cultural diversity.
2. All healthcare professions share the metaparadigm concepts of global society, family, person, and health.
3. One culture is not better than another culture; they are just different.
4. There are core similarities shared by all cultures.
5. There are differences within, between, and among cultures.
6. Cultures change slowly over time.
7. The variant cultural characteristics determine the degree to which one varies from the dominant culture.
8. If clients are coparticipants in their care and have a choice in health-related goals, plans, and interventions, their compliance and health outcomes will be improved.
9. Culture has a powerful influence on an individual's interpretation of and responses to health care.
10. Individuals and families belong to several subcultures.
11. Each individual has the right to be respected for his or her uniqueness and cultural heritage.
12. APNs need both cultural-general and cultural-specific information to provide culturally sensitive and culturally competent care.
13. Caregivers who can assess, plan, intervene, and evaluate in a culturally competent manner will improve the care of clients for whom they care.
14. Learning culture is an ongoing process that develops in a variety of ways, but primarily through cultural encounters (Campinha-Bacote, 2015).
15. Prejudices and biases can be minimized with cultural understanding.
16. To be effective, health care must reflect the unique understanding of the values, beliefs, attitudes, life ways, and worldview of diverse populations and individual acculturation patterns.
17. Differences in race and culture often require adaptations to standard interventions.
18. Cultural awareness improves the caregiver's self-awareness.
19. Professions, organizations, and associations have their own cultures, which can be analyzed using a grand theory of culture.
20. Every client encounter is a cultural encounter (Purnell, 2013, 2014).

Variant Cultural Characteristics

Major influences that shape individuals' worldview and the extent to which people identify with their cultural group of origin are called variant cultural characteristics and include the following: nationality, race, color, gender, age, religious affiliation, educational status, socioeconomic status, occupation, military experience, political beliefs, urban versus rural residence, enclave identity, marital status, parental status, physical characteristics, sexual orientation, gender issues, reason for migration (e.g., sojourner, immigrant, or undocumented status), length of time away from the country of origin, and hearing impairment. Moreover, immigration status also influences a person's worldview. For example, people who voluntarily immigrate generally acculturate and assimilate into a new society more easily. Conversely, sojourners who immigrate with the intention of remaining in their new homeland for only a short time or refugees who think they may return to their home country may not have the need or desire to acculturate or assimilate. Additionally, undocumented individuals (illegal immigrants) may have a different worldview from those who have arrived legally (Purnell, 2013). Some of these variant cultural characteristics change over time, while others do not. In addition, a stigma may occur for some, either the individual or the family, if they do change (e.g., changing religious affiliation from Judaism to Pentecostal).

Cultural Competence According to the Purnell Model

Cultural competence is multifactorial in nature. To be comprehensive, this term is defined as developing an awareness of one's own existence, sensations, thoughts, and environment, without letting those factors have an undue influence on persons from other backgrounds. It incorporates the following aspects of care:

1. Demonstrating knowledge and understanding of the client's culture, health-related needs, and culturally specific meanings of health and illness
2. Continuing to learn about the cultures of clients to whom one provides care
3. Recognizing that the primary and secondary characteristics of culture determine the degree to which clients adhere to the beliefs, values, and practices of their dominant culture
4. Accepting and respecting cultural differences in a manner that facilitates clients' and families' abilities to make decisions to meet their needs and beliefs
5. Not assuming that the healthcare provider's beliefs and values are the same as the client's
6. Resisting judgmental attitudes such as "different is not as good"
7. Being open to cultural encounters
8. Being comfortable with cultural encounters

9. Adapting care to be congruent with the client's culture
10. Engaging in cultural competence as a conscious process and not necessarily a linear one
11. Accepting responsibility for one's own education in cultural competence by attending conferences, reading professional literature, and observing cultural practices

Description of the Purnell Model

The Purnell model for cultural competence and its organizing framework can be used in all kinds of practice settings and by all kinds of healthcare providers. The model is depicted graphically as a series of circles, where the outlying rim represents global society, the second rim represents community, the third rim represents family, and the inner rim represents the person (see **Figure 23-1**). The interior of the circle is divided into 12 pie-shaped wedges depicting cultural domains (constructs) and their associated concepts. The dark center of the circle represents unknown phenomena. Along the bottom of the model is a jagged line representing the nonlinear concept of cultural consciousness.

The 12 cultural domains and their concepts provide the organizing framework. Each domain includes concepts that need to be addressed when assessing patients in various settings. Moreover, APNs can use these same concepts to better understand their own cultural beliefs, attitudes, values, practices, and behaviors. An especially important concept is the notion that no single domain stands alone; rather, all of the domains are inextricably interconnected. The 12 domains are (1) overview/heritage, (2) communications, (3) family roles and organization, (4) workforce issues, (5) biocultural ecology, (6) high-risk health behaviors, (7) nutrition, (8) pregnancy and the childbearing family, (9) death rituals, (10) spirituality, (11) healthcare practices, and (12) healthcare practitioners (see Figure 23-1).

The Purnell model has clarity, generality, empirical precision, and derivable consequences. The model in its entirety is complex. The practitioner would rarely complete a full assessment using all of the concepts in the 12 domains, especially in any one setting. This cultural model is one of the most thoroughly developed to date (Catalano, 2011).

Macro Aspects of the Purnell Model

The macro aspects of this interactional model include the metaparadigm concepts of global society, community, family, person, and conscious competence. The theory and model are conceptualized from foundations in biology, anthropology, sociology, economics, geography, history, ecology, physiology, psychology, political science, pharmacology, and nutrition, as well as theories from communication, family development, and social support. The model can be used in clinical practice, education, research, and the administration and management of healthcare services; it also can be used to analyze organizational culture.

Phenomena related to a global society include world communication and politics; conflicts and warfare; natural disasters and famines; international exchanges in education,

The Purnell Model for Cultural Competence

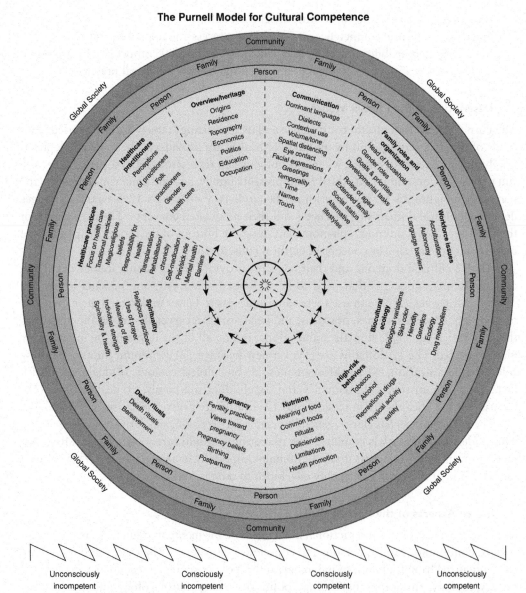

Variant cultural characteristics: age, generation, nationality, race, color, gender, religion, educational status, socioeconomic status, occupation, military status, political beliefs, urban versus rural residence, enclave identity, marital status, parental status, physical characteristics, sexual orientation, gender issues, and reason for migration (sojourner, immigrant, undocumented status).

Unconsciously incompetent: not being aware that one is lacking knowledge about another culture. Consciously incompetent: being aware that one is lacking knowledge about another culture. Consciously competent: learning about the client's culture, verifying generalizations about the client's culture, and providing culturally specific interventions. Unconsciously competent: automatically providing culturally congruent care to clients of diverse cultures.

Figure 23-1   The Purnell model for cultural competence.

Purnell model for cultural competence reprinted with permission of Larry D. Purnell, PhD, RN, FAAN.

business, commerce, and information technology; advances in health science; space exploration; and the expanded opportunities for people to travel around the world and interact with diverse societies. Information about global events that is widely disseminated by television, radio, satellite transmission, newsprint, and information technology affects all societies, either directly or indirectly. Such events create chaos while consciously and unconsciously forcing people to alter their life ways and worldviews.

In its broadest definition, *community* is a group of people having a common interest or identity; it goes beyond the physical environment. Community includes the physical, social, and symbolic characteristics that cause people to connect. Bodies of water, mountains, rural versus urban living, and even railroad tracks help people define their physical concept of community. Of course, technology and the Internet now allow people to readily expand their community beyond the physical boundaries that defined communities in the past. Economics, religion, politics, age, generation, and marital status delineate the social concepts of community. Moreover, sharing a specific language or dialect, lifestyle, history, dress, art, or musical interest are symbolic characteristics of a community. People actively and passively interact with the community, necessitating adaptation and assimilation for equilibrium and homeostasis in their worldview. Individuals may willingly change their physical, social, and symbolic community when it no longer meets their needs.

A *family* is two or more people who are emotionally connected. They may—but do not necessarily—live in close proximity to one another. Family may include physically and emotionally close and distant consanguineous relatives, as well as physically and emotionally connected and distant non-blood-related significant others. Family structure and roles change according to age, generation, marital status, relocation or immigration, and socio-economic status, requiring each person to rethink his or her individual beliefs and life ways.

A *person* is a bio-psycho-sociocultural being who is constantly adapting to his or her community. Human beings adapt biologically and physiologically with the aging process; psychologically in the context of social relationships, stress, and relaxation; socially as they interact with the changing community; and ethno-culturally within the broad global society. In Western cultures, a person is considered a separate physical and unique psychological being and a singular member of society; that is, the self remains separate from others. In contrast, in Asian and some other primarily collectivistic cultures, the individual is defined in relation to the family or other group, rather than as a basic unit of nature.

Health is a state of wellness as defined by the individual within his or her ethnocultural group. Health generally includes physical, mental, and spiritual states because group members interact with the family, community, and global society. The concept of health, which permeates all metaparadigm concepts of culture, is defined globally, nationally, regionally, locally, and individually. Thus, people can speak about their personal health status or the health status of the nation or community. Health also can be subjective or objective in nature (Purnell, 2013).

Domains of the Purnell Model and the Organizing Framework

The 12 domains in the Purnell model are listed in this section, along with the major concepts, key questions, and observations to make for each domain.

Overview and Heritage

The overview and heritage domain includes concepts related to the country of origin and current residence, such as the effects of the topography of the country of origin and the current residence on health, economics, politics, reasons for migration, educational status, and occupations. **Box 23-1** lists specific questions and a sample rationale that the APN should consider for this domain.

Communication

The communication domain includes concepts related to the dominant language, sign language, dialects, health literacy, and the contextual use of the language; paralanguage variations such as voice volume, tone, intonations, inflections, and willingness to share thoughts and feelings; nonverbal communications such as eye contact, gesturing, facial expressions, use of touch, body language, spatial distancing practices, and acceptable greetings; temporality in terms of past, present, and future orientation of worldview; clock versus social time; and the amount of formality in use of names. **Box 23-2** lists specific questions and a sample rationale that the APN should consider for this domain.

Box 23-1 Overview, Inhabited Localities, and Topography

The following are suggested questions, each accompanied by a sample rationale, that the APN can ask in a cultural assessment.

1. Where do you currently live? *Sample rationale:* Someone living in the inner city may be at increased risk for illnesses such as emphysema and asthma because of increased air pollution. American Indians living on reservations have increased tuberculosis rates owing to living conditions and lifestyle.
2. What is your ancestry? *Sample rationale:* Members of the Amish community have high rates of glutaric acidemia, dwarfism, cartilage-hair hypoplasia, and hemophilia B. Turks have high rates of helminthiasis owing to lifestyle and environment.
3. Where were you born? *Sample rationale:* Some studies of the Chernobyl (Russia) nuclear incident show an increase in genetic mutations and hereditary defects related to radioactive contamination.
4. How many years have you lived in the United States (or other country, as appropriate)? *Sample rationale:* May show degree of assimilation and acculturation.
5. Were your parents born in the United States (or other country, as appropriate)? *Sample rationale:* May show degree of assimilation and acculturation.

(Continues)

6. What brought you (your parents/ancestors) to the United States (or other country, as appropriate)? *Sample rationale:* Refugees may have post-traumatic stress disorders related to their stay in refugee camps.

7. Describe the land or countryside where you live. Is it mountainous? Swampy (and so on)? *Sample rationale:* People living in or around wooded areas and who have vague symptoms of fever, fatigue, and headache with or without skin rash may have Lyme disease. People emigrating from Panama may have a high risk for dengue fever.

8. Have you lived other places in the United States/world? *Sample rationale:* People immigrating from, or who have recently visited parts of, Central America or Africa and who present with fever, chills, headache, and fatigue may need to be assessed for malaria or dengue fever.

9. What was the land or countryside like when you lived there? *Sample rationale:* People who have lived near a contaminated (Superfund) site may be at risk for increased incidence of cancer.

10. What is your income level? *Sample rationale:* May provide information about the ability to afford prescription medication and other treatment aids such as dressings and prescriptive devices.

11. Does your income allow you to afford the essentials of life? *Sample rationale:* May have implications for the ability to purchase "fresh fruits and vegetables," affecting overall health.

12. Are you able to afford health insurance on your salary? *Sample rationale:* An individual may have the financial wherewithal to afford insurance, but some persons who have a present orientation may not see the value in obtaining health insurance.

13. Do you have health insurance? *Sample rationale:* If the patient does not have health insurance, he or she may be referred to social services for financial support.

14. What is your educational level (formal/informal/self-taught)? *Sample rationale:* May have implications for health literacy and teaching.

15. What is your current occupation? If the individual is retired, ask about previous occupations. *Sample rationale:* A person may currently work in the construction industry but previously have worked in coal mines, which increases the risk for radiation poisoning and black lung. Asbestosis may still be a concern for people working in the construction industry.

16. Have you worked in other occupations? What were they? *Sample rationale:* An individual may currently work in carpentry but previously have worked in welding and therefore have an increased risk for cataracts.

17. Are there (were there) any particular health hazards associated with your job(s)? *Sample rationale:* People who work in the ornamental nursery industry and farming are at high risk for health problems related to the use of pesticides.

Questions and observations related to the primary and secondary characteristics of culture not covered in the previous questions include the following:

1. Have you been in the military? If so, in which foreign countries were you stationed? *Sample rationale:* People who have served in Afghanistan are at high risk for water- and foodborne diseases. Veterans and their families who lived in Camp Lejeune, North Carolina, are at high risk for waterborne illnesses due exposure to benzene and other contaminants in drinking water.

2. Are you married? *Sample rationale:* Part of a standard assessment and may provide information about support.

3. How many children do you have? *Sample rationale:* Part of a standard assessment and may provide information about support.

Box 23-2 Communication

The following are suggested questions, each accompanied by a sample rationale, that the APN can ask in a cultural assessment.

1. What is your full name? *Sample rationale:* Part of a standard assessment. Complex naming can create difficulties for medical record keeping.
2. What is your legal name? *Sample rationale:* Hispanic/Latino individuals have an extended name format that includes a first name, middle name, father's last name, and mother's last name, with an additional last name of the husband if a woman is married. In these cases, a person selects any combination of last names for his or her legal name.
3. By which name do you wish to be called? *Sample rationale:* Helps establish trust and increases comfort level of the patient.
4. What is your primary language? *Sample rationale:* The primary language is usually best for patient education, but the APN should ask about the preferred language. Signing may be a concern because of the differences among Arabic sign languages, American Sign Language, and British Sign Language.
5. Do you speak a specific dialect? *Sample rationale:* A dialect-specific interpreter is preferred. For example, people from northern China speak a different dialect than people from southern China.
6. Which other languages do you speak? *Sample rationale:* May be helpful for interpretation if the preferred language interpreter is not available. For example, many Vietnamese persons speak French as a secondary language.
7. Do you find it difficult to share your thoughts, feelings, and ideas with family? Friends? Healthcare providers? *Sample rationale:* For people who find it difficult to share their feelings, additional time may be needed to establish trust and get full disclosure, especially with sensitive topics such as sexuality and substance use/misuse.
8. Do you mind being touched by friends? Strangers? Healthcare workers? *Sample rationale:* Reinforces the necessity to ask permission before touching. Always ask permission and explain the rationale for touching.
9. How do you wish to be greeted? Handshake? Nod of the head? Something else? *Sample rationale:* Preferred greetings help establish trust.
10. Are you usually on time for appointments? *Sample rationale:* A clear rationale can be given for intolerance of lateness; for example, some healthcare organizations will not see the patient if he or she is more than 15 minutes late and some still may charge for the visit.
11. Are you usually on time for social engagements? *Sample rationale:* Ask only if the question is pertinent.
12. Observe the client's speech pattern. Does the speech pattern demonstrate a high or low context? *Sample rationale:* Clients from highly contexted cultures place greater value on silence and may take more time to give a response.
13. Observe the client when physical contact is made. Does he or she withdraw from the touch or become tense? *Sample rationale:* Helps establish trust and reinforces the necessity of explaining the reason for touch.
14. How close does the client stand when talking with family members? With healthcare providers? *Sample rationale:* The APN should not take offense if a patient stands closer to or farther away than the distance to which the APN is accustomed. Spatial distancing is culture bound.
15. Does the client maintain eye contact when talking with the APN? *Sample rationale:* Some cultures avoid eye contact with people in hierarchal positions (the APN is in a hierarchal position in the healthcare setting) as a sign of respect.

Family Roles and Organization

The family roles and organization domain includes concepts related to the head of the household, gender/sex roles (a product of biology and culture), family goals and priorities, developmental tasks of children and adolescents, roles of the aged and extended family, individual and family social status in the community, and acceptance of alternative lifestyles such as single parenting, sexual orientations, childless marriages, and divorce. **Box 23-3** lists specific questions and a sample rationale that the APN should consider for this domain.

Box 23-3   Family Roles and Organization

The following are suggested questions, each accompanied by a sample rationale, that the APN can ask in a cultural assessment.

1. Who makes most of the decisions in your family? *Sample rationale:* If the decision maker is not accessed, no decision will be made and time will be wasted. In addition, the spokesperson for the family might not be the decision maker, as occurs among many Hispanic/Latino populations.
2. Which types of decisions do(es) the female(s) in your family make? *Sample rationale:* In many traditional families, the female makes decisions about the household and child care, but not always.
3. Which types of decisions do(es) the male(s) in your family make? *Sample rationale:* In many traditional families, the male is the primary decision maker regarding affairs outside the household, but not always.
4. What are the duties of the women in the family? *Sample rationale:* Understanding division of labor can become important when illness occurs.
5. What are the duties of the men in the family? *Sample rationale:* Understanding division of labor can become important when illness occurs.
6. What should children do to make a good impression for themselves and for the family? *Sample rationale:* Important to note in school health and family counseling. A child's behavior can bring shame upon or honor to the family.
7. What would children do that would *not* make a good impression for themselves and for the family? *Sample rationale:* Among traditional Chinese, children are to do well in school or shame may come to the family.
8. What are children forbidden to do? *Sample rationale:* Among traditional Germans and many other cultures, taboo behaviors include talking back to elders and touching another person's possessions.
9. What should young adults do to make a good impression for themselves and for the family? *Sample rationale:* Among most Koreans, one of the most important things young adults can do to bring pride to themselves and their families is to do well in school. Otherwise, shame can occur to the extent that many students have committed suicide.
10. What would young adults do that would *not* make a good impression for themselves and for the family? *Sample rationale:* Among traditional Mexican families, young adults should not dress in a provocative manner. Otherwise, shame can come to them or their family.

(Continues)

11. What are adolescents forbidden to do? *Sample rationale:* Taboo behaviors for young adults in Iran include using illicit drugs or engaging in sexual activity before marriage. This behavior can bring shame upon the family.

12. What are the priorities for your family? *Sample rationale:* For a lower-socioeconomic family, the priority may be having adequate food and shelter with stress on the present but still not forgetting the future. Health care and education may not be priorities if the basic needs are not met.

13. What are the roles of older adults in your family? Are they sought for their advice? *Sample rationale:* Among traditional Koreans, no decision is made until the advice of older adults has been sought, although the advice might not be followed.

14. Are there extended family members in your household? Who else lives in your household? *Sample rationale:* Being aware of the household membership is important for health teaching and adequacy of care for sick family members. Most members of traditional Asian cultures live in extended family arrangements. Some families might have children totally unrelated to the host family.

15. What are the roles of extended family members in this household? *Sample rationale:* In many Filipino families, extended family members provide significant financial and social support and are important resources for child care.

16. What gives you and your family status? *Sample rationale:* Among the Navajo, status is obtained by sharing what you have with others.

17. Is it acceptable to you for people to have children out of wedlock? *Sample rationale:* Among traditional Arab families, shame may occur if a pregnancy occurs outside of marriage.

18. Is it acceptable to you for people to live together and not be married? *Sample rationale:* Among many Asian cultures, if a man and a woman live together without being married, that relationship may cause them to be rejected by their families.

19. Are you accepting of gay, lesbian, or transgendered people? *Sample rationale:* Not all cultures and individuals are accepting of gay, lesbian, or transgendered populations. Do not disclose these relationships to family members.

20. What is your sexual preference/orientation? (Ask only if appropriate, and then later in the assessment after a modicum of trust has been established). *Sample rationale:* Important for health counseling if sexually active.

Workforce Issues

The workforce issues domain includes concepts related to autonomy, acculturation, assimilation, gender roles, ethnic communication styles, and healthcare practices of the country of origin. **Box 23-4** lists specific questions and a sample rationale that the APN should consider for this domain.

Biocultural Ecology

The biocultural ecology domain includes physical, biological, and physiological variations among ethnic and racial groups such as skin color (the most evident) and physical differences

Box 23-4   Workforce Issues

The following are suggested questions, each accompanied by a sample rationale, that the APN can ask in a cultural assessment.

1. Do you usually report to work on time? *Sample rationale:* For present-oriented people who are accustomed to a lack of timeliness in the workforce, the supervisor needs to be very clear about the importance of timeliness and any repercussions if timeliness becomes a concern, especially in individualistic cultures.
2. Do you usually report to meetings on time? *Sample rationale:* In some cultures, such as among Panamanians, a meeting starts when most people have arrived.
3. What concerns do you have about working with someone of the opposite gender? *Sample rationale:* Strict Muslim separation of the sexes means that there may be family disharmony if men and women are expected to work in close proximity.
4. Do you consider yourself a "loyal" employee? *Sample rationale:* In Japanese culture, an employer may expect absolute loyalty, and employees often remain with the same company for their entire lives.
5. How long do you expect to remain in your position? *Sample rationale:* May have implications for health insurance and seeking health care in the United States.
6. What do you do when you do not know how to do something related to your job? *Sample rationale:* Among many traditional Koreans, when an employee does not know how to do something, rather than going to a supervisor, a coworker of the same nationality (if available) is sought out.
7. Do you consider yourself to be assertive in your job? *Sample rationale:* Traditional Filipinos are frequently not considered as assertive as some U.S. employers would like.
8. What difficulty does English (or another language) give you in the workforce? *Sample rationale:* May have implications for accuracy in fulfilling job requirements, both verbally and in writing.

in body habitus; genetic, hereditary, endemic, and topographical diseases; psychological makeup of individuals; and the physiological differences that affect the way drugs are metabolized by the body. In general, most diseases and illnesses may be classified into one of three categories on the basis of their causes: environment, lifestyles, and genetics.

1. *Lifestyle causes* include cultural practices and behaviors that can generally be controlled—for example, smoking, diet, and stress.
2. *Environmental causes* refer to the external environment (e.g., air and water pollution) and situations over which the individual has little or no control (e.g., presence of malarial mosquitoes, exposure to chemicals and pesticides, access to care, and associated diseases).
3. *Genetic conditions* are caused by genes.

Box 23-5 lists specific questions and a sample rationale that the APN should consider for this domain.

Box 23-5 Biocultural Ecology

The following are suggested questions, each accompanied by a sample rationale, that the APN can ask in a cultural assessment.

1. Are you allergic to any medications? *Sample rationale:* Standard for any assessment.
2. What problems did you have when you took over-the-counter medications? *Sample rationale:* Looking for possible allergies and side effects is standard for any assessment. The APN should ask about medicines purchased in countries outside the United States. In Mexico and other countries, a wide variety of medicines can be purchased over the counter that would require a prescription in the United States.
3. What problems did you have when you took prescription medications? *Sample rationale:* Looking for possible allergies and side effects is standard for any assessment.
4. What are the major illnesses and diseases in your family? *Sample rationale:* Looking for opportunities for health promotion and teaching is standard for any assessment. In addition, many Asians and Pacific Islanders have high incidences of glucose-6-phosphate dehydrogenase deficiency and alpha-thalassemia.
5. Are you aware of any genetic diseases in your family? *Sample rationale:* Members of Amish, Jewish, and other populations have many hereditary and genetic illnesses, and heritage can be important for counseling.
6. What are the major health problems in the country from which you come (if appropriate)? *Sample rationale:* Vietnamese immigrants and people who have spent time in refugee camps have a high incidence of hepatitis A, tuberculosis, and other infectious diseases.
7. With which race do you identify? *Sample rationale:* May be important for organizational demographics for grants.
8. Observe skin coloration and physical characteristics. *Sample rationale:* To assess for rashes on people with dark skin, the APN may need to palpate the area rather than relying on visual cues.
9. Observe for physical handicaps and disabilities. *Sample rationale:* Part of standard assessment. Many people do not disclose handicaps or disabilities, especially learning disabilities, upon initial encounter unless specifically asked.
10. For clients who have undergone transgendered surgery, ask if they have all their organs. *Sample rationale:* Women who transgender to male usually still have ovaries and a uterus. Men who transgender to female usually still have a prostrate.

High-Risk Health Behaviors

The high-risk health behaviors domain includes substance use and misuse of tobacco, alcohol, and recreational drugs; lack of physical activity; increased calorie consumption; nonuse of safety measures such as seat belts, helmets, and safe driving practices; and not taking measures to prevent contracting HIV and sexually transmitted infections. **Box 23-6** lists specific questions and a sample rationale that the APN should consider for this domain.

Box 23-6 High-Risk Health Behaviors

The following are suggested questions, each accompanied by a sample rationale, that the APN can ask in a cultural assessment.

1. How many cigarettes per day do you smoke? *Sample rationale:* Standard for any assessment. Because smoking carries a stigma in some cultures, the APN should assess smoking with a nonjudgmental attitude.
2. Do you smoke a pipe (or cigars)? *Sample rationale:* Standard for any assessment. Because smoking carries a stigma in some cultures, the APN should assess smoking with a nonjudgmental attitude.
3. Do you chew tobacco? *Sample rationale:* In parts of rural Appalachia and other areas of the world, chewing tobacco is common; this increases the risk for oropharyngeal cancer.
4. For how many years have you smoked/chewed tobacco? *Sample rationale:* Part of a standard assessment if there is a history of tobacco use.
5. How much do you drink each day? Ask about wine, beer, spirits, coffee, sweet tea and other drinks high in sugar, and energy drinks. *Sample rationale:* Part of a standard assessment; important for follow-up with laboratory tests.
6. Which recreational drugs do you use? *Sample rationale:* Part of a standard assessment. The APN should ask this question in a nonjudgmental manner to encourage the patient to disclose this sensitive information.
7. How often do you use recreational drugs? *Sample rationale:* Part of a standard assessment for determining the degree of risk.
8. Do you exercise each day? What type of exercise? For how long? *Sample rationale:* Part of a standard assessment for health promotion and wellness.
9. Do you use seat belts/helmets? *Sample rationale:* Part of a standard assessment for injury prevention.
10. What precautions do you take to prevent getting a sexually transmitted infection/HIV? *Sample rationale:* Part of a standard assessment for health promotion and wellness, and illness and disease prevention.

Nutrition

The nutrition domain includes the meaning of food, common foods and rituals, nutritional deficiencies and food limitations, and the use of food for health promotion, restoration, illness, and disease prevention. **Box 23-7** lists specific questions and a sample rationale that the APN should consider for this domain.

Pregnancy and Childbearing Practices

The pregnancy and childbearing practices domain includes culturally sanctioned and unsanctioned fertility practices, views on pregnancy, and prescriptive, restrictive, and taboo practices related to pregnancy, birthing, and the postpartum period. **Box 23-8** lists specific questions and a sample rationale that the APN should consider for this domain.

Box 23-7 Nutrition

The following are suggested questions, each accompanied by a sample rationale, that the APN can ask in a cultural assessment.

1. Are you satisfied with your weight? *Sample rationale:* In many cultures, being overweight is seen as positive; members of these cultures do not adhere to the U.S. weight recommendations.
2. Which foods do you eat to maintain your health? *Sample rationale:* Food choices are seen as a means for promoting health. In the dominant U.S. culture, fresh fruits and vegetables are encouraged for health promotion.
3. Do you avoid certain foods to maintain your health? *Sample rationale:* Most Mexicans, as well as members of other cultures, try to avoid foods with high fat content.
4. Why do you avoid these foods? *Sample rationale:* People may avoid specific foods because they were not part of their diet when growing up, because they do not like the taste of the food, or because they do not like the appearance of the food. Recommending foods that the patient does not find pleasing diminishes the chance that the recommendations will be followed.
5. Which foods do you eat when you are ill? *Sample rationale:* In many cultures, common foods eaten when ill include toast and tea or ginger ale.
6. Which foods do you avoid when you are ill? *Sample rationale:* Recommending a food that the person culturally or personally avoids diminishes the chance that the recommendations will be followed.
7. Why do you avoid these foods (if appropriate)? *Sample rationale:* Foods may be avoided for a number of reasons.
8. For which illnesses do you eat certain foods? *Sample rationale:* In many cultures, people drink a "hot toddy" for a cold or minor illness. The ingredients for a hot toddy vary but generally include tea, lemon or lime, sugar or honey, and some type of liquor such as whiskey or rum.
9. Which foods do you eat to balance your diet? *Sample rationale:* Not all cultures adhere to the U.S. government's food pyramids because the food choices are not part of their cultural diet. Many Asians, Hispanics, and African Americans have lactose intolerance and, therefore, cannot follow the recommendations in these food pyramids.
10. Which foods do you eat every day? *Sample rationale:* Most people have specific foods that they eat on almost a daily basis. Incorporating these foods into dietary prescriptions will increase compliance with dietary instructions.
11. Which foods do you eat every week? *Sample rationale:* Most people have specific foods that they eat on almost a weekly basis. Incorporating these foods into dietary prescriptions will increase compliance with dietary instructions.
12. Which foods do you eat that are part of your cultural heritage? *Sample rationale:* Including culturally preferred foods into nutritional recommendations increases compliance.
13. Which foods are high-status foods in your family/culture? *Sample rationale:* High-status foods vary according to cost and availability. Among Panamanians, canned sausages are high-status foods; the same items are low-status foods in the United States. Lobster is low status in the Philippines because of its ready availability but is high status in the United States because of its cost.
14. Which foods are eaten only by men? Women? Children? Teenagers? Older people? *Sample rationale:* Among some Guatemalan highland indigenous populations, primarily men eat eggs for the added protein value. The belief is that because men do heavy labor, they need more protein. However, they are supposed to share the protein foods on their plates with children.

(Continues)

15. How many meals do you eat each day? *Sample rationale:* Not all cultures eat the standard U.S. three meals per day. Among many Turks, people eat four to six times per day, but they consume smaller amounts at these meals than do most European Americans.

16. What time do you eat each meal? *Sample rationale:* May have implications for medication administration.

17. Do you snack between meals? *Sample rationale:* Studies have demonstrated that young adults in Appalachia snack frequently without eating a regular meal.

18. Which foods do you eat when you snack? *Sample rationale:* Many snacks are not considered healthy food choices. The APN can recommend healthy snacks to replace less healthy food choices.

19. Which holidays do you celebrate? *Sample rationale:* Holidays are a time for special meals and a time when many people consume excessive amounts of calories. Among other celebrations, many Hispanic/Latino cultures celebrate all of the Catholic religious holidays, as well as the patron saint of their state or their province, their village, and their school.

20. Which foods do you eat on particular holidays? *Sample rationale:* Foods are an important part of maintaining one's culture, and diet is one measure of acculturation.

21. Who usually buys the food in your household? *Sample rationale:* Many times it is just as important for the APN to talk with the person who purchases the food as with the person who prepares the meals. In migrant worker camps, the person who purchases the foods is not the person who cooks for the group. If one member of the group needs a special diet (e.g., a diabetic individual), the purchaser of the food needs to be included in nutritional education.

22. Who does the cooking in your household? *Sample rationale:* The person who does the cooking should be included in dietary counseling and education for special diets.

23. Do you have a refrigerator? *Sample rationale:* For homeless persons and many living on remote reservations, proper food storage must be taken into consideration.

24. How do you cook your food? *Sample rationale:* Preparation practices can add significant calories to meals.

25. How do you prepare meat? *Sample rationale:* Preparation practices can add significant calories to meals.

26. How do you prepare vegetables? *Sample rationale:* Preparation practices can add significant calories to meals.

27. What do you drink with your meals? *Sample rationale:* Beverages can add significant calories to meals.

28. Do you drink special teas? *Sample rationale:* Teas are used by many people for health promotion and wellness and in times of illness.

29. Do you have any food allergies/intolerances? *Sample rationale:* Many African Americans and Asians have lactose intolerance. Encouraging milk and milk products in the diet would not be beneficial for these persons.

30. Are there certain foods that cause problems when you eat them? *Sample rationale:* Looking for allergies or food to avoid in dietary counseling.

31. How does your diet change with each season? *Sample rationale:* Most people's diet changes with the seasons. For those individuals who live in colder climates, fresh fruits and vegetables may be too expensive in the winter; these individuals must rely on frozen or canned vegetables that are high in sodium content.

32. Are your food habits different on days you work from when you are not working? *Sample rationale:* A common occurrence is for some people to eat less healthy foods during the busy workweek, especially those who are single.

Box 23-8   Pregnancy and Childbearing Practices

The following are suggested questions, each accompanied by a sample rationale, that the APN can ask in a cultural assessment.

1. How many children do you have? *Sample rationale:* Part of a standard assessment.
2. Have you ever had an abortion? Stillborn? Miscarriage? *Sample rationale:* Part of a standard obstetrical/gynecological assessment.
3. What do you use for birth control? *Sample rationale:* Each cultural and religious group has acceptable and unacceptable methods of birth control. Islamic jurists have ruled that the use of "reversible" forms of birth control is "undesirable but not forbidden."
4. What does it mean to you and your family when you are pregnant? *Sample rationale:* In some cultures, a woman is not a true woman and has not reached her potential until she becomes pregnant.
5. Which special foods do you eat when you are pregnant? *Sample rationale:* Although there are no specifically prescribed foods for a pregnant Polish woman, she is expected to eat for two.
6. Which foods do you avoid when you are pregnant? *Sample rationale:* Korean women who are pregnant avoid coffee, spicy foods, chicken, and crab. Among Haitians, women are restricted from eating spices that may irritate the fetus.
7. Which activities do you avoid when you are pregnant? *Sample rationale:* A belief among traditional Mexicans is that a pregnant woman should not walk in the moonlight for fear that the baby will be born with a cleft lip or palate.
8. Do you do anything special when you are pregnant? *Sample rationale:* A belief in many cultures is that a pregnant woman should not reach over her head for fear the cord will wrap around the baby's neck.
9. Do you eat nonfood substances when you are pregnant? *Sample rationale:* Eating nonfood substances is common among many cultural groups. Many African Americans eat clay in the belief that it has important minerals that the fetus needs.
10. Who do you want with you when you deliver your baby? *Sample rationale:* Most Filipino women prefer their mothers or another female family member, rather than husbands, to be present during the delivery.
11. In which position do you want to be when you deliver your baby? *Sample rationale:* Traditional Indian women in Guatemala prefer to deliver in a squatting position rather than in the supine position.
12. Which special foods do you eat after delivery? *Sample rationale:* Haitian women are encouraged to eat rice, porridge, plantains, and red beans after delivery to build up the blood.
13. Which foods do you avoid after delivery? *Sample rationale:* Chinese women avoid cold fruits and vegetables after delivery; instead, they eat cooked fruits and vegetables.
14. Which activities do you avoid after you deliver? *Sample rationale:* Russian women do no strenuous activity after delivery to prevent any complications.
15. Do you do anything special after delivery? *Sample rationale:* Traditional Haitian women have a series of three special baths that are given to them by family members.
16. Who will help you with the baby after delivery? *Sample rationale:* Looking for home support for the mother and rest of the family.
17. What bathing restrictions do you have after you deliver? *Sample rationale:* Many Arab women may be reluctant to bathe in a tub of water postpartum because they believe air may get into the mother and cause illness.

(Continues)

18. Do you want to keep the placenta? *Sample rationale:* Traditional Guatemalan women burn the placenta to keep away evil spirits. Other cultures may bury the placenta.
19. What do you do to care for the baby's umbilical cord? *Sample rationale:* A common practice among Central American Indians is to place a coin or metal object, held on with an abdominal binder, to prevent the umbilicus from protruding.

Death Rituals

The death rituals domain includes how an individual and society view death and euthanasia, rituals to prepare for death, burial practices, and bereavement behaviors. In most cultures, death rituals are slow to change. **Box 23-9** lists specific questions and a sample rationale that the APN should consider for this domain.

Spirituality

The spirituality domain includes formal religious beliefs related to faith and affiliation and the use of prayer, behavior practices that give meaning to life, and individual sources of strength. A person may be spiritual but not religious. **Box 23-10** lists specific questions and a sample rationale that the APN should consider for this domain.

Box 23-9   Death Rituals

The following are suggested questions, each accompanied by a sample rationale, that the APN can ask in a cultural assessment.

1. What special activities need to be performed to prepare for death? *Sample rationale:* When death is impending, Muslims want the bed to face toward Mecca.
2. Would you want to know about your impending death? *Sample rationale:* A belief among traditional Hindus is that people might give up hope if impending death is made known to them.
3. What is your preferred burial practice? Burial? Cremation? *Sample rationale:* The patient's wishes should be granted and the family should be encouraged to honor them.
4. How soon after death does burial occur? *Sample rationale:* For traditional Jews, burial should occur before sundown the next day, although there are exceptions.
5. How do men grieve in your culture? *Sample rationale:* A wide range of grieving practices exists, and all practices should be unconditionally accepted.
6. How do women grieve in your culture? *Sample rationale:* A wide range of grieving practices exists and all practices should be unconditionally accepted.
7. What does death mean to you? *Sample rationale:* According to Muslim beliefs, death is foreordained and worldly life is but a preparation for eternal life.
8. Do you believe in an afterlife? *Sample rationale:* Most Germans and German Americans believe that there is a better life after death.
9. Are children included in death rituals? *Sample rationale:* Members of Amish groups include children in all aspects of dying and burial.

Box 23-10   Spirituality

The following are suggested questions, each accompanied by a sample rationale, that the APN can ask in a cultural assessment.

1. What is your religion? *Sample rationale:* Traditional Judaism is more than a religion and prescribes male and female relationships as well as nutritional practices.
2. Do you consider yourself deeply religious? *Sample rationale:* Some people are religious but do not attend church on a regular basis.
3. How many times per day do you pray? *Sample rationale:* Islam requires prayer five times per day.
4. What items do you need to pray? *Sample rationale:* If possible, Muslims need a prayer rug.
5. Do you meditate? *Sample rationale:* Meditation may or may not be part of religious practice.
6. What gives strength and meaning to your life? *Sample rationale:* For some persons, religion is the most important thing in life; for others, the priority might be family or even work.
7. In which spiritual practices do you engage for your physical and emotional health? *Sample rationale:* For some people the key practice is prayer, for others meditation, and for others just having quiet time.

Healthcare Practices

The healthcare practices domain includes the focus of health care (acute versus preventive); traditional, magicoreligious, and biomedical beliefs and practices; individual responsibility for health; self-medicating practices; views on mental illness, chronicity, and rehabilitation; acceptance of blood and blood products; and organ donation and transplantation. **Box 23-11** lists specific questions and a sample rationale that the APN should consider for this domain.

Box 23-11   Healthcare Practices

The following are suggested questions, each accompanied by a sample rationale, that the APN can ask in a cultural assessment.

1. In what prevention activities do you engage to maintain your health? *Sample rationale:* A strong value in the dominant European American culture is to have regularly scheduled health checkups, including breast self-examinations and mammograms.
2. Who in your family takes responsibility for your health? *Sample rationale:* In many Hispanic/Latino cultures, the female in the family assumes the primary responsibility for the health of the family.
3. What over-the-counter medicines do you use? *Sample rationale:* Most cultural groups and individuals use over-the-counter medication, but some use them to the exclusion of prescription medicines. For many persons who have relatives in other countries, a large variety of prescription medications may be purchased and sent to family members in the United States.
4. Which herbal teas and folk medicines do you use? *Sample rationale:* Guatemalans, like members of many Hispanic/Latino populations, use a wide variety of herbal teas for many health conditions.
5. For which conditions do you use herbal medicines? *Sample rationale:* Many Panamanian men use "cat's claw" tea for prostate problems and delay going to a Western health professional.
6. What do you usually do when you are in pain? *Sample rationale:* Traditional Chinese individuals cope with pain by using externally applied treatments such as oils and massage.

(Continues)

7. How do you express your pain? *Sample rationale:* Many Filipinos view pain as part of living an honorable life and, therefore, may appear stoic and tolerate a high degree of pain.

8. How are people in your culture viewed or treated when they have a mental illness? *Sample rationale:* In many rural areas of Appalachia, rather than admitting that a person has a mental health illness, they are likely to say the person is "odd" or "quite turned."

9. How are people with physical disabilities treated in your culture? *Sample rationale:* In Haitian culture, people with a disability are seen as being as important as anyone else and are incorporated into all family and social activities.

10. What do you do when you are sick? Stay in bed, continue your normal activities, or something else? *Sample rationale:* Many people from an Eastern European heritage believe in the idea that "If you are not dead, take something for relief and continue with your daily routines."

11. What are your beliefs about rehabilitation? *Sample rationale:* Studies demonstrate that Germans are more accepting of rehabilitation than are other groups who have been studied. If rehabilitation is needed to function at maximum capacity, then all rehabilitation exercises are done.

12. How are people with chronic illnesses viewed or treated in your culture? *Sample rationale:* In cases of chronic illness among African Americans, close family and spiritual ties ensure that one's responsibilities are taken care of (by the family and even church members).

13. Are you averse to blood transfusions? *Sample rationale:* There is a religious prohibition against a Jehovah Witness receiving blood. In addition, many people do not want a blood transfusion for fear of contracting HIV/AIDS.

14. Is organ donation acceptable to you? *Sample rationale:* Jewish law views organ transplants from four perspectives: the recipient, the living donor, the cadaver donor, and the dying donor. Because life is sacred, if the recipient's life can be prolonged without considerable risk, then the transplant is favorably viewed.

15. Are you an organ donor? *Sample rationale:* Part of a standard health assessment. Many misconceptions exist about organ donations, and the APN can play a significant role in clarifying these misconceptions.

16. Would you consider having an organ transplant if needed? *Sample rationale:* Organ donation and transplantation among Koreans are rare, reflecting traditional attitudes toward integrity and purity. The APN can have a significant influence on Koreans' decisions about organ donation and transplantation by providing factual information.

17. Are healthcare services readily available to you? *Sample rationale:* APNs need to be aware of access problems for health care.

18. Do you have transportation problems in trying to access needed healthcare services? *Sample rationale:* Many organizations provide vouchers for public transportation if necessary.

19. Can you afford health care? *Sample rationale:* If the patient does not have adequate resources for health care, a social worker should be contacted for assistance.

20. Do you feel welcome when you see a healthcare professional? *Sample rationale:* If the answer is no, determine the reason. Just greeting the patient in a preferred manner, such as being formal with older African Americans, can make them feel welcome.

21. Which traditional healthcare practices do you use? Acupuncture, acupressure, *cai gao*, moxibustion, aromatherapy, coining/cupping, or something else? *Sample rationale:* If the APN is familiar with traditional practices in the culture, more specific information can be obtained.

22. Which home difficulties do you have that might prevent you from receiving health care? *Sample rationale:* Lack of support at home for child care may mean that a mother might not obtain regularly scheduled preventive care such as mammograms or Pap smears.

Box 23-12   Healthcare Practitioners

The following are suggested questions, each accompanied by a sample rationale, that the APN can ask in a cultural assessment.

1. Which healthcare providers do you see when you are ill? Physicians? Nurses? Folk traditional healers? *Sample rationale:* Not all patients see Western allopathic practitioners for illnesses, at least not as the first contact. The APN should also determine which treatments have been recommended by complementary alternative practitioners.
2. Do you prefer a same-sex healthcare provider for routine health problems? For intimate care? *Sample rationale:* Among traditional Islamic patients, a male healthcare provider should not tend to a female patient unless it is an emergency.
3. Which healers do you use in addition to physicians and nurses? *Sample rationale:* If the APN is familiar with the specific culture, he or she can ask more informed questions. Among many Hispanic/Latino groups, traditional healers include *curanderos, yerberos, masajistas, sacerdotes, sobadores,* and *espiritistas.*
4. For which conditions do you use healers? *Sample rationale:* Many Hispanics/Latinos use a variety of traditional healers. APNs who are caring for these populations should familiarize themselves with the specific groups' traditional healers and be able to ask the question in a nonjudgmental manner. Being able to integrate traditional healers with allopathic professionals will increase compliance with recommendations.

Healthcare Practitioners

The healthcare practitioners domain includes the status, use, and perceptions of traditional, magicoreligious, and biomedical healthcare providers and the gender of the healthcare provider. **Box 23-12** lists specific questions and a sample rationale that the APN should consider for this domain.

INDIVIDUAL PROFESSIONAL CULTURAL COMPETENCE

Much debate, especially in the last decade, has focused on the process of objectively measuring individual competence. Most tools for measuring cultural competence are self-reported and subjective in nature. A number of tools have been developed to assess individual and organizational cultural competence (Purnell, 2016). Some of these tools have been validated and are specific to a discipline or area of practice, whereas others are more general in nature. Most of these tools are available online. The Office of Minority Health has published a document on cultural competence standards (http://minorityhealth.hhs.gov/).

Cultural competence is a journey, rather than a skill mastered once and then used in an unchanging manner for the remainder of one's career. Its success relies on the willingness and ability of an individual to deliver culturally congruent and acceptable health and nursing care to clients. Individual cultural competence can be arbitrarily divided among cultural-general approaches, the clinical encounter, and language.

Cultural-General Competence

APNs need a cultural-general framework for assessment, as well as culturally specific knowledge about the clients to whom care is provided. Some cultural-general concepts follow:

1. Developing an awareness of one's own existence, sensations, thoughts, and environment without letting these factors have an undue influence on people from other backgrounds
2. Continuing to learn about the cultures of clients to whom one provides care
3. Demonstrating knowledge and understanding of the client's culture, health-related needs, and meanings of health and illness
4. Accepting and respecting cultural differences in a manner that facilitates the client's and family's ability to make decisions to meet their needs and beliefs
5. Recognizing that the APN's beliefs and values may not be the same as the client's
6. Resisting judgmental attitudes such as "different is not as good"
7. Being open to new cultural encounters
8. Recognizing that the variant characteristics of culture determine the degree to which clients adhere to the beliefs, values, and practices of their dominant culture
9. Having contact and experience with the communities from which clients come
10. Being willing to work with clients of diverse cultures and subcultures
11. Accepting responsibility for one's own education in cultural competence by attending conferences, reading the literature, and observing cultural practices
12. Promoting respect for individuals by discouraging racial and ethnic slurs among coworkers
13. Intervening with staff behavior that is insensitive, lacks cultural understanding, or reflects prejudice

The Clinical Encounter

Some principles and guidelines for APNs in the clinical encounter follow:

1. Adapting care to be congruent with the client's culture
2. Responding respectively to all clients and their families (including addressing clients and family members in the manner that they prefer, either formally or informally)
3. Collecting cultural data on assessments
4. Forming generalizations as a method for formulating questions rather than stereotyping
5. Recognizing culturally based healthcare beliefs and practices
6. Knowing the most common diseases and illnesses affecting the unique population to whom care is provided
7. Individualizing care plans to be consistent with the client's cultural beliefs
8. Having knowledge of the communication styles of clients to whom you provide care
9. Accepting varied gender roles and childrearing practices from clients to whom you provide care

10. Having a working knowledge of the religious and spiritual practices of clients to whom you provide care
11. Having an understanding of the family dynamics of clients to whom you provide care
12. Using faces and language pain scales in the ethnicity and preferred languages of the clients
13. Recognizing and accepting traditional, complementary, and alternative practices of clients to whom you provide care
14. Incorporating clients' cultural food choices and dietary practices into care plans
15. Incorporating clients' health literacy into care plans and health education initiatives

Language

Language ability has been determined to be one of the most important aspects in APNs' abilities to obtain an adequate assessment for many culturally diverse patients. Some guidelines for language follow:

1. Developing skills and using interpreters (includes sign language) with clients and families who have limited English proficiency
2. Providing clients with educational documents that are translated into their preferred language
3. Providing discharge instructions at a level that the client and family understand and in the language that the client and family prefer
4. Providing medication and treatment instruction in the language that the client prefers
5. Using pain scales in the language of the client

ORGANIZATIONAL CULTURAL COMPETENCE

Individual cultural competence is not sufficient to ensure the delivery of culturally competent care; the organization delivering the care must also demonstrate a commitment to cultural competence. Several things must be in place for an organization to demonstrate cultural competence. A list of attributes of culturally competent organizations, organized arbitrarily by governance and administration, education and orientation, and language, follows (Purnell et al., 2011; Purnell, 2013).

Governance and Administration

1. The organization has a mission statement and policies that address diversity.
2. The board of governance includes members of the ethnicity of the community that the organization serves.
3. A committee for cultural competence exists and includes staff, managers, administrators, chaplains, and members who are representative of the community.
4. The organization engages in community diversity fairs.
5. The organization seeks resources from federal, state, and private agencies to continually upgrade and integrate cultural competence into its care.

6. The organization partners with diverse community agencies.
7. The organization networks with diverse community leaders.
8. Administrators, managers, and staff are encouraged to be active in developing public policy for the client base to whom they deliver care.
9. Policy statements include efforts to eliminate bias and prejudice on the part of both clients and staff.
10. Programs reflect the needs of the diverse community.
11. The organization's programs are advertised in community newspapers and on the radio and television in the languages of the community.
12. There is a willingness to support a mentoring program to entice recruitment into the health professions.
13. Data collected include race, ethnicity, culture, and language preferences of the staff and client base.
14. Patient rights documents are available in the major languages of the community.
15. Cultural and linguistic standards are adhered to by all members of the organization.
16. Fiscal resources are available for interpretation and translation.
17. Strategic planning reflects the needs of the community.
18. Input on research priorities is sought from consumers.
19. Researchers are reflective of the staff, clients, and community.
20. Human resources recruitment and hiring activities reflect the diversity of the community.
21. The job analysis procedure includes scoring for ethnocultural and language ability.
22. Position descriptions and evaluation practices reflect cultural competence.
23. Conflict and grievance procedures reflect the language of the staff.
24. The organization actively recruits bilingual staff.
25. Staff members are compensated for bilingual ability and certification.
26. The ethics committee includes members who are reflective of the staff and clients.
27. The hours of operation of clinics are adjusted to meet the needs of the community.
28. Pictures and posters are reflective of the client base.
29. Food choices are reflective of the client and staff preferences.
30. The holiday calendar represents the holidays recognized by the client population base.
31. Intake forms reflect cultural assessment.
32. Pain scales are available in the diverse languages used by the population served.
33. Culturally appropriate toys are available (e.g., Hispanic Santa, African American dolls).
34. If staff members are used as interpreters or if professional interpretation is available, a plan is in effect to address their job duties while interpreting for patients and staff (also a requirement established by The Joint Commission).
35. Education and orientation diversity are addressed as part of new employees' orientation, in-service, and continuing education programs.

36. Nursing care delivery systems, the U.S. system of insurance reimbursement, and issues related to culture and autonomy are discussed.
37. Mentoring programs exist for diverse student and staff populations.
38. Diversity of the health professions is included in orientation.
39. All employees are offered education on both general cultural topics and the culture-specific needs of populations for whom they provide care.
40. Cultural celebrations are reflective of the staff and clients.
41. Resources are available to staff both the clinical unit and the library.
42. Staff members are trained in language interpretation.
43. Health classes are offered to clients whom the community serves.
44. Certification in culture for staff is offered at various levels.
45. Pharmacists, nurses, and physicians are educated in ethnopharmacology.
46. Lunch-and-learn series support the ongoing development of cultural competence.

Language

1. There are mechanisms in place for translation of written materials in the preferred language of the client.
2. Policies address interpretation (including sign language) and translation services.
3. Resources are available for translation of educational materials and discharge instructions in the languages of the client population.
4. The organization engages in activities that address the health literacy of the population whom it serves.
5. Written documents undergo a cultural sensitivity review.
6. Consent and procedure forms are translated into the languages of the population served.
7. English as a second language classes exist for staff.
8. Language classes are offered to clients and family (in English and the language of the population served).
9. Waiting areas have literature in the language of the population served.
10. Directions to referral facilities are in the languages of the client base.
11. Videos are in the language of the client base and have pictures reflective of the client base.
12. Diverse language includes sign language.
13. The need for an interpreter is determined ahead of time whenever possible.
14. The telephone system prompts are in the languages of the community.
15. Television programs are available in the languages of the community.
16. Satisfaction surveys are available in the languages of the community.
17. Staff surveys are available in the languages of the employees.
18. Audiovisual materials for staff and clients are available in their preferred languages.
19. Wellness and health promotion classes are offered in the languages of the client base.

SUMMARY

APNs—whether they work in clinical practice, education, research, policy, or administration and management—will inevitably work with multicultural patients and with diverse disciplines. When one considers the cultures of the patient, the APN, the profession, and the organization with a diverse workforce, culture competence becomes exceedingly complex. Even though the APN may have exceedingly excellent clinical practice skills, if he or she does not understand and include patients' culture into the nursing process, recommendations will not be followed.

APNs have a crucial role in helping eliminate health disparities, addressing social justice, collaborating with other health disciplines, advancing policy formulation, and participating in or conducting research. The Graduate Cultural Competencies developed by the AACN clearly outline APN core competencies:

- Prioritize the social and cultural factors that affect health in designing and delivering care across multiple contents.
- Construct socially and empirically derived cultural knowledge of people and populations to guide practice and research.
- Assume leadership in developing, implementing, and evaluating culturally competent nursing and other healthcare services.
- Transform systems to address social justice and health disparities.
- Provide leadership to educators and members of the healthcare or research team in learning, applying, and evaluating continuous cultural competence development.
- Conduct culturally competent scholarship that can be utilized in practice (AACN, 2011).

To this end, culturally competent care is not a luxury for APNs; it is a necessity.

The Purnell model for cultural competence provides a comprehensive guide for developing culturally competent health and nursing care. To date, this model has been used in organizational cultural competence with administration and management as well as research (Purnell et al., 2011).

REFERENCES

American Association of Colleges of Nursing. (2011). Toolkit for cultural competence in master's and doctoral nursing education. Retrieved from http://www.aacn.nche.edu/education-resources/Cultural_Competency_Toolkit_Grad.pdf

American Nurses Association. (2015). *Nursing: Scope and standards of practice* (3rd ed.). Silver Spring, MD: Author.

Berlin, E. A., & Fowkes, W. C. (1983). A teaching framework for cross-cultural health care: Application in family practice. *Western Journal of Medicine, 139*(12), 93–98.

Black-Lattanzi, J., & Purnell, L. (2006). *Developing cultural competence in physical therapy practice.* Philadelphia, PA: F. A. Davis.

Braithwaite, A. (2003). Selection of a conceptual model/framework for guiding research interventions. *Internet Journal of Advanced Nursing Practice, 6*(1), 73–93.

Campinha-Bacote, J. (2015). Transcultural C.A.R.E. Associates. Retrieved from http://transculturalcare .net/a-biblically-based-model-of-cultural-competence/

Catalano, J. T. (2011). *Nursing now: Today's issues, tomorrow's trends* (3rd ed.). Philadelphia, PA: F. A. Davis.

Crandall, S. J., George, G., Marion, G. S., & Davis, S. (2003). Applying theory to the design of cultural competency training for medical students: A case study. *Academic Medicine, 78*(6), 588–594.

Douglas, M., Pierce, J., Rosenkoetter, M., Clark Callister, L., Hattar-Pollara, M., Lauderdale, J., . . . Purnell, L. (2014). Guidelines for implementing culturally competent nursing care. *Journal of Transcultural Nursing, 25*(2), 109–121.

Fawcett, J., & DeSanto-Madeya, S. (2012). *Contemporary nursing knowledge: Analysis and evaluation of nursing models and theories.* Philadelphia, PA: F. A. Davis.

Giger, J. (2012). *Transcultural nursing: Assessment and intervention* (6th ed.). Philadelphia, PA: Elsevier.

Giger, J., Davidhizar, R., Purnell, L., Harden, J., Phillips, J., & Strickland, O. (2007). American Academy of Nursing Expert Panel report: Developing cultural competence to eliminate health disparities in ethnic minorities and other vulnerable populations. *Journal of Transcultural Nursing, 18*(2), 95–102.

Intercultural education of Nurses in Europe. (2016). Training plan. Retrieved from http://www .ieneproject.eu/teaching.php

Jeffreys, M. (2010). *Teaching cultural competence in nursing and health care: Inquiry, action, and innovation.* New York, NY: Springer.

Leonardo da Vinci Partnership Project. (2012). The Papadopoulos, Tilki and Taylor model for developing cultural competence. Retrieved from http://www.ieneproject.eu/download/Outputs /intercultural%20model.pdf

McFarland, M. R., & Wehbe-Alamah, H. B. (2015). Culture care diversity and universality: A worldwide nursing theory (3rd ed.). Burlington, MA: Jones & Bartlett Learning.

Nayar, S., & Tse, S. (2006). Cultural competence and models in mental health: Working with Asian service users. *International Journal of Psychosocial Rehabilitation, 10*(2), 79–87.

Purnell, L. (2000). A description of the Purnell model for cultural competence. *Journal of Transcultural Nursing, 11*(1), 40–46.

Purnell, L. (2003a, March–August). *Cultural diversity for older Americans: Cultural competence for the physical therapist working with clients with alternative lifestyles* [Monograph]. American Physical Therapy Association.

Purnell, L. (2003b). The Purnell model for cultural competence: A model for all healthcare providers. *Medical Network, 1*(1), 8–17.

Purnell, L. (2013). *Transcultural health care: A culturally competent approach* (3rd ed.). Philadelphia, PA: F. A. Davis.

Purnell, L. (2014). *Guide to culturally competent health care.* Philadelphia, PA: F. A. Davis.

Purnell, L. (2016). Scholarly dialogue: Are we really measuring cultural competence? *Nursing Science Quarterly: Theory, Research, and Practice, 19*(2), 124–127.

Purnell, L., Davidhizar, R., Giger, J., Strickland, O., Fishman, D., & Allison, D. (2011). Guide to culturally competent organizations. *Journal of Transcultural Nursing, 22*(1), 5–14.

Rickles, D., Hawe, P., & Shiell, A. (2007). A simple guide to chaos and complexity. *Journal of Epidemiology and Community Health, 61*, 933–937.

Spector, R. (2013). *Cultural diversity in health and illness* (8th ed.). Upper Saddle River, NJ: Pearson Prentice Hall.

StudyBlue. (2016). Theories/Nursing Theories/Values. Retrieved from https://www.studyblue.com/notes/note/n/theories-nursing-theories-values-in-nursing/deck/1333724?blurry=e&ads=true

U.S. Department of Health and Human Services. (n.d.). Effective Communication Tools for Health Care Professionals. Retrieved from http://pilot.train.hrsa.gov/uhc/pdf/modules/03/Module03JobAidModelBATHE.pdf

Chapter 24

The Praxis Theory of Suffering

Janice M. Morse

INTRODUCTION

The praxis theory of suffering provides a way to conceptualize an individual's and family's emotional response to the losses that occur because of accidental injury or illness, or during dying and bereavement. What a patient and their family *feel* is evident in their behavior. Nurses, in turn, can "read" or interpret these cues or signals of distress—whether they be signs of pain or discomfort, or emotions such as feeling scared, frightened, or terrified—and quickly respond with comforting strategies. These nursing responses may take the form of an appropriate behavioral or verbal interaction, or a nursing intervention intended to reduce the physical or emotional distress. The nurse then immediately reevaluates the patient's signals of distress and either continues with the comforting strategy or changes to a different intervention.

Thus the *praxis* part of the praxis theory of suffering refers to pragmatic interventions—that is, the nursing strategies that ease and relieve the suffering (i.e., comfort patients and families). This theory is clinically useful: Nursing assessments and interventions often take place within an interaction. As such, nurses, by recognizing behavioral cues and instantly responding, serve as the "front line" of intervention.

People often ask how it is possible to "intervene" if the problem is not known. In fact, it is not necessary to know details of the "problem," at least initially, and rarely does a nurse have more than a brief account before taking action. What the nurse sees is the person's emotional behavior—in this case, the suffering behaviors—and then responds to it. To recognize the state of suffering, the nurse does not need to know the *reasons* or the details of the cause—just as when a person enters a room full of laughing people, the person does not need to know the reason for their happiness, or to have heard the joke, to recognize that they are happy. What is important, in the case of suffering, is that the person approaching the suffering person reads the person's behavioral cues and responds accordingly. The "intervener" (in this case, the nurse) must take his or her cues from the person who is suffering, must provide behavioral responses that match those cues, and must change those responses as the sufferer's behavioral cues change. In this way, the interaction is dynamic and, ideally, the suffering diminishes as the comforting continues.

THE PRAXIS THEORY OF SUFFERING

The Development of the Praxis Theory of Suffering

The *praxis theory of suffering* is a qualitatively derived theory; it has been developed from a synthesis of three decades of qualitative studies (see **Table 24-1**). In the 1980s, master's-level students were conducting research on various illness experiences using grounded theory, and some of these studies were published in *The Illness Experience: Dimensions of Suffering* (Morse & Johnson, 1991). The final chapter of the Morse and Johnson book provides a synthesis of the commonalities in all of these chapters. Titled the *illness-constellation model*, it depicts the individual and his or her family's response to illness. The publication of this theory was one of the first qualitative metasyntheses. The illness-constellation model became a part of undergraduate curricula in Europe (e.g., in the Netherlands and Belgium) and is still used in the United States in some physical therapy programs.

About this time, Morse received a 3-year foreign award from the National Institute of Nursing Research (NINR) to delineate comfort and comfort concepts (1991–1994) and to develop the comfort interaction model. A 5-year continuation grant then enabled the identification of comforting strategies during trauma care:

- The Comfort Talk Register—a linguistic register used by nurses to assist patients in excruciating pain to endure and cooperate with trauma care, thereby expediting and increasing its safety (Morse & Proctor, 1998; Proctor, Morse, & Khonsari, 1996)
- A comparison of successful and unsuccessful attempts at nasogastric tube insertion, noting ways that nurses facilitated patient endurance and decreased distress during the procedure (Morse, Penrod, Kassab, & Dellasega, 2000; Penrod, Morse, & Wilson, 1999)
- Integration of the family into trauma resuscitation, classification of their suffering behaviors, and identification of helpful and unhelpful interactions with staff (Morse & Pooler, 2002)

Morse and colleagues also identified a model of "preserving self" with burn patients (Morse, 1997; Morse & O'Brien, 1995) and analyzed their disembodying language as they spoke about their bodies when in agonizing pain (Morse & Mitcham, 1998). Morse and colleagues interviewed emergency department/trauma room nurses about suffering and identified *compathy*—the physical equivalent to empathy, referring to the contagion of pain. They delineated this concept and developed a model of compathetic caregiving

Table 24-1   Research Program for the Development of the Praxis Theory of Suffering: Components, Progress, and Funding Received

1. Background (1985–1991)

Goal: To develop grounded theories of illness experience/trajectory of suffering: e.g., trajectories of myocardial infarction, hysterectomy, discharge form psychiatric hospital adolescent abortion, impact of chemotherapy on the family

Funding: Small grants

Publications: See references 1–9 in Appendix 24–1

Metasynthesis: The illness experience: dimensions of suffering[10]

2. Delineation of comfort and comforting (1991–1994)

Goal: To delineate the concepts inherent in comforting

Concepts: Caring, empathy, trust, social support, reciprocity, compathy; patterns of touch (infants)

Funding: NRC NIH R01 (3-year foreign award)

Publications: See references 11–26 in Appendix 24–1

3. Identification of role of suffering in comforting (1994–1996)

Goal: Identification of role of suffering in comforting

Strategies: Comfort talk register, nasogastric tube insertion, family presence in trauma care, pain dialogues, normalization

Funding: NINR NIH R01 continuation grant (5 years)

Publications: See references 27–36 in Appendix 24–1

4. Explication of suffering behaviors (1997–2001)

Goal: Development of praxis theory of suffering

Model of 'preserving self'; development of praxis theory of suffering; model of reformulated self

Funding: NINR NIH R01 (continuation)

Publications: See references 37–56 in Appendix 24–1

5. Identification of patterns of suffering (2001–2006)

Identification of patterns of suffering and further development of the praxis theory of suffering; facial coding system for expressions of suffering; synchrony of suffering; patterns of suffering during breast cancer diagnosis

Funding: CIHR, Canadian Breast CA FDN

Publications: See references 57–62 in Appendix 24–1

6. Anticipated outcomes of this application (2010–2015)

Verified theory

Compendium of enduring behaviors

Clinical implementation model

(Morse & Mitcham, 1997; Morse, Mitcham, & van der Steen, 1998). By 1996, with Barbara Carter, Morse recognized that there were two primary behavioral states in suffering: enduring (in which the emotions were suppressed) and emotional suffering (in which the emotions were released) (Morse 2000a; Morse & Carter, 1996). Finally, Morse developed (2001) and refined (2005) the model known as the praxis theory of suffering. According to this model, a suffering individual exits the suffering state as the reformulated self, with a new perspective on life (Carter, 1994; Morse & Carter, 1996; see **Figure 24-1**).

In 2001, the investigation continued with a 3-year grant from the Canadian Institutes of Health to further delineate the behaviors of suffering. As part of this study, Morse and colleagues video recorded interviews with patients who had been critically ill and relatives of patients who had died (Morse, Beres, Spiers, Mayan, & Olson, 2003). They conducted qualitative ethology of these recorded interviews, exploring the transitions between the states of enduring and emotional suffering. They used Ekman's Emotional Facial Action Coding System (EMFACS), which is a modified version of the Facial Action Coding System (Ekman & Friesen, 1978; Ekman, Irwin, & Rosenberg, 1994). Morse and colleagues described facial expressions of enduring and emotional suffering in the interviews, and

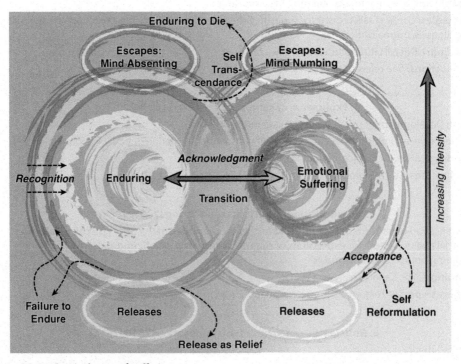

Figure 24-1 Praxis theory of suffering.

they recorded patterned behavioral indices of transitions between enduring and emotional suffering, which lasted from 7.5 to 35 seconds.

More recently, Morse and colleagues interviewed women who were awaiting a diagnosis (either positive or negative) of breast cancer and who had negative results to determine further patterns of suffering. Funding from the Alberta Cancer Foundation enabled them to determine whether women who were in the state of enduring must enter a state of emotional suffering to release the suppressed emotions (while enduring) to exit the suffering model, or whether they exited directly from enduring (see Figure 24-1). Morse and colleagues found that some exited directly from enduring, releasing emotions as relief and laughter; others exited the model by transitioning through emotional suffering in a torrent of tears; and still others remained either in enduring or in emotional suffering, believing that the negative results were an error and that the physician simply had not found the cancer yet.

The Components of the Praxis Theory of Suffering

The praxis theory of suffering is a *state* theory: Suffering is an emotional experience; emotion is reflected in, and evidenced in, the suffering person's behaviors. However, while these emotions are observable in distinctive behaviors, they may also be "covered" or concealed. Suffering is a patient-centered, patient-led, dynamic model, and the responses to suffering are individualized and may vary according to a given person's way of responding to loss, the context, cultural and social norms, and the amount of privacy afforded.

Suffering is defined as a basic human response to a threat to one's physical or psychosocial integrity (such as occurs in illness or disability, pain, or the death of a loved one), or to untenable life situations (such as abuse or accident). The suffering response may vary in intensity from slight to severe, according to the significance of the loss to the person. It is an emotional response that is manifested behaviorally, that occurs in response to a perceived, threatened (anticipated), or actual loss. The goal of the suffering response is to "shut down" the body or mind to protect the self.

Suffering consists of two major states: enduring and emotional suffering. *Enduring* is a state in which a person's emotions are suppressed and the person focuses on the present. In this situation, the past, which has resulted in the loss, is too painful to recall, and the altered future is too painful to contemplate. Suffering persons are aware that if they respond emotionally to the loss, they might "break down"; that is, they would be unable to function in daily activities and do whatever needs to be done. The emotional suppression is visible and evident in the person's posture, facial expression, interaction with others, and speech. The person who is enduring stands erect, has a mask-like expression, and moves "like a robot" with a lumbering gait that is devoid of spontaneous movement. These people stand apart from one another, tend to be silent, and respond to any attempt at conversation with a single word, nod, or gesture.

When a person is "ready to take it"—that is, to accept whatever is being suffered—he or she transitions into emotional suffering. This shift in state occurs when an individual acknowledges the actuality of his or her loss. The emotional resources can no longer be controlled and are manifested as states of despair, grief, and sorrow.

Emotional suffering is a state in which the emotions of distress are released and a person acknowledges the incomprehensible past, the altered present, and the anticipated future. Persons who are in a state of emotional suffering may cry or weep and have a sorrowful expression. They often want to talk incessantly about the loss to whoever will listen; they have a hunched posture that invites others to hold and comfort them.

These states—enduring and emotional suffering—do not occur simultaneously, nor is the praxis theory of suffering a stage model. Instead, a person may flip back and forth between enduring and emotional suffering. Eventually, when a person has "suffered enough," hope seeps in and the emotions change. The person gains a new perspective about the experience of suffering—that is, *reformulates* (see "self-reformulation" in Figure 24-1; Carter, 1994; Morse & Carter, 1996). Individuals who have suffered reevaluate the experience and their altered lives. They are able to consider whatever has made them suffer in a new light, even valuing the experience. Suffering has given them a new appreciation for living, and they leave the states of suffering with a new perspective.

Enduring

Enduring (see Figure 24-1) is defined as a response to the actual or threatened loss that causes feelings of chaos. When individuals speak of the antecedents to enduring, they describe feeling "blown away," of having "the wind knocked out of them," of being "devastated" or "crushed"—feelings of shock as they learn of, or experience, the loss. This antecedent event is something that is unavoidable, incomprehensible, and, if anticipated, dreaded. In the face of this loss, individuals respond by attempting to control the internal chaos by containing chaotic emotional responses. "Shutting down" emotionally allows a person to "hold on" or "last through" the threat to the self.

Attributes of Enduring

As a concept, enduring consists of attributes, or characteristics, that are common to all instances of enduring: (1) maintaining control of self, (2) living in the present moment, (3) removing oneself from the situation, and (4) being aware of the danger or consequences of emotional disintegration.

Maintaining Control of Self

How do those who are enduring hold on? Enduring is attained by *maintaining control of self*, primarily by deliberately suppressing the emotions of despair, grief, terror, or panic.

Based on interview data, the initial response to an intrusive event appears to be one of shock, horror, terror, panic, or feeling very scared. When learning their diagnosis, fear may "grip at the heart." People in this state instinctively suppress their emotions so that they may remain in control, until the diagnosis is *real*, and they may think of what to do and who to tell, when and where and how. Enduring requires deliberate effort and focus to keep going, to do what is required to get through each day, and to bear whatever must be endured.

How do individuals suppress these emotions? They refuse to let the sorrow show in their face for fear of upsetting others. They refuse to cry; if they do cry, they conceal their tears. Cognitively, they refuse to weep, moan, complain, and "break down." They suppress their feelings to the extent that they may feel calm, competent, and believe they are "managing" well, maintaining normality. Aware that a display of emotions would be distressing to others, they conceal any signals of distress.

This suppression of emotions may be so extreme that it inhibits motor movement in a form of forced self-composure. People in the enduring state feel it is important to maintain dignity: They stand erect but sometimes literally "hold themselves together" by standing with their arms crossed over their chest, clasping the opposite upper arm. They have a distinctive facial expression—one characterized by the lack of movement, a blank unfocused stare. Even if asked a question, they will respond with a monosyllable or a barely perceptible nod. These people do not initiate conversation. Their gait loses spontaneous movement, and they lumber from side to side as they walk. They stand apart from others, and family members may stand at each side flanking the suffering person. They walk in a line, or stand apart from each other, with spaces between. The implicit cue sent out from the enduring person is, "I am okay. Leave me alone." and "Do not touch me."

Living in the Present Moment

Individuals in the enduring state are present focused, concentrating on what is happening now and unable to think about their past or contemplate their future. They feel overwhelmed and are unable to consider several tasks at once, focusing on one small thing at a time instead. They hope to get through the next hour—or sometimes only the next minute—and are unable to comprehend what must be done in a whole day.

For instance, trauma victims narrow their perception by focusing on breathing in and out in an attempt to maintain control; burn victims in the intensive care unit watch the hands of the clock move or count the tiles of the roof or the number of treatments. Those bereaving take "one step at a time." All state that they cannot see the big picture and instead focus on simply getting through the next minute, hour, or day.

Removing Oneself from the Situation

Individuals may remove themselves physically from situations where whatever is being suffered would be publicly acknowledged—for instance, by not going to church or to the store, where others may offer condolences. Such acknowledgment brings whatever is being suffered to the fore and may result in a rush of emotions—the emotions that the individual has been trying to hold in check. For this reason, sympathy cards are valued by those who are enduring, because they may be read when the person is ready to handle the emotions.

Cognitively, individuals put whatever is being endured deliberately at the back of their mind. They may refuse to let thoughts that may cause suffering enter their consciousness. They work hard, focusing intensely and concentrating on work or on special tasks they have set themselves.

Those who are ill may focus on their therapies—for example, counting pills or tests, so that therapy itself becomes the distraction. Nurses' "small talk" becomes important, psychologically removing the person from the sick bed to the life "outside." Patients grab onto the smallest, most feeble joke they hear, repeating it endlessly. Finally, it is no accident that so many jigsaw puzzles can be found in rehabilitation facilities; they are there to distract disabled patients and to remove patients, albeit temporarily, from their present situation.

Being Aware of the Danger and Consequences of Emotional Disintegration

Persons who are enduring resist crying and report they are afraid to cry—afraid they will not be able to stop, afraid they will not be there to do what needs to be done, and metaphorically afraid that they will break down and will not be there for others. They resist sympathetic or empathetic interactions, avoiding those who may offer condolences, because such responses "break through" the stoicism of enduring.

Recognizing Facial Expressions of Enduring

When assessed using Ekman's EMFACS (Ekman & Friesen, 1978; Ekman et al., 1994), the suppressed emotion gives the face a blank appearance. Facial muscles lack tone and shape. The lips and mouths move only slightly during speech, the eyes are unfocused and rarely blink, and the gaze is centered in the distance, away from the interviewer (see **Figure 24-2**; Morse et al., 2003).

Escaping from Enduring

When enduring, individuals use *escapes* to vent suppressed emotions. These escapes are *mind-absenting strategies*, or actions that occupy individuals so they do not have to think about whatever it is they are enduring. They include tactics such as keeping busy, concentrating on work, or doing puzzles. Occasionally the suppressed energy cannot be controlled or contained, however; it is then released as anger, fury, excessive exercise, or hysterical laughter. While releases remove the emotional pressure and help individuals remain in control, exhaustion and the fatigue of illness without a release may also weaken an individual's ability to endure (i.e., contain the emotions) and cause him or her to lose control.

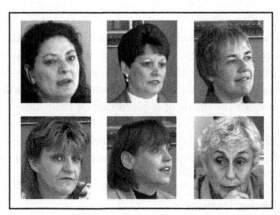

Figure 24-2 Faces of enduring.

Republished with permission of Sage Publications, from Identifying signals of suffering by linking verbal and facial cues, Janice M. Morse, Melanie A. Beres, Judith A. Spiers, Maria Mayan, & Karin Olson, *Qualitative Health Research,* *13*(8), 2003; permission conveyed through Copyright Clearance Center, Inc.

Conceptual Boundaries of Enduring

A conceptual boundary separates what enduring is and what it is not. Enduring has not occurred (*fails to endure*) when an individual in the trauma room shifts to an out-of-control state. Out-of-control behavior is an event in which an individual resists care and fights caregivers. Persons in this state shout, swear, and may vocalize nonsensically instead of being able to articulate their emotions and thoughts (see "failure to endure" in Figure 24-1).

Styles of Enduring

Styles of enduring differ according to (1) role expectations (with males more prone than females to endure), (2) culturally sanctioned behaviors, and (3) context. In Japan, for example, and with the American and Canadian native peoples, enduring is a "public" response and emotional suffering remains largely a private behavior. In other cultures, emotional suffering is likely to be sanctioned culturally but would be expected behavior at funerals, for instance.

Releases from Enduring

A person cannot remain in a state of enduring indefinitely; the suppressed energy must go somewhere. The emotions emerge and break through explosively as anger or hysterical laughter. If anger emerges, it is usually targeted toward someone "safe" who will not jeopardize care. For example, if it occurs in the emergency department, relatives are more likely to kick the soda machine than to shout at the physician who is providing care.

Transition

The transition from a state of enduring into the state of emotional suffering is usually deliberate and can be resisted by "fighting" the rising emotions. Most often, a person moves into emotional suffering when he or she feels emotionally ready. As mentioned previously, Morse et al. (2003) studied this transition by conducting video recorded interviews, asking people to tell their story of the death of a loved one or their illness. As participants told their story, they relived the emotions experienced at that time ("emotional reenactment"; see Morse & Pooler, 2002). Thus, the states of enduring and emotional suffering, and the transitions between the two states, could be microanalyzed, and the dialogue simultaneously analyzed (see **Figure 24-3**).

Facial Expression During Transition

Transitioning from enduring to emotional suffering tended to take from 7.5 seconds to 35 seconds (mean, 18 seconds). The first indicator of transition from enduring to emotional suffering was the movement of participants' eyes, which made frequent and rapid undirected movements. Their eyes would dart around the room yet remained unseeing and unfocused. Then, as their emotions "broke through" their neutral facial expressions, participants frowned, with their inner forehead raised and their middlebrow lowered. As they lost control, their lips quivered, causing them to tighten and raise their chin to attempt to control the quivering and increasing expression of emotion. Often, at this point participants placed their hands over their mouths. If they continued talking, their upper lips and cheeks began to rise, and lips would begin to stretch as they tried to control their lower face and mouth to keep talking (see **Figure 24-4**; Morse et al., 2003).

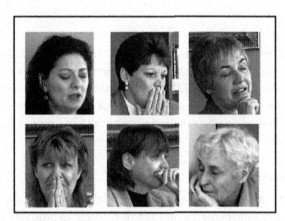

Figure 24-3 Faces of transition.

Republished with permission of Sage Publications, from Identifying signals of suffering by linking verbal and facial cues, Janice M. Morse, Melanie A. Beres, Judith A. Spiers, Maria Mayan, & Karin Olson, *Qualitative Health Research, 13*(8), 2003; permission conveyed through Copyright Clearance Center, Inc.

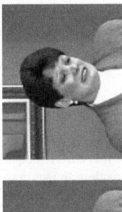
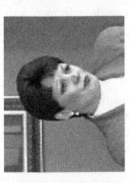
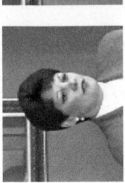

State	Enduring (suppressing emotions)	Transition	Releasing (Emotional suffering)
AU's	eye movements ⟶ nodding ⟶	tilts head left head down (slightly) eyes blinking–(eyes down) ⟶ 14+24 ⟶ 10+14+24 ⟶ 1+4 ⟶ breath in ⟶	10+20+ ⟶ 10+14+24 ⟶ 10+20+24/10+14+24 ⟶ 20+24+25 ⟶ 10+14+24 ⟶ 1+4+7 ⟶ hard swallow ⟶
Text	and, um, within hours Dr. X called and asked if I could have my Dad at 3 o'clock (Pause ——————————	—————————)And,	when Dr. X got up and hugged my dad

Seconds

0   5   10   15   20   24

Key: EMFACS Codes (Ekman, Irwin & Rosenberg, 1994)

Action Unit (AU)	Corresponding Action	Action Unit (AU)	Corresponding Action	Action Unit (AU)	Corresponding Action
1	inner brow raise	12	lip corner pull	17	chin raise
4	brow lower	14	dimpler	23	lip tight
10	upper lip raise	15	lip corner depress	24	lip press

Figure 24-4 The transition from enduring (emotional suppression) to releasing (emotional suffering).

Republished with permission of Sage Publications, from Identifying signals of suffering by linking verbal and facial cues, Janice M. Morse, Melanie A. Beres, Judith A. Spiers, Maria Mayan, & Karin Olson, Qualitative Health Research, 13(8), 2003; permission conveyed through Copyright Clearance Center, Inc.

The Process of Transition

The Morse et al. video recordings of 19 participants' stories of suffering revealed 28 transitions, ranging from 1 to 8 transitions per interview. Transitions from 9 participants were microanalyzed (Morse et al., 2003).

Facial expression and interview text were interdependent. In almost every case, the movement from enduring and reference to self and the future ramifications of the event being suffered was evident, with tearing or crying indicating the onset of emotional releasing.

In the preceding text, notice how the language changes from "John" to "I" or "me" as the person transitions into emotional suffering.

Emotional Suffering

Emotional suffering occurs when the individual acknowledges the actuality of the loss. The emotional resources can no longer be controlled and become manifested as states of despair, grief, and sorrow. During emotional suffering, individuals release emotions to mourn the lost past and altered future. They may cry, weep, or sob; they have a hunched posture and a sorrowful expression. Their posture and their tears touch others emotionally, who are moved to step forward and console the suffering person. Sufferers seek others to be there with them. They talk about the event and their loss incessantly to whoever will listen, psychologically working through and mourning their lost past and their altered future. They accept touch, sympathy, and empathy. When the pain of emotionally suffering is too much to bear, these individuals use escapes—mind-numbing strategies, such as watching television or sleeping incessantly (Morse, 2001)—to dull the emotional pain of suffering.

Recognizing Facial Expressions of Emotional Suffering

When emotionally suffering, participants revealed a furrowed brow, the corners of their mouths dimpled, and they raised their chins as they pressed their lips together. Verbally, they moved the conversation to the self ("I" or "me"), and their speech was marked with swallowing, cracking of the voice, pausing, and uneven pacing (see **Figure 24-5**; Morse et al., 2003).

The Synchrony of Suffering

Of importance to nursing is the synchrony of enduring and emotional suffering in family groups. Individuals within family groups move from enduring to suffering, and back to enduring, in a synchronized manner. Emotional suffering is often a private behavior that is concealed from others. We may watch family members endure as they walk down the corridor and into the cubical where their ill relative rests. Because they recognize that their own emotional suffering may cause distress in the sick person, family members endure while in the presence of the sick person, making jovial small talk and so forth. Then, after

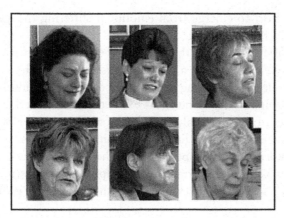

Figure 24-5 Faces of emotional suffering.

Republished with permission of Sage Publications, from Identifying signals of suffering by linking verbal and facial cues, Janice M. Morse, Melanie A. Beres, Judith A. Spiers, Maria Mayan, & Karin Olson, *Qualitative Health Research,* *13*(8), 2003; permission conveyed through Copyright Clearance Center, Inc.

the visit, and as family members walk back to the family room, they may transition into emotional suffering, sobbing in the family room or the bathroom.

In family groups, family members take turns enduring and "holding the family together," acting as comforter and taking care of others. When family members are emotionally suffering, one may become the endurer, remaining strong enough to comfort and support those who are emotionally suffering. Later, they may switch roles.

In their studies, Morse et al. were able to explore the patterns of interactions between those who were enduring and those who were suffering by examining the video recordings of family groups as they entered the trauma room and visited their injured or ill family member (Morse & Pooler, 2002). In emergency situations, families are usually in shock, trying to grapple with what has happened. As such, the family members are usually in states of enduring, standing apart from one another and trying to hold themselves together. As the crisis passes, they move into suffering, with one member remaining in enduring to hold and comfort the others, talk to the staff, and make decisions.

Coming Out of Suffering

Once a person has been able to accept what has happened and envision a new and altered future, hope seeps in. Using techniques of theoretical coalescence in their studies, Morse et al. were able to "open" the concepts and examine processes of emotional suffering and hope and document the interaction of these two concepts. They were able to identify the linkage of these two concepts (the process of hope initially links to emotional suffering in the despair associated with emotional suffering) and to show how hoping enables an individual to make the effort to emerge from emotional suffering (Mayan, Morse, & Eldershaw, 2006; Morse & Penrod, 1999).

If the person who is suffering is dying, the outcome of emotional suffering is resolution of the suffering as *transcendence*; in such a case, the person does not have the energy to emotionally suffer and "fades away," dying in a state of enduring ("enduring to die"). If the person is in rehabilitation or is not ill, he or she exits emotional suffering as a *reformulated self*. Using techniques of concept analysis, Morse et al. (2014) are able to show that transcendence is reached by using hope to find new meaning in a situation. *Reformulation* takes longer than transcendence, with the person living the renewed perspective by giving back to others—for instance, by volunteering for self-help groups or assisting in a cancer unit. In this state, people reevaluate their lives and change their values and goals accordingly.

Enduring to Die

Facing one's own death when receiving palliative care, Morse et al. (2014) reasoned, must be extraordinarily distressful. Therefore, they expected that extensive emotional suffering would be apparent in palliative care settings. "Not so," the nurses reported. Some patients did become distraught now and then (and this distress usually occurred in private). Very occasionally they had a patient who was "often" distressed, but by and large the patients manifested behaviors that could be described as enduring.

To investigate this matter further, Morse et al. conducted a study interviewing patients and nurses (Olson, Morse, Smith, Mayan, & Hammond, 2000–2001) about emotions in palliative care. During this study, the patients' emotional states were, indeed, aptly described as enduring. As patients became increasingly sick and nearer to death, enduring behaviors continued, until the patients simply "faded away" as they became increasingly unaware, lost consciousness, and died. An important relationship was discovered between fatigue and emotional suffering; namely, "to emotionally suffer," energy is required. Palliative patients simply did not have the energy to emotionally suffer and, to conserve energy, maintained a state of enduring.

Is It Possible to Exit the Model from Enduring?

By 2000, it was clear that assumptions of the praxis theory of suffering needed to be further explored. The original model was not linear, but rather dynamic. Persons could vary in intensity of enduring and emotional suffering and could move through the transition into suffering and then return to enduring; they could even move into a transitional state from enduring and then resist emotional suffering and return to enduring. What was uncertain was, except in the scenario of "enduring to die," whether a person must exit the model through emotional suffering to release the suppressed emotions of enduring. *Was it possible to exit the model directly from enduring in situations other than dying?*

Morse et al. (2014) designed a study to explore this question, examining the release of enduring when the condition being endured was removed. They chose the instance of undergoing diagnostic tests for breast cancer—specifically, instances in which the mammography was initially indicative of cancer but the result of the breast biopsy was later found to be negative for cancer.

Suffering Breast Cancer Diagnosis

Morse et al. (2014) deliberately selected a situation in which maximal enduring was required to "get through" but in which the conditions necessary to endure were then removed. Women have described discovering a breast lump or having a suspicious mammogram, and subsequently waiting for the diagnosis, as "the worst experience of their lives." When a subsequent breast biopsy revealed that the lesion was benign, Morse et al. (2014) conjectured that when the woman was informed that she did not have cancer, she would then enter emotional suffering to release the suppressed emotions of enduring, rather than moving directly from enduring without emotional release.

Morse et al.'s (2014) first assumption, that women would be *intensely* enduring, proved only partly correct. Some women did endure the threat of cancer; others were able to endure only partially and did emotionally suffer on occasions, switching back and forth between enduring and suffering as they contemplated their future cancer and death. A third group of women were not able to endure well and almost constantly displayed emotional suffering while waiting for their test results, already convinced that they had cancer.

Indeed, when told they did not have cancer, some women did enter emotional suffering and then displayed relief. The physician reported that it is these patients, "who do not have cancer, who cry at this time." Others exited enduring directly to a state of relief, laughing and celebrating. Surprisingly, despite the negative results, a third group continued enduring and emotionally suffering. They did *not* believe that they did not have cancer; they were certain that they did have cancer and that the physician had simply not found it yet. Perhaps listening to the tentative nature of the physicians' request for long-term follow-up and mammograms at 6-month intervals supported their skepticism.

Nevertheless, the implications for the development of the praxis theory of suffering were that it was clear that the suppressed energy from enduring could be released directly from enduring as other emotions. The person did not have to enter emotional suffering, although this was certainly a path selected by some participants in the study.

Learning to Recognize Behavioral States of Suffering

This model is titled the *praxis* theory because it has clear implications for nursing practice. By learning to read the behavioral cues of those who are suffering, nurses can determine if a person is enduring or emotionally suffering—a critical consideration because nurses' interactions with a person who is enduring are very different from the interventions that should be used with a person who is emotionally suffering.

When a person is enduring, the role of the nurse should be to support the enduring behaviors. People in this state are grappling and cognitively struggling to come to terms with whatever has happened to cause them to endure, or they may be enduring by moving the events to the back of their mind so they do not have to face or handle them at that particular moment. Because they are suppressing emotions, any empathetic expression or the use of comforting touch could bring the negative events to the fore and give them something else to endure. These people respond best to the caregiver *being with* them in silence, standing apart, and being available should they need anything. They may not converse. They will not respond well to questions about how they *feel*; they may withdraw if touched. Later, they may respond to distractions, grabbing onto any conversation that is about anything other than what is being endured, and struggle to maintain a normal appearance to the household routine.

In contrast, persons who are emotionally suffering send a message to caregivers that they need to be comforted. They respond to touch, being held, being stroked, and being listened to. They accept empathetic and comforting words, and need (and will accept) assistance.

Ideally, all nurses should learn to read bodily cues to discover individuals' states of mind (Morse, 2000a). The way a nurse interacts with a patient, for example, is determined by that individual's state. A nurse responds to a patient who is enduring by standing apart from that patient and providing concrete information in a factual manner. A nurse responds to a patient in emotional suffering quite differently: The nurse may express condolences, touch the person, or even place an arm around the individual.

The praxis theory of suffering is a forgiving model: If a nurse makes a mistake—for instance, uses touch inappropriately with a person who is enduring—that person will instantly withdraw. Sensing this rejection, the nurse can immediately apologize and correct his or her approach. However, if the nurse does not attend to patients' cues of withdrawal and continues with the touch approach, he or she may cause persons to collapse because empathetic statements and comforting touch *confirm* that the "worst has happened." Persons are then eligible for all of the social supports that are offered to individuals in crisis, hence forcing persons to accept what has happened before they are cognitively able to accept the event.

For nursing, the praxis theory of suffering is interlaced with comforting interventions. Comforting is the intervention to ease suffering: It enables enduring, and it relieves emotional suffering.

Using this perspective on suffering (i.e., that the suffering experience is observable) means that the nurse can assess a patient's state without using instruments, questionnaires, or interviews. The nurse can also determine a patient's state of suffering—and identify the patient's comfort needs—both quickly and accurately (Morse, 2000a). *Does the nurse need to know the details of what is being suffered?* Often nurses do not; they must move in to assist before they have that information, or perhaps to obtain that information. In fact, nurses must often move toward comforting a distressed person to find out "what the matter is" so that comfort begins before assessment is complete.

Degrees of Enduring/Modes of Enduring

The preceding model incorporates two major states, enduring and emotional suffering. It would be naïve to suggest that there are only two behavioral states in patients. We can also identify degrees of the two states—for instance, emotional suffering ranging from sad to distraught.

While conducting research in the trauma care, Morse et al. (2014) listened to nurses' descriptions of patients and then assessed these *emic* categorizations of behavioral states and characteristics displayed by patients and the modes of comforting interaction by nurses. Each of these states may be conceptualized in the praxis theory of suffering as evidence of a certain degree of either enduring or failure to endure.

Scared

Patients who are scared are relatively quiet and, if spoken to, may respond with a single word or a silent nod. Verbalizations are not offered spontaneously, but rather are given only in response to direct questions. For example, the patient responds with such words as "what?" "yes," and "no" and uses vocalizations such as "mm" and "huh, huh":

Volume, or loudness of the voice, can range from soft to normal. Voice modulation can range from normal to some quivering. These patients are generally quiet and are absorbing everything that is going on, so that the quiet, minimal behavior is pragmatically functional. They appear to listen intently to whatever is being said about them.

Scared patients do not have any spontaneous movements and lie very still ("scared stiff"). If a nurse moves their arm, they will keep that arm in that position until the nurse moves it again. If they cry, the tear will roll out of the corner of their eyes without being wiped away.

Comforting interactions with these patients include *being there*, with the nurse sometimes providing a "running commentary" of what he or she is doing: "I am here, just behind your head, changing your IV."

Anxious

In contrast to scared patients, anxious patients are often hyperverbal and produce a continuous flow of words, perhaps in an attempt to control their anxiety. This hyperverbal behavior is manifested by constant talking; patients provide more information than is needed. Caregivers tend to interrupt them to move the assessment along. Anxious patients' affects may vary; these patients may present with joking, flirting, frequent excessive praising of the staff, or comments to minimize their injury. At the same time, they may constantly verbalize their concern about their injury, the treatment, or general concern about others involved in the accident. The essential feature is that patients keep talking: "Oh I'm, I'm okay. I tell you, you girls are doing a great job with me. Great job."

Patients' volume is normal with efforts to control the levels of intensity; this attempted control may give the voice a restrained quality. When the restraint threatens to be lost, a tremulous quality is reflected in the voice. Some patients may exhibit whining behavior, particularly in children ("Mommmy" or "I, I, I, I'm, I'm, sooooo thirsty"). It seems that the children's alternative to hyperverbalization is this whining.

Frightened

The critical and distinctive features of being frightened are complaining, moaning, groaning, whimpering, and begging interspersed with rapid questioning ("What are you doing?"), repeated requests, and demands for changes in care practices.

Frightened patients are not reticent about letting the staff know when procedures are painful or when their level of discomfort is unbearable. Their speech is peppered with expressions such as "ouch," "ooh," and "stop," vocalized in a commanding voice quality.

Patients who are frightened speak at moderate volume, which seems to be used as a mechanism to reduce their fear. When they are verbalizing, the content has an unsteady quality in that they produce longer chunks of language before the nurse hears a break in the voice. In all age groups, crying can be heard. This is the only behavioral state in which crying with vocalization occurs.

Frightened patients may withdraw from care and treatments, although if nurses and other staff hold their hands, they will not pull away from care and do not need to be restrained. They watch—monitor—all staff movements very carefully.

Terrified

In the terrified state, patients vocalize in short phrases or short sentences, during which they loudly protest, swear, shout, and beg the staff. These short sentences or phrases are usually up to five words in length. These patients vacillate between loud intensity and a moderate volume, and they include vocalizations that take the form of loud protestations ("Noooooo," "Please, oh God. Please, God!"). Vocal modulation has an emphatic and exclamatory nature, and a lot of anger and hostility is often evident. Note that these patients are irrationally refusing care despite the urgent nature of the care. Physically, they may struggle to get up from the gurney, are restless, may be combative and fight caregivers, and may have to be restrained. (The numbers in the following comments and in other places in this chapter represent the line numbers, the time, or the seconds from the interview transcriptions.)

Both frightened and terrified patients respond to a nurse being there for them and *talking them through* the experience (Morse & Proctor, 1998; Proctor et al., 1996). More recently, this response has been proven effective with frightened patients in second-stage labor (Bergstrom, Richards, Morse, & Roberts, 2010; Bergstrom et al., 2009). Talking them through as a nursing intervention is discussed in more detail later in this chapter.

Out of Control

Out-of-control patients exhibit hysterical, screaming, bellowing behavior. They are beyond coherent verbalizations, although occasionally a single word may be intelligible. Some attempts to verbalize are characterized by babbling, and short verbalizations will often be heard between screams.

The sound ranges from very loud to piercing and continuous. Voice modulation is erratic and inconsistent. This piercing and vacillating voice quality is accompanied by guttural sounds, such as "Aghuh gh gh gh gh" or "Aghuhuhhuh Owww Owwww Owwww." This kind of volatile patient often loses the ability to modulate his or her voice and produces maximum volume, yelling and screaming at the highest possible level. Staff interaction with these patients ceases, and it is difficult when a patient is out of control to communicate or to stop the vocalizations.

Out-of-control patients must be restrained so that emergency care can be administered, or they must be anesthetized as quickly as possible. They can be so distraught that they lose the ability to speak and vocalize shouts of rage. At this point, any discourse with the patient stops and caregivers go ahead, attending to the person's injuries.

Nurses can identify other behavioral states in the clinical areas and select the most appropriate modes of nursing interactions with those patients. There is much work to do in this area. Nurses see severe suffering on a daily basis, but they also see the suffering resulting from minor discomforts—for example, from a sore back from lying in bed, from nausea, from worries about how the family is managing at home while the mother is in the hospital. Nurses become adept at quickly and easily recognizing the cues that indicate something is not quite right. Sometimes comforting is providing an analgesic, giving a back rub, talking, listening, or just being there.

COMFORT AND COMFORTING

What, then, is comfort? *Comfort* is a concept that incorporates the caring focus of nursing—which enables us to see the cues and signals of suffering and motivates us to comfort—and a comforting action or task (Morse, 2000b). Note that when comfort is the central concept for nursing, nursing care is focused on the patient; in contrast, when *caring* is the central concept, nursing care is focused on the nurse. Within this framework, nurses' use of touch and talk are not indicators of caring per se; rather, they are comforting strategies that are responses to *signals of suffering*. They are *strategies for alleviating suffering* (Morse, 1992). Comfort, therefore, cannot be separated from suffering.

Comforting is not a "one-shot" intervention; it is a process that occurs in many iterative steps within the interaction and the developing relationship. During the *comforting interaction loop* in which a comforting action occurs, the patient is reevaluated and another comforting action is provided, and so forth. Examples of the comforting interaction loop follow:

- The nurse observes that the patient appears to be in pain (noting the signal of suffering or cues of distress), verifies the pain with the patient (action), administers an analgesic action (comforting action), and observes signs that the pain was subsequently alleviated.
- The nurse observes that the patient appears cold and is shivering (noting the behavioral cue), fetches a warm blanket (comforting action), and observes that the patient appears more relaxed and warmer.

As nursing tasks increase in complexity, so do the comforting actions:

- During childbirth, the nurse observes that the patient is becoming distressed (signal of suffering) and uses his or her voice (comforting interaction, "talking through") to assist in synchronizing the second-stage labor until the woman regains control (Bergstrom et al., 2010).
- In the trauma room during resuscitation, a patient is scared but lying still (caring observation). The nurse provides a "running commentary" by talking constantly, describing everything that he or she and the trauma team are doing. Later, the patient reports that she "just listened to that nurse's voice and held on."
- During trauma resuscitation, the nurse observes that the patient is terrified (signal of suffering). He or she uses the *comfort talk register* to enable the patient to hold on, and hold still (comforting action) until the analgesics take effect (Morse & Proctor, 1998; Proctor et al., 1996).

Comforting continues until it is no longer needed or demanded by the patient. Thus, comfort is defined as a relative and optimal state of well-being that may occur during any stage of the illness–health continuum. Responding to signals of suffering by making the patient comfortable is the goal of nursing (Morse, 1992).

The Comforting Interaction

The *comforting interaction* comprises the patient cue or a signal of distress from the patient, the cue or signal observed by the nurse, and the nurse's assessment of the patient and provision of a comfort strategy (Morse, Havens, DeLuca, & Wilson, 1997). The nurse then assesses the effectiveness of the strategy and, if the need has not been resolved, provides another strategy. This cycle may be slow and deliberate or as quick and almost subconscious as an interaction. As the comforting interactions accrue, the trust in the nurse–patient relationship builds. The relationship itself changes from a clinical relationship to a therapeutic relationship, then to a connected relationship (Morse, 1991); the patient feels safe and relinquishes himself or herself to the nurse's care (Morse, 1992).

The comforting interaction is patient led. In Morse et al.'s observations of postoperative infants, for example, comforting always occurred in response to the infant's cues. If the infant did not, or could not, "demand" a comforting strategy, it was usually not provided. For instance, because the infants were intubated, they cried silently, unable to vocalize their distress. As a result, nurses rarely used their voices to comfort the infants (Morse, Solberg, & Edwards, 1993; Solberg & Morse, 1991).

The nurse needs to provide care that is appropriate to the patient's state, and each state is associated with a different compendium of comforting strategies. If the nurse provides the wrong strategy, then the patient's state escalates. Ideally, the nurse will immediately correct the error and change the comforting intervention (Morse et al., 1997).

How important are these comforting interventions? Did you know that the way a nurse talks to the patient while inserting a nasogastric tube affects the success of the procedure (Morse et al., 2000; Penrod et al., 1999)? If the nurse, either by using technical talk (talk that focuses solely on what the patient should do) or by using solely caring terms of endearment, is overly receptive to the patient's cues of distress and does not include instructions for the patient, then the nurse will require more trials to place the tube correctly. The optimal way to talk to patients is a blend of technical and caring talk. Morse et al.'s research has shown that when the nurse uses the optimal style of talking, the nasogastric tube is successfully inserted with the smallest number of trials.

How important is comfort talk in trauma care? Trauma patients may be highly anxious, terrified, or out of control. Out of control is a very dangerous state. These patients could be irrational and try to fight the caregivers, and such effort both slows the delivery of emergency care and exacerbates injuries.

Can you imagine how pushing off caregivers and fighting care increases intracranial pressure? If the patient has a head injury, such actions could produce a large amount of cerebral damage. In the window of time before the patient can be given analgesics, the nurse assists the patient in maintaining control. The nurse talks the patient through the experience, using the *comfort talk register* (Morse & Proctor, 1998; Proctor et al., 1996), positions himself or herself over the patient's head, and holds his or her gaze (see **Figure 24-6**). The nurse then talks to the patient using a high "sing-song" register with distinct verbal contours. The nurse immediately interrupts any patient utterances and cries, urges the patient to "hold on," constantly warns the patient of painful procedures, and informs the patient how much longer the procedures will last.

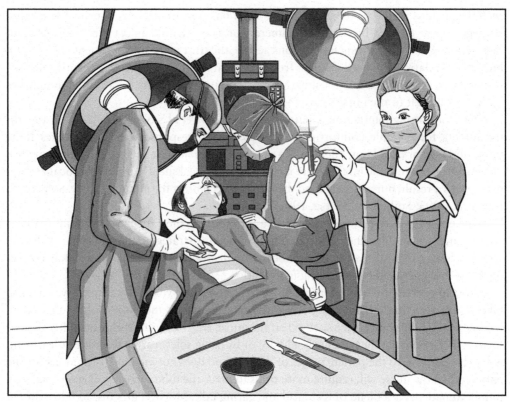

Figure 24-6   Posturing in "talking through" using the comfort talk register.

The practice of talking through also serves other important functions in trauma care. All communications to and from the patient go through the nurse. The nurse receives and communicates information about the patient's condition; he or she provides explanations, and the nurse's explanations then pace the trauma team. Procedures are performed one at a time, and only once the patient has been told what will happen. For instance, the nurse might say, "You will feel a finger in your bum, okay? Okay? *Okay*?" Only then is the rectal examination conducted. Without this information and pacing, the patient is very likely to lose control.

In a trauma situation, comfort is clearly a combination of touching, talking, posturing, and being immediately available to the patient. This approach assists the patient in maintaining control and is essential for the provision of safe care. These states in which care is given are known as *relinquishment to care* (Morse, 2000b). Types of relinquishment are described as follows:

• *Complete relinquishment:* The patient is unconscious or the patient cedes control totally to the nurse, urging the nurse to do "whatever is necessary."

- *Relaxed relinquishment:* The patient passively lies or dozes and lets the nurse give care. The patient trusts the nurse and senses the degree of vigilance, "watching over," and monitoring of the patient's condition, as with scared states.
- *Guarded relinquishment:* The patient watches what the nurse does and follows the nurse's action with his or her eyes. The patient holds still and permits care but does not trust the nurse or has limited trust.
- *Conditional relinquishment:* Bargaining takes place between the patient and the caregiver: The patient demands information about the procedure, sometimes in great detail. This behavior is often seen in children or highly anxious patients.
- *Reluctant relinquishment:* After bargaining, the patient continues to protest throughout the procedure. The patient often must be persuaded with a bribe.
- *Forced relinquishment:* The patient protests, refuses care, and must be held down. Patients constantly try to pull away, shout, or beg the nurse to "Hurry!" These patients are often terrified.

In trauma care, for instance, patients who feel in control relinquish to care; that is, they are responsive, cooperative, and receptive. Despite the pain, they try to remain passive and hold still, to "take it," to "bear it," and not to cry out. They work with staff; the patient who has completely relinquished realizes that care is necessary and submits to "whatever needs to be done." The result is that care is given quickly and safely. Again, the comfort level is a dynamic continuum, and patients generally fall somewhere between complete relinquishment and forced relinquishment (Morse, 2000b, p. 36). Nevertheless, the nurse–patient relationship is complex, and the patient does not immediately move to complete relinquishment, unless the patient's needs are great and life threatening.

The Patient's Comfort Level

Interestingly, nursing is just beginning to develop a solid theoretical base for providing comfort. When in the clinical areas, nurses would be well advised to listen for the ways that other nurses talk about patient states and communicate information about the patient's comfort states. Often, nurses will hear references to the patient's *comfort* level (Sasano & Morse, 2006). The comfort level is actually not a level of comfort, but rather the level of *distress* and the extent to which pain (or whatever is causing the distress) is being tolerated. For instance, a nurse may ask, "What is the patient's comfort level?" and be told, "He is tolerating it quite well"—which means that the patient is enduring the procedure, and it is not necessary to provide an analgesic immediately. Conversely, the nurse may reply, "He is really scared" or "He is out of control—we really need a hand in the trauma room!" Again, the comfort level is not the amount of pain that is being experienced, but rather how well it is being tolerated. Description of this level enables the rapid communication of the patient's behavioral state of suffering.

Compendium of Comforting Strategies

Comforting strategies available to nurses are numerous, and only some have been mentioned thus far. It is beyond the scope of this chapter to list them all. A brief classification of comforting strategies—by no means complete—is provided here.

Some strategies are present in the everyday interaction, without premeditation, as we console, or commiserate. Other strategies are used thoughtfully, and with care, such as providing empathy or formal counseling strategies. Some comforting strategies are prescribed, such as administering an analgesic. Some are standardized as a part of excellent nursing care, such as a back rub, position change, or bed bath. Some are in the control of nursing but are not routine, such as placing a patient on an air mattress. Some are indirect, such as controlling the environment—noise level or temperature, for example. The point is that all of these strategies are intended to enhance enduring, to help the patient "get through," and to reduce or to minimize the patient's suffering.

SUMMARY

Developed first from a synthesis of many research projects, and later by systematic research to test conjectures or to fill gaps, the praxis theory of suffering links myriad patient emotional states with comforting strategies. The model is patient led. With the nurse being responsive to patients' needs and the effects of nursing interventions, the model is dynamic and provides a means by which the nurse can systematically provide comfort. It is a malleable model, so that if a nurse provides an inappropriate strategy and the patient withdraws or has a negative response, the nurse may immediately change the strategy and move again toward comforting.

Is the model culturally bound? Can it be used cross-culturally? Because the nurse follows a patient's cues and signals of distress, this theory may be used to provide interventions with any culture.

Is the model limited to acute care or to trauma care? While most of the observational work has been done in areas of extreme distress, this model could be used in any setting, in home care, in clinics, in nursing homes—indeed, in any caregiving situation. Because the nurse "reads" the patient's behavior, the praxis theory of suffering offers many benefits over other models in which assessment is much slower, is more complex, or requires psychometric instruments. This model is compatible with actual patient care, bereavement, and rehabilitation.

A significant amount of work remains to be done on this theory, such as identification of patient states, signals and cues of distress, and comforting strategies, as well as development of the model. For instance, much work remains to be done on the state of enduring, on styles of enduring, and on the ways in which people self-console. We need to be able to develop and apply the model clinically: Can nurses, for instance, teach strategies of enduring, and if so, will those strategies decrease the length of time spent in rehabilitation?

DISCUSSION QUESTIONS

1. Search the Web for groups of people who are suffering. If you use "suffering" as the search term, for example, you will retrieve great works of art, depicting emotional suffering. But if you search for current events that have caused suffering—earthquakes, floods, fires, accidents, and so forth—you will get very interesting pictures from which you can easily identify states of enduring or emotional suffering. Examine both the person whom the photographer has targeted and the states of the people in the background. Often the target person is emotionally suffering and those in the background are enduring. Why do photographers target those who are emotionally suffering rather than enduring? Examine the proximal relationships of groups of people. Who are the supporters and who is releasing emotions? Who are the comforters? Note the states (enduring or emotional suffering) of each person.

2. Examine photographs of formal ceremonies, such as funerals. Do you think conventions and ceremonies support enduring or emotional suffering behaviors in the bereaved? How? Why?

3. Both enduring and emotional suffering trigger emotions in observers. How do these emotions differ? Which kinds of responses in the observer do they elicit?

REFERENCES

Bergstrom, L., Richards, L., Morse, J., & Roberts, J. (2010). How caregivers manage pain and distress in second stage labor. *Midwifery, 55*(1), 38–45.

Bergstrom, L., Richards, L., Proctor, A., Bohrer-Avila, L., Morse, J., & Roberts, J. (2009). Birth talk in second stage labor. *Qualitative Health Research, 19*, 954–964.

Carter, B. J. (1994). Surviving breast cancer. *Cancer Practice, 2*(2), 135–140.

Ekman, P., & Friesen, W. V. (1978). *Facial action coding system: A technique for the measurement of facial movement.* Palo Alto, CA: Consulting Psychologists.

Ekman, P., Irwin, W., & Rosenberg, E. (1994). *EMFACS: Coders instructions (EMFACS-8).* San Francisco, CA: University of California, San Francisco.

Mayan, M., Morse, J. M., & Eldershaw, L. P. (2006). Developing the concept of self-reformulation. *QHW: International Journal of Qualitative Studies on Health and Well-being, 1*(1), 20–26.

Morse, J. M. (1991). Negotiating commitment and involvement in the patient–nurse relationship. *Journal of Advanced Nursing, 16*, 455–468.

Morse, J. M. (1992). Comfort: The refocusing of nursing care. *Clinical Nursing Research, 1*, 91–113.

Morse, J. M. (1997). Responding to threats to integrity of self. *Advances in Nursing Science, 19*(4), 21–36.

Morse, J. M. (2000a). Responding to the cues of suffering. *Health Care for Women International, 21*, 1–9.

Morse, J. M. (2000b). On comfort and comforting. *American Journal of Nursing, 100*(9), 34–38.

Morse, J. M. (2001). Toward a praxis theory of suffering. *Advances in Nursing Science, 24*(1), 47–59.

Morse, J. M. (2005). Creating a qualitatively-derived theory of suffering. In U. Zeitler (Ed.), *Clinical practice and development in nursing* (pp. 83–91). Aarhus, Denmark: Center for Innovation in Nurse Training.

Morse, J. M., Beres, M., Spiers, J., Mayan, M., & Olson, K. (2003). Identifying signals of suffering by linking verbal and facial cues. *Qualitative Health Research, 13*(8), 1063–1077.

Morse, J. M., & Carter, B. (1996). The essence of enduring and the expression of suffering: The reformulation of self. *Scholarly Inquiry for Nursing Practice, 10*(1), 43–60.

Morse, J. M., Havens, G., DeLuca, A., & Wilson, S. (1997). The comforting interaction: Developing a model of nurse–patient relationship. *Scholarly Inquiry for Nursing Practice, 11*(4), 321–343.

Morse, J. M., & Johnson, J. L. (Eds.). (1991). *The illness experience: Dimensions of suffering.* Newbury Park, CA: Sage.

Morse, J. M., & Mitcham, C. (1997). Compathy: The contagion of physical distress. *Journal of Advanced Nursing, 26,* 649–657.

Morse, J. M., & Mitcham, C. (1998). The experience of agonizing pain and signals of disembodiment. *Journal of Psychosomatic Research, 44*(6), 667–680.

Morse, J. M., Mitcham, C., & van der Steen, V. (1998). Compathy or physical empathy: Implications for the caregiver relationship. *Journal of Medical Humanities, 19*(1), 51–65.

Morse, J. M., & O'Brien, B. (1995). Preserving self: From victim, to patient, to disabled person. *Journal of Advanced Nursing, 21,* 886–896.

Morse, J. M., & Penrod, J. (1999). Linking concepts of enduring, suffering, and hope. *Image: Journal of Nursing Scholarship, 31*(2), 145–150.

Morse, J. M., Penrod, J., Kassab, C., & Dellasega, C. (2000). Evaluating the efficiency and effectiveness of approaches to nasogastric tube insertion during trauma care. *American Journal of Critical Care, 9*(5), 325–333.

Morse, J. M., & Pooler, C. (2002). Patient–family–nurse interactions in the trauma resuscitation room. *American Journal of Critical Care, 11*(3), 240–249.

Morse, J. M., & Proctor, A. (1998). Maintaining patient endurance: The comfort work of trauma nurses. *Clinical Nursing Research, 7*(3), 250–274.

Morse, J. M., Solberg, S., & Edwards, J. (1993). Caregiver–infant interaction: Comforting the postoperative infant. *Scandinavian Journal of Caring Sciences, 7,* 105–111.

Olson, K., Morse, J. M., Smith, J., Mayan, M., & Hammond, D. (2000–2001). Linking trajectories of illness and dying. *Omega, 42*(4), 293–308.

Penrod, J., Morse, J. M., & Wilson, S. (1999). Comforting strategies used during nasogastric tube insertion. *Journal of Clinical Nursing, 8,* 31–38.

Proctor, A., Morse, J. M., & Khonsari, E. S. (1996). Sounds of comfort in the trauma center: How nurses talk to patients in pain. *Social Sciences and Medicine, 42,* 1669–1680.

Sasano, P., & Morse, J. (2006). *What is a patient's comfort level? Defining a nursing concept.* Unpublished paper, University of Alberta, Canada.

Solberg, S., & Morse, J. M. (1991). The comforting behaviors of caregivers toward distressed post-operative neonates. *Issues in Comprehensive Pediatric Nursing, 14*(2), 77–92.

APPENDIX: REFERENCE LIST FOR TABLE 24-1

1. Morse, J. M. (1983). An ethnoscientific analysis of comfort: A preliminary investigation. *Nursing Papers/Perspectives in Nursing, 15*(1), 6–19.
2. Johnson, J. L., & Morse, J. M. (1990). Regaining control: The process of adjustment following myocardial infarction. *Heart and Lung, 19*(2), 126–135.
3. Wilson, S., & Morse, J. M. (1991). Living with a wife undergoing chemotherapy: Perceptions of the husband. *Image: Journal of Nursing Scholarship, 23*(2), 78–84.
4. Thomas, A., & Morse, J. M. (1991). Managing urinary incontinence. *Journal of Gerontological Nursing, 17*(6), 9–14.
5. Côté, J. J., Morse, J. M., & James, S. G. (1991). The pain experience of the post-operative newborn. *Journal of Advanced Nursing, 16*, 378–387.
6. Morse, J. M. (1991). Negotiating commitment and involvement in the patient–nurse relationship. *Journal of Advanced Nursing, 16*, 455–468.
7. Solberg, S., & Morse, J. M. (1991). The comforting behaviors of caregivers toward distressed post-operative neonates. *Issues in Comprehensive Pediatric Nursing, 14*(2), 77–92.
8. Morse, J. M. (1991). The structure and function of gift-giving in the patient–nurse relationship. *Western Journal of Nursing Research, 13*, 597–615.
9. Solberg, S., & Morse, J. M. (1991). The comforting behaviors of caregivers toward distressed post-operative neonates. *Issues in Comprehensive Pediatric Nursing, 14*(2), 77–92.
10. Morse, J. M., & Johnson, J. L. (Eds.). (1991). *The illness experience: Dimensions of suffering.* Newbury Park, CA: Sage.
11. Morse, J. M., Bottorff, J., Neander, W., & Solberg, S. (1991). Comparative analysis of the conceptualizations and theories of caring. *Image: Journal of Nursing Scholarship, 23*(2), 119–126.
12. Morse, J. M. (1992). Comfort: The refocusing of nursing care. *Clinical Nursing Research, 1*, 91–113.
13. Estabrooks, C., & Morse, J. M. (1992). Toward a theory of touch: The touching process and acquiring a touching style. *Journal of Advanced Nursing, 17*, 448–456.
14. Morse, J. M., Bottorff, J., Anderson, G., O'Brien, B., & Solberg, S. (1992). Beyond empathy: Expanding expressions of caring. *Journal of Advanced Nursing, 17*, 809–821.
15. Morse, J. M., Anderson, G., Bottorff, J., Yonge, O., O'Brien, B., Solberg, S., & McIlveen, K. (1992). Exploring empathy: A conceptual fit for nursing practice? *Image: Journal of Nursing Scholarship, 24*(4), 274–280.
16. Morse, J. M., Solberg, S., & Edwards, J. (1993). Caregiver–infant interaction: Comforting the postoperative infant. *Scandinavian Journal of Caring Sciences, 7*, 105–111.
17. Laskiwski, S., & Morse, J. M. (1993). The spinal cord injured patient: The modification of hope and expressions of despair. *Canadian Journal of Rehabilitation, 6*(3), 143–153.
18. Morse, J. M., Solberg, S., & Edwards, J. (1993). Caregiver–infant interaction: Comforting the postoperative infant. *Scandinavian Journal of Caring Sciences, 7*, 105–111.
19. Morse, J. M., Bottorff, J. L., & Hutchinson, S. (1994). The phenomenology of comfort. *Journal of Advanced Nursing, 20*, 189–195.
20. Siegl, D., & Morse, J. M. (1994). Tolerating reality: The experiences of parents with HIV positive sons. *Social Science and Medicine, 38*, 959–971.

21. Bottorff, J. L., & Morse, J. M. (1994). Identifying types of attending: Patterns of nurses' work. *Image: Journal of Nursing Scholarship*, 26(1), 53–60.

22. Morse, J. M., Bottorff, J. L., & Hutchinson, S. (1994). The phenomenology of comfort. *Journal of Advanced Nursing*, 20, 189–195.

23. Morse, J. M., Miles, M. W., Clark, D. A., & Doberneck, B. M. (1994). Sensing patient needs: Exploring concepts of nursing insight and receptivity used in nursing assessment. *Scholarly Inquiry for Nursing Practice*, 8(3), 233–254.

24. Morse, J. M., Bottorff, J. L., & Hutchinson, S. (1995). The paradox of comfort. *Nursing Research*, 44(1), 14–19.

25. Applegate, M., & Morse, J. M. (1994). Personal privacy and interaction patterns in a nursing home. *Journal of Aging Studies*, 8(4), 413–434.

26. McIlveen, K. M., & Morse, J. M. (1995). The role of comfort in nursing care: 1900–1980. *Clinical Nursing Research*, 4(2), 127–148.

27. Morse, J. M., & Carter, B. J. (1995). Strategies of enduring and the suffering of loss: Modes of comfort used by a resilient survivor. *Holistic Nursing Practice*, 9(3), 33–58. Reprinted in Danish: N. Gress (Ed.), *Klinisk Sygrpleje, bd 1,11, og 111, 2000.*

28. Morse, J. M., & O'Brien, B. (1995). Preserving self: From victim, to patient, to disabled person. *Journal of Advanced Nursing*, 21, 886–896.

29. Miles, M., & Morse, J. M. (1995). Utilizing the concepts of transference and countertransference in the consultation process. *Journal of the American Psychiatric Nurses Association*, 1(2), 42–47.

30. Hyland, L., & Morse, J. M. (1995). Orchestrating comfort: The role of funeral directors. *Death Studies*, 19, 453–474.

31. Hupcey, J. E., & Morse, J. M. (1995). Family and social support: Application to the critically ill patient. *Journal of Family Nursing*, 1(3), 257–280.

32. Morse, J. M., & Doberneck, B. M. (1995). Delineating the concept of hope. *Image: Journal of Nursing Scholarship*, 27(4), 277–285.

33. Dewar, A., & Morse, J. M. (1995). Unbearable incidents: Failure to endure the experience of illness. *Journal of Advanced Nursing*, 22(5), 957–964.

34. Proctor, A., Morse, J. M., & Khonsari, E. S. (1996). Sounds of comfort in the trauma center: How nurses talk to patients in pain. *Social Sciences and Medicine*, 42, 1669–1680.

35. Hogan, N., Morse, J. M., & Tasón, M. C. (1996). Toward an experiential theory of bereavement. *Omega*, 33(1), 43–65.

36. Morse, J. M., & Carter, B. (1996). The essence of enduring and the expression of suffering: The reformulation of self. *Scholarly Inquiry for Nursing Practice*, 10(1), 43–60.

37. Morse, J. M., & Mitcham, C. (1997). Compathy: The contagion of physical distress. *Journal of Advanced Nursing*, 26, 649–657.

38. Morse, J. M. (1997). Responding to threats to integrity of self. *Advances in Nursing Science*, 19(4), 21–36.

39. Penrod, J., & Morse, J. M. (1997). Strategies for assessing and fostering hope: The Hope Assessment Guide. *Oncology Nurses Forum*, 24(6), 1055–1063.

40. Morse, J. M., & Mitcham, C. (1998). The experience of agonizing pain and signals of disembodiment. *Journal of Psychosomatic Research*, 44(6), 667–680.

41. Penrod, J., Morse, J. M., & Wilson, S. (1999). Comforting strategies used during nasogastric tube insertion. *Journal of Clinical Nursing, 8*, 31–38.
42. Morse, J. M., Havens, G., DeLuca, A., & Wilson, S. (1997). The comforting interaction: Developing a model of nurse–patient relationship. *Scholarly Inquiry for Nursing Practice, 11*(4), 321–343.
43. Morse, J. M., Mitcham, C., & van der Steen, V. (1998). Compathy or physical empathy: Implications for the caregiver relationship. *Journal of Medical Humanities, 19*(1), 51–65.
44. Wilson, S., Morse, J. M., & Penrod, J. (1998). Developing reciprocal trust in the caregiving relationship. *Qualitative Health Research, 8*, 446–465.
45. Morse, J. M., & Proctor, A. (1998). Maintaining patient endurance: The comfort work of trauma nurses. *Clinical Nursing Research, 7*(3), 250–274.
46. Morse, J. M. (2000). On comfort and comforting. *American Journal of Nursing, 100*(9), 34–38.
47. Wilson, S., Morse, J. M., & Penrod, J. (1998). Absolute involvement: The experience of mothers of ventilator-dependent children. *Health and Social Care, 6*(4), 224–233.
48. Hupcey, J. E., Penrod, J., & Morse, J. M. (2000). Establishing and maintaining trust during acute care hospitalizations. *Scholarly Inquiry for Nursing Practice: An International Journal, 14*(3), 227–242.
49. Morse, J. M. (2000). Responding to the cues of suffering. *Health Care for Women International, 21*, 1–9.
50. Morse, J. M., & Penrod, J. (1999). Linking concepts of enduring, suffering, and hope. *Image: Journal of Nursing Scholarship, 31*(2), 145–150.
51. Morse, J. M., Penrod, J., Kassab, C., & Dellasega, C. (2000). Evaluating the efficiency and effectiveness of approaches to nasogastric tube insertion during trauma care. *American Journal of Critical Care, 9*(5), 325–333.
52. Morse, J. M., Wilson, S., & Penrod, J. (2000). Mothers and their disabled children: Refining the concept of normalization. *Health Care for Women International, 21*(8), 659–676.
53. Olson, K., Morse, J. M., Smith, J., Mayan, M., & Hammond, D. (2000–2001). Linking trajectories of illness and dying. *Omega, 42*(4), 293–308.
54. Morse, J. M. (2001). Toward a praxis theory of suffering. *Advances in Nursing Science, 24*(1), 47–59. [Italian: Verso una teoria della prassi della sofferenza, (traduzione di Luca Mori). *Salute e Società, 1*, a cura di Enzo Giorgo e Willem Tousijn, FrancoAngeli, 2003, pp. 169–185; Commentary: Mori, L. l'osserfvzione della sofferenza nel lavoro di Janice Morse, pp. 186–189].
55. Hupcey, J., Penrod, J., Morse, J., & Mitcham, C. (2001). An exploration and advancement of the concept of trust. *Journal of Advanced Nursing, 36*(2), 282–293.
56. Morse, J. M., & Pooler, C. (2002). Patient–family–nurse interactions in the trauma-resuscitation room. *American Journal of Critical Care, 11*(3), 240–249.
57. Morse, J. M., Beres, M., Spiers, J., Mayan, M., & Olson, K. (2003). Identifying signals of suffering by linking verbal and facial cues. *Qualitative Health Research, 13*(8), 1063–1077.
58. Mayan, M., Morse, J. M., & Eldershaw, L. P. (2006). Developing the concept of self-reformulation. *QHW: International Journal of Qualitative Studies on Health and Well-being, 1*(1), 20–26.
59. Weaver, K., Morse, J. M., & Mitcham, C. (2008). Ethical sensitivity in practice: Concept analysis. *Journal of Advanced Nursing, 62*(5), 607–618.

60. Bergstrom, L., Richards, L., Proctor, A., Bohrer-Avila, L., Morse, J., & Roberts, J. (2009). Birth talk in second stage labor. *Qualitative Health Research, 19,* 954–964.
61. Bergstrom, L., Richards, L., Morse, J., & Roberts, J. (2009). How caregivers manage pain and distress in second stage labor. *Midwifery, 55*(1), 38–45.
62. Morse, J. M., Konrad, S. J., Pooler, C., & Mott, R. (2014). Awaiting the diagnosis of breast cancer: Strategies of enduring for preserving self. *Oncology Nursing Forum, 41*(4), 350–359.

V

Tools for Integrating and Disseminating Knowledge in Advanced Nursing Practice

Chapter 25

Theory Testing and Theory Evaluation*

Jacqueline Fawcett

INTRODUCTION

The focus of this chapter is the science and art of theory development and evaluation. The chapter begins with a definition of theory and a description of the process of theory development and continues with a discussion of the critical thinking that is required for the evaluation of theories. The emphasis in this chapter is theory development and evaluation activities that are required for advanced practice nursing. The content of this chapter is especially relevant to two of the American Association of Colleges of Nursing's Essentials of Doctoral Education for Advanced Nursing Practice: *Essential I, Scientific Underpinnings for Practice*, and *Essential III, Clinical Scholarship and Analytical Methods for Evidence-Based Practice*.

THE SCIENCE AND ART OF THEORY DEVELOPMENT

The term *theory* is used to refer to diverse works, ranging from very abstract and general conceptual models to less abstract and general grand theories, to relatively concrete and specific middle-range theories, to very concrete and specific narrow-range situation-specific theories. Despite the lack of consensus about the meaning of theory, King and Fawcett (1997) found considerable agreement about the existence of levels of abstraction for theoretical work. In this chapter, the term refers to middle-range theories and situation-specific theories. The term *conceptual model* refers to the very abstract and general work from which theories are derived.

---

*Portions of this chapter are adapted from Fawcett, J., & Garity, J. (2009). *Evaluating research for evidence-based nursing practice*. Philadelphia, PA: F. A. Davis. Used with permission.

Theories

A theory is made up of concepts and propositions about a phenomenon. A *concept* is a word or phrase that captures the essence of something, such as adjustment or distress. It may have one or more dimensions. An example of a single-dimensional concept is resiliency. An example of a multidimensional concept is perceived stigma, the six dimensions of which are fear of contagion, healthcare neglect, negative self-perception, social isolation, verbal abuse, and workplace stigma (Mwangi, 2013).

A *proposition* is a statement about one or more concepts. A proposition about one concept is a definition or a description of the concept; *resiliency*, for example, is defined as "The capacity to return to a restorative level of functioning using compensatory/coping mechanisms; the ability to bounce back quickly after an insult" (American Association of Critical Care Nurses, 2014, p. 1). A proposition about two or more concepts states an association between the concepts, including the relation between the concepts or the effect of one concept on one or more other concepts. An example of a statement of the relation between two concepts is, "Socio-demographic characteristics are related to perceived stigma" (Mwangi, 2013). An example of a statement about the effect of a concept on other concepts, which typically involves the effect of some intervention on some outcomes, is, "Information about walking exercise has a positive effect on symptoms, fatigue, emotional distress, and physical function" (Mock et al., 2007)

Nursing theories usually focus on experiences of health conditions and health-related events. Examples of health conditions include such medical diagnoses as congestive heart failure cancer, and diabetes. Examples of health-related events include pregnancy, childbirth, the postpartum period, and aging. The health condition or health event of interest provides a context for a theory. For example, the concepts of exercise intervention, fatigue, and emotional distress and the propositions about those concepts could make up a theory about the effects of an exercise intervention on fatigue and emotional distress experienced by men with colon cancer. Alternatively, the concepts of fatigue and emotional distress might make up a theory about the relation between fatigue and emotional distress during the postpartum period.

Types of Theories

Three types of theories are descriptive, explanatory, and predictive. *Descriptive theories* simply describe some phenomenon. They typically comprise one concept and one proposition that is a definition or description of the concept. An example of a descriptive theory is the theory of fatigue. In this case, the theory concept is fatigue. The theory proposition asserts that fatigue is a multidimensional concept defined as behavioral, sensory, and affective experiences (Piper et al., 1998).

Explanatory theories specify how concepts are related to each other and, therefore, provide explanations for phenomena. They consist of two or more concepts, the propositions that are definitions or descriptions of each concept, and the propositions that specify the relation(s) between the concepts. An example is the theory of chronic pain (Tsai, Tak, Moore, & Palencia, 2003). The theory concepts are chronic pain, physical disability, social support, age, gender, perceived daily stress, and depression. The propositions that are definitions of each concept are as follows:

- Chronic pain is defined as the frequency and severity of pain (Tsai et al., 2003).
- Physical disability is defined as the frequency and extent of mobility, walking, bending, and hand and finger function (Tsai et al., 2003).
- Social support is defined as "perceived levels of social support . . . [including] (a) provision of attachment/intimacy, (b) social integration, (c) opportunity for nurturant behavior, (d) reassurance of worth, and (e) availability of informational, emotional, and material help" (Tsai et al., 2003, p. 162).
- Age is defined as age in years (Tsai et al., 2003).
- Gender is defined as male or female (Tsai et al., 2003).
- Perceived daily stress is defined as "the degree to which older persons experience daily stress from irritating, frustrating, or repeated occurrences in their lives" (Tsai et al., 2003, p. 162).
- Depression is defined as the frequency of depressed mood symptoms within the past week (Tsai et al., 2003).

The following theory proposition specifies the relations between the concepts: Chronic pain, physical disability, social support, age, and gender are related to perceived daily stress, which is related to depression.

Predictive theories specify how a concept affects one or more other concepts. They are made up of two or more concepts, the propositions that are definitions or descriptions of each concept, and the propositions that specify the effect(s) of one concept on one or more other concepts. An example is the theory of the effects of simulated conflict management training (Pines et al., 2014). The theory concepts are simulated conflict management training exercises, stress resiliency, psychological empowerment, and conflict management style. The propositions that are definitions of each concept are as follows:

- Simulated conflict management training exercises are defined as "didactic and simulated training using a variety of scenarios for learning resiliency skills, enhancing perceptions of empowerment and increasing knowledge of personal styles of conflict management" (Pines et al., 2014, p. 87).
- Stressr resiliency is defined as "the ability of an individual to adjust to adversity, maintain equilibrium, retain some control over the environment, and move in a positive direction" (Pines et al., 2014, p. 86).

- Psychological empowerment is defined as "the individual's perceived sense of meaning and purpose, competence, self-determination, and impact on the work role" (Pines et al., 2014, p. 86).
- Conflict management style is defined as "[depending] on the situation and the parties involved and [involving] a choice of methods to manage a situation. . . . [The five] conflict management styles [are] accommodating, avoiding, collaborating, competing, and compromising. Accommodating is unassertive and cooperative and allows the other person to dominate. Avoiding is both uncooperative and unassertive and is characterized by the individual's avoidance of taking any action. Collaborating is assertive and cooperative and represents an attempt to find a solution to the conflict. Competing is assertive and uncooperative. Finally, compromising is intermediate in both assertiveness and cooperativeness and partially satisfies the needs of each party. With competing, [an individual] assertively pursues personal concerns at the expense of the concerns of another. In compromising, the object is to find a mutually agreeable solution that partially satisfies both parties. Resiliency and empowerment reflect application of the appropriate strategy/style in response to the situation" (Thomas & Kilmann, as cited in Pines et al., 2014, p. 86).

The following theory proposition specifies effects: Simulated conflict management training exercises have a positive effect on stress resiliency, psychological empowerment, and conflict management style (Pines et al., 2014).

Empirical Indicators and Other Empirical Methods

Most theory concepts and propositions cannot be directly observed or measured. Instead, each concept must be connected to an *empirical indicator*, which serves as a real-world proxy—or substitute—for a concept. Empirical indicators that are particularly useful for advanced practice nurses are assessment tools and intervention protocols. *Assessment tools* include various types of questionnaires, such as checklists and rating scales, which contain one or more items. For example, postpartum mood disorder is assessed by the 21-item Neuman Postpartum Mood Questionnaire (Fashinpaur, 2002), or as a one-item rating scale that asks the woman to indicate, on a scale of 0 to 10, the extent to which she feels depressed. One-item assessment tools are particularly useful in advanced practice nursing because they do not impose a burden on patients, which may occur when a tool with many items is used. One-item assessment tools also are useful because they do not impose an undue burden on the advanced practice nurse, which may occur with use of a multi-item tool that requires calculation of a score.

Intervention protocols are explanations of procedures that are administered to or engaged in by patients; they are analogous to the experimental and control treatments of experimental research and to the procedures included in clinical guidelines or a hospital procedure manual. An example is the explanation for all procedures used to administer simulated conflict management training exercises (Pines et al., 2014). Other empirical methods that are part of nursing practice and research include the number of times and the ways in which the assessment tool and intervention protocol are applied (the research design and data collection procedures), the number of patients who are assessed and receive the intervention (the sample of research participants), and the ways in which the results of the assessment and outcomes of the interventions are analyzed for quality improvement initiatives (the data analysis techniques).

Conceptual Models

Theories are developed through a melding of science and art in the form of creative conversion of ideas stemming from provocative facts (Levine, 1966; 1991) observed in practice and in the literature. These facts are noticed because they fit with the observer's frame of reference about nursing, which also is called a *conceptual model* of nursing. Among the best-known conceptual models are Levine's Conservation Model, Neuman's Systems Model, Orem's Self-Care Framework, and Roy's Adaptation Model. Overviews of these and other conceptual models of nursing are found in Appendix N-1 of *Taber's Cyclopedic Medical Dictionary* (Fawcett, 2013). A comprehensive analysis and evaluation of each of these and other conceptual models of nursing is given in Fawcett and DeSanto-Madeya's (2013) book *Contemporary Nursing Knowledge: Analysis and Evaluation of Nursing Models and Theories*.

Each conceptual model of nursing is made up of concepts and propositions that are more abstract and general than those of a theory. Examples of concepts from Roy's adaptation model include stimuli and adaptation. For example, the following proposition defines a conceptual model concept: Adaptation is defined as "the process and outcome whereby thinking and feeling people, as individuals and in groups, use conscious awareness and choice to create human and environment integration" (Roy, 2009, p. 26). An example of a proposition that links the concepts of stimuli and adaptation is as follows: Stimuli are related to the physiological, self-concept, role function, and interdependence modes of adaptation (Fawcett, 2003).

Conceptual–Theoretical–Empirical Structures for Theory Development

Theory development involves specification of a conceptual–theoretical–empirical (C-T-E) structure made up of three components:

1. A conceptual model
2. A theory
3. Empirical indicators and other empirical methods

Theory development is the product of research, which is a systematic process of inquiry (Fawcett & Garity, 2009). Thus, every study is explicitly or implicitly designed to develop a theory by means of generation of new theory or testing of an existing theory. Theory-generating research is descriptive research, the findings of which are new descriptive theories. Theory testing research can be descriptive, correlational, or experimental research. The findings of descriptive theory-testing research determine the empirical adequacy of an existing descriptive theory. The findings of correlational theory-testing research determine the empirical adequacy of an existing explanatory theory. The findings of experimental theory-testing research determine the empirical adequacy of an existing predictive theory. Although the conduct of research typically is thought of as a rigorous scientific process, it is also a creative endeavor involving an appreciation of the beauty of logical reasoning and the "aha" moments that come when developing elegant C-T-E structures, designing studies, and interpreting data.

Conceptual–Theoretical–Empirical Structures for Theory Generation

Theory-generating research involves inductive reasoning from specific observations of a phenomenon to a general concept and one or more propositions about the concept. As can be seen in **Figure 25-1**, the C-T-E structure for theory-generating research proceeds from the conceptual model to the empirical indicators and other empirical methods to the concepts and propositions of a new theory.

Creating Conceptual–Theoretical–Empirical Structures for Theory Generation

Advanced practice nurses can create C-T-E structures for their own studies designed to generate a new theory, or they can prepare a diagram of the C-T-E structure for an existing study. The C-T-E structure begins with the identification of the conceptual model concept that guides the selection of the empirical indicator used to collect data. This structure is completed when the theory concept and any concept dimensions are identified (see Figures 25-1).

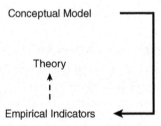

Figure 25-1   Conceptual–theoretical–empirical (C-T-E) structure for theory generation: from conceptual model to empirical indicators to theory.

Conceptual–Theoretical–Empirical Structures for Theory Testing

Theory-testing research involves deductive reasoning from one or more general concepts and propositions to a specific set of concepts and propositions. As can be seen in **Figure 25-2**, the C-T-E structure for theory-testing research proceeds from the conceptual model to the theory and then to the empirical indicators and other empirical methods. **Figure 25-3** is an example of a C-T-E structure for theory testing. This example was constructed from the report of a study designed to test a theory of the efficacy of a self-care intervention to improve cancer pain management (Rustøen et al., 2014). The study was guided by Orem's Self-Care Framework. As can be seen in Figure 25-3, Orem's Self-Care Framework concept of nursing systems was linked with the theory concept of psychoeducational intervention. The two dimensions of psychoeducational intervention are the PRO-SELF Pain Control

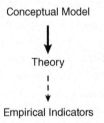

Figure 25-2 C-T-E structure for theory testing: from conceptual model to theory to empirical indicators.

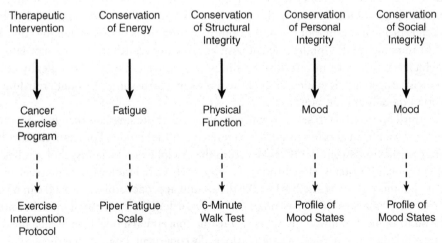

Figure 25-3   C-T-E structure for Rustøen et al.'s theory-testing study.

Program and a control intervention, each of which was implemented by means of the empirical indicators that specified the precise intervention protocols. Orem's Self-Care Framework concept of self-care behaviors was linked with the theory concept of cancer pain management behaviors. Some dimensions of cancer pain management behaviors are pain intensity, pain frequency, and breakthrough pain, which were measured by documentation in a diary that included a numeric rating scale, as well as pain location, which was measured by a body diagram. Another dimension of cancer pain management behaviors is total doses of and prescription changes for opioid analgesics, which was measured by documentation in a diary.

Creating Conceptual–Theoretical–Empirical Structures for Theory Testing

Advanced practice nurses can create C-T-E structures for their own studies designed to test an existing theory, or they can prepare a diagram of the C-T-E structure for an existing study. The most important aspect of creating C-T-E structures for theory testing is the linkage of a conceptual model to a theory. Three approaches have been identified.

The first approach is the selection of the conceptual model of nursing and the direct derivation of a theory from that conceptual model. For example, two theories of family health have been directly derived from King's conceptual system (Doornbos, 1995, 2000; Wicks, 1995, 1997). This approach ensures a logical linkage between the conceptual model and the theory. The logic is ensured because the philosophical assumptions undergirding the conceptual model and the theory are the same.

The second approach is to select a conceptual model of nursing and then link an existing nursing theory to that conceptual model. For example, a researcher might want to link the nursing theory of uncertainty in illness (Mishel, 1990) to Roy's Adaptation Model. This approach is problematic in that the philosophical assumptions undergirding the conceptual model of nursing and the philosophical assumptions undergirding the conceptual model from which the theory of uncertainty in illness was derived may not be logically congruent. Logical congruence is evident only if the philosophical assumptions undergirding both conceptual models are the same.

The third approach is to select a conceptual model of nursing and then link an existing theory borrowed from another discipline to that conceptual model. For example, the theory of planned behavior (Ajzen, 1991), taken from the discipline of social psychology, has been linked to Neuman's Systems Model and with Orem's Self-Care Framework (Villarruel, Bishop, Simpson, Jemmott, & Fawcett, 2001). Like the second approach, this approach can be problematic in that the philosophical assumptions undergirding the conceptual model of nursing and the philosophical assumptions undergirding the conceptual model from which the theory of planned behavior was derived may not be logically congruent. Logical congruence is evident only if the philosophical assumptions undergirding both conceptual models are the same.

Latham (2002) rejected the third approach on the grounds that it does not contribute to the advancement of the discipline of nursing. She declared the following:

> Grafting a particular borrowed theory onto a nursing conceptual model may be a questionable exercise. . . . Rather the emphasis could be placed on creating distinctive cognitive approaches with the parameters of nursing. . . . Nursing research will not advance knowledge if it continues to hang on the coattails of other disciplines. (p. 264)

The C-T-E structure for theory testing is completed when the theory concepts are linked to empirical indicators (see Figures 25-2 and 25-3).

Partnerships for Theory Development

Advanced practice nurses certainly may construct C-T-E structures and conduct research independently, but they may be more successful if they form partnerships with nurse researchers who are fully prepared to conduct research through research training from a doctor of philosophy or other research-intensive educational program. Such partnerships integrate the clinical expertise of the advanced practice nurse with the research expertise of the nurse researcher. An example of a successful partnership that brought together student nurses, staff nurses, advanced practice nurses, and nurse researchers is an international multisite study designed to test a theory of women's perceptions of and responses to cesarean birth that was guided by Roy's Adaptation Model (Fawcett et al., 2005; Fawcett et al., 2011).

THE SCIENCE AND ART OF THEORY EVALUATION

Many different sets of criteria for evaluating theories are found in the nursing literature (e.g., Barnum, 1998; Duffy & Muhlenkamp, 1974; Fawcett, 2005; Fawcett & DeSanto-Madeya, 2013; Parse, 2005). However, only one set of criteria includes the three components of C-T-E structures—conceptual model, theory, empirical indicators (Fawcett & Garity, 2009).

Evaluating C-T-E structures for theory generation and theory testing is a five-step process that requires thinking critically and making judgments about the extent to which the information about each component of the C-T-E structure satisfies a certain set of criteria. Critical thinking and making judgments is a primarily scientific endeavor grounded in the criteria, but it also involves the art of grasping the meaning of what is intended in the linkages among the C-T-E structural components and appreciating the beauty of the elegance of those linkages in a nonscientific, intuitive manner.

Step 1: Evaluation of the Conceptual–Theoretical–Empirical Linkages

The first step in evaluation of C-T-E structures focuses on the conceptual model (C) component. The two criteria are specification adequacy and linkage adequacy.

Box 25-1 Example of Narrative Content Required for the Criteria of Conceptual Model Specification Adequacy and Linkage Adequacy

Specification Adequacy

The study was guided by Orem's Self-Care Framework. This conceptual model of nursing draws attention to individuals' motivation and capability for care of self, including universal, developmental, and health-deviation self-care requisites. When individuals are not able to care for self, nurses develop wholly compensatory, partly compensatory, or supportive-educative nursing systems using various methods of helping—acting for or doing for the patient, guiding the patient, supporting the patient, providing a developmental environment for the patient, and teaching the patient.

Linkage Adequacy

As can be seen in Figure 25-3, Orem's Self-Care Framework concept of nursing systems was represented by psychoeducational intervention, which was implemented by means of empirical indicators that specified precise PRO-SELF pain control program and control intervention protocols. Orem's Self-Care Framework concept of self-care behaviors was represented by cancer pain management behaviors, which were measured by documentation in a diary that included a numeric rating scale and a body diagram.

Data from Rustøen, T., Valeberg, B. T., Kolstad, E., Wist, E., Paul, S., & Miaskowski, C. (2014). A randomized clinical trial of the efficacy of a self-care intervention to improve cancer pain management. *Cancer Nursing, 37*, 34–43.

Specification Adequacy

Specification adequacy refers to the amount of information about the conceptual model that is used to construct the C-T-E structure. This criterion requires that the conceptual model be identified explicitly and also requires that the content of the conceptual model that is relevant to the C-T-E structure be described clearly and concisely. An example of the content required for specification adequacy is given in **Box 25-1**.

Linkage Adequacy

Linkage adequacy refers to the clarity of the connections between the conceptual model, the theory, and the empirical indicators. This criterion requires those connections to be stated explicitly and completely. An example of the content required for linkage adequacy is given in Box 25-1, and Figure 25-3 is a diagram of the complete C-T-E structure.

Step 2: Evaluation of the Theory

The second step in evaluation of C-T-E structures focuses on the theory (T) component. The four criteria in this step are significance, internal consistency, parsimony, and testability.

Significance of the Theory

Significance refers to the extent to which the theory is socially important (social significance) and theoretically important (theoretical significance). This criterion requires that the theory be about a topic that society currently regards as practically important. This criterion also requires that the theory offer new, compelling, and nontrivial insights into the topic.

Internal Consistency of the Theory

Internal consistency refers to the extent to which the concepts of the theory are comprehensible. This criterion requires that the theory concepts be explicitly identified and clearly defined. This criterion also requires that the same terms be consistently used for the same concepts. For example, it is not appropriate to refer to the concept of mood as both "mood" and "depression." An example of a narrative for internal consistency is given in **Box 25-2**.

Parsimony of the Theory

Parsimony refers to the extent to which content of the theory is stated as concisely as possible. It requires that the theory be made up of as few concepts and propositions as necessary to clearly convey the meaning of each concept and proposition. An example of parsimony is evident in Figure 25-3. Rustøen et al.'s (2014) review of the literature about the effects of psychoeducational intervention led these researchers to identify a parsimonious set of concepts that they regarded as plausible effects of the psychoeducational intervention—namely,

Box 25-2 Example of Narrative Content Required for the Criterion of Theory Internal Consistency

The two concepts of Rustøen et al.'s (2014) theory are psychoeducational intervention and cancer pain management behaviors. Each concept is theoretically defined by its dimensions.
 	
    Psychoeducational intervention is defined as a PRO-SELF Pain Control Program and a control intervention. The dimensions of the psychoeducational intervention are described in detail as operational definitions that state how the two dimensions were to be implemented, rather than as theoretical definitions.
 	
    Cancer pain management behaviors are defined as pain intensity, pain frequency, pain location, breakthrough pain, and opioid analgesic intake. The dimensions of cancer pain management behaviors are pain intensity, pain frequency, pain location, breakthrough pain, and opioid analgesic intake. These dimensions are defined operationally rather than theoretically. For example, pain intensity was defined as ratings on a numeric rating scale of the least, worst, and average pain experienced each day as recorded in a diary; and pain frequency was operationally defined as the number of hours per day of significant pain as recorded in the diary.

Data from Rustøen, T., Valeberg, B. T., Kolstad, E., Wist, E., Paul, S., & Miaskowski, C. (2014). A randomized clinical trial of the efficacy of a self-care intervention to improve cancer pain management. *Cancer Nursing, 37*, 34–43.

cancer pain management behaviors encompassing pain intensity, pain frequency, pain location, breakthrough pain, and opioid analgesic intake. Furthermore, propositions that specified the operational definition of each concept and propositions that specified effects of the psychoeducational intervention on cancer pain management behaviors were stated relatively concisely.

Testability of the Theory

Testability refers to the extent to which the theory can be empirically tested. Each concept of the theory must be empirically measurable, which is accomplished when each concept is explicitly linked to an empirical indicator. Figure 25-3 provides an example of the linkage of theory concepts and empirical indicators; the narrative supporting testability is evident in the linkage adequacy section of Box 25-1, in which each theory concept is explicitly linked to its respective empirical indicator.

Step 3: Evaluation of the Empirical Research Methods

The third step in the evaluation of C-T-E structures research focuses on the empirical indicators and other empirical methods. The criterion in this step is operational adequacy.

Operational adequacy refers to the appropriateness of the empirical indicators as measures of the theory concepts. When the empirical indicator used to measure a theory concept yields qualitative data—that is, data that are words—it should be dependable and credible. Dependability of qualitative data requires that the study be replicated (that is, completely repeated using the same methods and another sample from the same population), which very rarely is done, or that an inquiry audit is used, which means that another independent researcher, who was not involved in the study, reviews the process of data analysis and the study findings and then agrees or disagrees with the findings as proposed by the researchers who conducted the study. Credibility of the data requires that the researcher conveys confidence in the study findings by means of one or more activities, including prolonged engagement with or immersion in the relevant literature, persistent observation, triangulation, peer debriefing, member checks, or negative case analysis.

When the empirical indicator used to measure a theory concept yields quantitative data—that is, data that are numbers—it should be reliable and valid. Reliability of an instrument requires that the items consistently measure the theory concept, whereas validity means that the instrument measures the concept it is supposed to measure. The many approaches to estimating reliability and validity are explained in Fawcett and Garity's *Evaluating Research for Evidence-Based Nursing Practice* (2009), as well as in other research textbooks.

Examples of the narrative content needed to meet the criterion of operational adequacy for empirical indicators yielding qualitative and quantitative data are given in **Box 25-3**. Note that operational adequacy also refers to the appropriateness of the research design,

Box 25-3   Example of Narrative Content Required for the Criterion of Operational Adequacy

Operational Adequacy of an Empirical Indicator Yielding Qualitative Data
Cummings (2011) explained that word data obtained from in-depth interviews were analyzed using an interpretive phenomenological research approach, which is a type of content analysis. She described the research as follows:

> The following steps were taken to achieve rigor; preconceived notions and beliefs were put aside about the phenomenon under study. A holistic reading was done of each transcript to get a sense of it as a whole and then read again to see what statements or phrases seems to best represent the experience of the participants. . . . Each of the statements or phrases was listed in categories that seemed to be related. After repeatedly reviewing and dwelling with the data, five essential themes were identified, after determining that the phenomenon would lose its meaning without the inclusion of these themes. (Cummings, 2011, p. 188)

> With regard to dependability, Cummings (2011) explained that as she read the interview transcripts, she made notes "in the margins, using different color highlighters for what appeared to be different categories of statements. Each of the statements or phrases was listed in categories that seemed to be related." She went on to state that she "collaborated with two professional colleagues and expert qualitative researchers who reviewed transcripts and findings; each had more than 20 years of experience in qualitative research. A journal was kept to record additional observations and personal reflections" (p. 388). The transcript margin notes, the journal, and the results of the data analysis then were used by other independent researchers to conduct the inquiry audit. Cummings (2011) explained that she and the other researchers agreed about the study findings: "There was intersubjective agreement on themes between the [principal investigator] . . . and expert qualitative researchers" (p. 388).

> With regard to credibility, Cummings's (2011) statement that "Findings were presented and clarified with participants to assess whether the transcripts were accurate and whether the identified themes resonated with them" indicates that she used member checks as one activity to estimate credibility. Her use of "professional colleagues and expert qualitative researchers" (p. 388) to review findings indicates that she used peer debriefing as another activity to estimate credibility. Her statement that "There was intersubjective agreement on themes between the [principal investigator], participants, and expert qualitative researchers" indicates that the study findings are credible (Cummings, 2011, p. 388).

Operational Adequacy of an Empirical Indicator Yielding Quantitative Data
The 10-item version of the Center for Epidemiological Studies of Depression (CESD) scale was used to measure depression. Tsai et al. (2003) describe the CESD as follows:

> The 10-item version of the CESD scale uses a four-point scale ranging from 0 (none of the time) to 3 (most of the time). Respondents were asked to indicate how often in "the past week" they experienced each of the 10 descriptions of depressed mood. Higher scores reflect a higher level of depression. The possible range of scores is 0–30, with cutoff scores for depression at ≥ 10. Alpha coefficient was 0.86 in past studies . . . and 0.69 for this study. The scale's validity has been reported as adequate. (p. 162)

the sample, the data collection procedures, the procedures used to protect research participants, and the data analysis techniques (Fawcett & Garity, 2009).

Step 4: Evaluation of the Research Findings

The fourth step in evaluation of C-T-E structures again focuses on the theory (T) component. The criterion in this step is empirical adequacy.

Empirical adequacy refers to the extent to which the data from a study designed to generate or test a theory agree with the theory concepts and propositions. If the data are not completely congruent with theory concepts and propositions, the theory cannot be regarded as empirically adequate. Such a result could mean that the theory is more or less parsimonious than initially proposed. Alternatively, such a result could mean that the theory has no merit and should be discarded. An example of an empirically adequate theory is Tsai et al.'s (2003) theory of chronic pain. The data from their correlational study revealed that "The hypothesized model was supported by data showing that pain, disability, and social support resulted in perceived daily stress that in turn predicted depression" (Tsai et al., 2003, p. 164).

Step 5: Evaluation of the Utility and Soundness of the Conceptual Model

The fifth step in evaluation of C-T-E structures focuses on the conceptual model (C) component. The criterion in this step is legitimacy.

Legitimacy refers to the extent to which research findings support the usefulness of the conceptual model as a guide for construction of C-T-E structures for theory generation and theory testing, as well as the soundness of its content. The research findings cannot reveal any major flaws in the conceptual model concepts and propositions. Discovery of any flaws indicates that revisions in the content of the conceptual model are required or that the conceptual model should be discarded. Examples of narratives addressing legitimacy of a conceptual model appear in **Box 25-4**.

Box 25-4   Example of Narrative Content for the Criterion of Legitimacy

Example From a Theory-Generating Study

According to Cummings, her 2011 study of sharing a traumatic event "revealed a collaborative, adaptive process between listener and storyteller, consistent with Roy's Adaptation Model" (Cummings, 2011, p. 390). Cummings (2011) went on to state, "Participant's [sic] individual patterns of adaptation and individual attempts at coping were illuminated providing a deeper understanding of the lived experience of these individuals" (p. 390). The first statement addresses the soundness of the conceptual model, and the second statement addresses the utility of the conceptual model as a guide for the study.

(Continues)

Example From a Theory-Testing Study

Tsai et al. (2003) describe their efforts to test a theory of chronic pain as follows:

> This study was the first step in validating a middle-range theory of chronic pain derived from the RAM [Roy Adaptation Model] in a sample of older people with arthritis, and we found that daily stress is a very important factor leading to depression in older people with arthritis. To treat depression properly, health care providers need not only to use antidepressants for symptom control but also to understand the influence of daily stress for individuals and develop a strategy to minimize its impact. The nursing discipline struggles to be professional and distinct from that of medicine. The medical model has been criticized because it neglects psychosocial-behavioural influences on health. On the other hand, nursing emphasizes the influence of environment, both internal and external, on health, as evidenced in the work of Roy . . . and other theorists. This study supports the above proposition about the nursing discipline and provides evidence of the importance of psychosocial-behavioral issues for personal health. This middle-range theory also yields more specific hypotheses in relation to stress and adaptation processes in older people with arthritis than the RAM. Thus, the findings of this study will be more appropriate to explaining stress and adaptation processes in older people with arthritis. They advance our knowledge in using the RAM in clinical practice to deal with older people with arthritis experiencing pain, stress and depression. Similarly, the specific focus of this middle-range theory on older people with arthritis makes it more applicable in clinical practice. (Tsai et al., 2003, p. 165)

Reproduced from Tsai, P.F., Tak, S., Moore, C., & Palencia, I. (2003). Testing a theory of chronic pain. *Journal of Advanced Nursing, 43*(2), 158-169. Republished with permission of John Wiley and Sons, Inc. Permission conveyed through Copyright Clearance Center, Inc.

SUMMARY

This chapter's focus is on the C-T-E structures that need to be constructed for systematic theory generation and theory testing. The chapter also presented a discussion of criteria used to evaluate C-T-E structures. These go beyond the norm for theory evaluation theories by including criteria to evaluate conceptual models and empirical indicators.

REFERENCES

Ajzen, I. (1991). The theory of planned behavior. *Organizational Behavior and Human Decision Processes, 50*, 179–211.

American Association of Critical Care Nurses. (2014). *Synergy Model: Basic information about the ACCN Synergy Model for Patient Care*. Retrieved from https://www.aacn.org/nursing-excellence /aacn-standards/synergy-model

Barnum, B. J. S. (1998). *Nursing theory: Analysis, application, evaluation* (5th ed.). Philadelphia, PA: Lippincott.

Cummings, J. (2011). Sharing a traumatic event: The experience of the listener and the storyteller within the dyad. *Nursing Research, 60,* 386–392.

Doornbos, M. M. (1995). Using King's systems framework to explore family health in the families of the young chronically mentally ill. In M. A. Frey & C. L. Sieloff (Eds.), *Advancing King's systems framework and theory of nursing* (pp. 192–205). Thousand Oaks, CA: Sage.

Doornbos, M. M. (2000). King's systems framework and family health: The derivation and testing of a theory. *Journal of Theory Construction and Testing, 4,* 20–26.

Duffy, M., & Muhlenkamp, A. F. (1974). A framework for theory analysis. *Nursing Outlook, 22,* 570–574.

Fashinpaur, D. (2002). Using the Neuman Systems Model to guide nursing practice in the United States: Nursing prevention interventions for postpartum mood disorders. In B. Neuman & J. Fawcett (Eds.), *The Neuman Systems Model* (4th ed., pp. 74–89). Upper Saddle River, NJ: Prentice Hall.

Fawcett, J. (2003). The Roy Adaptation Model: A program of nursing research. *Japanese Journal of Nursing Research, 36*(1), 67–73.

Fawcett, J. (2005). Criteria for evaluation of theory. *Nursing Science Quarterly, 18,* 131–135.

Fawcett, J. (2013). Appendix N-1: Conceptual models and theories of nursing. In D. Venes (Ed.), *Taber's cyclopedic medical dictionary* (22nd ed., pp. 2629–2660). Philadelphia, PA: F. A. Davis.

Fawcett, J., Aber, C., Haussler, S., Weiss, M., Myers, S. T., Hall, J. L., . . . Silva, V. (2011). Women's perceptions of caesarean birth: A Roy international study. *Nursing Science Quarterly, 24,* 352–362.

Fawcett, J., Aber, C., Weiss, M., Haussler, S., Myers, S. T., King, C., . . . & Silva, V. (2005). Adaptation to cesarean birth: Implementation of an international multisite study. *Nursing Science Quarterly, 18,* 204–210.

Fawcett, J., & DeSanto-Madeya, S. (2013). *Contemporary nursing knowledge: Analysis and evaluation of nursing models and theories* (3rd ed.). Philadelphia, PA: F. A. Davis.

Fawcett, J., & Garity, J. (2009). *Evaluating research for evidence-based nursing practice.* Philadelphia, PA: F. A. Davis.

King, I. M., & Fawcett, J. (1997). *The language of nursing theory and metatheory.* Indianapolis, IN: Sigma Theta Tau International Center Nursing Press.

Latham, L. (2002). Letter to the editor. *Nursing Science Quarterly, 15,* 264.

Levine, M. E. (1991). The conservation principles: A model for health. In K. M. Schaefer & J. B. Pond (Eds.), *Levine's conservation model: A framework for nursing practice (pp. 1–11).*

Mishel, M. H. (1990). Reconceptualization of the uncertainty in illness theory. *Image: Journal of Nursing Scholarship, 22,* 256–262.

Mock, V., Krumm, S., Belcher, A., Stewart, K., DeWeese, T., Shang, J., & Hall, S. (2007). Exercise during prostate cancer treatment: Effects on functional status and symptoms. *Oncology Nursing Forum, 34,* 189–190. [Abstract]

Mwangi, R. N. (2013). *Kenyan women living with HIV/AIDS: A mixed methods study* (Doctoral dissertation). Retrieved from ProQuest Dissertations and Theses Full Text (ProQuest document ID 1430545502).

Parse, R. R. (2005). Fawcett's criteria for evaluation of theory with a comparison of Fawcett's and Parse's approaches. *Nursing Science Quarterly, 18,* 135–137.

Pines, E. W, Rauschhuber, M. L., Cook, J. D., Norgan, G. H., Canchosa, L., Richardson, C., & Jones, M. E. (2014). Enhancing resilience, empowerment, and conflict management among baccalaureate students: Outcomes of a pilot study. *Nurse Educator, 39,* 85–90.

Piper B. F., Dibble S. L., Dodd M. J., Weiss M. C., Slaughter R. E. & Paul S. M. (1998). The revised Piper Fatigue Scale: Psychometric evaluation in women with breast cancer. *Oncology Nursing Forum 25,* 677–684.

Roy, C. (2009). *The Roy adaptation model* (3rd ed.). Upper Saddle River, NJ: Pearson.

Rustøen, T., Valeberg, B. T., Kolstad, E., Wist, E., Paul, S., & Miaskowski, C. (2014). A randomized clinical trial of the efficacy of a self-care intervention to improve cancer pain management. *Cancer Nursing, 37,* 34–43.

Tsai, P. F., Tak, S., Moore, C., & Palencia, I. (2003). Testing a theory of chronic pain. *Journal of Advanced Nursing, 43,* 158–169.

Villarruel, A. M., Bishop, T. L., Simpson, E. M., Jemmott, L. S., & Fawcett, J. (2001). Borrowed theories, shared theories, and the advancement of nursing knowledge. *Nursing Science Quarterly, 14,* 158–163.

Wicks, M. N. (1995). Family health as derived from King's framework. In M. A. Frey & C. L. Sieloff (Eds.), *Advancing King's systems framework and theory of nursing* (pp. 97–108). Thousand Oaks, CA: Sage.

Wicks, M. N. (1997). A test of the Wicks family health model in families coping with chronic obstructive pulmonary disease. *Journal of Family Nursing, 3,* 189–212.

Chapter 26

Using Theory in Evidence-Based Advanced Nursing Practice[*]

Jacqueline Fawcett

INTRODUCTION

This chapter is focused on the use of theory as evidence in advanced nursing practice. It begins with a discussion of the equivalence of theory and evidence and a description of translational research, which is used to translate research findings into practical actions. The chapter continues with a presentation of the steps to follow and the criteria to be met to translate theories, in the form of research findings, into evidence-based best practices for advanced nursing practice. This chapter's content is especially relevant to three of the American Association of Colleges of Nursing's Essentials of Doctoral Education for Advanced Nursing Practice: *Essential I, Scientific Underpinnings for Practice*; *Essential III, Clinical Scholarship and Analytical Methods for Evidence-Based Practice*; and *Essential VIII, Advanced Nursing Practice*.

THEORY AND EVIDENCE

Theories are typically thought of as formulations that are not relevant for practice, which is the source of the so-called *theory–practice gap*. Yet, "nothing is quite so practical as a good theory" (Lewin, as cited in Van de Ven, 1989, p. 486). A central point of this chapter is that a theory does not *lead* to evidence but rather *is* the evidence. Thus, when we talk and write about evidence-based practice, we are actually talking and writing about theory-based

---

[*]Portions of this chapter are adapted from Fawcett, J., & Garity, J. (2009). *Evaluating research for evidence-based nursing practice*. Philadelphia, PA: F. A. Davis. Used with permission.

practice. Accordingly, no gap exists between theory and practice, as can be seen in the definition of evidence-based nursing practice given here: "Evidence-based nursing practice is the deliberate and critical use of theories about human beings' health-related experiences to guide [nursing] actions" (Fawcett & Garity, 2009, p. 8).

Of course, it is possible that no theory exists that can serve as evidence for a practical action. In this case, the evidence may be the tenacious beliefs of one or more individuals ("We always have done the procedure this way"), an authority ("The nurse manager said to do the procedure this way" or "The procedure manual [or textbook] said to do the procedure this way"), or common sense ("It seems reasonable to do the procedure this way") (Fawcett & Garity, 2009). Inasmuch as theory is regarded as the very best evidence, any nursing action that is not based on theory requires the generation of a new theory.

TRANSLATIONAL RESEARCH

Interest in translating theories into practical actions—such as assessment of health-related experiences and interventions used to promote positive responses to those experiences—has increased dramatically during the last several years in conjunction with an increased emphasis on evidence-based practice. *Translational research* is a research process used to determine which conditions, costs, and resources are required to progress from theory generation and theory testing to evidence-based practice. The goal of translational research is to decrease the time required for translation of theories into assessment tools and intervention protocols that will improve people's health-related quality of life.

TYPES OF THEORIES, RESEARCH, AND PRACTICE TOOLS

Five types of theories have been identified as what Carper (1978) and White (1995) referred to as the *fundamental patterns of knowing* in nursing: (1) empirical theories (the science of nursing), (2) aesthetic theories (the art of nursing), (3) ethical theories (the ethics of nursing), (4) personal knowing theories (the interpersonal relationships of nursing), and (5) sociopolitical theories (the policies and politics of nursing). Collectively, the five types of theories constitute evidence for nursing practice. The five types are integrated in nursing practice, although one type of theory may be more obvious than another in a given situation. For example, if an advanced practice nurse is caring for a patient who is experiencing shortness of breath, the best empirical theory about the most appropriate nursing intervention is applied. However, at the same time, the nurse will not neglect application of the other four types of theories.

Almost all contemporary discussions about evidence-based practice focus on empirical theories. Three primary types of empirical theories and research designs are (1) *descriptive theories* generated and tested by descriptive research, (2) *explanatory theories* tested by correlational research, and (3) *predictive theories* tested by experimental research. Most researchers and clinicians agree that predictive theories can be translated into intervention

Table 26-1   Types of Theories, Research Designs, and Practice Tools

Type of Theory	Type of Research Design	Type of Practice Tool
Descriptive theories	Descriptive research	Assessment tools
Explanatory theories	Correlational research	Comprehensive assessment tools
Predictive theories	Experimental research	Intervention protocols

protocols. Nevertheless, few researchers or clinicians understand that descriptive and explanatory theories also have practical uses when translated into assessment tools.

Table 26-1 lists types of theories and research designs, as well as the types of practice tools that can be developed when research findings for each type of theory are translated for practice. As can be seen in the table, descriptive theories, which are generated or tested by descriptive research, can be translated into assessment tools. An example is the Coping and Adaptation Processing Scale (CAPS), an assessment tool that was designed to measure the descriptive theory of coping and adaptation processing, which was derived from the Roy Adaptation Model (Alkrisat & Dee, 2014).

Explanatory theories, which are tested by correlational research, can be translated into comprehensive assessment tools. For example, Heelan (2015) tested an explanatory theory of the relations of power, attitudes regarding intermittent fetal monitoring, and perceived barriers to research utilization to labor and delivery nurses' attitudes toward patient advocacy. The theory, which Heelan derived from Rogers's science of unitary human beings, can be translated into a comprehensive assessment tool that includes one or more questions about each concept (power, attitudes regarding intermittent fetal monitoring, perceived barriers to research utilization, and attitudes toward patient advocacy); alternatively, the research instruments Heelan used—the Power as Knowing Participation in Change Tool, the Attitudes Regarding Intermittent Fetal Monitoring Instrument, the Barriers to Research Utilization Scale, and the Attitudes Toward Patient Advocacy Scale—could be evaluated for use as practice tools. **Box 26-1** is a summary of factors to take into account when considering the use of a research instrument as a practice tool.

Predictive theories that are tested by experimental research can be translated into intervention protocols. For example, Shah et al. (2015) tested the predictive theory of the effects of a virtual reality–based stress management program that they derived from the Neuman Systems Model. Shah et al. (2015) operationalized the theory as an individualized tertiary prevention as intervention protocol (the VR DE-STRESS Program) and questionnaires measuring stress, depression, anxiety, perceived relaxation, and knowledge. The protocol encompassed daily 1-hour in-person psychoeducational sessions and virtual reality–guided relaxation delivered via videos for 3 days. The findings of their quasi-experimental pre-test, post-test study revealed that the participants, all of whom experienced mood disorders,

Box 26-1   Guidelines for Evaluating the Use of Research Instruments as Practice Tools

What is the length of the research instrument?
- Is the research instrument made up of one or many items?
  - Fewer items impose less burden on patients.
  - Fewer items also may impose less burden on the nurse when administering and scoring the tool and interpreting the patients' responses.

What is the reading level of the research instrument?
- No more than an eighth-grade reading level is recommended for use with patients.
- If the patient cannot read, can the instrument be administered orally by the nurse?

Is the research instrument written in English or in the patient's native language?
- If the instrument must be translated into the patient's native language, is the translation and back-translation technique used? (See Varricchio, 2004.)
- If the instrument must be translated into the patient's native language, is cultural equivalence—including content equivalence, semantic equivalence, technical equivalence, criterion equivalence, and conceptual equivalence—documented? (See Cha, Kim, & Erlen, 2007, and Flaherty et al., 1988.)
  - *Content equivalence* refers to the relevance of each item to the culture of interest.
  - *Semantic equivalence* refers to the extent to which the connotative meaning of each item is the same in the original culture and the culture for which the instrument is being translated.
  - *Technical equivalence* refers to the extent to which the way the data were collected—such as interviews or survey questionnaires—is similar in each culture.
  - *Criterion equivalence* refers to the extent to which the interpretation of the data is similar across cultures.
  - *Conceptual* equivalence refers to the extent to which the researcher is able to measure the same middle-range theory concept in each culture.

How easy are the research instrument items to complete?
- Open-ended questions:
  - The patient has to write his or her response, or the nurse has to record the patient's response.
  - Example: How are you feeling physically?
- Visual analog scales:
  - The patient has to make a mark on a scale line. The scale line has to be 100 mm, and the nurse has to measure from one end of the line to the location of the patient's mark.
  - Example: Physically, I feel

  Dreadful ←————————————→ Great

- Rating scales:
  - The patient has to circle a number, or the nurse has to circle the number for the patient.
  - Example: On a scale of 1 to 10, where 1 = dreadful and 10 = great: Physically, I feel

  1   2   3   4   5   6   7   8   9   10

reported less stress, depression, and anxiety, and greater perceived relaxation and knowledge following administration of the protocol (Shah et al., 2015).

TRANSLATING THEORIES INTO PRACTICAL ACTIONS

Translation of theories into evidence-based assessment tools, intervention protocols, and any other practical actions follows a seven-step sequence. The seven steps identified in this chapter are adapted from the work of Melnyk, Fineout-Overholt, Stillwell, and Williamson (2010).

First Step

The first step, which might seem obvious, is to identify a practice problem for which evidence is needed. This step requires an awareness of the problem and the possibility of a new way of assessing the problem or intervening to help people overcome it. Awareness may be catalyzed by something a patient experiences, an article in a nursing journal, a presentation at a workshop or conference, or a position statement from a government agency or professional society. An example of a problem is uncertainty about the effectiveness of self-instructional guidelines about child trafficking on students' knowledge of and attitudes about child trafficking (Bist & Tomar, 2015).

Second Step

The second step is to use the PICOT format to ask a question about the problem, which may be a way to assess people or an intervention. This format takes into account the patient population (P), an assessment or intervention (I), group comparisons (C), the desired outcome (O), and time (T) (Melnyk et al., 2010).

The following is an example of a PICOT question about *assessment*:

- **P:** For women who have had a cesarean delivery
- **I:** who complete the Inventory of Functional Status After Childbirth
- **C:** compared with the same women who complete the Karnofsky Performance Scale,
- **O:** what is the average level of functional status
- **T:** at 3 weeks postpartum?

The following is an example of a PICOT question about *intervention*:

- **P:** For children with asthma,
- **I:** does use of an asthma action plan shared with the school nurse
- **C:** compared with parental management only
- **O:** reduce the incidence and severity of asthma attacks
- **T:** by the end of the school year?

Third, Fourth, and Fifth Steps

The third, fourth, and fifth steps focus on the available evidence about the problem. The third step is a search of the published literature about the problem. Reference materials at university, hospital, and public libraries can provide invaluable assistance with the search for relevant literature.

Literature reviews focus primarily on the theory component of conceptual–theoretical–empirical (C-T-E) structures, may include the empirical methods component (E), and also should include the conceptual model component (C). As Popper (1968) explained, "Theories are nets cast to catch what we call 'the world': to rationalize, to explain, and to master it. We endeavour to make the mesh ever finer and finer" (p. 59). Extrapolating from Popper's (1968) argument, the content of the conceptual model should be the net used to catch the relevant literature for the review, including literature encompassing empirical, aesthetic, ethical, personal knowing, and sociopolitical patterns of knowing (Carper, 1978; White, 1995). That is, the concepts and propositions of the conceptual model should be used to guide the search for and classification of the empirical and nonempirical literature to be reviewed. The Roy Adaptation Model, for example, could be used as a search term.

Other search terms can be drawn from the PICOT format (Melnyk et al., 2010). For example, search terms drawn from the examples of the PICOT format given in the discussion of the second step in translating theory into practical action might include the following: cesarean delivery, functional status, and instruments for the PICOT assessment question; and children, asthma, management, and action plan for the PICOT intervention question. The search can be narrowed when the name of the conceptual model is added as a search term.

The search terms also may include the type of paper, such as a review article (including systematic reviews and state-of-the-science papers), practice guidelines, and best practices. *Best practice guidelines* are "systematically developed statements to assist health care practitioners' decisions about appropriate health care for specific clinical circumstances" (Wallin, 2005, pp. 248–249). *Best practices* refer to "the organizational use of evidence to improve practice" (Driever, 2002, p. 593). These evidence-based practices include not only the actions required for assessment or intervention, but also specification of the most efficient and effective uses of human resources and equipment to attain the best possible patient outcomes. Advanced practice nurses could take advantage of existing resources for evidence-based practice. Although most of these resources do not explicitly identify a conceptual model that guided the work or a theory that was generated or tested, they provide a summary of research findings, which advanced practice nurses will recognize as theories. Two especially useful resources are the practice guidelines available from the National Guideline Clearinghouse (http://www.guideline.gov/) and the best practices information sheets available from the Joanna Briggs Institute (http://joannabriggs.org); these documents contain brief summaries of best practices gleaned from systematic reviews of research.

A scoping review of literature is recommended to determine the amount of literature available about a topic. Cacchione (2016), who explained that a universal definition of a scoping review does not yet exist, offered three of the various definitions found in the literature:

- "Scoping reviews aim to map rapidly the key concepts underpinning a research area and the main sources and types of evidence available" (Arksey & O'Malley, as cited in Cacchione, 2016, p. 115).
- "Scoping reviews involve the synthesis and analysis of a wide range of research and non-research materials to provide a greater [theoretical] clarity about a specific topic or field of evidence" (Davis, Drey, & Gould, as cited in Cacchione, 2016, p. 115).
- "Scoping revises aim to provide a map of what evidence has been produced from disparate or heterogeneous sources as opposed to seeking only the best evidence to answer a particular question related to policy or practice" (Joannna Briggs Institute, as cited in Cacchione, 2016, p. 115).

A worksheet typically is used to systematically record details about literature that is retrieved. **Figures 26-1** and **26-2** are examples of worksheets for recording literature details. Note that the quality of the study column would not be used for scoping reviews.

The fourth step in the process of translating theory into practical actions involves a critical evaluation of the literature. A realist review of literature is recommended as an efficient and effective approach to integrating and critically evaluating the available literature that was identified in the scoping review. The question asked when conducting a realist review is, "What works for whom under what circumstances, how, and why?" (Wong, Greenhalgh, Westhorp, Buckingham, & Pawson, 2013, p. 1006). Thus, a realist review "seeks to unpack the context-mechanism-outcome relationship, thereby explaining examples of success, failure, and various eventualities in between" (Wong et al., 2013, p. 1006). The conceptual and theoretical perspectives evident in the literature are of particular interest in a realist review. Indeed, Pawson, Greenhalgh, Harvey, and Walshe (2005) regard assessments and interventions as theories that are derived from conceptual models. Elaborating on this point, Pawson et al. (2005) explained that assessments and interventions "are always based on a hypothesis that postulates: if we deliver [an assessment or intervention] in this way or we manage services like so, then this will bring about some improved outcome" (p. 22).

Realist reviews of the literature involve appraisal, integration, and evaluation of theory-generating research, theory-testing research, or both. *Metasynthesis* (Sandelowski & Barroso, 2003) and *metasummary* (Sandelowski, Barroso, & Voils, 2007) are techniques used to integrate qualitative theory-generating research. *Meta-analysis* is a technique used to integrate quantitative theory-testing research (Rosenthal, 1991). *Critical interpretative synthesis* is a technique used to integrate both qualitative theory-generating and quantitative theory-testing research (Fleming, 2010).

Citation Author(s)/ Year	Name of Conceptual Model	Name of Theory/ Concepts	Sample Size/ Name of Characteristics	Instruments	Results	Effect Size (If Available)	Quality of the Study

Figure 26-1 Example 1 of a literature review worksheet.

	Conceptual Model Concept₁	Conceptual Model Concept₂	Conceptual Model Concept₃	Conceptual Model Conceptₙ
Citation				
Purpose				
Type of Theory/ Name of Theory Concept				
Sample Size/ Characteristics				
Instruments				
Results				
Effect Size (if applicable)				
Quality of the Study (if applicable)				

Directions

1. List all of the concepts of the conceptual model or theory across the top of the page or make a separate page for each concept.
2. As the literature is reviewed, enter the citation (journal article, book chapter, book) and notes about the study in the rows under the relevant conceptual model concept. Note that any one citation may have information about more than one concept.
3. List the full citation on a separate page so that the reference list/bibliography will be completed when the literature review is done.

Figure 26-2 Example 2 of a literature review worksheet.

The worksheets shown in Figures 26-1 and 26-2, including the quality of the study column, are examples of how the results of a realist review can be recorded. A typical levels-of-evidence schema is shown in **Box 26-2**. Fawcett and Garity (2009) explained that the quality of a study is rated using a levels-of-evidence schema that includes "ratings for various types of research designs and even expert opinion, although the best ratings are typically assigned to integrated reviews of experimental research, especially RCTs [randomized controlled trials]" (p. 268). They stated, furthermore, that "levels of evidence [schemas] . . . ignore the different contributions of each type of research—descriptive, correlational, experimental—to practice" (p. 268). (See Table 26-1.)

The fifth step in the translation of theory into practical actions is the use of the literature to inform all elements required for evidence-based practice—assessments and interventions; the context of care delivery; patient and family preferences, values, and needs; and the

Box 26-2 Example of a Levels-of-Evidence Schema to Rate Each Study Included in a Literature Review
1++: High-quality meta-analyses, systematic reviews of randomized controlled trials (RCTs), or RCTs with a very low risk of bias
1+: Well-conducted meta-analyses, systematic reviews of RCTs, or RCTs with a low risk of bias
1−: Meta-analyses, systematic reviews of RCTs, or RCTs with a high risk of bias
2++: High-quality systematic reviews of case control or cohort studies; high-quality case-control or cohort studies with a very low risk of confounding or bias and a high probability that the relationship is causal
2+: Well-conducted case-control or cohort studies with a low risk of confounding or bias and a moderate probability that the relationship is causal
2−: Case-control or cohort studies with a high risk of confounding or bias and a significant risk that the relationship is not causal
3: Nonanalytic studies (e.g., case reports, case series)
4: Expert opinion

Scottish Intercollegiate Guidelines Network (SIGN). (2003, July). *Cutaneous melanoma: A national clinical guideline* (SIGN Publication No. 72), Edinburgh, Scotland: Author. Reprinted by permission.

nurse's expertise and clinical judgment (Fawcett, 2012). All five types of theories (empirical, aesthetic, ethical, personal knowing, sociopolitical) constitute the best evidence for assessments and interventions, although empirical theories tend to be the most obviously useful (Fawcett, 2012). Sociopolitical theories are the best evidence for the context of care delivery, which requires consideration of the policies and politics of the healthcare delivery system, including the extent to which healthcare resources are available and allocated for use by advanced practice nurses, in which the patient and nurse are located, such as the patient's home, a community health center, an outpatient clinic, an inpatient tertiary or rehabilitation hospital, or a long-term care facility.

Sociopolitical, aesthetic, and empirical theories provide the evidence for recognition of and accounting for patient and family preferences, values, and needs. These three types of theories sensitize the advanced practice nurse to consideration of the patient's and the family's culture, which has a major influence on the patient's and family's health-related beliefs, values, and life ways (McFarland & Wehbe-Alamah, 2015) and on family dynamics regarding preferences for a particular approach to assessment and a specific intervention. These three types of theories also guide the nurse to consider the influence of social media (e.g., Facebook and Twitter) and public media (e.g., print and electronic news stories, advertisements, and television and radio talk shows) on patient and family preferences and values.

Aesthetic, ethical, personal knowing, and empirical theories are the evidence for the nurse's expertise and clinical judgment. Aesthetic theories guide the advanced practice nurse's understanding of the meaning of the individual patient's behavior and needs. Ethical theories are the guides to what the nurse should do in practice. Personal knowing theories undergird the nurse's understanding of how he or she expresses authentic caring with patients. Empirical theories tell the nurse what to expect when applying a particular assessment tool or intervention. The nurse's expertise and clinical judgment are the mechanisms by which all elements of evidence-based practice are integrated (Melnyk & Fineout-Overholt, 2015).

Although there is no magic formula for weighting, as Melnyk et al. (2010) noted, integration of all elements (assessments and interventions; context of care delivery; patient and family preferences, values, and needs; and the nurse's expertise and clinical judgment) and, we can add, all types of theories (empirical, aesthetic, ethical, personal knowing, sociopolitical) that need to be taken into account when considering implementing a new evidence-based practical action can be guided by the criterion of pragmatic adequacy of a theory. *Pragmatic adequacy* refers to the extent to which a theory serves as the evidence for practical actions, including assessment tools and interventional protocols. Theories that are judged to be pragmatically adequate are socially meaningful, are compatible with a particular practice setting, are feasible in the real world of practice, are consistent with patients' preferences for and expectations about care, and lead to actions that are within the legal scope of nursing practice (Fawcett & Garity, 2009).

Evaluating the social meaningfulness of a theory requires consideration of the extent to which translation of the theory into a new assessment tool or intervention protocol would yield desired outcomes that are consistent with patient needs. Desired outcomes include comprehensive assessments of health-related experiences and positive effects of interventions, such as reduction in the incidence of symptom distress and increased quality of life. Radwin, Washko, Suchy, and Tyman (2005), for example, identified five desired outcomes of oncology nursing care:

1. *Sense of well-being:* "the patient's positive emotional state"
2. *Trust:* "the patient's confidence that care was appropriate and reliable and would be as successful as possible"
3. *Fortitude:* "the patient's strength and willingness to bear the effects of cancer treatments and the symptoms of the disease"
4. *Optimism:* "the patient's belief that he or she had made appropriate choices regarding treatment and the patient's feelings of hopefulness about treatment outcomes"
5. *Authentic self-representation:* "the patient's sense of genuine self-portrayal" (p. 93)

Social meaningfulness of qualitative theory-generating research depends on how confident the reader is that the new theory will be meaningful for practice and can be translated into a new assessment tool. The social meaningfulness of theory-testing research depends on both the statistical significance and the clinical significance of the research findings. Statistical significance is determined by the p value. A caveat applies, however: "Statistical significance does not guarantee clinical significance and more to the point, the magnitude of the p value (.05, .01, .001, .00029, or whatever) is no guide to clinical significance" (Slakter, Wu, & Suzuki-Slakter, 1991, p. 249).

Clinical significance is determined by the magnitude of the findings, which is calculated as an effect size. Effect sizes for different statistical tests can be classified according to whether the frequency of occurrence of a phenomenon, the relation between variables, or the difference between groups is small, medium, or large (Cohen, 1992). Tulman and Fawcett (1996), for example, found small and medium effect sizes for the relationships between the concepts of their explanatory theory of biobehavioral correlates of functional status in women with breast cancer. Clinical significance also may take into account the cost-effectiveness of use of a new assessment tool or intervention (Leeman, Jackson, & Sandelowski, 2006). For example, Mock and colleagues (2004) pointed out that a home-based walking exercise intervention was "low-cost . . . and well received" by women receiving treatment for breast cancer (p. 475).

Evaluating the compatibility of the theory with a particular practice situation draws attention to the context of the situation and requires consideration of the demographic and health-related characteristics of the research participants and the setting in which the research took place. The theory that was generated or tested should be compatible with a particular practice specialty setting, a particular health condition, and particular ages or developmental phases of the people for whom the new assessment tool or intervention protocol is intended. Mock et al. (2004), for example, claimed that their predictive theory of the effects of a home-based walking exercise program on fatigue is "widely applicable . . . to many women with breast cancer" (p. 475).

Evaluating the feasibility of translating the theory into practical actions in a particular practice setting involves making clinical judgments about the complexity of implementing a new assessment tool or intervention protocol. Complexity is determined by considering the following factors:

- The type of training and the time needed to learn how to use the new practice tool or intervention protocol
- The number, type, and expertise of personnel required for all aspects of the design and implementation of the new practice tool or intervention protocol
- The number of contacts and amount of time for each contact required to use the new tool or to deliver and evaluate the new intervention
- The cost of in-service or other continuing education, salaries, and equipment

Feasibility also takes into consideration the willingness of those who control resources to utilize those resources. If they are not willing to surrender those resources to implement the new assessment tool or intervention protocol, the complexity of that practical action does not matter. However, it may be easier to convince whoever controls the resources to allocate them if the new assessment tool or intervention protocol has minimal cost and requires little training and a short time to learn how to use it, few personnel to implement it, and few contacts of short duration.

Furthermore, feasibility requires determining the willingness of nurses or other healthcare personnel to use a new tool or protocol. Making time to search and critically evaluate the literature and translate the theory that was generated or tested into a new assessment tool or intervention protocol can be especially difficult given ever-increasing patient acuity, ever-higher risks, and the ever–more rapid pace of healthcare settings. Advanced practice nurses have to be leaders in fostering evidence-based practice. They can do so by forming partnerships with nurse researchers to conduct research. An advanced practice nurse also can form a partnership with a nursing faculty member whose students have clinical experiences in the setting in which the advanced practice nurse works. The faculty member may be willing to develop a student assignment that focuses on a scoping or a realist review addressing a problem identified by the advanced practice nurse.

Evaluation of pragmatic adequacy also involves determining the extent to which the theory is consistent with patients' preferences for and expectations about care. For example, Mock et al. (2004) noted that implementation of their predictive theory about the effects of a home-based walking exercise program was "acceptable" to many women with breast cancer (p. 475). Their comment, coupled with their finding that almost three-fourths (72%) of the women in the experimental treatment group adhered to the walking exercise intervention, indicates that walking-type exercise was consistent with the women's preferences for and expectations about nursing care.

If the new assessment tool or intervention protocol is not consistent with patient preferences or expectations, it should not be used or patients should be helped to change their preferences and expectations for care. Johnson's (1974) words of more than 40 years ago remain relevant today: "Current . . . practice is not entirely what it might become and [thus patients] might come to expect a different form of practice, given the opportunity to experience it" (p. 376). Suppose, for example, that a researcher found that listening to music the day before surgery reduced patients' anxiety on the morning of the surgery, and an advanced practice nurse decided to implement the music intervention as part of routine preoperative preparation. Some patients might be receptive to this intervention, whereas others might indicate that they did not want or expect to be asked to listen to music the day before their surgery. The advanced practice nurse would then have to explain the research results and the evidence base supporting the music intervention.

Evaluation of the pragmatic adequacy of a theory must also take into account whether the use of a particular assessment tool or intervention protocol is within the legal scope of advanced nursing practice. For example, prescribing medications has not always been included in the scope of advanced nursing practice.

The outcome of evaluation of pragmatic adequacy is a decision about translating the theory into a practical action. Fawcett and Garity (2009) identified four possible decisions:

- A call for additional research (what requires additional study)
- Advocacy for translating a theory into a new assessment tool or intervention protocol and adoption of the tool or protocol in advanced nursing practice (what should be done)
- A trial of a new tool or protocol in a practice setting (what could be tried)
- Discontinuation of a currently used tool or protocol or abandonment of a new tool or protocol (what should not be done)

Furthermore, as Fawcett and Garity (2009) explained:

> If the decision is to translate the theory into [a practical action]—What Should Be Done or What Could Be Tried—the how, when, and where of implementation of the new tool or protocol also need to be considered. How refers to the procedures to follow to actually use the tool or protocol. When refers to the time during an individual's experience in the healthcare system the tool or protocol is used, such as when the person initially seeks treatment, during the time that treatment is being received, or at the end of treatment. Where refers to the location in which the new tool or protocol will be used, such as in a hospital or at home. (p. 265)

Sixth Step

The sixth step in the process of translating theory into practical action involves evaluation of the innovative action, which occurs after the innovation has been implemented in practice. Evaluation may be done by means of a formal research project or through a quality improvement project. An example of a formal research project is the evaluation of the Common Journey Breast Cancer Support Group sponsored by a small community hospital in a rural New England state (Zeigler, Smith, & Fawcett, 2004). An example of a quality improvement project is a multidisciplinary group discharge teaching plan to increase patients' heart failure self-care management, which was guided by Orem's Self-Care Framework (Ryan, Aloe, & Mason-Johnson, 2009).

Seventh Step

The seventh step is dissemination of the results of the evaluation of the innovation. This means that the results of the evaluation of the innovation should be presented publicly—for example, at agency-based nursing rounds and at local, regional, national, and international conferences. In addition, results should be published because the widest audience is made up of the readers of general and specialty journals. Presentations and publications are the necessary final step in translating theories into practical actions of evidence-based practice. As noted by Melnyk et al. (2010), "Clinicians can achieve wonderful outcomes for their patients through [evidence-based practice], but they often fail to share their experiences with colleagues and their own or other healthcare organizations. This leads to needless duplication of effort, and perpetuates clinical approaches that are not evidence based" (p. 53).

SUMMARY

All nurses must have the skills needed to review current findings and evaluate if these findings are applicable for their setting (LaPierre, Ritchey, & Newhouse, 2004). The outcome of evaluating the applicability of research findings to a particular setting is a major element when nurses evaluate the pragmatic adequacy of a theory. Evidence-based nursing practice calls for advanced practice nurses to be leaders in evaluating the pragmatic adequacy of nursing theories and translating the theory, in the form of research findings, into evidence-based practice guidelines and best practices. Advanced practice nurses also need to take the lead in helping all nurses understand that evidence-based practice is equivalent to theory-based practice.

REFERENCES

Alkrisat, M., & Dee, V. (2014). The validation of the Coping and Adaptation Processing Scale based on the Roy Adaptation Model. *Journal of Nursing Measurement, 22*, 368–380.

Bist, L. S., & Tomar, N. (2015). Effectiveness of self instructional guidelines on child trafficking in terms of knowledge and attitude of students studying in selected rural school of Bisrakh, Greater Noida. *International Journal of Nursing Education, 7*(2), 34–37.

Cacchione, P. Z. (2016). Editorial: The evolving methodology of scoping reviews. *Clinical Nursing Research, 25*, 115–119.

Carper, B. A. (1978). Fundamental patterns of knowing in nursing. *Advances in Nursing Science, 1*(1), 13–23.

Cha, E. S., Kim, K. H., & Erlen, J. A. (2007). Translation of scales in cross-cultural research: Issues and techniques. *Journal of Advanced Nursing, 58*, 386–395.

Cohen, J. (1992). A power primer. *Psychological Bulletin, 112*, 135–159.

Driever, M. J. (2002). Are evidence-based practice and best practice the same? *Western Journal of Nursing Research, 24*, 591–597.

Fawcett, J. (2012). Thoughts about evidence-based nursing practice. *Nursing Science Quarterly, 25*, 199–200.

Fawcett, J., & Garity, J. (2009). *Evaluating research for evidence-based nursing practice*. Philadelphia, PA: F. A. Davis.

Flaherty, J. A., Gaviria, F. M., Pathak, D., Mitchell, T., Wintrob, R., Richman, J. A., & Birz, S. (1988). Developing instruments for cross-cultural psychiatric research. *Journal of Nervous and Mental Diseases, 176*, 257–263.

Fleming, K. (2010). Synthesis of quantitative and qualitative research: An example using critical interpretive synthesis. *Journal of Advanced Nursing, 66*, 201–207.

Heelan, L. (2015). Exploring the relationships of power, attitudes regarding intermittent fetal monitoring, and perceived barriers to research utilization with a labor and delivery nurse's attitude toward patient advocacy (Doctoral dissertation). Retrieved from ProQuest Dissertations and Theses Global (ProQuest document ID 1430545502).

Johnson, D. E. (1974). Development of a theory: A requisite for nursing as a primary health profession. *Nursing Research, 23*(5), 372–377.

Lapierre, E., Ritchey, K., & Newhouse, R. (2004). Barriers to research use in PACU. *Journal of Perianesthesia Nursing, 19*(2), 78–83.

Leeman, J., Jackson, B., & Sandelowski, M. (2006). An evaluation of how well research reports facilitate the use of findings in practice. *Journal of Nursing Scholarship, 38,* 171–177.

McFarland, M. R., & Wehbe-Alamah, H. B. (2015). *Leininger's culture care diversity and universality: A worldwide nursing theory* (3rd ed.). Burlington, MA: Jones and Bartlett Learning.

Melnyk, B., & Fineout-Overholt, E. (2015). *Evidence-based practice in nursing and healthcare: A guide to best practice* (3rd ed.). Philadelphia, PA: Wolters Kluwer/Lippincott Williams & Wilkins.

Melnyk, B. M., Fineout-Overholt, E., Stillwell, S. B., & Williamson, K. M. (2010). The seven steps of evidence-based practice. *American Journal of Nursing, 110*(1), 51–53.

Mock, V., Frangakis, C., Davidson, N. E., Ropka, M. E., Pickett, M., Poniatowski, B., . . . McCorkle, R. (2004). Exercise manages fatigue during breast cancer treatment: A randomized controlled trial. *Psycho-Oncology, 14,* 464–477.

Pawson, R., Greenhalgh, T., Harvey, G., & Walshe, K. (2005). Realist review: A new method of systematic review designed for complex policy interventions. *Journal of Health Services Research and Policy, 10*(Suppl. 1), 21–34.

Popper, K. R. (1968). *The logic of scientific discovery.* New York, NY: Harper Torchbooks.

Radwin, L. E., Washko, M., Suchy, K. A., & Tyman, K. (2005). Development and pilot testing of four desired health outcomes scales. *Oncology Nursing Forum, 32,* 92–96.

Rosenthal, R. (1991). *Meta-analytic procedures for social research* (rev. ed.). Newbury Park, CA: Sage.

Ryan, M., Aloe, K., & Mason-Johnson, J. (2009). Improving self-management and reducing hospital readmission in heart failure patients. *Clinical Nurse Specialist: The Journal of Advanced Nursing Practice, 23,* 216–223.

Sandelowski, M., & Barroso, M. (2003). Toward a metasynthesis of qualitative findings on motherhood in HIV-positive women. *Research in Nursing and Health, 26,* 153–170.

Sandelowski, M., Barroso, J., & Voils, C. I. (2007). Using qualitative metasummary to synthesize qualitative and quantitative descriptive findings. *Research in Nursing and Health, 30,* 99–111.

Shah, L. B. I., Torres, S., Kannusamy, P., Chang, C. M. L., He, H.-G., & Klainin-Yobas, P. (2015). Efficacy of the virtual reality-based stress management program on stress-related variables in people with mood disorders: The feasibility study. *Archives of Psychiatric Nursing, 29,* 6–13.

Slakter, M. J., Wu, Y. W. B., & Suzuki-Slakter, N. S. (1991). *, **, and ***: Statistical nonsense at the .00000 level. *Nursing Research, 40,* 248–249.

Tulman, L., & Fawcett, J. (1996). Lessons learned from a pilot study of biobehavioral correlates of functional status in women with breast cancer. *Nursing Research, 45,* 356–358.

Van de Ven, A. H. (1989). Nothing is quite so practical as a good theory. *Academy of Management Review, 14,* 486–489.

Varricchio, C. G. (2004). Measurement issues concerning linguistic translations. In F. Frank-Stromborg & S. J. Olsen (Eds.), *Instruments for clinical health-care research* (3rd ed., pp. 56–64). Sudbury, MA: Jones and Bartlett Publishers.

Wallin, L. (2005). Clinical practice guidelines in nursing. *AWHONN Lifelines, 9,* 248–251.

White, J. (1995). Patterns of knowing: Review, critique, and update. *Advances in Nursing Science, 17*(4), 73–86.

Wong, G., Greenhalgh, T., Westhorp, G., Buckingham, J., & Pawson, R. (2013). RAMESES publication standards: Realist syntheses. *Journal of Advanced Nursing, 69,* 1005–1022.

Zeigler, L., Smith, P. A., & Fawcett, J. (2004). Breast cancer: Evaluation of the Common Journey Breast Cancer Support Group. *Journal of Clinical Nursing, 13,* 467–478.

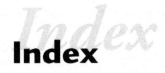

Index

Note: Page numbers followed by *b*, *f*, or *t* indicate material in boxes, figures, or tables, respectively.